# McCance and Widdowson's
# The Composition of Foods

Ministry of Agriculture, Fisheries and Food

Medical Research Council

McCance and Widdowson's

# The Composition of Foods

Fourth revised and extended edition
of MRC Special Report No 297

By A. A. Paul and D. A. T. Southgate

London
HER MAJESTY'S STATIONERY OFFICE

Amsterdam New York Oxford
ELSEVIER/NORTH-HOLLAND BIOMEDICAL PRESS

First published 1940
Second edition 1946
Third edition 1960
Reprinted with amendments 1967
Fourth edition 1978

*Sole distributors outside the UK and Eire*
Elsevier/North-Holland Biomedical Press
335 Jan van Galenstraat, PO Box 211
Amsterdam, The Netherlands

*Sole distributors for the USA and Canada*
Elsevier/North-Holland Inc
52 Vanderbilt Avenue
New York, NY 10017, USA



Typographic design by HMSO

ISBN HMSO 0 11 450036 3*
ISBN Elsevier/North-Holland 0 444 80027 1

# Preface to the fourth edition

This edition is the result of collaboration between the Ministry of Agriculture, Fisheries and Food and the Medical Research Council, with the analytical work and method development carried out by the Laboratory of the Government Chemist. This work was supported by a grant from the Department of Education and Science, the Department of Health and Social Security, the Ministry of Defence and the Ministry of Agriculture, Fisheries and Food from March 1971 to April 1975, and from the Ministry of Agriculture, Fisheries and Food from April 1975 onwards.

The work began in 1969 under the Ministry's Inter-departmental Committee on Food Composition acting through a Steering Panel. The members of this panel were as follows:

| | |
|---|---|
| Dr D. A. T. Southgate | Medical Research Council (Convener) |
| Miss A. A. Paul<br>Miss J. Robertson | Ministry of Agriculture, Fisheries and Food (Joint Secretaries) |
| Mr A. A. Christie | Laboratory of the Government Chemist |
| Mrs M. M. Disselduff | Department of Health and Social Security |
| Mr D. Kimber | Ministry of Agriculture, Fisheries and Food |
| Mrs G. M. Mann | Ministry of Defence (until December 1975) |
| Miss J. W. Marr | Medical Research Council |
| Dr E. M. Widdowson | Medical Research Council |

The Steering Panel acted as an advisory group with a working group at the Dunn Nutritional Laboratory, Cambridge, consisting of Miss Paul and Dr Southgate, who were responsible for reviewing the literature, the preparation of the sampling and analytical protocols and the final compilation of the book, with advice from Dr Widdowson as the work progressed. The analytical work was carried out at the Laboratory of the Government Chemist under the supervision of Mr Christie. Mrs J. Thorn (Ministry of Agriculture, Fisheries and Food) joined the working group in Cambridge for short periods and helped in the revision of certain sections, notably the recipes for the cooked dishes. Miss J. Russell (Ministry of Agriculture, Fisheries and Food) has been responsible for the computerisation of the tables.

The sections dealing with cereals, milk and milk products, meat and fish have been extensively revised. Other sections have required a more limited revision, especially the sections on fruits, vegetables and nuts, where it has been possible to use a large amount of the information from earlier editions. In all, some 400 foods have been analysed either completely or partially for this edition. The recipes used in the calculations of the composition of cooked dishes have been converted to metric units and the composition of the dishes recalculated. At the same time a number of new dishes have been included. The tables giving the values for vitamins have been revised and extended. The amino acid tables have similarly been expanded. A new part giving the fatty acid composition of foods has been included and tables giving cholesterol values have also been added. The arrangement of the tables of vitamins, amino acids and fatty acids has been made similar to that used for the proximate constituents.

Committee on Food Composition
Ministry of Agriculture, Fisheries and Food
Horseferry Road, London SW1P 2AE

Medical Research Council
Park Crescent, London W1N 4AL

*November 1976*

# Contents

Contents *continued*

# Note from the compilers

Anyone who sets about the task of revising a standard work such as 'McCance and Widdowson' is bound to approach the work with a certain amount of awe and we are no exception. In our revision we have had the great advantage of being able to build on a very firm foundation. We have tried to retain all the features of the earlier editions which have proved themselves in over 35 years of use. Most of the changes in this edition have been necessary because of changes in methods of food production and food technology and because of an increased awareness of the importance of nutrients not included in earlier editions.

We have received advice and encouragement from many sources. This advice was often conflicting and we, as compilers, with the help of the Steering Panel have made some compromises which will not necessarily suit all the users of these tables. In the preparation of the final text and tables we have had to use a considerable amount of judgement and we alone must be held responsible for any errors in this respect. In this we have some comfort in Dr Widdowson's remark: 'The man who makes no mistakes does not usually make anything—he certainly does not make food tables.'

A. A. Paul
D. A. T. Southgate
MRC Dunn Nutrition Unit
Dunn Nutritional Laboratory
Cambridge

# Acknowledgements

A revision such as this would not have been possible without the collaboration, assistance and advice received from a large number of people. Miss D. F. Hollingsworth and Dr J. P. Greaves played an important role in the initiation of the work in 1969.

The major part of the sampling of the meat and its cooking and preparation was carried out by domestic science and dietetic students under the direction of Miss J. C. Currie (Glasgow and West of Scotland College of Domestic Science), Miss M. M. Jamieson (The Polytechnic of North London), Miss B. M. Llewelyn (Llandaff College of Education, Cardiff), Mrs J. Powell (City of Bath Technical College), Miss A. P. Robotham (Northern Counties College, Newcastle upon Tyne) and Miss M. Waterworth (City of Liverpool F. L. Calder College of Education). Miss M. Cameron, Mrs E. D. Davies, Mrs B. H. Lake, Mrs M. L. McLeod, Mrs J. R. Salfield and Miss B. Waugh were also involved at the colleges in various parts of the meat study. Insulated boxes for transporting the samples were kindly loaned by the Army Medical Directorate. The preparation and cooking of fish and vegetable samples was carried out under the direction of Mrs N. Parker (Cambridgeshire College of Arts and Technology). Other samples were obtained by Mrs H. S. Butler, Miss E. O. Ellis, Miss S. Hunt, Miss P. Mumford, Mrs I. M. Leppington and Dr J. O'Hara May. The Indian dishes and recipes were prepared by Miss P. Gill. To each of these people we tender our sincere thanks for undertaking the large amount of work that was involved.

Many individuals have given us much advice and in addition have willingly supplied us with unpublished data. Special thanks are due to Dr J. W. G. Porter and Dr S. Y. Thompson (National Institute for Research in Dairying), Dr R. M. Love (Torry Research Station), Mr A. Cuthbertson (Meat and Livestock Commission), Dr R. W. Pomeroy and Mr J. M. Harries (Meat Research Institute), Dr R. A. Barton (Massey University, New Zealand), Mr P. J. Harkett and Miss M. B. Groom (Food Research Institute), Mr R. A. Knight (Flour Milling and Baking Research Association), Dr J. N. Davies (Glasshouse Crops Research Institute), Dr J. D. Henshall and Mr D. J. Cook (The Campden Food Preservation Research Assocation), Dr I. H. Burger (British Food Manufacturing Industries Research Association), Dr A. Sinclair (Zoological Society of London), the Milk Marketing Board, the Herring Industry Board and the Wine and Spirit Association of Great Britain. To all the others who are not mentioned by name thanks are no less due for help in many aspects of the work.

The collection of material on manufactured foods was greatly assisted by the cooperation of manufacturers in providing information on their products.

These included Batchelor's Foods Ltd, Beecham Products Ltd, Birds Eye Foods Ltd, Bovril Ltd, Cadbury Schweppes Ltd, The Cocoa, Chocolate and Confectionery Alliance, the Coca-Cola Export Corporation, Energen Foods Co. Ltd, Express Dairies Ltd, General Foods Ltd, H. J. Heinz Co. Ltd, Mars Ltd, Nabisco Ltd, R. Paterson & Sons Ltd, Quaker Oats Ltd, Rank Hovis McDougall Ltd, Unilever Research Laboratory, Van den Berghs and Jurgens Ltd, A. Wander Ltd and Weetabix Ltd. Useful correspondence and discussions have also been held with a number of other companies.

We would also like to thank the members of the staff of the Laboratory of the Government Chemist, the Dunn Nutritional Laboratory and the Ministry of Agriculture, Fisheries and Food for their part in the analytical work, calculations, provision of library facilities and typing.

Thanks are also due to the large number of dietitians who replied to the questionnaires sent out in the early stages of the revision.

All the values in the tables are expressed in metric units ; the imperial equivalents are as follows :

| | |
|---|---|
| 1 ounce (oz) = 28.35 g | 100 g = 3.53 oz |
| 1 pound (lb) = 453.6 g | 1 kg = 2.2 lb (2lb 3oz) |
| 1 pint (pt) = 568 ml | 1 litre = 1.76 pt |

# General introduction

A knowledge of the composition of foods is essential in the dietary treatment and management of disease and in most quantitative studies of human nutrition.

The first edition *The Chemical Composition of Foods* in 1940 arose from a need to provide investigators, particularly those in Great Britain, with this information for a wide range of foods. The first edition was mostly compiled from a number of previous studies of the composition of foods made by Professor McCance and Dr Widdowson and their colleagues and especially from the study of meat and fish by McCance and Shipp (1933) and of fruits, vegetables and nuts by McCance, Widdowson and Shackleton (1936). The second edition, published in 1946, included some of the more important wartime and postwar foods but was otherwise little changed.

Some changes were made in the third edition, published in 1960 under the title *The Composition of Foods*. The range of nutrients was increased by the inclusion of sections giving values for vitamins and amino acids. The values for the vitamins were drawn mainly, but not exclusively, from the literature and were based on a very comprehensive search through and a critical appraisal of the literature by the late Dr W. I. M. Holman, compiled by Miss I. M. Barrett. The values for amino acids were compiled by Dr B. P. Hughes using a similar approach supplemented by analytical work.

The preparation of a fourth edition has followed the general principles used in the preparation of the third edition, that is using a combination of direct analysis and selection of values published in the literature. The approach adopted for this revision, however, has resulted in some changes in the way the book has been prepared. This is described in the following section because knowledge of the way in which the tables were prepared will help the reader to make the best use of the values in them.

The proximate composition, energy value, inorganic constituent and vitamin tables, the amino acid tables, the fatty acid tables and the cholesterol tables are also available in a form suitable for input to computers. The data from the tables are held on a paper tape file, which has been prepared using the International Reference Version of the ISO 7-bit coded character set, thereby making it internationally acceptable. While every effort has been made to include as much of the information from the tables as possible on the paper tape some parts, such as the footnotes, have had to be omitted. Where this has happened, indicators to refer users to the printed tables have been included. A booklet specifying the layout, contents, copyright position etc accompanies the paper tape file. The paper tape and booklet can be ordered from the Ministry of Agriculture, Fisheries and Food (Publications).

# Method of preparing the fourth edition

The process of revision can be considered under a number of headings, although in practice the various aspects are interrelated.

**Examination of the existing values**

This involved a detailed consideration of the values published in the third edition. All the values were examined in relation to recent published data for comparable foods, wherever these were available. It is worth noting, however, that for many foods and constituents the values recorded in the third edition are the only ones available. This survey showed which of the published values should be checked and possibly updated by analyses of a new sample. A few little used items have not been reprinted in this edition. The examination also showed that a large amount of the material in the third edition was still valid and nearly half of the values in this fourth edition have been taken directly from the third edition, particularly those for the fruits and vegetables.

**Selection of new foods for inclusion**

Views were sought from dietitians (Paul and Southgate, 1970), the food manufacturers and many nutrition workers and food scientists about new foods that should be included. The number of items suggested by these major users of the tables was very large, amounting to over 500; however, many of these were closely related foods. The most frequently requested items from this list were selected. Other items from this list were selected because of their importance in the national diet according to statistics on food consumption collected by the Ministry of Agriculture, Fisheries and Food and the retail food trade, and by consultation with specialists (usually food scientists) working with particular groups of foodstuffs. This approach ensured that most items of importance would be covered by the tables and in addition that the tables would provide information on the composition of the range of foods within different food groups.

The selection of manufactured and processed foods for inclusion was difficult. Many products undergo frequent changes in formulation and it was considered undesirable that foods of this type should be included in food composition tables which might be printed several years after the sample was collected and analysed, and remain in print for a number of years. The manufactured food items have therefore been restricted to those with an established and stable composition. In general, proprietary names have only been used where the designation of the food without the use of these names would have been difficult. The inclusion of a proprietary name does not imply that the particular brand has any special nutritional value.

Some food items which form an important part of the diets of various groups of immigrants have also been included. As data on many of these foods can be found in the tables compiled by Platt (1962) only a few raw foods have been included. A number of cooked and canned items were however analysed.

**Choice of nutrients to be covered**

Guidance in the choice of which nutrients should be included in the fourth edition was obtained from dietitians and nutrition workers in industry and in academic and research fields. These views showed that only a very few of the constituents given in the third edition were not used. They also indicated that there was a need for tables giving the fatty acid composition of foods and for improving the coverage of vitamins and amino acids. Many requests were also received for cholesterol values and for trace elements, especially zinc.

## Selection of values from the literature

A detailed examination of the published literature was first undertaken to establish whether or not reliable values were available for the food or the nutrients in question. Unpublished values for the composition of the food were also considered. Preference was given to values where the publication gave full details of the sample, its method of preparation and analysis, and where the results were presented in a detailed and acceptable form. The complete list of criteria which were used in assessing the published values are summarised in table 1 (Southgate, 1974). Only rarely, however, did the published sources meet all these criteria. It was also rare to find complete analyses, and in many cases it has been necessary to consider values for different nutrients obtained on different samples.

**Table 1** *Details considered in the evaluation of compositional data*

| | |
|---|---|
| Name of food | Common name, with local synonyms<br>Systematic name with variety where known |
| Origin | Plants:<br>Locality, with details of soil conditions and fertiliser treatments |
| | Animals:<br>Locality and method of husbandry and slaughter (where applicable) |
| Sampling | Place and time of collection<br>Number of samples<br>How obtained<br>Nature of sample (e.g. raw, prepared, deep frozen, prepacked etc) |
| Treatment of samples before analysis | Conditions and length of storage<br>Preparative treatment, including details of material discarded as waste<br>Method of cooking (where applicable) |
| Analysis | Details of material analysed<br>Methods used, with appropriate references and details of any modifications |
| Method of expression of results | Statistical treatment of analytical values<br>Whether expressed on an 'as purchased', 'edible matter' or 'dry matter' etc basis |

All the reported values for each nutrient in each item were collated and considered in detail and, on the basis of this review, selected values for each nutrient were chosen. These selected values are not necessarily the mean of all published values and depend very greatly on the judgement of the compilers in their interpretation of the results obtained by different analysts, sometimes using different methods.

If the review of the literature showed that little or no information on the composition of a food was available, or that the values given in the third edition were not representative of present-day foods, arrangements were made for the direct analysis of the food, either completely or for a restricted number of nutrients.

**Analysis**

Detailed sampling and analytical protocols were devised for each item for which analyses were required. The scope of the sampling scheme varied with the importance of the food, for example meats and meat products were collected in six regional centres, whereas other foods were collected only in Cambridge and London as there was reasonable confidence that this would be representative of the country as a whole. In the case of flour use was made of samples which were collected on a national scale in the Voluntary Flour Sampling Scheme.

The samples have been analysed at the Laboratory of the Government Chemist for all the constituents except the unavailable carbohydrates (=dietary fibre) and a few other constituents where a confirmatory analysis for an item already in the tables was required. These additional analyses were carried out at the Dunn Nutritional Laboratory, Cambridge (Southgate, Bailey, Collinson and Walker, 1976).

The details of the methods used in the analysis of foods for this and previous editions are given in appendix 1 (p 313).

# Arrangement of the tables

**General features of the fourth edition**

The tables are arranged in four sections. In the first three sections the same general arrangement has been used and throughout the tables the code number of a food is the same each time it appears. These code numbers are not the same as those used in previous editions. The first section contains the descriptions of the foods and gives values for the proximate constituents, energy value, inorganic constituents and vitamins in the foods. The values are given per 100g. The second section gives the amino acid compositions and these are given as mg amino acid per g nitrogen. The third section gives values for fatty acid composition as g fatty acids per 100g total fatty acids. The fourth section contains some subsidiary tables giving values for some constituents in a more limited range of foods. The section contains tables of values for the cholesterol and phytic acid in foods and notes on the iodine and organic acids in foods.

Within each section the foods are arranged in the following groups: cereals and cereal foods; milk and milk products; eggs; fats and oils; meat and meat products; fish and fish products; vegetables; fruits; nuts; sugars, preserves and confectionery; beverages and alcoholic beverages; sauces, soups and miscellaneous foods. The cooked dishes are included in the appropriate food groups and not given in separate sections as in previous editions.

This classification is practical rather than scientific and may appear rather arbitrary in some cases. This is inevitable, whatever system of grouping is used, and a full index is provided so that any food can be located easily.

In each food group related foods are listed together. In most cases an alphabetical order of listing within these subgroups has been used but in some cases some other arrangement has seemed more appropriate.

## Conventions and symbols used in the tables

Throughout the tables a number of conventions have been adopted and a number of symbols are used which have a precise meaning.

*Expression of values*

All the values in the tables apply to the edible part of the food and are expressed per 100 g. In the amino acid and fatty acid sections the values are expressed on nitrogen and total fatty acid bases respectively. Where a food is usually served with the inedible matter as an integral part of the food (for example, a chop with its bone) a separate series of values is given which apply to the composition of 100 g of the food weighed with its inedible matter.

*Edible matter*

Where the food is purchased or served with inedible material a factor is given which shows the proportion of the edible matter in the food. In the case of cooked foods this proportion also takes into account any changes in weight in cooking and gives the proportion of cooked edible material derived from the corresponding original raw item. The proportional factor is simply the percentage value given in previous editions divided by 100. The use of this factor is described later (p 32). Where the factor is greater than one (for example, stewed dried fruit) there is a gain in weight in cooking.

*Selected values*

Where the compositional values have been derived from the literature, they are not usually the average of all published values but represent the result of a critical assessment of the literature. This assessment involved consideration of the nature and origins of the samples, the method of cooking or other preparation and finally the analytical methods used. The values used in the tables are therefore designated selected values.

*Ranges*

Wherever possible, ranges are given in parentheses for some nutrients, particularly vitamins. These are mainly for important foods and for those where an appreciable amount of the constituent is present. The values given for the range show the usual extent of variation and extreme values have been discounted. These ranges are given for guidance in order to help the user assess the confidence which should be given to values for intakes of these nutrients calculated from the tables. In many cases there is insufficient information for a range to be given, but this does not mean that the nutrient composition is constant or any less variable than that of a nutrient for which a range is given.

*Symbols*

0 In the tables 0 signifies that virtually none of the constituent is known to be present in the food.

Tr This indicates that a trace is known to be present. In some cases a measurement has been made, and in other cases the literature indicates that a small amount is probably present but usually below the limits of the method used for analysis. The use of Tr indicates that the amount of the nutrient in the food in most cases is not known to be of quantitative dietetic significance and the value zero may be used in data processing.

( ) Figures in parentheses are estimates taken from related foods or, more rarely, tentative values based on a limited number of published sources.

— A dash shows that no information is available, either from direct analysis or by inference from the literature, to enable a value for the nutrient to be given in the tables. *This symbol should not be assigned the value zero in data processing: rather a value from a related food should be used with qualification.*

**Food code number**

The items in section 1 have been numbered from 1, Arrowroot, through to 969, Yeast, bakers, dried. In the other sections the code numbers are prefixed 2—amino acid composition; 3—fatty acid composition and 4—cholesterol.

Where the sample analysed for amino acids, fatty acids or cholesterol corresponded exactly with the item given in section 1, this is indicated by the code number assigned to the values in these sections.

For example:
Turkey, raw, meat only, has the code number 340 in section 1; 2340 in section 2; 3340 in section 3 and 4340 in section 4. The amino acid composition 2340, however, applies to all turkey entries and similarly 3340 gives the fatty acid composition of all fat in turkey entries.

Many values in sections 2 and 3 were obtained on grouped samples which do not appear in section 1; in these cases the base number (that is, the last three digits) is not used in section 1 but appears with its appropriate prefix in the other sections. These grouped values may apply to many different items in section 1.

For example:
The base number 123 is not used in section 1 because the amino acid composition of the protein in all cows' milk products is virtually the same and the values given under 2123 apply to all cows' milk products; similarly 3123 gives the composition of the fat in all cows' milk products.

In section 1, cows' milk, fresh, whole; cows' milk, fresh, whole, Channel Island; and single, double and whipping creams have been given two numbers to allow for different vitamin values in summer and winter milks.

**Description and number of samples**

The information given under this heading describes the number and nature of the samples taken for analysis. The sources of values not based on direct analysis that have been derived either from the literature or by calculation are also indicated under this heading. The description of the sample also includes the method of cooking where appropriate. Where the calculated composition of a cooked dish is given, the corresponding recipe and details of the cooking method are given in appendix 4. For most foods a number of samples were purchased at different shops, supermarkets or other retail outlets. The samples were not analysed separately but, as in previous editions, pooled before analysis. When the composite sample was made up from a number of different brands of a food, the numbers of the individual brands purchased was related to the relative shares of the retail market held by those brands. The different brands may or may not have been purchased at the same shop.

**Blank pages**

In section 1 a set of blank pages has been inserted between each major food group so that additional foods may be entered by the user if required.

# Modes of expression and determination of constituents

This section is mainly concerned with indicating the principles which are used in the determination of the constituents and in describing the modes of expression used in the tables. Details of the analytical procedures used for this and previous editions are given in appendix 1.

## Proximate constituents

The classical nutritional terminology has been adopted to describe the major constituents of a food, that is the water, protein, fat and carbohydrates. In the third edition the term 'calorific constituents' was used but it did not seem appropriate in this edition to use the corresponding term derived from the approved SI unit.

*Water*

Water is usually measured as the loss after drying either in an oven or at a lower temperature under reduced pressure. The water content of food containing volatile constituents, such as essential oils or alcohol, cannot be measured in this way and in the case of the alcoholic beverages values for total solids are given instead.

The water content of many foods, especially those of plant origin, can vary over fairly wide limits and differences in the water content of different samples are frequently a cause of analytical discrepancies. Many of these are eliminated if compositions are given on a dry-weight basis, but it is inappropriate to use this method of expression in tables of food composition.

*Total nitrogen*

Total nitrogen is measured by a variant of the Kjeldahl method. In previous editions attempts were made for some foods to estimate the non-protein nitrogen. This has not been possible in the present edition except where significant amounts were known to be present in the form of urea, purine or pyrimidine derivatives in mushrooms, beverages and a few fishes.

*Protein*

Protein has been calculated from the total nitrogen values by the use of factors. In the case of foods containing urea, purine and pyrimidine derivatives the total nitrogen value has been corrected before applying the factor. The factors used in this edition are those suggested by the FAO/WHO Committee on Energy and Protein Requirements (FAO/WHO, 1973)—see table 2.

**Table 2** *Factors for converting total nitrogen in foods to protein*

| | Factor (per gN) | | Factor (per gN) |
|---|---|---|---|
| Cereals | | Nuts | |
| Wheat | | Peanuts, Brazil nuts | 5.41 |
| Wholemeal | 5.83 | Almonds | 5.18 |
| Flours, except wholemeal | 5.70 | All other nuts | 5.30 |
| Macaroni | 5.70 | | |
| Bran | 6.31 | Milk and milk products | 6.38 |
| Rice | 5.95 | | |
| | | Gelatin | 5.55 |
| Barley, oats, rye | 5.83 | | |
| Soya | 5.71 | All other foods | 6.25 |

The proportion of non-protein nitrogen is high in many foods, notably fish, fruits and vegetables. In most of these, however, this non-protein nitrogen is amino acid in nature and therefore little dietetic error is involved in the use of a factor applied to the total nitrogen, although protein in the strict sense is overestimated.

A few other foods (notably Bovril and Marmite) contain a high proportion of non-protein nitrogen, which is again mainly amino acid and peptide nitrogen. In these foods total nitrogen (minus purine-N) has also been multiplied by 6.25 to give a value for 'protein'. For nutritional purposes this seemed justifiable and means that the energy values for these foods are now, more correctly, considerably higher than in previous editions.

*Fat*

Fat in most foods is a mixture of triglycerides, phospholipids, sterols and related compounds. For this edition it was decided that, where possible, the standard procedure for estimating fat in each class of foodstuffs would be used and the values given refer to total lipid.

The value for the fat in a food is extremely dependent on the analytical method used in its measurement and even officially approved methods have given very conficting results in some cases. In general the observations recorded in earlier editions have been confirmed, that is that the Soxhlet procedure gives incomplete extraction of the fat from many foods and values obtained by this method are almost invariably lower than those obtained using more recent methods involving acid hydrolysis or mixed solvent extraction.

*Carbohydrates*

Carbohydrates (including sugars and starch) are in all cases expressed as *monosaccharides* and throughout the tables all values for carbohydrate are *available carbohydrate*: that is, the sum of the free sugars (glucose, fructose, sucrose, lactose, maltose and higher maltose homologues), dextrins, starch and glycogen expressed as monosaccharides. These are the carbohydrates which are digested and absorbed by man and which are glucogenic in man. In the tables the headings are as follows:

*Sugars* include free monosaccharides and disaccharides.

*Lactose* is also expressed as monosaccharide, which is equivalent to lactose measured as the monohydrate.

*Starch* includes starch and dextrins hydrolysed by amyloglucosidase enzyme preparations and excludes glucofructans and fructans that are not hydrolysed by this enzyme.

On hydrolysis a disaccharide such as sucrose gives 105 g monosaccharide per 100 g and a polysaccharide such as starch gives 110 g of the monosaccharide glucose per 100 g. This means that white sugar (item 843) for example contains 105 g of carbohydrate (expressed as monosaccharide) per 100 g of sugar. To convert the carbohydrate expressed as monosaccharide to the forms present in the food, the monosaccharides derived from disaccharides should be divided by 1.05 and those from polysaccharides by 1.10.

*Dietary fibre*

The term 'dietary fibre' has been used instead of the '*unavailable carbohydrates*' of earlier editions; for all practical purposes these two terms are synonymous. Dietary fibre is defined as the sum of the polysaccharides and lignin which are not digested by the endogenous secretions of the human gastrointestinal tract. This fraction has a variable composition as it is made up of several different types of polysaccharide (pectic substances, hemicelluloses and cellulose) and the non-carbohydrate lignin.

The values given in this edition for cereals and cereal foods and some vegetables and fruit are based on direct analyses; the remainder are based on the values taken from earlier editions, where an indirect but equally valid method of measurement was used.

*Alcohol*

The values for alcohol are given as g/100ml of alcoholic beverages. Pure ethyl alcohol has a specific gravity of 0.790 and these values can be converted to alcohol, by volume (that is ml/100ml), by dividing by 0.79 (see p28).

**Energy value**

The energy values of the foods are given as both kilocalories (kcal) and kilojoules (kJ). These energy values have been calculated from the amounts of protein, fat, carbohydrate and alcohol in the foods using energy conversion factors.

The third edition of these tables included a note by Dr E M. Widdowson, which has been reprinted in appendix 2, on the calculation of the calorific values of foods and of diets. This note gave an account of the historical background to the various systems of energy conversion factors and the reasons behind the choice of the factors for that edition, which were 4.1 kcal/g protein, 9.3 kcal/g fat and 3.75 kcal/g carbohydrate (available, expressed as monosaccharides).

In this edition the conversion factors used are as follows: protein 4 kcal/g; fat 9 kcal/g; carbohydrate (available, expressed as monosaccharides) 3.75 kcal/g and alcohol 7 kcal/g.

These factors permit the calculation of the metabolisable energy of a mixed diet of the type eaten in the United Kingdom with an accuracy which is equal to, or greater than, the accuracy one could reasonably expect in dietary work using tables of food composition (Southgate and Durnin, 1970).

In the calculation of energy values in terms of kilojoules the factors recommended by the Committee on Metrication in the Nutritional Sciences of the Royal Society (1972) have been used: that is, protein 17 kJ/g; fat 37 kJ/g; carbohydrate (available, expressed as monosaccharides) 16 kJ/g and alcohol 29 kJ/g. The factors have been applied directly to the amounts of protein, fat, carbohydrate and alcohol in the foods. If the energy values in kJ are calculated from the kcal values directly using the conversion factor 4.184 kJ/kcal, numerically different values are obtained. The differences are small, being at the most of the order of 1–2 per cent and frequently less; furthermore they are of no dietetic significance.

For consistency, however, it is preferable that the calculation should be carried out in the manner adopted in these tables. The kilojoule factors are in fact closer to the factors calculated from the studies of Southgate and Durnin (1970) and indeed of Atwater himself (Merrill and Watt, 1955) than are the conventional 4, 9 and 3.75 kcal factors. Table 3 summarises the energy conversion factors used in the present edition; the table also includes factors for organic acids and glycerol based on the heats of combustion of these substances. The contribution of organic acids and glycerol to the energy has not, however, been included for the relevant foods in this edition because of lack of suitable analytical data.

*Changes due to the use of new factors in this edition*

The energy values in the present edition are slightly lower than values given in the previous editions for foods with identical compositions. The differences

**Table 3** *Energy conversion factors*

| | kcal/g | kJ/g |
|---|---|---|
| Protein | 4 | 17 |
| Fat | 9 | 37 |
| Carbohydrate[a] | 3.75 | 16 |
| Ethyl alcohol | 7 | 29 |
| Glycerol | 4.31[b] | 18.0[b] |
| Acetic acid | 3.49[b] | 14.6[b] |
| Citric acid | 2.47[b] | 10.3[b] |
| Lactic acid | 3.62[b] | 15.1[b] |
| Malic acid | 2.39[b] | 10.0[b] |

[a] Value for available carbohydrate expressed as monosaccharide
[b] Values derived from heat of combustion

are due principally to the use of a lower factor for the energy value of fat. Again the differences are small (less than 1 per cent for most foods) and are of little true dietetic significance.

*Contribution of unavailable carbohydrates*

Any contribution to the metabolisable energy arising from the bacterial degradation of unavailable carbohydrates in the large intestine is discounted by the method of calculation of energy values. The products of degradation are mainly short-chain fatty acids and it is not clear how well these are absorbed. In any case their energy contribution would be small. Any effect of the unavailable carbohydrates or dietary fibre on the absorption of other energy-yielding nutrients has also been discounted.

**Inorganic constituents**

The values for the inorganic constituents are given in the tables as mg per 100 g. They appear in the order sodium (Na); potassium (K); calcium (Ca); magnesium (Mg); phosphorus (P); iron (Fe); copper (Cu); zinc (Zn); sulphur (S) and chloride (Cl).

*Sodium* and *potassium* are now usually measured by flame photometry or atomic absorption spectrophotometry. Common salt is one of the most frequently used food additives and consequently the values for sodium are likely to be much more variable than for potassium. The calculation of sodium intakes from food tables is therefore prone to error, particularly if salt is used in cooking. Accurate values for sodium intakes can only be obtained by analysis of replicates of the diet. Nevertheless the values given should provide a reliable guide for planning low-sodium diets. If the values for these elements are required in millimoles (milliequivalents) then the values in mg should be divided by 23 and 39 for Na and K respectively.

*Calcium* can be measured chemically or by atomic absorption spectrophotometry. The calcium content of a particular food varies within fairly narrow limits. There are, however, several major uses of calcium salts as additives. These are first to wheat flour, where there is a statutory addition in the United Kingdom to all wheat flours except wholemeal. The raising agents in self-raising flour and in some baking powders also contain calcium. The latter are very rich sources of calcium and their use increases the calcium content of the food considerably.

Contamination of the edible portion of meat and fish by pieces of bone also causes variation in the calcium content; this is especially evident in the case of fish where the very fine bones are frequently eaten. Contamination from particles of bone is common in many foods where the carcase of the animal has been cut with a saw or scissors (for example brain).

The tap water in many areas contains appreciable amounts of calcium (and other inorganic salts) and foods which have been cooked in hard tap water may have their calcium contents enhanced from this source. However, vegetables, fruits and soups in the tables were cooked in distilled water, and and the beverages were also prepared with distilled water.

*Magnesium* is now usually measured by atomic absorption spectrophotometry. The concentration of magnesium in a particular food varies within narrow limits.

*Phosphorus* is usually measured colorimetrically as the phosphate. Polyphosphates are becoming increasingly used as food additives, particularly in meat products, and occasionally in evaporated canned milks. The amounts used are small and only minor increases in the total phosphate content result from the use of these compounds. Phosphates are used as raising agents, and some baking powders are rich sources of phosphorus. The values expressed as mg P can be converted to mg $PO_4$ by multiplying by 3.06.

*Iron, copper and zinc* may be measured colorimetrically or by atomic absorption spectrophotometry. The elements, as well as being derived from constituents occurring naturally in foods, may also be derived from metallic contamination either from processing machinery, kitchen knives, pots and pans or from particles of soil. The contamination of foods from one source or another is probably a major cause of variation but, even so, wide ranges of values are often reported in the literature under circumstances where precautions had been taken to avoid contamination. Iron compounds are added to a number of important foods; there is a statutory addition in the UK to all wheat flours except wholemeal, and many proprietary breakfast cereals and baby foods contain added iron. Copper and zinc compounds are rarely used as food additives *per se* and elevated values for copper and zinc are usually evidence of metallic contamination. Iron and copper salts are frequently used in animal feeding and these often result in elevated levels in some tissues used as foods. Marine organisms, specially molluscs and crustaceans, accumulate quite high concentrations of inorganic constituents.

*Sulphur* in foods is mostly derived from the sulphur-containing amino acids, cysteine and methionine, and the nitrogen:sulphur ratio in many groups of foods has been shown to give a reasonable prediction of the sulphur content from the total nitrogen. The sulphur in foods is usually estimated after oxidation of the sulphur to sulphate but a range of techniques have been studied in order to establish the best methods for the foods analysed for this edition (see p318). Sulphur dioxide is widely used as preservative and its use results in high observed values for total sulphur, but this is almost certainly unavailable.

*Chloride* is measured by titration. The chloride in foods is mainly associated with the alkali metals and generally varies with the sodium. The variations in the use of added common salt that are responsible for the variations in the sodium content of foods also produce great variability in the chloride contents. The values expressed as mg can be converted to millimoles (milliequivalents) by dividing by 35.5.

## Vitamins

The vitamins for each food are given on two pages; the first gives figures for retinol, carotene, vitamin D, thiamin, riboflavin, nicotinic acid, vitamin C and vitamin E, and the second for vitamin $B_6$, vitamin $B_{12}$, folic acid, pantothenic acid and biotin. The figures given on the second page are based on more limited data than those given on the first and calculations using them should be interpreted accordingly. The second page also includes a panel containing notes which apply to the vitamins on both pages.

The comments below on methodology refer in the main to the criteria used in assessing values in the literature; the methods used for the analyses undertaken for this edition are given in appendix 1 (p318).

*Vitamin A: retinol and carotene*

In the third edition values for vitamin A potency were calculated as the sum of the preformed vitamin and the contribution from any carotenoids present. In this edition these two constituents have been expressed separately as μg retinol and carotene respectively. The values for the latter in most foods are for β-carotene. Where no information is available on the proportions of the different carotenoids in the food, the value given is for total carotene. In these cases the total vitamin A activity will be slightly overestimated, but the error introduced in this way is only small. Calculation of the total vitamin A potency in terms of μg retinol equivalents can be made by applying a divisor to the carotene values. The numerical value of this divisor depends on the types of carotenoids present and is a measure of the relative efficiency with which the carotenoids are converted to retinol in the body. For the total carotenoids in the diet, experimental studies have shown that 6 is the best value to use for the divisor so that:

$$\text{Vitamin A potency } (\mu\text{g retinol equivalents}) = \mu\text{g retinol} + \frac{\mu\text{g } \beta\text{-carotene}}{6}$$

Very few studies of individual foods have been made which enable one to propose the correct divisor for each food. It is more correct to calculate the retinol equivalents contributed by carotenoids from the total dietary carotenoids, and values for retinol equivalents are not given in the tables for individual foods (see p33). Values reported in international units have been recalculated according to the definition that one international unit of vitamin A potency is equal to 0.3μg retinol or 0.6μg β-carotene.

Retinol is estimated spectrophotometrically after saponification, extraction and chromatographic separation; carotenes are usually measured spectrophotometrically after extraction and chromatographic separation.

*Vitamin D*

In most foodstuffs the concentration of vitamin D is too low for measurement by chemical techniques and biological assay is the only method available for these foods at present. Values from the older literature using the rat have been used in the tables but very few recent reports of the amounts of vitamin D in foods are available. In foods where there are high concentrations naturally or where vitamin D has been added, some values obtained by gas–liquid chromatographic methods have been given. These are limited to concentrations of the order of that found in fatty fish. The values are expressed as μg cholecalciferol per 100g. Values reported in international units have been recalculated on the basis that 1 i u = 0.025μg cholecalciferol.

*Thiamin*

The values given are based on chemical measurements by the thiochrome method and microbiological assay using *Lactobacillus viridescens* (ATCC

12706) or *L. fermenti* (ATCC 9338). These procedures give similar results provided that the appropriate extraction technique has been used to release the thiamin from the coenzyme. The values are expressed as mg per 100g.

*Riboflavin*

Preliminary acid or enzymatic hydrolyses using proteolytic and amylolytic enzymes are required to release riboflavin from the bound forms, riboflavin mononucleotide and flavin adenine dinucleotide, which occur in foods. Provided that the appropriate preliminary treatment has been used, fluorimetric methods and microbiological assay using *Lactobacillus casei* (ATCC 7469) or *Streptococcus zymogenes* (ATCC 10100) give similar results. The values are expressed as mg per 100g.

*Nicotinic acid*

A preliminary acid or enzymatic hydrolysis of the food samples is required to release the nicotinic acid from its bound forms. The values given are based on measurements which include both nicotinic acid and nicotinamide determinations. The method of determination is either by the colorimetric reaction with cyanogen bromide or by microbiological assay using *Lactobacillus plantarum* (ATCC 8014). The values are expressed as mg nicotinic acid per 100g and no attempt has been made to separate the bound and probably unavailable forms of nicotinic acid in cereals (see p33).

The calculation of nicotinic acid equivalents, which includes the contribution from tryptophan, should be made on the total diet as follows:

$$\text{mg nicotinic acid equivalents} = \text{mg nicotinic acid} + \frac{\text{mg tryptophan}}{60}$$

The conversion of tryptophan to nicotinic acid takes place in the body with varying efficiency and the factor of 60 is an approximation based on a limited number of studies. There are no data on which to judge whether this factor applies equally to all foods; thus nicotinic acid equivalents are not given for individual foods, but the potential contribution from the tryptophan in the food, calculated as mg tryptophan divided by 60, is given for guidance (see p33).

*Vitamin C*

This term has been preferred for the sum of ascorbic acid and dehydroascorbic acid, as both forms are active. In fresh foods the reduced form is the major one present and the proportions present as the dehydro-form are increased during cooking and processing. Values given refer to total ascorbic acid, that is reduced plus dehydroascorbic acid, wherever possible.

The values considered from the literature are based on a variety of methods. For foods where only the reduced form was judged to be present, values based on the titration with 2,6-dichlorophenolindophenol have been used together with those based on the more specific 2,4-dinitrophenylhydrazine method and the more recent fluorimetric method, which measure total ascorbic acid.

*Vitamin E*

The various forms of tocopherols found in foods have different biological activities. In most animal products the α-form is the only one present but in plant products, especially seeds and the oils from seeds, other forms are present. β-tocopherol has an activity of around 30 per cent, γ-tocopherol 15 per cent, and α-tocotrienol (ζ-tocopherol) 30 per cent of the α-form respectively. The other forms have activities of 5 per cent or less of α-tocopherol. In the column headed 'Vitamin E' the values are for α-tocopherol and information is given in the notes about the other major active forms where the data are available.

The figures given in the tables are based on methods involving chromatographic separation of the various tocopherols and colorimetric measurements and occasionally on more recent gas–liquid chromatography methods. The values are expressed as mg per 100 g.

*Vitamin $B_6$*

The various forms of pyridoxine, pyridoxal, pyridoxamine and their phosphates and some other conjugated forms all contribute to the vitamin $B_6$ activity in a food. A preliminary treatment with acid in an autoclave is usually necessary to achieve complete extraction. Values obtained by microbiological assay using *Saccharomyces carlsbergensis* (ATCC 9080), which measures all forms, have been used. The values are expressed as mg per 100 g.

*Vitamin $B_{12}$*

Values obtained by microbiological assay with *Lactobacillus leichmanni* (ATCC 7830) have been preferred. The values are given as μg per 100 g.

*Folic acid*

Values for folic acid are given as the amounts for free and total folic acid present. These are respectively the folic acid activity measured microbiologically with *L. casei* (ATCC 7649) before and after treatment with conjugase. Values reported in the literature before the use of ascorbic acid as an antioxidant in the extraction medium have not been used, as folic acid activity is underestimated if it is not protected during extraction.

The availability of the various forms and conjugates of folic acid is poorly understood at the present time and it is not clear whether the organisms used in its assay respond to the same forms that are available to man. Many foods contain conjugases which will degrade the higher conjugates quite rapidly during the normal course of the storage and preparation of foods for consumption or analysis. This means that values for free folate are very variable and of doubtful significance. It is therefore probable that the estimates of the folic acid in foods given in this edition will need revision in the future and they should therefore be used with this in mind when the amounts of folic acid in a diet are being assessed. The values are given as μg per 100 g.

*Pantothenic acid*

These data are based on values obtained by microbiological assay using *L. plantarum* or *S. carlsbergenis*, after release from the bound form in which it occurs by the double enzyme treatment, usually avian liver and pig intestinal phosphatase. The values are expressed as mg per 100 g.

*Biotin*

These values are also based on microbiological determinations using *L. plantarum* after acid hydrolysis to release the bound forms. Recent improvements in techniques have resulted in lower amounts of biotin found and these are believed to be more correct than the older ones. The values are given as μg per 100 g.

**Amino acids**

The amino acid compositions are given in section 2 of the tables, in which the foods are arranged in the same groups as in section 1. In this section the values are given as mg amino acid per g nitrogen. This method of expression means that a single series of figures can be given which applies to all the foods containing proteins with the same amino acid composition. For example a single entry suffices for all types of beef. Values for the amounts of amino acids in 100 g of food can be calculated using the total nitrogen values given in section 1 (see appendix 5); this calculation has been included in the computer tape version of these tables.

The amino acids are listed in the tables under their recognised three-letter abbreviations. These are as follows:

| *Essential* | | *Non-essential* | |
|---|---|---|---|
| Isoleucine | Ile | Arginine | Arg |
| Leucine | Leu | Histidine | His |
| Lysine | Lys | Alanine | Ala |
| Methionine | Met | Aspartic acid | Asp |
| Cystine | Cys | Glutamic acid | Glu |
| Phenylalanine | Phe | Glycine | Gly |
| Tyrosine | Tyr | Proline | Pro |
| Threonine | Thr | Serine | Ser |
| Tryptophan | Trp | | |
| Valine | Val | | |

A wider space between columns separates the essential amino acids—that is, those required for the maintenance of nitrogen balance in adult man—from the non-essential. Cystine and tyrosine have been included in the former group because of their sparing effects on the requirements for methionine and phenylalanine respectively.

In assessing the values reported in the literature results obtained both by microbiological methods and by ion-exchange chromatography have been considered, although most recent analyses have been by chromatographic methods. It is interesting to note that despite the virtually complete automation in this field, and the fact that these analyses can be carried out very rapidly, the actual number of reliable analyses which have been reported for even major foodstuffs is still quite small.

In assessing the values in the literature the description of the conditions used for the hydrolyses of the proteins and the measurement of hydrolytic losses were frequently inadequate and preference has been given, where possible, to results reported by authors who have carried out serial hydrolyses to determine the optimum length of hydrolysis and who give estimates of the hydrolytic losses. Unfortunately many authors do not describe their hydrolytic conditions, the most critical part of amino acid analysis, in sufficient detail, and it is often not possible to decide whether the discrepancies between reported values are genuine or are analytical artefacts.

The values for the sulphur amino acids (cystine and methionine) have been taken from analyses where the intact protein has been oxidised with performic acid before hydrolysis.

The values for tryptophan are derived in the main from separate colorimetric analyses and, more rarely, from the results obtained by the ion-exchange chromatography of alkaline hydrolysates.

**Fatty acids**

The tables giving the fatty acid composition of foods are contained in section 3. The values are expressed as g of the individual fatty acids per 100 g total fatty acids. Not all the fatty acids present in trace amounts are given in the tables and therefore the sum of the values may be less than 100. The foods are arranged in the same groups as in section 1, although some condensation has been possible because foods with the same fatty acid composition can be covered by a single series of values.

The values given in the tables are virtually all based on gas–liquid chromatographic analysis, usually of the methyl esters of the fatty acids prepared from the total extracted lipid, and they include the fatty acids derived from both triglycerides and phospholipids.

Occasional difficulties were met in the interpretation of values in the literature where these were expressed in an unusual way and insufficient data were given to enable recalculation to the basis adopted. Values have therefore been preferred which were reported in terms of fatty acids per 100 g total fatty acids or as methyl esters per 100 g total methyl esters. These two methods of expression are very similar for most individual foods.

The fatty acids are listed under their carbon number and number of double bonds in the usual way (table 4). The common names for the most frequently occurring fatty acids are also given in this table. In each food group the most appropriate arrangement of the column headings in the tables has been used. For example the tables for milk have more headings for the shorter-chain fatty acids and those for fish more headings to cover the long-chain polyunsaturated acids present. The fatty acids are grouped into saturated, mono-unsaturated and polyunsaturated groups, and at the end of each table the column headed 'Others' gives values for fatty acids, other than those listed, that are present in measurable amounts. A trace in these tables usually means that less than 0.1 g/100 g total fatty acids was present. The value 0 usually means that the fatty acid in question was not reported and it has been assumed that none was present.

**Table 4** *The most common fatty acids in foods*

| Carbon : Double bonds | Common name |
|---|---|
| *Saturated* | |
| C4 : 0 | Butyric |
| C6 : 0 | Caproic |
| C8 : 0 | Caprylic |
| C10 : 0 | Capric |
| C12 : 0 | Lauric |
| C14 : 0 | Myristic |
| C16 : 0 | Palmitic |
| C18 : 0 | Stearic |
| C20 : 0 | Arachidic |
| C22 : 0 | Behenic |
| C24 : 0 | Lignoceric |
| *Mono-unsaturated* | |
| C16 : 1 | Palmitoleic |
| C18 : 1 | Oleic |
| C20 : 1 | Eicosenoic |
| C22 : 1 | Erucic |
| *Polyunsaturated* | |
| C18 : 2 | Linoleic |
| C18 : 3 | Linolenic |
| C20 : 4 | Arachidonic |

When the fatty acids provided by a given weight of food are being calculated allowance must be made for the fact that the total fat in a food includes triglycerides, of which a proportion is glycerol (that is, not fatty acid), phospholipids and unsaponifiable components such as sterols.

In foods where the total fat is virtually all triglyceride a correction factor based on the average chain length of the fatty acids present is adequate. The factors for food containing appreciable amounts of phospholipids and unsaponifiable matter depend on the class of foodstuff. Some suggested values for these factors are given in table 5.

**Table 5** *Conversion factors to be applied to total fat to give values for total fatty acids in the fat*

| | | | |
|---|---|---|---|
| Wheat, barley and rye [a] | | Beef [c] lean | 0.916 |
| whole grain | 0.72 | fat | 0.953 |
| flour | 0.67 | Lamb, take as beef | |
| bran | 0.82 | Pork [d] lean | 0.910 |
| Oats, whole [a] | 0.94 | fat | 0.953 |
| Rice, milled [a] | 0.85 | Poultry | 0.945 |
| Milk and milk products | 0.945 | Brain [d] | 0.561 |
| Eggs [b] | 0.83 | Heart [d] | 0.789 |
| Fats and oils | | Kidney [d] | 0.747 |
| all except coconut | 0.956 | Liver [d] | 0.741 |
| coconut | 0.942 | Fish, fatty [e] | 0.90 |
| | | white [e] | 0.70 |
| | | Vegetables and fruit | 0.80 |
| | | Avocado pears | 0.956 |
| | | Nuts | 0.956 |

[a] Weihrauch, Kinsella and Watt (1976)
[b] Posati, Kinsella and Watt (1975)
[c] Anderson, Kinsella and Watt (1975)
[d] Anderson (1976)
[e] Exler, Kinsella and Watt (1975)

These factors are used as in the following examples.

Palmitic acid in 100 g goats milk containing 4.5 g fat:
$4.5 \times 0.945 = 4.25$ g total fatty acids
$4.25 \times \frac{27}{100} = 1.15$ g palmitic acid

Stearic acid in 100 g whole egg containing 10.9 g fat:
$10.9 \times 0.83 = 9.05$ g total fatty acids
$9.05 \times \frac{9.3}{100} = 0.84$ g stearic acid

The fatty acids per 100 g of food have been calculated on the computer tape version of these tables for all foods for which appropriate fatty acid data are available (see appendix 5).

# Notes on food groups

## Cereals and cereal products

The items in the cereals section are arranged in the following groups: grains, flours and starches; bread and rolls; breakfast cereals; biscuits; cakes, buns and pastries; and puddings.

The first group includes foods which are not strictly of cereal origin such as tapioca and soya. The wheat flour and breads are arranged in order of descending extraction rate but otherwise an alphabetical arrangement has been followed. Some groups include items whose composition has been calculated from recipes in addition to items which have been analysed as purchased. The 'pudding' group consists almost entirely of items calculated from recipes.

*Moisture content*

The composition of many cereals seems to be relatively constant and the major cause of variation is the moisture content. Most air-dry grains and flours have moisture contents of 10 to 14 per cent and, furthermore, above 15 per cent most cereals deteriorate on storage. Many proprietary breakfast cereals are packed at a moisture content of around 2 per cent but rapidly absorb some moisture once the packet has been opened. The values given refer to packets purchased in the usual way which were opened and mixed just before analysis.

*Fortification*

Wheat flours (other than wholemeal) are fortified with calcium, iron, thiamin and nicotinic acid in the UK at the present time. Self-raising flours are exempt from the requirement to add creta (calcium carbonate) if a calcium acid phosphate raising agent is used. The values given for flours are for those available in the UK; the composition of unfortified flours are given in the notes. Nicotinic acid is expressed as the total content and the question of availability of the nicotinic acid present naturally in these foods is discussed on p 33.

*Carbohydrates*

Many cereals contain glucofructans, at concentrations around 1 per cent in wheat for example. These polysaccharides are very readily hydrolysed and should probably be regarded as available carbohydrate. They are thus included in the 'sugars' in the tables.

*Vitamin losses on cooking*

Average losses of vitamins have been used to calculate the composition of cooked items. These are shown in table 6.

**Table 6** *Percentage losses of vitamins in cereals during cooking*

| | Boiling | Baking | | Boiling | Baking |
|---|---|---|---|---|---|
| Thiamin | 40 | 25* | Folic acid (free) | 90 | 50 |
| Riboflavin | 40 | 15 | (total) | 50 | 50 |
| Nicotinic acid | 40 | 5 | Biotin | 40 | 0 |
| Vitamin $B_6$ | 40 | 25 | Pantothenic acid | 40 | 25 |

* 15% in breadmaking
(For other vitamins the losses have been assumed to be zero)

## Milk and milk products

This group includes milk, butter, cream, cheese and yogurt. The milks are arranged in a sequence which is not strictly alphabetical. The first item—milk, fresh, whole—provides the basic figures from which the composition of a number of milk products is derived by calculation.

No separate values are given for infant milk formulations. This is because of the present state of flux concerning these foods (Department of Health and Social Security, 1974) and it was considered unwise to include products which were likely to be superseded before or shortly after the tables were published.

In the cheese group the items are grouped according to their types, with a few individual cheeses which do not fall strictly within these classifications given separately. This was done because the variations observed for a named cheese were of the same order as those within the group type.

*Modes of expression*

The values are expressed per 100g edible portion. A very small error is involved if these values are applied to liquid unconcentrated milks measured by volume, that is per 100ml. Milk has a specific gravity of about 1.03 so that 100ml = 103g.

*Non-protein nitrogen*

Milks contain some non-protein nitrogen but no allowance for this has been made in the calculated protein values in the tables.

*Values for fat-soluble vitamins*

The vitamin content of milk fat shows a seasonal variation with regard to the fat-soluble vitamins (retinol, carotene, vitamin D and vitamin E). Two sets of values are given for these vitamins in whole milk and cream to allow for the seasonal differences. In the heading 'summer' refers to milks between May and October and 'winter' between November and April. In the case of processed milk and milk products, where the values for the fat-soluble vitamins have been calculated from the fat content of these items, an average value for the vitamins in milkfat has been used. The one exception is cheese, for which the summer values have been used.

The values used were as follows:

*Fat-soluble vitamins µg/g fat*

| Non-Channel Island breeds | Retinol | Carotene | Vitamin D | Vitamin E |
|---|---|---|---|---|
| Summer | 9.3 | 5.8 | 0.0078 | 25 |
| Winter | 6.8 | 3.3 | 0.0038 | 19 |
| Average | 8.1 | 4.6 | 0.0058 | 22 |
| Channel Island breeds | | | | |
| Summer | 7.9 | 12.8 | 0.0078 | 25 |
| Winter | 5.8 | 7.3 | 0.0038 | 19 |

*Vitamin losses on heat treatment*

The values given for the vitamins in milks which have been heat treated have been calculated from the values for raw milk using measured losses reported in the literature. The values for the percentage losses used were as shown in table 7. The amounts of the vitamins in other forms of processed milk were measured directly. The other vitamins show little or no loss under these conditions.

**Table 7** *Percentage losses of vitamins on processing milk*

| | Thiamin | Riboflavin | Vitamin $B_6$ | Vitamin $B_{12}$ | Folic acid | Vitamin C | Vitamin E |
|---|---|---|---|---|---|---|---|
| Pasteurisation | 10 | 0 | 0 | 0 | 5 | 25 | 0 |
| Sterilization | 20 | 0 | 20 | 20 | 30 | 60 | 0 |
| Ultra-high temperature (UHT) | 10 | 0 | 10 | 5 | 20 | 30 | 0 |
| UHT stored 3 months | 10 | 0 | 35 | 20 | $>50$ | 100 | 0 |
| Boiled (from pasteurised milk) | 0 | 10 | 10 | 5 | 20 | 30–70 | 20 |

For other vitamins the losses have been assumed to be zero.

*B vitamins in cheese*

The values for the B vitamins in cheeses show great variability. This is due to the synthesis of these vitamins by the microorganism involved in cheese production. The values therefore vary according to the stage of maturity of the cheese and, particularly for the soft cheeses, with the proportion of rind incorporated in the sample, because the concentration of many B vitamins is very much higher in the rind than in the body of the cheese.

## Eggs

The values for whole egg are taken in the main from the large study described by Tolan *et al.* (1974). The average values for the composition of eggs obtained in this study were very similar to those reported in previous editions. The values for cooking losses are shown in table 8.

**Table 8** *Percentage losses of vitamins in eggs during cooking*

| | Boiled | Fried | Poached | Omelette | Scrambled |
|---|---|---|---|---|---|
| Thiamin | 10 | 20 | 20 | 5 | 5 |
| Riboflavin | 5 | 10 | 20 | 20 | 20 |
| Vitamin $B_6$ | 10 | 20 | 20 | 15 | 15 |
| Folic acid | 10 | 30 | 35 | 30 | 30 |
| Pantothenic acid | 10 | 20 | 20 | 15 | 15 |

For other vitamins the losses have been assumed to be zero.

## Fats and oils

This group includes the major fats and oils; the values for butter have been repeated in this group as a comparison with other fats is frequently made. The proximate section for this group is rather simple as most of these foods are virtually pure triglyceride and the amounts of nitrogen and inorganic constituents are very low. This, however, is not the case in the fatty acid section, where the compositions of the different oils are given separately. But it is important to bear in mind that most oils show a very wide range of fatty acid composition depending on variety, growing conditions and maturity of the oil seed.

*Composition of compounded fats including margarines*

These fats are mixtures prepared by the manufacturer to have the desired physical and other properties. In several cases these properties can be achieved by several different blends and it is normal commercial practice to adjust the blending according to the availability of the different oil ingredients, which will alter the fatty acid composition of the product. If accurate fatty acid data are required for specific products it is usually better to consult the manufacturer if analytical facilities are not at one's disposal.

## Meat and meat products

The items are arranged in the following groups: bacon; beef; lamb; pork; veal; poultry and game; offal; and meat products and dishes. This last group includes the items whose compositions are derived from recipes and which were given in a separate section in previous editions. Within these groupings the foods are arranged alphabetically.

*Sources of values*

The values for the composition of an average dressed carcase which are given in the bacon, beef, lamb and pork sections are derived by calculation from dissection data from the Meat and Livestock Commission (see appendix 6) and other information, including the new analytical values for raw meats described below.

For the most part the values given in this section are based on the results of new analyses of a large number of samples which were collected from different parts of the country (Paul and Southgate, 1977). Samples were purchased at six centres (London, Bath, Cardiff, Liverpool, Newcastle and Glasgow). Each centre purchased six samples of each item, three at each centre were cooked and three were used to provide the raw samples for analysis. Where two methods of cooking were used the number of cuts or products purchased was increased accordingly. The bacon and carcase meats were separated into lean, separable fat and inedible matter. The lean meat from each particular item was pooled for analysis and the separable fat was combined in a similar way to provide the fat sample for analysis. Some meat products were not available at all the regional centres and in these cases the number of samples purchased was usually increased at the centres where they were available to provide a sample of sufficient size. In the case of liver additional samples were purchased in London to assess the importance of seasonal factors for vitamin A content and for the losses of vitamin C during cooking.

*The lean-to-fat ratio in meat*

The major variable affecting the composition of meat is the proportion of lean to fat and it is extremely difficult to define the average degree of the fatness for a particular joint, or to be sure that this would be very helpful to the user of the tables who is concerned with the food and nutrient intake of an individual. For this reason values for 'lean only' and 'lean and fat' are given for virtually all the items in the bacon, beef, lamb and pork groups. The percentage of separable lean in the edible portion of the different cuts analysed is given in the description of the sample. If the meat consumed has a different percentage of lean then its composition should be computed from the 'lean only' values and the values for 'fat, average, raw or cooked'.

In the sampling scheme, care was taken to select typical cuts with regard to degree of fatness and the lean and fat values should provide a reasonable guide to the average composition of an item. However, for accurate use of the tables it is essential to measure the lean and fat separately in any bacon or carcase meat consumed.

*Composition of processed meats*

Meat technology in this area is in a particularly rapid state of development at the present time. In the case of bacon it has been possible to cover some of the very recent changes in a small subsidiary study. When the values for processed meats are being used it is essential to bear in mind that the composition of some of these products may have changed considerably over the interval between analysis and publication of these tables.

*Effect of cooking on vitamins*

For many of the items purchased and analysed for this edition, it has been possible to derive values for the percentage losses of vitamins on cooking. These observed values have been used to calculate losses in foods for which direct values were not available. The observed losses are summarised in table 9.

**Table 9** *Percentage losses of vitamins in meat during cooking (average loss with range)*

| | Roasting, frying and grilling | Stewing and boiling* |
|---|---|---|
| Thiamin | 20 (0–40) | 60 (40–70) |
| Riboflavin | 20 (0–30) | 30 (0–40) |
| Nicotinic acid | 20 (10–30) | 50 (30–70) |
| Vitamin $B_6$ | 20 (0–40) | 50 (30–60) |
| Pantothenic acid | 20 | 40 (30–50) |
| Folic acid (free) | — | 30 } liver and kidney only† |
| (total) | — | 30 } liver and kidney only† |
| | All methods | |
| Vitamin $B_{12}$ | 20 (10–50) | |
| Biotin | 10 (0–30) | |
| Vitamin C | 20 (0–30) liver only | |
| Vitamin A | 0 | |
| Vitamin E | 20 (0–40) | |

* These losses refer to the meat alone: the water-soluble vitamins are leached into the gravies and liquors, which means that if these are used the overall losses with these methods of cooking are smaller.

† The content of folic acid in other meats is too low to make meaningful calculations of losses.

*B vitamins in fat*

In most cases the separable fat samples were not analysed for the B vitamins. The technical problems associated with these measurements in the presence of large amounts of fat are quite considerable and it is often very difficult to obtain good replicate analyses. The values for the B vitamins in the lean and fat items may therefore be slight underestimates of the true amounts present. In most cases the contribution from the B vitamins in the fat would be less than 10 per cent.

*Cooking losses in sausages*

The composition of cooked sausages can be affected by the cooking procedure. Losses of water and to a certain extent fat are reduced if the sausage is not pricked during cooking and is cooked slowly to prevent bursting or extrusion at the ends. The figures in these tables refer to sausages that were cooked after pricking.

## Fish and fish products

In considering the values for fish it is important to bear in mind that at present fish are drawn from a wild population. They are in fact one of the few remaining foods which are obtained by what is in effect hunting. This means that their composition is probably more variable than that of foods drawn from domesticated inbred stock whose nutrition has been closely controlled.

The fish section in the previous editions was very extensive and included a large number of species which are rarely eaten. There is, however, considerable variation in composition within one species and this variation is often considerably greater than that between species. In the fourth edition only the fish species which constitute the major part of fish landing in the UK have been included and in many cases combined values for groups of species are given. The systematic names for fish are given in appendix 3.

The items are arranged in several groups: white fish, fatty fish, cartilagenous fish, crustacea, molluscs and fish products and dishes. Many items have been retained from the previous edition, and particular attention was given to those fish which were cooked by being dipped in batter and breadcrumbs and fried. A limited number of comparative analyses have shown that the shape and size of the portion of fish fried has a much greater effect on its composition than the composition of the batter (with or without the crumbs) and thus these older items were considered to be reasonable ones to retain.

### *Fat content*

The fat contents of many fish show considerable seasonal changes and it is difficult to assign definite values. The actual fat content of fish normally landed and consumed shows less variation because the fish tend to be caught during a limited part of the annual cycle; the values used are therefore based on the fat content of the fish during the period when the major landings of the species are made.

### *Calcium and phosphorus values*

In fish with fine bones it is often difficult to remove the bones completely, whether before analysis or before consumption. The calcium and phosphorus content of these fish is thus more variable than in a fish which can be boned easily. The values in the tables are based on samples which have been prepared for consumption in the normal way.

### *Accumulation of metals*

The crustaceans and molluscs tend to accumulate many cations from their environment, and the concentration of iron, copper and zinc reported in these fish shows very wide variation, depending on the source of the samples and the levels of metallic contamination to which they have been exposed.

### *Vitamin content*

There is a general scarcity in the literature of values for the vitamin content of fish. Very often the sources of the samples are not well documented and many of the values cited in the literature are based on a very small number of analyses. The compilations prepared by other authors have been considered when the values given in these tables were being selected, but where the source of the data used in the compilation could not be examined directly the values have been used in only a few instances. There is a special need for work in this area, particularly on vitamin levels in crustacea and molluscs, about which there seems to be little information.

*Effects of cooking on vitamins*

Table 10 gives the cooking losses which were used to calculate the vitamin content of cooked fish. They are based mainly on the losses found in the samples of cod analysed for this edition. The values are thus more tentative than those given for other food groups and should be used only as a guide. No information on vitamin losses during frying (apart from those analysed for this edition) are available.

**Table 10** *Percentage losses of vitamins during cooking fish*

| | Poaching | Baking | Frying/grilling |
|---|---|---|---|
| Thiamin | 10 | 30 | 20 |
| Riboflavin | 0 | 20 | 20 |
| Nicotinic acid | 10 | 20 | 20 |
| Vitamin $B_6$ | 0 | 10 | 20 |
| Pantothenic acid | 20 | 20 | 20 |
| Folic acid (free) | 50 | 30 | 0 |
| (total) | 0 | 20 | 0 |
| Vitamin $B_{12}$ | 0 | 10 | 0 |
| Biotin | 10 | 10 | 10 |
| Vitamin C | — | — | 20* |
| Vitamin E | (0) | 0 | 0 |

* Used for roe

## Vegetables

The vegetable section is based for the most part on the values published in earlier editions. All the figures have been compared with those in more recent published work; this comparison has shown that the values given in the previous edition are still representative.

New analyses have been carried out to provide values for a few additional foods and for a selected number of nutrients in foods already included. These selected analyses have been designed to provide additional values for dietary fibre ('unavailable carbohydrates' in previous editions) and for some vitamins and the effects of cooking on those vitamins. The new items include frozen peas, instant potato powder, sweet corn, peppers and some vegetables especially important for immigrants. Some cooked pulse dishes are given (calculated from recipes) and for these the general term 'dahl' has been used.

The vegetables are arranged in alphabetical order (as in previous editions) as it was found that subgrouping them was impracticable. The systematic names for vegetables are given in appendix 3.

*Edible matter as a proportion of the weight purchased*

The amount of inedible material removed from a vegetable before it is cooked depends on a number of factors: the condition of the vegetable, damage during harvesting, contamination of leaves with soil and not least the personal idiosyncracies of the person preparing the vegetable. The values given are those measured in the samples described, which were usually purchased at a variety of retail outlets. Where a vegetable is purchased 'prepacked' much of the waste has already been removed and the edible matter will usually represent a higher proportion of the weight purchased than that given in the tables.

*Moisture*

The water content is the major variable affecting the proximate composition of vegetables. This will depend on the conditions under which the vegetable has been stored. It is difficult to give figures which will allow for possible variations in water content due to storage, and the user of the tables should bear in mind that a wilted vegetable will have a lower moisture content than that shown.

*Protein*

Part of the total nitrogen in vegetables is non-protein nitrogen and is largely made up of free amino acids and their amides. For nutritional purposes it is therefore reasonable to consider all the total nitrogen as if it were in the form of protein.

*Vitamins*

The full range of vitamins was not measured in the new items and in most cases the vitamin values in these items were taken from the literature. The vitamins measured were thiamin, riboflavin, nicotinic acid, vitamin C and folic acid (that is, carotenes, biotin, pantothenic acid and vitamin $B_{12}$ were not measured). Losses of vitamins under different cooking methods are given in table 11.

**Table 11** *Percentage losses of vitamins in vegetables during cooking*

| | Root vegetables | Leafy vegetables | Seeds |
|---|---|---|---|
| Carotene | 0 | 0 | 0 |
| Thiamin | 25 | 40 | 30 |
| Riboflavin | 30 | 40 | 30 |
| Nicotinic acid | 30 | 40 | 30 |
| Vitamin C | 40 | 70 | 50 |
| Vitamin E | 0 | 0 | 0 |
| Vitamin $B_6$ | 40 | 40 | 40 |
| Folic acid (free) | 90 | 90 | 90 |
| (total) | 50 | 20–40 | 50 |
| Pantothenic acid | 30 | 30 | 30 |
| Biotin | 30 | 30 | 30 |

These are representative values and actual losses depend on:

(*a*) volume of water used to cook the vegetables
(*b*) time of cooking
(*c*) state of division of the food

*Vitamin C*

Where sufficient information was available ranges are given to provide guidance to the user. The values for vitamin C in potatoes are dependent on the time that the tuber has been stored and, in the cooked potato, on the method of cooking. The vitamin C values for potatoes are given as a range, the lowest representing the value for a potato stored for 8–9 months and cooked with the greatest loss; the higher value represents the value in a freshly harvested tuber cooked with the minimum of loss.

*Folic acid*

In many vegetables the value for free folate (that is, measured before conjugase treatment) is higher in the raw than in the cooked state. This is probably due to the fact that conjugases present in the vegetable are inactivated during cooking whereas in the raw vegetable they are active during the extraction of the plant tissues.

*Inorganic constituents*

The concentration of inorganic constituents in vegetables is affected by soil and fertiliser treatment during growth and in the cooked vegetable by leaching into the cooking water. The variations due to cultural conditions affect the trace elements more than the major inorganic constituents. The data in the literature, however, were insufficient for values representing the effects of this variable to be given. Losses during cooking are increased if the vegetable is cut into small pieces or cooked in a large volume of water for a long time. The values given apply to the samples cooked as described. Vegetables may also acquire constituents from tap water, for example Ca, Mg, Fe and trace metals Fe, Cu, Zn and Al from pots and pans. These effects are extremely variable and if accurate intakes of inorganic constituents are required all cooking should be carried out in distilled water in glass or stainless steel vessels and if possible the calculations should be supplemented by analyses.

*Amino acids and fatty acids*

Values for the amino acids and fatty acids in vegetables have been drawn almost completely from the literature. The amino acid data in particular are very limited indeed. This is particularly unfortunate because these foods are widely used in low protein diets and a more extensive knowledge of their amino acid composition would be useful for those involved in this type of diet therapy.

**Fruit**

The values for fruits are based on the values published in previous editions; as was the case with the vegetables, recently published values showed that the values given in earlier editions were still representative. Some additional canned fruits have been included together with values for some 'tropical' fruits which are becoming more common. The systematic names of the fruits are given in appendix 3.

*Stewed fruits*

The values given for the stewed fruits have been recalculated using additional experimental values for the proportion of water added to the fruit and making a correction for the evaporative losses in stewing (10 per cent). All fruits were stewed in the minimum of water and the composition of the cooked fruit was calculated, as in previous editions, on the basis of measured values for the ratio of cooked to raw weights. The ratio of cooked weight (including inedible stones) to raw weight was 1.05:1 for loganberries and raspberries; 2:1 for dried figs and prunes; 3:1 for dried apricots and peaches; and 1.3:1 for all other fruits.

The earlier editions included fruit stewed without sugar. In this edition values are also given for fruit stewed with a given amount of sugar (12 g per 100 g fruit). The amount of sugar added will vary with personal preference and the fruit being cooked but it was felt that these new inclusions would be useful for the 'average' user, although where control of carbohydrate intake is essential the 'stewed without sugar' values are still required by the user.

*Vitamin C*

Where information was available ranges for this vitamin are given in addition to the selected value. The vitamin C in fruits is extremely variable and is dependent on the level of illumination that the individual fruit has received. This means that appreciable variation can occur in fruit from the same tree or bush and within the same fruit.

*Amino acids and fatty acids*

The comments in the vegetable section apply to the fruits with even more force.

**Nuts**

The values for nuts are with one exception derived from the previous edition. The new item is peanut butter, although an estimate of the salt in salted peanuts has also been made. The systematic names for the nuts are given in appendix 3.

**Sugars, preserves and confectionery**

Here the items are arranged according to the three subgroups. Many values have been taken from the third edition as most of the sweets were analysed for that edition.

The items analysed for this edition include lemon curd (starch-based) as purchased, mincemeat and chocolate. The composition of the other items appears to be still representative and falls within the ranges reported in the literature or obtained from evidence provided by the manufacturers.

*Carbohydrate*

The values are given in terms of monosaccharides and this means that white sugar, which is virtually pure sucrose, has a value of 105 g/100 g carbohydrate because one molecule of water is taken up on hydrolysis to give glucose and fructose. Many products in this group contain 'glucose syrup', which contains glucose, maltose and higher maltose homologues. These higher oligosaccharides will analyse as sugar in most methods but in others they appear in the starch fraction. Nutritionally there are only minor differences between these higher oligosaccharides and starch but the user should be aware that these products may yield analytical anomalies.

*Water*

It is particularly difficult to obtain values for the water content of products very rich in sugar and some, such as boiled sweets, contain water of crystallisation, which may or may not be considered as part of the water content of the food.

**Beverages**

These have been arranged in two subgroups. The first includes the concentrated powders, which are usually diluted with milk or water before consumption; the second comprises the soft drinks, and fruit and vegetable juices that are either diluted with water or are purchased ready for consumption. The values are expressed on a 100 g basis, as accurate measurement by volume is difficult with both effervescent and syrupy beverages.

The first subgroup includes coffee and tea and infusions made from them. Values for the diluted concentrated powders have not been given because of the wide range of methods recommended and because many nutritional workers are concerned with total milk intake, which is often considered separately.

*Dietary fibre*

Coffee and cocoa products seem to contain high concentrations of dietary fibre and in particular a 'high' apparent lignin content. This is due to the presence of the ill-defined component humic acid which analyses as lignin. It seems improbable that these products will prove to be useful sources of dietary fibre.

*Fruit drinks*

Only one example is given as the type of fruit used has little or no influence on its composition.

*Vitamin C*

Many beverages which are ostensibly fruit-based contain little or no vitamin C unless it is added during their manufacture. The user should check the label of any beverage of this sort to establish whether or not vitamin C has been added.

**Alcoholic beverages**

The items in this group are arranged into a number of subgroups: beers, ciders, wines, liqueur wines (in other words fortified wines), vermouths, liqueurs and spirits.

All values (with the exception of specific gravity) are given as g per 100 ml (w/v). The specific gravities are given so that calculations can be made if the beverages are measured by weight.

It has not been possible to cover all the different vintages or types of wine available and the values for the wines were obtained on typical examples. They should provide a reasonable guide for nutritional purposes but should not be regarded as a definitive one for the composition of wines.

The alcoholic strengths of beverages can be expressed in several different ways. The common method on the European continent is to use degrees Gay-Lussac, which are the percentage alcohol by volume (v/v). In the United Kingdom the proof system is used; in this, proof spirit is defined as having a specific gravity ($SG^{20}_{20}$) of 0.91702 and contains 49.276 per cent alcohol (w/w) or 57.155 per cent (v/v) (that is, about 45.2 g per 100 ml).

The approximate alcohol contents of various proof strengths are as follows (Customs and Excise, 1954):

| °Proof | Alcohol (g/100 ml) |
|---|---|
| 10 | 4.6 |
| 20 | 9.1 |
| 30 | 13.6 |
| 40 | 18.2 |
| 50 | 22.7 |
| 60 | 27.2 |
| 70 | 31.7 |

**Sauces, pickles, soups, condiments and miscellaneous foods**

This group includes in addition to the major named items a few miscellaneous items which are difficult to assign to other food groups. The first subgroup, sauces and pickles, includes items whose composition has been calculated from recipes and others which have been analysed directly. Some values have been retained from the third edition and others have been analysed for this edition.

The second subgroup, soups, includes many new items and a few whose composition has been calculated. The concentrated (condensed) and dried soups are given as purchased and as diluted ready for consumption. In the calculation of the composition of the dilutions of dried soups, a correction for evaporative losses has been made.

The third subgroup includes condiments, ingredients and a number of items such as yeast, Marmite, Bovril and Oxo. These last three items contain a large amount of non-protein nitrogen, which is largely in the form of amino acids and peptides. Nutritionally these behave as protein and it is therefore appropriate to multiply the total amino nitrogen by 6.25 to get some measure of their weight. This is not 'protein' in the strict sense but no nutritional errors are involved in treating it as such.

## The composition of cooked dishes

The compositions of a range of cooked dishes are included in the tables. In contrast to the previous editions these are now given with the major food groups rather than in separate sections. For the fourth edition a complete revision of all the items based on calculations from recipes has been made. Some items have been deleted and a number of items with very similar compositions have been combined, for example milk puddings. About twenty new dishes have been added including some foreign dishes such as pizza, moussaka and cheesecake.

The composition of these cooked dishes has been calculated, as in previous editions, from the recipes, the composition of the ingredients and the change in weight on cooking. The change in weight on cooking has been assumed to be due either to the evaporation of water or to a gain by absorption. The composition of dishes where the method of preparation involves a change in fat content in addition to water content cannot be calculated directly in this way and in these cases the cooked dishes were analysed for fat and water before the calculations were made.

All the recipes are given in metric quantities and the calculations have been made using the compositions of the ingredients given in this edition. The composition of the new items has been based on experimentally determined changes in weight on cooking. The dishes have been prepared on at least two occasions and the average of these two sets of data has been used in the calculations.

The composition of the items given in the third edition have been recalculated from the metricated recipes on the assumption that the final consistency, and therefore water content, would be the same as that found previously.

Where flour was used as an ingredient, plain flour was used and baking powder was added for cakes and some puddings. The baking powder used was a proprietary preparation whose composition is given in the tables (item 956). This preparation contains calcium acid phosphate, sodium bicarbonate, sodium pyrophosphate and flour; the use of another raising agent (for example sodium bicarbonate) will result in a different composition in the cooked dish with respect to Na, Ca and P. Margarine fortified with vitamins A and D was used in the preparation of the dishes. The use of an unfortified margarine or other fat would affect the values for these two vitamins.

In the calculations an egg has been assumed to weigh 50 g; a level teaspoon refers to the standard 5 ml spoon and has been taken to hold 5 g salt and 3.5 g baking powder.

The recipes are given in appendix 4 and their numbering corresponds to the numbering of the item in the tables.

*Calculation of the composition of dishes prepared from other recipes*
The method of calculation is as follows. The weights of the raw ingredients are used to calculate the total amounts of nutrients in the dish. A correction for wastage due to ingredients left on utensils and in the vessels used in preparation is made at this stage. The weight of the raw dish is then measured, using a scale weighing to about 1 g (a less accurate scale may be used if the total weight of ingredients is over 500g). The dish is then cooked and the dish reweighed. (A minor correction to allow for the difference between weighing the dish hot and at room temperature is not usually necessary.) The difference in weight is taken as being accounted for by water and the composition of the cooked dish is calculated as follows. Divide the total nutrients in the dish calculated from the raw ingredients by the weight of the cooked dish and multiply by 100. The water content of the raw ingredients *less* the loss in weight on cooking divided by the weight of the cooked dish gives the water content of the cooked dish if it is required. An example is:

**Egg Custard**

| Ingredient | Amount in recipe g | Amounts contributed Protein g | Fat g | Carbohydrate etc. g |
|---|---|---|---|---|
| Milk | 500 | 16.5 | 19.0 | 23.5 |
| Egg | 100 | 12.3 | 10.9 | Tr |
| Sugar | 30 | 0 | 0 | 31.5 |
| Vanilla essense | to taste | Ignored for calculation | | |
| Total in recipe (a) | 630 | 28.8 | 29.9 | 55.0 |
| Cooked weight | 500 | | | |
| Composition of cooked dish (per 100g) (b) | — | 5.8 | 6.0 | 11.0 |

(a) = sum of nutrients in ingredients
(b) = (a) divided by cooked weight × 100

If some of the ingredients are left in the mixing bowl or not used then the (a) values should be multiplied by weight used divided by weight of total ingredients.

# Using the tables

Tables of food composition are used for many different purposes and this section is intended to guide the reader in the use of the tables and to give some idea of the accuracy of calculations based on the values in them.

The first of the main uses of tables of food composition is the calculation of nutrient intakes from records of food consumption. These calculations may be for large groups of people such as the population of a country, where the records of food consumption are derived from food supplies measured in raw commodities at the wholesale level, or for the individual, where food intake has been measured as consumed in the prepared state. In the United Kingdom at least there are several different levels of calculation using food consumption data between these two extremes.

The second major use is the formulation of diets or food supplies that will provide a specified intake of nutrients. Again, calculations are made at several different levels ranging from an international agency's estimates of the desirable food supplies for a country or region to the dietitian's formulation of a diet for an individual according to the prescription of a physician.

Another use is the calculation of the nutrient composition of a manufactured food from its ingredients.

Each of these types of usage has its own requirements for food items and range of nutrients in the food tables and, furthermore, requires a different level of accuracy from the calculations. It is, however, extremely difficult to cover all these requirements in a single compilation and the tables in this book are designed to provide information from which the users must make their own selection.

### Variation in composition of foods

The first point that the user must bear in mind is that very few foods have a constant composition. Anyone who uses a table of food composition as an oracle is misleading himself. Foods are biological materials and as such show a considerable variation in composition. Manufactured foods are usually subjected to quality control, which may apply to some aspects of their composition, and they might therefore be expected to have a more constant composition. All manufacturers, however, permit some tolerances and in practice manufactured foods may show as much variation in composition as some unprocessed foods. These variations in composition depend on the type of foodstuff and the nutrient in question. The main features of the variations in the concentrations of different nutrients have been described in the section on modes of expression.

The values in the tables are in the main analytical results obtained from the analysis of representative samples of the food items. One should therefore expect them to reflect the average composition of the food; isolated samples on the other hand may well have a different composition. This means that calculations from food composition data should intrinsically be more accurate when they are concerned with large groups of people (although not necessarily where they are drawn from one institution for example). Where studies involving individuals are concerned one should achieve an improvement in accuracy by extending the period of study and thus in effect increasing the size of the food sample consumed. This is borne out by comparisons of calculated and analysed values for the composition of mixed diets, where agreement between these two is better for a collection taken over seven days than for a single meal.

### Probable levels of accuracy using food tables

The variations in the composition of foods thus have a considerable influence on the level of accuracy that one can expect from food tables. Accuracy will also depend to a certain extent on the appropriateness of the items in the tables. Guidance in this area can only be given in a general fashion because the number of experimental studies where this accuracy has been tested experimentally is very limited.

In general, when comparisons are made over a period of several days for an individual's diet under metabolic balance conditions the agreement between calculated and analysed values for protein, carbohydrate, energy, K, Ca, Mg and P is usually within 5–10 per cent. Calculated fat intakes often show a great discrepancy but this is sometimes attributable to the method of analysis used for fat (see p8). Calculated intakes of sodium and iron may differ greatly from analysed values owing to variations in added salt and contamination respectively. Little information is available concerning the vitamins except for vitamin C, where intakes calculated from tables can be rather inaccurate. The amino acid composition of a diet, however, is quite accurately estimated by calculation (Hughes, 1959). No information is available for comparisons of fatty acid compositions.

## The calculation of nutrient intakes

The first stage in the calculation of nutrient intakes is deciding which item in the tables corresponds with the item consumed, a process often known as 'coding'. This is a procedure that needs to be approached with thought and is one reason why these tables include a fairly detailed description of the samples used to obtain the values. Difficulties arise where there is no corresponding item in the tables or where the description of either the food consumed or the item in the tables is inadequate and the coder cannot be sure that these two do in fact correspond.

In the usual dietary calculation (where a food item is part of a diet) the best procedure is to use a related food for items that are not listed. The user should, however, first check in the index (p407 *et seq.*) because the food may be listed under a synonym or it may be included in another food group. The choice of the related food can be guided by texture or consistency if no other information is available. Where there is uncertainty about whether items correspond, in most calculations little error is involved by assuming that they do (except for foods which may or may not contain added constituents such as salt).

The number of manufactured foods included in this edition is limited for reasons discussed earlier (p2), and the user is advised to consult the manufacturer concerned if a food forms an important part of the diet or accurate control of sugar or sodium intakes, for example, is essential.

## Cooked dishes

Many users have felt in the past that because they used different recipes the composition of their cooked dishes would be very different from those given in the tables. This may be true but often these differences are quite small. However, if different recipes are used regularly it may be useful to calculate the composition of dishes from these recipes. The procedure is relatively simple and is described at the end of the section on the recipes (p334).

## Calculation from 'as purchased' weights

All the values in the tables refer to the composition of the edible matter and where consumption data are available on the basis of food 'as purchased' it is necessary to correct these weights before making calculations (see p5).

For all foods where there is a loss through wastage or a change in weight during cooking, the column headed 'Edible matter, proportion of weight purchased' gives a factor by which the 'as purchased' weight should be multiplied to give the weight of edible matter.

For example:

100g streaky bacon rashers as purchased will give
100 × 0.85 = 85g edible raw bacon and
100 × 0.51 = 51g edible cooked (fried) bacon

### Vitamin equivalents

Over recent years it has become customary to express most vitamin values in terms of the weight of the pure vitamin rather than in 'international units'.

In the case of two vitamins, vitamin A and nicotinic acid, where activity can come from more than one substance having different activities, a system of weight equivalents has been suggested.

In the present UK recommendations for nutrient intakes (Department of Health and Social Security, 1969) the recommended intakes for these two vitamins are expressed in equivalents and the user may need to make calculations on these terms in order to compare nutrient intakes with the recommendations.

The method of calculating retinol equivalents is given on p12. The divisor of 6, which is used to calculate the retinol equivalents from the β-carotene, is an average value for mixed diets. Many foods should have different divisors, depending on the carotenes present in the food. The DHSS report (Department of Health and Social Security, 1969) specifically recommends that the β-carotene in milk and milk products should be divided by 2, while the FAO/WHO recommendation (FAO/WHO, 1965) is to use the divisor of 6 for all foods. Until sufficient information is available on individual foods, it is better to use the divisor of 6 for the sum of the β-carotenes in the diet as this has some experimental justification.

If one needs to calculate retinol equivalents for direct comparison with the DHSS recommendations the calculation is as follows:

$$\mu\text{g retinol equivalents} = \mu\text{g retinol} + \frac{\mu\text{g } \beta\text{-carotene from milk and milk products}}{2} + \frac{\mu\text{g } \beta\text{-carotene from other foods}}{6}$$

In practice the use of a divisor of 2 rather than 6 for milk and milk products gives a difference of about 100 µg (7 per cent of the total retinol equivalents) in the average British diet.

The method for calculating the potential contribution of tryptophan to the nicotinic acid equivalents in the diet has general agreement and is described on p13. In the DHSS recommendations, however, it is suggested that the nicotinic acid naturally occurring in cereals should be discounted because it is probably unavailable.

Direct comparison with the DHSS recommended intakes of nicotinic acid should therefore be made using the following calculations.

$$\text{Nicotinic acid equivalents (mg)} = \left[\text{Total nicotinic acid (mg)} - \text{Nicotinic acid naturally present in cereals (mg)}\right] + \frac{\text{mg tryptophan}}{60}$$

The naturally occurring nicotinic acid in cereals contributes about 2 mg nicotinic acid to the average British diet (about 7 per cent of the total intake of nicotinic acid equivalents: Paul, 1969).

### Availability of nutrients

The values given in the tables have been obtained by chemical or microbiological analyses and give the total amount of the constituent in the food. With the exception of carbohydrate and the calculated energy content no attempt has been made to give any estimate of availability.

In the case of carbohydrate, the 'available carbohydrates' consist of carbohydrates which are chemically distinct from the 'unavailable carbohydrates'. The energy values are for metabolisable energy (p 9) and make allowance for losses of energy-yielding constituents in urine and faeces. Many foods contain unavailable forms of some nutrients, of which the best documented are iron, nicotinic acid and lysine. As nutritional studies progress, however, it is becoming apparent that the question of availability should be extended to many other nutrients, especially amino acids and the trace elements. The availability of many inorganic constituents is also influenced by other constituents of the diet. It is difficult to devise analytical procedures that can be used to measure availability because it is essentially a physiological concept. Furthermore, the availability of iron, for example, depends on the iron status of the individual and it would therefore not be possible to give a meaningful value for available iron in the tables which would apply to any individual.

Each nutrient poses special problems and it was not considered that there were enough experimentally based data to give values for 'available nutrients' in this edition of the tables. But the user must be aware that differences in availability do exist and that the total chemical (or microbiological) values given in these tables may, for many nutrients, represent the maximum that could be available to the body, and that the actual amount may be much smaller.

**Conclusion: the need for the combined use of tables and text**

It is extremely difficult to present in the tables themselves all the various factors that should be considered when the tabulated values are used. This could be done only by the use of an inordinate number of qualifying footnotes, which would make the tables difficult to use. This means that it is important to be thoroughly familiar with the text and to use tables and text together. It is especially important for the user to be familiar with the symbols and conventions. This approach to the tables should lead to a more accurate use of the data and resolve many of the problems which appear to have arisen with the previous editions. Certainly many of the inquiries that have been received relating to the earlier editions would not have arisen had the text been referred to first.

## References to text

Anderson, B. A. (1976) Comprehensive evaluation of fatty acids in foods. VII. Pork products. *J. Amer. diet. Ass.*, **69**, 44–49

Anderson, B. A., Kinsella, J. A., and Watt, B. K. (1975) Comprehensive evaluation of fatty acids in foods. II. Beef products. *J. Amer. diet. Ass.*, **67**, 35–41

Customs and Excise (1954) *Specific gravity of spirits.* HMSO, London

Department of Health and Social Security (1969) *Recommended intakes of nutrients for the United Kingdom.* Reports on Public Health and Medical Subjects, No. 120. HMSO, London

Department of Health and Social Security (1974) *Present day practice in infant feeding.* Reports on Health and Social Subjects, No. 9. HMSO, London

Exler, J., Kinsella, J. E., and Watt, B. K. (1975) Lipids and fatty acids of important finfish. New data for nutrient tables. *J. Amer. Oil Chem. Soc.*, **52**, 154–159

FAO/WHO (1967) *Requirements of vitamin A, thiamine, riboflavine and niacin.* Report of a Joint FAO/WHO Expert Group. FAO Nutrition Meeting Report Series, No. 41; WHO Technical Report Series, No. 362

FAO/WHO (1973) *Energy and protein requirements.* Report of a Joint FAO/WHO *Ad Hoc* Expert Committee. FAO Nutrition Meetings Report Series, No. 52; WHO Technical Report Series, No. 522

Hughes, B. P. (1959) The amino-acid composition of three mixed diets. *Brit. J. Nutr.*, **13**, 330–337

McCance, R. A., and Shipp, H. L. (1933) *The chemistry of flesh foods and their losses on cooking.* Medical Research Council Special Report Series, No. 187. HMSO, London

McCance, R. A., Widdowson, E. M., and Shackleton, L. R. B. (1936) *The nutritive value of fruits, vegetables and nuts.* Medical Research Council Special Report Series, No. 213. HMSO, London

Merrill, A. L., and Watt, B. K. (1955) *Energy value of foods—basis and derivation.* US Department of Agriculture, Agriculture Handbook No. 74. Washington, DC

Paul, A. A. (1969) The calculation of nicotinic acid equivalents and retinol equivalents in the British diet. *Nutrition, Lond.*, **23**, 131–136

Paul, A. A., and Southgate, D. A. T. (1970) Revision of *The composition of foods.* Some views of dietitians. *Nutrition, Lond.*, **24**, 21–24

Paul, A. A., and Southgate, D. A. T. (1977) A study of the composition of retail meat: dissection into lean, separable fat and inedible portion. *J. hum. Nutr.* **31**, 259–272

Platt, B. S. (1962) *Tables of representative values of foods commonly used in tropical countries.* Medical Research Council Special Report Series, No. 302. HMSO, London

Posati, L. P., Kinsella, J. E., and Watt, B. K. (1975) Comprehensive evaluation of fatty acids in foods. III. Eggs and egg products. *J. Amer. diet. Ass.*, **67**, 111–115

Royal Society (1972) *Metric units, conversion factors and nomenclature in nutritional and food sciences.* Report of the subcommittee on metrication of the British National Committee for Nutritional Sciences

Southgate, D. A. T. (1974) *Guide lines for the preparation of tables of food composition.* S. Karger, Basel

Southgate, D. A. T., and Durnin, J. V. G. A. (1970) Calorie conversion factors: an experimental reassessment of the factors used in the calculations of the energy value of human diets. *Brit. J. Nutr.*, **24**, 517–535

Southgate, D. A. T., Bailey, B., Collinson, E., and Walker, A. F. (1976) A guide to calculating of intakes of dietary fibre. *J. hum. Nutr.*, **30**, 303–313

Tolan, A., Robertson, J., Orton, C. R., Head, M. J., Christie, A. A., and Millburn, B. A. (1974) Studies on the composition of food. 5. The chemical composition of eggs produced under battery, deep litter and free range conditions. *Brit. J. Nutr.*, **31**, 185–200

Weihrauch, J. L., Kinsella, J. E., and Watt, B. K. (1976) Comprehensive evaluation of fatty acids in foods. VI. Cereal products. *J. Amer. diet. Ass.*, **68**, 335–340

# The tables

*Symbols* (see p 5)

Tr Trace

( ) Estimated value

— No information available

---

## Section I
## Description of foods, proximate composition, energy value, inorganic constituents and vitamins (per 100 g)

All carbohydrate values are for available carbohydrate as monosaccharides

Note: A set of blank pages has been inserted between each major food group so that additional foods may be entered by the user if required.

| No | Food | Description and number of samples | Water g | Sugars g | Starch and dextrins g | Dietary fibre g | Total nitrogen g |
|---|---|---|---|---|---|---|---|
| | ***Grains, flours and starches*** | | | | | | |
| 1 | **Arrowroot** | 2 samples from different shops | 12.2 | Tr | 94.0 | — | 0.07 |
| 2 | **Barley** pearl, raw | 2 samples from different shops | 10.6 | Tr | 83.6 | 6.5 | 1.35 |
| 3 | boiled | 2 samples from different shops, boiled in water | 69.6 | Tr | 27.6 | 2.2 | 0.46 |
| 4 | **Bemax** | Stabilized wheat germ; mixed sample | 6.0 | 16.0 | 28.7 | — | 4.54 |
| 5 | **Bran** wheat | Analytical and literature sources | 8.3 | 3.8 | 23.0 | 44.0 | 2.24 |
| 6 | **Cornflour** | 3 samples from different shops | 12.5 | Tr | 92.0 | — | 0.09 |
| 7 | **Custard powder** | Taken as cornflour, except for Na and Cl | 12.5 | Tr | 92.0 | — | 0.09 |
| 9 | **Flour** wholemeal (100%) | Data from Voluntary Flour Sampling | 14.0 | 2.3[a] | 63.5 | 9.6 | 2.26 |
| 10 | brown (85%) | Scheme, 1974–5, Ministry of | 14.0 | 1.9[a] | 66.9 | 7.5 | 2.25 |
| 11 | white (72%) breadmaking | Agriculture, Fisheries and Food; cake | 14.5 | 1.5[a] | 73.3 | 3.0 | 1.98 |
| 12 | household, plain | and biscuit flour are similar in composi- | 13.0 | 1.7[a] | 78.4 | 3.4 | 1.72 |
| 13 | self-raising | tion to household plain flour | 13.0 | 1.4[a] | 76.1 | 3.7 | 1.63 |
| 14 | patent (40%) | Mixed sample | 14.1 | 1.4[a] | 76.6 | — | 1.89 |
| 15 | **Macaroni** raw | 2 samples from different shops | 10.4 | Tr | 79.2 | — | 2.41 |
| 16 | boiled | 2 samples from different shops, boiled in water | 71.5 | Tr | 25.2 | — | 0.75 |
| 17 | **Oatmeal** raw | Coarse, medium and fine; 2 samples of each | 8.9 | Tr | 72.8 | 7.0 | 2.12 |
| 18 | **Porridge** | 60g oatmeal and 2 level teaspoons salt per 500ml water | 89.1 | Tr | 8.2 | 0.8 | 0.24 |

[a] Includes the glucofructan levosin

| No | Food | Energy value | | Protein (see p7) | Fat | Carbo-hydrate | mg | | | | | | | | | |
|---|---|---|---|---|---|---|---|---|---|---|---|---|---|---|---|---|
| | | kcal | kJ | g | g | g | Na | K | Ca | Mg | P | Fe | Cu | Zn | S | Cl |
| | ***Grains, flours and starches*** | | | | | | | | | | | | | | | |
| 1 | **Arrowroot** | 355 | 1515 | 0.4 | 0.1 | 94.0 | 5 | 18 | 7 | 8 | 27 | 2.0 | 0.22 | — | 2 | 7 |
| 2 | **Barley** pearl, raw | 360 | 1535 | 7.9 | 1.7 | 83.6 | 3 | 120 | 10 | 20 | 210 | 0.7 | 0.12 | (2.0) | 110 | 110 |
| 3 | boiled | 120 | 510 | 2.7 | 0.6 | 27.6 | 1 | 40 | 3 | 7 | 70 | 0.2 | 0.04 | (0.7) | 36 | 36 |
| 4 | **Bemax** | 347 | 1465 | 26.5 | 8.1 | 44.7 | 4 | 1000 | 17 | 300 | 930 | 10.0 | 1.20 | — | — | 80 |
| 5 | **Bran** wheat | 206 | 872 | 14.1 | 5.5 | 26.8 | 28 | 1160 | 110 | 520 | 1200 | 12.9 | 1.34 | 16.2 | 65 | 150 |
| 6 | **Cornflour** | 354 | 1508 | 0.6 | 0.7 | 92.0 | 52 | 61 | 15 | 7 | 39 | 1.4 | 0.13 | Tr | 1 | 71 |
| 7 | **Custard powder** | 354 | 1508 | 0.6 | 0.7 | 92.0 | 320 | 61 | 15 | 7 | 39 | 1.4 | 0.13 | Tr | 1 | 480 |
| 9 | **Flour** wholemeal (100%) | 318 | 1351 | 13.2 | 2.0 | 65.8 | 3 | 360 | 35 | 140 | 340 | 4.0 | 0.40 | 3.0 | — | 38 |
| 10 | brown (85%) | 327 | 1392 | 12.8 | 2.0 | 68.8 | 4 | 280 | 150[a] | 110 | 270 | 3.6[a] | 0.35 | 2.4 | — | 45 |
| 11 | white (72%) breadmaking | 337 | 1433 | 11.3 | 1.2 | 74.8 | 3 | 130 | 140[b] | 36 | 130 | 2.2[b] | 0.22 | 0.9 | 110 | 62 |
| 12 | household, plain | 350 | 1493 | 9.8 | 1.2 | 80.1 | 2 | 140 | 150[b] | 20 | 110 | 2.4[b] | 0.17 | 0.7 | — | 45 |
| 13 | self-raising | 339 | 1443 | 9.3 | 1.2 | 77.5 | 350[c] | 170 | 350[c] | 42 | 510[c] | 2.6[b] | 0.15 | 0.6 | — | 45 |
| 14 | patent (40%) | 347 | 1480 | 10.8 | 1.3 | 78.0 | 3 | 100 | 110 | 19 | 89 | 1.7 | 0.11 | — | 110 | 60 |
| 15 | **Macaroni** raw | 370 | 1574 | 13.7 | 2.0 | 79.2 | 26 | 220 | 26 | 57 | 150 | 1.4 | 0.07 | (1.0) | 95 | 31 |
| 16 | boiled | 117 | 499 | 4.3 | 0.6 | 25.2 | 8 | 67 | 8 | 18 | 47 | 0.5 | 0.02 | (0.3) | 29 | 10 |
| 17 | **Oatmeal** raw | 401 | 1698 | 12.4 | 8.7 | 72.8 | 33 | 370 | 55 | 110 | 380 | 4.1 | 0.23 | (3.0) | 160 | 73 |
| 18 | **Porridge** | 44 | 188 | 1.4 | 0.9 | 8.2 | 580 | 42 | 6 | 13 | 43 | 0.5 | 0.03 | (0.3) | 18 | 890 |

[a] These are values for fortified flour. Unfortified brown flour would contain about 20 mg Ca and 2.5 mg Fe per 100 g

[b] These are values for fortified flour. Unfortified white flour would contain about 15 mg Ca and 1.5 mg Fe per 100 g

[c] The amount present will depend on the nature and level of the raising agent used

| No | Food | Retinol µg | Carotene µg | Vitamin D µg | Thiamin mg | Riboflavin mg | Nicotinic acid mg | Potential nicotinic acid from tryptophan mg Trp ÷ 60 | Vitamin C mg | Vitamin E mg |
|---|---|---|---|---|---|---|---|---|---|---|
| | ***Grains, flours and starches*** | | | | | | | | | |
| 1 | **Arrowroot** | 0 | 0 | 0 | (Tr) | (Tr) | (Tr) | 0.1 | 0 | (Tr) |
| 2 | **Barley** pearl, raw | 0 | 0 | 0 | 0.12 | 0.05 | 2.5 | 2.3 | 0 | 0.2[a] |
| 3 | boiled | 0 | 0 | 0 | Tr | Tr | (0.9) | 0.8 | 0 | Tr |
| 4 | **Bemax** | 0 | 0 | 0 | 1.45 | 0.61 | 5.8 | 5.3 | 0 | 11.0[b] |
| 5 | **Bran** wheat | 0 | 0 | 0 | 0.89 | 0.36 | 29.6 | 3.0 | 0 | 1.6[c] |
| 6 | **Cornflour** | 0 | 0 | 0 | (Tr) | (Tr) | (Tr) | 0.1 | 0 | 0 |
| 7 | **Custard powder** | 0 | 0 | 0 | (Tr) | (Tr) | (Tr) | 0.1 | 0 | 0 |
| 9 | **Flour** wholemeal (100%) | 0 | 0 | 0 | 0.46 | 0.08 | 5.6 | 2.5 | 0 | 1.0[d] |
| 10 | brown (85%) | 0 | 0 | 0 | 0.42[e] | 0.06 | 4.2[e] | 2.6 | 0 | (Tr) |
| 11 | white (72%) breadmaking | 0 | 0 | 0 | 0.31[f] | 0.03 | 2.0[f] | 2.3 | 0 | Tr |
| 12 | household, plain | 0 | 0 | 0 | 0.33[f] | 0.02 | 2.0[f] | 2.0 | 0 | Tr |
| 13 | self-raising | 0 | 0 | 0 | 0.28[f] | 0.02 | 1.5[f] | 1.9 | 0 | Tr |
| 14 | patent (40%) | 0 | 0 | 0 | (0.32[f]) | (0.02) | (2.0[f]) | 2.2 | 0 | Tr |
| 15 | **Macaroni** raw | 0 | 0 | 0 | 0.14 | 0.06 | 2.0 | 2.8 | 0 | (Tr) |
| 16 | boiled | 0 | 0 | 0 | 0.01 | 0.01 | 0.3 | 0.9 | 0 | (Tr) |
| 17 | **Oatmeal** raw | 0 | 0 | 0 | 0.50 | 0.10 | 1.0 | 2.8 | 0 | 0.8[g] |
| 18 | **Porridge** | 0 | 0 | 0 | 0.05 | 0.01 | 0.1 | 0.3 | 0 | (0.1) |

| No | Food | Vitamin $B_6$ mg | Vitamin $B_{12}$ µg | Folic acid Free µg | Folic acid Total µg | Pantothenic acid mg | Biotin µg |
|---|---|---|---|---|---|---|---|
| | ***Grains, flours and starches*** | | | | | | |
| 1 | **Arrowroot** | (Tr) | 0 | Tr | Tr | (Tr) | (Tr) |
| 2 | **Barley** pearl, raw | 0.22 | 0 | 9 | 20 | 0.5 | — |
| 3 | boiled | Tr | 0 | Tr | (3) | (0.2) | (Tr) |
| 4 | **Bemax** | 0.95 | 0 | (260) | (330) | (1.7) | — |
| 5 | **Bran** wheat | 1.38 | 0 | 130 | 260 | 2.4 | 14 |
| 6 | **Cornflour** | (Tr) | 0 | Tr | Tr | (Tr) | (Tr) |
| 7 | **Custard powder** | (Tr) | 0 | Tr | Tr | (Tr) | (Tr) |
| 9 | **Flour** wholemeal (100%) | 0.50 | 0 | 25 | 57 | 0.8 | 7 |
| 10 | brown (85%) | (0.30) | 0 | 23 | 51 | (0.4) | (3) |
| 11 | white (72%) breadmaking | 0.15 | 0 | 14 | 31 | 0.3 | 1 |
| 12 | houshold, plain | 0.15 | 0 | 14 | 22 | 0.3 | 1 |
| 13 | self-raising | 0.15 | 0 | 11 | 19 | 0.3 | 1 |
| 14 | patent (40%) | (0.10) | 0 | (5) | (10) | (0.3) | (1) |
| 15 | **Macaroni** raw | 0.06 | 0 | 4 | 11 | (0.3) | (1) |
| 16 | boiled | (0.01) | 0 | Tr | (2) | (Tr) | (Tr) |
| 17 | **Oatmeal** raw | 0.12 | 0 | 11 | 60 | 1.0 | 20 |
| 18 | **Porridge** | 0.01 | 0 | 1 | 6 | 0.1 | (2) |

Notes

[a] Also contains 0.3 mg β-tocopherol and 1.2 mg α-tocotrienol per 100 g.

[b] α-tocopherol constitutes about half the total tocopherols present.

[c] Also contains 1.0 mg β-tocopherol and 1.1 mg α-tocotrienol per 100 g.

[d] Also contains 0.7 mg β-tocopherol and 0.4 mg α-tocotrienol per 100 g. There is a loss of tocopherols on storage of about 60% over 13 weeks.

[e] These are levels for fortified flour. Unfortified flour would contain 0.30 mg thiamin and 1.7 mg nicotinic acid per 100 g.

[f] These are levels for fortified flour. Unfortified flour would contain 0.10 mg thiamin and 0.7 mg nicotinic acid per 100 g.

[g] Also contains 0.1 mg γ-tocopherol and 1.0 mg α-tocotrienol per 100 g.

| No | Food | Description and number of samples | Water g | Sugars g | Starch and dextrins g | Dietary fibre g | Total nitrogen g |
|---|---|---|---|---|---|---|---|
| | ***Grains, flours and starches** contd* | | | | | | |
| 19 | **Rice** polished, raw | 5 samples from different shops | 11.7 | Tr | 86.8 | 2.4 | 1.09 |
| 20 | boiled | 5 samples from different shops, boiled in water | 69.9 | Tr | 29.6 | 0.8 | 0.37 |
| 21 | **Rye** flour (100%) | Commercial grist of all-English rye | 15.0 | Tr | 75.9 | — | 1.40 |
| 22 | **Sago** raw | 2 samples from different shops | 12.6 | Tr | 94.0 | — | 0.04 |
| 23 | **Semolina** raw | 2 samples from different shops, coarse and fine | 14.0 | Tr | 77.5 | — | 1.87 |
| 24 | **Soya** flour, full fat | Mixed sample | 7.0 | 11.2 | 12.3 | 11.9 | 6.45 |
| 25 | low fat | Mixed sample | 7.0 | 13.4 | 14.8 | 14.3 | 7.94 |
| 26 | **Spaghetti** raw | 6 samples from different shops | 10.5 | 2.7 | 81.3 | — | 2.39 |
| 27 | boiled | 6 samples from different shops, boiled in water | 71.7 | 0.8 | 25.2 | — | 0.74 |
| 28 | canned in tomato sauce | 6 large cans from different shops | 83.1 | 3.4 | 8.8 | — | 0.30 |
| 29 | **Tapioca** raw | 4 varieties, medium pearl, seed pearl, coarse and flake | 12.2 | Tr | 95.0 | — | 0.07 |
| | ***Bread and Rolls*** | | | | | | |
| | **Bread** | | | | | | |
| 30 | wholemeal | Analytical and calculated values, mixed samples | 40.0 | 2.1 | 39.7 | 8.5 | 1.51 |
| 31 | brown | Calculated from brown flour | 39.0 | 1.8 | 42.9 | 5.1 | 1.56 |
| 32 | Hovis | Bulked sample | 40.0 | 2.4 | 42.7 | 4.6 | 1.70 |
| 33 | white | Analytical and calculated values, mixed samples | 39.0 | 1.8 | 47.9 | 2.7 | 1.40 |

| No | Food | Energy value kcal | Energy value kJ | Protein (see p7) g | Fat g | Carbo-hydrate g | Na mg | K mg | Ca mg | Mg mg | P mg | Fe mg | Cu mg | Zn mg | S mg | Cl mg |
|---|---|---|---|---|---|---|---|---|---|---|---|---|---|---|---|---|
| | ***Grains, flours and starches contd*** | | | | | | | | | | | | | | | |
| 19 | **Rice** polished, raw | 361 | 1536 | 6.5 | 1.0 | 86.8 | 6 | 110 | 4 | 13 | 100 | 0.5 | 0.06 | 1.3 | 78 | 27 |
| 20 | boiled | 123 | 522 | 2.2 | 0.3 | 29.6 | 2 | 38 | 1 | 4 | 34 | 0.2 | 0.02 | 0.4 | 27 | 9 |
| 21 | **Rye** flour (100%) | 335 | 1428 | 8.2 | 2.0 | 75.9 | (1) | 410 | 32 | 92 | 360 | 2.7 | 0.42 | (2.8) | — | — |
| 22 | **Sago** raw | 355 | 1515 | 0.2 | 0.2 | 94.0 | 3 | 5 | 10 | 3 | 29 | 1.2 | 0.03 | — | 1 | 13 |
| 23 | **Semolina** raw | 350 | 1489 | 10.7 | 1.8 | 77.5 | 12 | 170 | 18 | 32 | 110 | 1.0 | 0.15 | — | 92 | 71 |
| 24 | **Soya** flour, full fat | 447 | 1871 | 36.8 | 23.5 | 23.5 | 1 | 1660 | 210 | 240 | 600 | 6.9 | — | — | — | — |
| 25 | low fat | 352 | 1488 | 45.3 | 7.2 | 28.2 | 1 | 2030 | 240 | 290 | 640 | 9.1 | — | — | — | — |
| 26 | **Spaghetti** raw | 378 | 1612 | 13.6 | 1.0 | 84.0 | 5 | 160 | 23 | 35 | 120 | 1.2 | 0.27 | (1.0) | 97 | 63 |
| 27 | boiled | 117 | 499 | 4.2 | 0.3 | 26.0 | 2 | 50 | 7 | 11 | 37 | 0.4 | 0.08 | (0.3) | 30 | 20 |
| 28 | canned in tomato sauce | 59 | 250 | 1.7 | 0.7 | 12.2 | 500 | 130 | 21 | 11 | 30 | 0.4 | 0.13 | — | — | 800 |
| 29 | **Tapicoa** raw | 359 | 1531 | 0.4 | 0.1 | 95.0 | 4 | 20 | 8 | 2 | 30 | 0.3 | 0.07 | — | 4 | 13 |
| | ***Bread and rolls*** | | | | | | | | | | | | | | | |
| | **Bread** | | | | | | | | | | | | | | | |
| 30 | wholemeal | 216 | 918 | 8.8 | 2.7 | 41.8 | 540 | 220 | 23 | 93 | 230 | 2.5 | 0.27 | 2.0 | 81 | 860 |
| 31 | brown | 223 | 948 | 8.9 | 2.2 | 44.7 | 550 | 210 | 100 | 75 | 190 | 2.5 | 0.23 | 1.6 | 85 | 880 |
| 32 | Hovis | 228 | 968 | 9.7 | 2.2 | 45.1 | 580 | 210 | 150 | 60 | 190 | 4.5 | 0.18 | — | 88 | 790 |
| 33 | white | 233 | 991 | 7.8 | 1.7 | 49.7 | 540[a] | 100 | 100 | 26 | 97 | 1.7 | 0.15 | 0.8 | 79 | 890[a] |

[a] Batch loaves contain 610mg Na and 1000mg Cl per 100g

| No | Food | Retinol µg | Carotene µg | Vitamin D µg | Thiamin mg | Riboflavin mg | Nicotinic acid mg | Potential nicotinic acid from tryptophan mg Trp ÷ 60 | Vitamin C mg | Vitamin E mg |
|---|---|---|---|---|---|---|---|---|---|---|
| | ***Grains, flours and starches*** *contd* | | | | | | | | | |
| 19 | **Rice** polished, raw | 0 | 0 | 0 | 0.08 | 0.03 | 1.5 | 1.5 | 0 | 0.3[a] |
| 20 | boiled | 0 | 0 | 0 | 0.01 | 0.01 | 0.3 | 0.5 | 0 | (0.1) |
| 21 | **Rye** flour (100%) | 0 | 0 | 0 | 0.40 | 0.22 | 1.0 | 1.6 | 0 | 0.8[b] |
| 22 | **Sago** raw | 0 | 0 | 0 | (Tr) | (Tr) | (Tr) | Tr | 0 | (Tr) |
| 23 | **Semolina** raw | 0 | 0 | 0 | (0.10) | (0.02) | (0.7) | 2.2 | 0 | (Tr) |
| 24 | **Soya** flour, full fat | 0 | — | 0 | 0.75 | 0.31 | 2.0 | 8.6 | 0 | — |
| 25 | low fat | 0 | — | 0 | 0.90 | 0.36 | 2.4 | 10.6 | 0 | — |
| 26 | **Spaghetti** raw | 0 | 0 | 0 | 0.14 | 0.06 | 2.0 | 2.8 | 0 | — |
| 27 | boiled | 0 | 0 | 0 | 0.01 | 0.01 | 0.3 | 0.9 | 0 | — |
| 28 | canned in tomato sauce | 0 | Tr | 0 | (0.01) | (0.01) | (0.3) | 0.4 | Tr | — |
| 29 | **Tapioca** raw | 0 | 0 | 0 | (Tr) | (Tr) | (Tr) | 0.1 | 0 | (Tr) |
| | ***Bread and Rolls*** | | | | | | | | | |
| | **Bread** | | | | | | | | | |
| 30 | wholemeal | 0 | 0 | 0 | 0.26 | 0.06 | 3.9 | 1.7 | 0 | (0.2) |
| 31 | brown | 0 | 0 | 0 | 0.24 | 0.06 | 2.9 | 1.8 | 0 | (Tr) |
| 32 | Hovis | 0 | 0 | 0 | 0.52 | 0.10 | 3.9 | 2.0 | 0 | — |
| 33 | white | 0 | 0 | 0 | 0.18 | 0.03 | 1.4 | 1.6 | 0 | Tr |

| No | Food | Vitamin $B_6$ mg | Vitamin $B_{12}$ µg | Folic acid Free µg | Folic acid Total µg | Pantothenic acid mg | Biotin µg |
|---|---|---|---|---|---|---|---|
| | ***Grains, flours and starches*** *contd* | | | | | | |
| 19 | **Rice** polished, raw | 0.30 | 0 | 15 | 29 | 0.6 | 3 |
| 20 | boiled | (0.05) | 0 | 3 | (6) | (0.2) | (1) |
| 21 | **Rye** flour (100%) | 0.35 | 0 | 31 | 78 | 1.0 | 6 |
| 22 | **Sago** raw | (Tr) | 0 | (Tr) | (Tr) | (Tr) | (Tr) |
| 23 | **Semolina** raw | (0.15) | 0 | (20) | (25) | (0.3) | (1) |
| 24 | **Soya** flour, full fat | 0.57 | 0 | — | — | 1.8 | — |
| 25 | low fat | 0.68 | 0 | — | — | 2.1 | — |
| 26 | **Spaghetti** raw | 0.06 | 0 | 4 | 13 | (0.3) | (1) |
| 27 | boiled | (0.01) | 0 | Tr | (2) | (Tr) | (Tr) |
| 28 | canned in tomato sauce | (0.01) | 0 | Tr | (2) | (Tr) | (Tr) |
| 29 | **Tapioca** raw | (Tr) | 0 | (Tr) | (Tr) | (Tr) | (Tr) |
| | ***Bread and Rolls*** | | | | | | |
| | **Bread** | | | | | | |
| 30 | wholemeal | 0.14 | 0 | 22 | 39 | 0.6 | 6 |
| 31 | brown | 0.08 | 0 | 21 | 36 | 0.3 | 3 |
| 32 | Hovis | 0.09 | 0 | — | 20 | 0.3 | 2 |
| 33 | white | 0.04 | 0 | 6 | 27 | 0.3 | 1 |

Notes

[a] Also contains 0.3 mg γ-tocopherol per 100 g.

[b] Also contains 0.4 mg β-tocopherol, 0.3 mg γ-tocopherol and 1.5 mg α-tocotrienol per 100 g.

| No | Food | Description and number of samples | Water g | Sugars g | Starch and dextrins g | Dietary fibre g | Total nitrogen g |
|---|---|---|---|---|---|---|---|
| | ***Bread** contd* | | | | | | |
| 34 | white, fried | Mean of 3 pooled samples | 4.0 | 1.7 | 49.6 | (2.2) | 1.33 |
| 35 | toasted | Mean of 3 pooled samples | 24.0 | 2.1 | 62.8 | (2.8) | 1.69 |
| 36 | dried crumbs | Mean of several samples | 9.7 | 2.6 | 74.9 | (3.4) | 2.03 |
| 37 | currant | 4 samples from different shops | 37.7 | 13.0 | 38.8 | (1.7) | 1.12 |
| 38 | malt | 3 varieties | 39.0 | 18.6 | 30.8 | — | 1.46 |
| 39 | soda | Recipe p 334 | 34.2 | 3.0 | 53.3 | 2.3 | 1.37 |
| 40 | **Rolls** brown, crusty | Mean of 3 pooled samples | 28.6 | 2.1 | 55.1 | (5.9) | 2.02 |
| 41 | soft | 1 pooled sample | 31.0 | 1.9 | 46.0 | (5.4) | 2.05 |
| 42 | white, crusty | Mean of 5 pooled samples | 28.8 | 2.1 | 55.1 | (3.1) | 2.04 |
| 43 | soft | Mean of 6 pooled samples | 28.8 | 1.9 | 51.7 | (2.9) | 1.72 |
| 44 | starch reduced | 5 samples from different shops (Energen) | 8.5 | 1.6 | 44.1 | (2.0) | 7.72 |
| 45 | **Chapatis** made with fat | 6 samples | 28.5 | 1.8 | 46.5 | 3.7 | 1.42 |
| 46 | made without fat | Analysed and calculated values | 45.8 | 1.6 | 42.1 | (3.4) | 1.28 |
| | ***Breakfast cereals*** | | | | | | |
| 47 | **All-Bran** | 6 packets of the same brand (Kellogg's) | 2.3 | 15.4 | 27.6 | 26.7 | 2.40 |
| 48 | **Cornflakes** | 6 packets of the same brand (Kellogg's) | 3.0 | 7.4 | 77.7 | 11.0 | 1.38 |
| 49 | **Grapenuts** | 6 packets of the same brand (General Foods) | 3.9 | 9.5 | 66.4 | 7.0 | 1.85 |
| 50 | **Muesli** | 10 packets, 4 brands | 5.8 | 26.2 | 40.0 | 7.4 | 2.21 |
| 51 | **Puffed Wheat** | 6 packets of the same brand (Quaker) | 2.5 | 1.5 | 67.0 | 15.4 | 2.44 |
| 52 | **Ready Brek** | 6 packets of the same brand (Lyons) | 6.3 | 2.2 | 67.7 | 7.6 | 2.12 |
| 53 | **Rice Krispies** | 6 packets of the same brand (Kellogg's) | 3.8 | 9.0 | 79.1 | 4.5 | 0.99 |

| No | Food | Energy value kcal | Energy value kJ | Protein (see p7) g | Fat g | Carbo-hydrate g | mg Na | K | Ca | Mg | P | Fe | Cu | Zn | S | Cl |
|---|---|---|---|---|---|---|---|---|---|---|---|---|---|---|---|---|
| | ***Bread** contd* | | | | | | | | | | | | | | | |
| 34 | white, fried | 558 | 2326 | 7.6 | 37.2[a] | 51.3 | 500 | 100 | 90 | 22 | 79 | 1.8 | 0.13 | (0.8) | 75 | 820 |
| 35 | toasted | 297 | 1265 | 9.6 | 1.7 | 64.9 | 640 | 130 | 110 | 28 | 100 | 2.2 | 0.16 | (0.8) | 95 | 1040 |
| 36 | dried crumbs | 354 | 1508 | 11.6 | 1.9 | 77.5 | 760 | 150 | 130 | 34 | 120 | 2.8 | 0.20 | (0.9) | 110 | 1140 |
| 37 | currant | 250 | 1063 | 6.4 | 3.4 | 51.8 | 160 | 250 | 90 | 25 | 120 | 2.7 | 0.09 | (0.8) | 59 | 280 |
| 38 | malt | 248 | 1054 | 8.3 | 3.3 | 49.4 | 280 | 380 | 94 | 78 | 250 | 3.6 | 0.06 | (0.8) | 110 | 530 |
| 39 | soda | 264 | 1122 | 8.0 | 2.3 | 56.3 | 410 | 270 | 150 | 20 | 110 | 1.7 | 0.13 | 0.6 | — | 480 |
| 40 | **Rolls** brown, crusty | 289 | 1229 | 11.5 | 3.2 | 57.2 | (640) | 240 | 120 | 86 | 220 | 3.2 | 0.26 | 1.8 | 170 | (1030) |
| 41 | soft | 282 | 1194 | 11.7 | 6.4 | 47.9 | (620) | 220 | 120 | 80 | 200 | 2.5 | 0.24 | 1.7 | 190 | (990) |
| 42 | white, crusty | 290 | 1231 | 11.6 | 3.2 | 57.2 | (630) | 120 | 120 | 30 | 110 | 2.1 | 0.17 | 0.9 | 150 | (1040) |
| 43 | soft | 305 | 1291 | 9.8 | 7.3 | 53.6 | (630) | 110 | 120 | 28 | 100 | 1.8 | 0.16 | 0.9 | 130 | (1040) |
| 44 | starch reduced | 384 | 1631 | 44.0 | 4.1 | 45.7 | 650 | 130 | 47 | 63 | 190 | 4.0 | 0.52 | — | — | (980) |
| 45 | **Chapatis** made with fat | 336 | 1415 | 8.1 | 12.8 | 50.2 | 130 | 160 | 66 | 41 | 130 | 2.3 | 0.20 | 1.1 | — | 250 |
| 46 | made without fat | 202 | 860 | 7.3 | 1.0 | 43.7 | 120 | 150 | 60 | 37 | 120 | 2.1 | 0.20 | 1.0 | — | 230 |
| | ***Breakfast cereals*** | | | | | | | | | | | | | | | |
| 47 | **All-bran** | 273 | 1156 | 15.1 | 5.7 | 43.0 | 1670 | 1070 | 74 | 370 | 900 | 12.0 | 1.2 | 8.4 | — | 2440 |
| 48 | **Cornflakes** | 368 | 1567 | 8.6 | 1.6 | 85.1 | 1160 | 99 | 3 | 14 | 47 | 0.6 | 0.03 | 0.3 | — | 1780 |
| 49 | **Grapenuts** | 355 | 1510 | 10.8 | 3.0 | 75.9 | 660 | 270 | 37 | 78 | 240 | 5.2 | 0.25 | 2.1 | — | 1080 |
| 50 | **Muesli** | 368 | 1556 | 12.9 | 7.5 | 66.2 | 180 | 600 | 200 | 100 | 380 | 4.6 | 0.41 | 2.2 | — | 330 |
| 51 | **Puffed Wheat** | 325 | 1386 | 14.2 | 1.3 | 68.5 | 4 | 390 | 26 | 140 | 350 | 4.6 | 0.56 | 2.8 | — | 50 |
| 52 | **Ready Brek** | 390 | 1651 | 12.4 | 8.7 | 69.9 | 23 | 390 | 64 | 120 | 420 | 4.9 | 0.41 | 2.7 | — | 66 |
| 53 | **Rice Krispies** | 372 | 1584 | 5.9 | 2.0 | 88.1 | 1110 | 160 | 7 | 50 | 150 | 0.7 | 0.12 | 1.1 | — | 1700 |

[a] The fat content depends on the conditions of frying; thin slices pick up more fat than thick ones

| No | Food | Retinol µg | Carotene µg | Vitamin D µg | Thiamin mg | Riboflavin mg | Nicotinic acid mg | Potential nicotinic acid from tryptophan mg Trp ÷ 60 | Vitamin C mg | Vitamin E mg |
|---|---|---|---|---|---|---|---|---|---|---|
| | ***Bread** contd* | | | | | | | | | |
| 34 | white, fried | 0 | 0 | 0 | — | — | — | 1.6 | 0 | —[a] |
| 35 | toasted | 0 | 0 | 0 | (0.17) | (0.04) | (1.8) | 2.0 | 0 | Tr |
| 36 | dried crumbs | 0 | 0 | 0 | (0.20) | (0.04) | (2.1) | 2.4 | 0 | Tr |
| 37 | currant | 0 | 0 | 0 | (0.18) | (0.03) | (1.4) | 1.3 | 0 | Tr |
| 38 | malt | 0 | 0 | 0 | — | — | — | 1.7 | 0 | — |
| 39 | soda | 10 | 10 | 0.01 | (Tr) | 0.06 | 1.3 | 1.7 | 0 | Tr |
| 40 | **Rolls** brown, crusty | 0 | 0 | 0 | 0.23 | 0.12 | 2.6 | 2.4 | 0 | (Tr) |
| 41 | soft | 0 | 0 | 0 | 0.23 | 0.15 | 2.7 | 2.4 | 0 | (Tr) |
| 42 | white, crusty | 0 | 0 | 0 | 0.23 | 0.07 | 1.5 | 2.4 | 0 | Tr |
| 43 | soft | 0 | 0 | 0 | 0.25 | 0.08 | 1.4 | 2.0 | 0 | Tr |
| 44 | starch reduced | 0 | 0 | 0 | — | — | — | 9.0 | 0 | — |
| 45 | **Chapatis** made with fat | — | — | — | 0.26 | 0.04 | 1.7 | 1.7 | 0 | — |
| 46 | made without fat | 0 | 0 | 0 | 0.23 | 0.04 | 1.5 | 1.5 | 0 | Tr |
| | ***Breakfast cereals*** | | | | | | | | | |
| 47 | **All-bran** | 0 | 0 | 0 | 0.75 | 2.8 | 49.0 | 3.2 | 0 | 2.0[c] |
| 48 | **Cornflakes** | 0 | 0 | 0 | 1.8[b] | 1.6[b] | 21.0[b] | 0.9 | 0 | 0.4 |
| 49 | **Grapenuts** | 1330[f] | 0 | 3.5[f] | 1.2 | 1.6 | 17.0 | 2.2 | 0 | 1.6[d] |
| 50 | **Muesli** | 0 | 0 | 0 | 0.33 | 0.27 | 2.7 | 3.0 | Tr | 3.2 |
| 51 | **Puffed Wheat** | 0 | 0 | 0 | Tr | 0.06 | 5.2 | 2.9 | 0 | 1.7[e] |
| 52 | **Ready Brek** | 0 | 0 | 0 | 1.5 | 0.09 | 9.4 | 2.8 | 0 | 1.2 |
| 53 | **Rice Krispies** | 0 | 0 | 0 | 2.3 | 1.7 | 24.0 | 1.3 | 0 | 0.6 |

| No | Food | Vitamin $B_6$ mg | Vitamin $B_{12}$ µg | Folic acid Free µg | Folic acid Total µg | Pantothenic acid µg | Biotin µg |
|---|---|---|---|---|---|---|---|
| | ***Bread** contd* | | | | | | |
| 34 | white, fried | — | 0 | — | — | — | — |
| 35 | toasted | — | 0 | — | — | (0.4) | (2) |
| 36 | dried crumbs | — | 0 | — | — | — | — |
| 37 | currant | (0.04) | 0 | (6) | (30) | (0.3) | (1) |
| 38 | malt | — | 0 | — | — | — | — |
| 39 | soda | 0.09 | 0 | 6 | 9 | 0.3 | 1 |
| 40 | **Rolls** brown, crusty | 0.15 | 0 | (21) | (36) | (0.3) | (3) |
| 41 | soft | 0.14 | 0 | (21) | (36) | (0.3) | (3) |
| 42 | white, crusty | 0.06 | 0 | (7) | (27) | (0.3) | (1) |
| 43 | soft | 0.06 | 0 | (7) | (27) | (0.3) | (1) |
| 44 | starch reduced | — | 0 | — | — | — | — |
| 45 | **Chapatis** made with fat | (0.21) | 0 | 9 | 15 | (0.3) | (2) |
| 46 | made without fat | (0.19) | 0 | 8 | 14 | (0.3) | (2) |
| | ***Breakfast cereals*** | | | | | | |
| 47 | **All-bran** | 0.83 | 0 | 27 | 100 | — | — |
| 48 | **Cornflakes** | 0.03 | 0 | 6 | 7 | — | — |
| 49 | **Grapenuts** | 2.81 | 5[f] | 30 | 41 | — | — |
| 50 | **Muesli** | 0.14 | 0 | 11 | 48 | — | — |
| 51 | **Puffed Wheat** | 0.14 | 0 | 16 | 19 | — | — |
| 52 | **Ready Brek** | 1.5 | 0 | 10 | 53 | — | — |
| 53 | **Rice Krispies** | 0.19 | 0 | 6 | 14 | — | — |

Notes

[a] The vitamin E content will depend on the fat used for frying.

[b] These cornflakes are fortified. Unfortified cornflakes contain a trace of thiamin, 0.03 mg riboflavin and 0.6 mg nicotinic acid per 100 g.

[c] Also contains 1.6 mg γ-tocopherol per 100 g.

[d] Also contains 0.6 mg γ-tocopherol per 100 g.

[e] Also contains 2.5 mg γ-tocopherol per 100 g.

[f] Data supplied by the manufacturer.

| No | Food | Description and number of samples | Water g | Sugars g | Starch and dextrins g | Dietary fibre g | Total nitrogen g |
|---|---|---|---|---|---|---|---|
| | ***Breakfast cereals** contd* | | | | | | |
| 54 | **Shredded Wheat** | 6 packets of the same brand (Nabisco) | 7.6 | 0.4 | 67.5 | 12.3 | 1.81 |
| 55 | **Special K** | 6 packets of the same brand (Kellogg's) | 2.7 | 9.6 | 68.6 | 5.5 | 3.15 |
| 56 | **Sugar Puffs** | 6 packets of the same brand (Quaker) | 1.8 | 56.5 | 28.0 | 6.1 | 1.01 |
| 57 | **Weetabix** | 6 packets of the same brand (Weetabix) | 3.8 | 6.1 | 66.5 | 12.7 | 1.96 |
| | ***Biscuits*** | | | | | | |
| 58 | **Chocolate** full coated | 7 different kinds | 2.2 | 43.4 | 24.0 | 3.1 | 1.00 |
| 59 | **Cream crackers** | 6 packets | 4.3 | Tr | 68.3 | (3.0) | 1.66 |
| 60 | **Crispbread** rye | 8 packets of the same brand (Ryvita) | 6.4 | 3.2 | 67.4 | 11.7 | 1.61 |
| 61 | wheat, starch reduced | 8 packets of the same brand (Energen) | 4.9 | 7.4 | 29.5 | 4.9 | 7.94 |
| 62 | **Digestive** plain | 3 brands | 4.5 | 16.4 | 49.6 | (5.5) | 1.68 |
| 63 | chocolate | 10 packets, 5 plain chocolate, 5 milk chocolate | 2.5 | 28.5 | 38.0 | 3.5 | 1.17 |
| 64 | **Ginger nuts** | 10 packets, 6 brands | 3.4 | 35.8 | 43.3 | 2.0 | 0.98 |
| 65 | **Home made** | eg Easter, Imperial; basic recipe p334 | 8.4 | 26.8 | 38.7 | 1.7 | 1.10 |
| 66 | **Matzo** | 6 packets, Rakusens, Superfine, tea | 6.7 | 4.2 | 82.4 | 3.9 | 1.85 |
| 67 | **Oatcakes** | 6 packets, 4 brands | 5.5 | 3.1 | 59.9 | 4.0 | 1.71 |
| 68 | **Sandwich** | 10 packets, custard creams and similar types | 2.6 | 30.2 | 39.0 | 1.2 | 0.87 |
| 69 | **Semi-sweet** | 10 packets, Osborne, Rich Tea, Marie | 2.5 | 22.3 | 52.5 | 2.3 | 1.18 |
| 70 | **Short-sweet** | 10 packets, shortcake, Lincoln | 2.6 | 24.1 | 38.1 | 1.7 | 1.08 |
| 71 | **Shortbread** | Recipe p334 | 5.0 | 17.2 | 48.3 | 2.1 | 1.08 |
| 72 | **Wafers** filled | 9 packets, assorted | 2.3 | 44.7 | 21.3 | 1.6 | 0.82 |
| 73 | **Water biscuits** | 3 brands | 4.5 | 2.3 | 73.5 | (3.2) | 1.89 |

| No | Food | Energy value kcal | Energy value kJ | Protein (see p7) g | Fat g | Carbo-hydrate g | Na mg | K mg | Ca mg | Mg mg | P mg | Fe mg | Cu mg | Zn mg | S mg | Cl mg |
|---|---|---|---|---|---|---|---|---|---|---|---|---|---|---|---|---|
| | ***Breakfast cereals** contd* | | | | | | | | | | | | | | | |
| 54 | **Shredded Wheat** | 324 | 1378 | 10.6 | 3.0 | 67.9 | 8 | 330 | 38 | 130 | 340 | 4.2 | 0.40 | 2.3 | — | 53 |
| 55 | **Special K** | 388 | 1650 | 18.0[a] | 2.5 | 78.2 | 880 | 190 | 42 | 52 | 190 | 20.0 | 0.26 | 1.9 | — | 1460 |
| 56 | **Sugar Puffs** | 348 | 1482 | 5.9 | 0.8 | 84.5 | 9 | 160 | 14 | 55 | 140 | 2.1 | 0.23 | 1.5 | — | 41 |
| 57 | **Weetabix** | 340 | 1444 | 11.4 | 3.4 | 70.3 | 360 | 420 | 33 | 120 | 300 | 7.6 | 0.54 | 2.1 | — | 570 |
| | ***Biscuits*** | | | | | | | | | | | | | | | |
| 58 | **Chocolate** full-coated | 524 | 2197 | 5.7 | 27.6 | 67.4 | 160 | 230 | 110 | 42 | 130 | 1.7 | 0.25 | 0.8 | — | 250 |
| 59 | **Cream crackers** | 440 | 1857 | 9.5 | 16.3 | 68.3 | 610 | 120 | 110 | 25 | 110 | 1.7 | — | (0.6) | 87 | 830 |
| 60 | **Crispbread** rye | 321 | 1367 | 9.4 | 2.1 | 70.6 | 220 | 500 | 50 | 100 | 310 | 3.7 | 0.38 | 3.1 | — | 370 |
| 61 | wheat, starch reduced | 388 | 1642 | 45.3 | 7.6 | 36.9 | 610 | 210 | 60 | 61 | 220 | 5.4 | 0.47 | 2.8 | — | 980 |
| 62 | **Digestive** plain | 471 | 1981 | 9.8 | 20.5 | 66.0 | 440 | 160 | 110 | 32 | 130 | 2.0 | 0.23 | (0.6) | 72 | 430 |
| 63 | chocolate | 493 | 2071 | 6.8 | 24.1 | 66.5 | 450 | 210 | 84 | 41 | 130 | 2.1 | 0.24 | 1.0 | — | 410 |
| 64 | **Ginger nuts** | 456 | 1923 | 5.6 | 15.2 | 79.1 | 330 | 220 | 130 | 25 | 87 | 4.0 | 0.16 | 0.5 | — | 320 |
| 65 | **Home made** | 469 | 1971 | 6.4 | 22.0 | 65.5 | 220 | 88 | 82 | 12 | 84 | 1.5 | 0.11 | 0.5 | — | 340 |
| 66 | **Matzo** | 384 | 1634 | 10.5 | 1.9 | 86.6 | 17 | 150 | 32 | 20 | 100 | 1.5 | 0.16 | 0.7 | — | 80 |
| 67 | **Oatcakes** | 441 | 1855 | 10.0 | 18.3 | 63.0 | 1230 | 340 | 54 | 100 | 420 | 4.5 | 0.37 | 2.3 | — | 1290 |
| 68 | **Sandwich** | 513 | 2151 | 5.0 | 25.9 | 69.2 | 220 | 120 | 100 | 13 | 82 | 1.6 | 0.07 | 0.5 | — | 290 |
| 69 | **Semi-sweet** | 457 | 1925 | 6.7 | 16.6 | 74.8 | 410 | 140 | 120 | 17 | 84 | 2.1 | 0.08 | 0.6 | — | 520 |
| 70 | **Short-sweet** | 469 | 1966 | 6.2 | 23.4 | 62.2 | 360 | 110 | 87 | 15 | 85 | 1.8 | 0.11 | 0.6 | — | 490 |
| 71 | **Shortbread** | 504 | 2115 | 6.2 | 26.0 | 65.5 | 270 | 91 | 97 | 13 | 75 | 1.5 | 0.12 | 0.5 | — | 440 |
| 72 | **Wafers** filled | 535 | 2242 | 4.7 | 29.9 | 66.0 | 70 | 160 | 73 | 22 | 83 | 1.6 | 0.16 | 0.6 | — | 150 |
| 73 | **Water biscuits** | 440 | 1859 | 10.8 | 12.5 | 75.8 | 470 | 140 | 120 | 19 | 87 | 1.6 | 0.08 | (0.6) | 100 | 680 |

[a] N × 5.7

| No | Food | Retinol µg | Carotene µg | Vitamin D µg | Thiamin mg | Riboflavin mg | Nicotinic acid mg | Potential nicotinic acid from tryptophan mg Trp ÷ 60 | Vitamin C mg | Vitamin E mg |
|---|---|---|---|---|---|---|---|---|---|---|
| | ***Breakfast cereals** contd* | | | | | | | | | |
| 54 | **Shredded Wheat** | 0 | 0 | 0 | 0.27 | 0.05 | 4.5 | 2.1 | 0 | 1.0[a] |
| 55 | **Special K** | 0 | 0 | 0 | 1.7 | 1.9 | 21.0 | 3.7 | 0 | 0.5[b] |
| 56 | **Sugar Puffs** | 0 | 0 | 0 | Tr | 0.03 | 2.5 | 1.2 | 0 | 0.2[c] |
| 57 | **Weetabix** | 0 | 0 | 0 | 1.0 | 1.5 | 12.0 | 2.3 | 0 | 1.8[d] |
| | ***Biscuits*** | | | | | | | | | |
| 58 | **Chocolate** full coated | 0 | Tr | 0 | 0.03 | 0.13 | 0.5 | 1.2 | 0 | 1.3[e] |
| 59 | **Cream crackers** | 0 | 0 | 0 | (0.13) | (0.08) | (1.5) | 1.9 | 0 | — |
| 60 | **Crispbread** rye | 0 | 0 | 0 | 0.28 | 0.14 | 1.1 | 1.8 | 0 | 0.5 |
| 61 | wheat, starch reduced | 0 | 0 | 0 | 0.15 | 0.10 | 3.9 | 9.3 | 0 | 0.5 |
| 62 | **Digestive** plain | 0 | 0 | 0 | (0.13) | (0.08) | (1.5) | 2.0 | 0 | — |
| 63 | chocolate | 0 | Tr | 0 | 0.08 | 0.11 | 1.3 | 1.4 | 0 | 1.0[f] |
| 64 | **Ginger nuts** | 0 | 0 | 0 | 0.10 | 0.03 | 0.9 | 1.1 | 0 | 1.5 |
| 65 | **Home made** | 240 | 0 | 2.18 | 0.14 | 0.06 | 1.0 | 1.0 | 0 | 2.2 |
| 66 | **Matzo** | 0 | 0 | 0 | 0.11 | 0.03 | 0.9 | 2.2 | 0 | Tr |
| 67 | **Oatcakes** | 0 | 0 | 0 | 0.32 | 0.09 | 0.7 | 2.3 | 0 | 2.0[g] |
| 68 | **Sandwich** | 0 | 0 | 0 | 0.14 | 0.13 | 1.1 | 1.0 | 0 | 3.4 |
| 69 | **Semi-sweet** | 0 | 0 | 0 | 0.13 | 0.08 | 1.5 | 1.4 | 0 | 1.4 |
| 70 | **Short-sweet** | 0 | 0 | 0 | 0.16 | 0.04 | 0.9 | 1.3 | 0 | 1.3 |
| 71 | **Shortbread** | 230 | 140 | 0.23 | 0.15 | 0.01 | 1.1 | 1.3 | 0 | 0.6 |
| 72 | **Wafers** filled | 0 | 0 | 0 | 0.09 | 0.08 | 0.5 | 1.0 | 0 | 1.9 |
| 73 | **Water biscuits** | 0 | 0 | 0 | (0.11) | (0.03) | (0.9) | 2.2 | 0 | — |

| No | Food | Vitamin $B_6$ mg | Vitamin $B_{12}$ µg | Folic acid Free µg | Folic acid Total µg | Pantothenic acid mg | Biotin µg |
|---|---|---|---|---|---|---|---|
| | ***Breakfast cereals** contd* | | | | | | |
| 54 | **Shredded Wheat** | 0.24 | 0 | 10 | 29 | — | — |
| 55 | **Special K** | 0.16 | 0 | 11 | 37 | — | — |
| 56 | **Sugar puffs** | 0.05 | 0 | 8 | 12 | — | — |
| 57 | **Weetabix** | 0.24 | 0 | 14 | 50 | — | — |
| | ***Biscuits*** | | | | | | |
| 58 | **Chocolate** full coated | 0.04 | 0 | — | — | — | — |
| 59 | **Cream crackers** | (0.06) | 0 | (13) | — | — | — |
| 60 | **Crispbread** rye | 0.29 | 0 | (17) | (40) | (1.1) | (7) |
| 61 | wheat, starch reduced | 0.22 | 0 | — | — | — | — |
| 62 | **Digestive**, plain | (0.06) | 0 | (8) | — | — | — |
| 63 | chocolate | 0.08 | 0 | — | — | — | — |
| 64 | **Ginger nuts** | 0.07 | 0 | (8) | — | — | — |
| 65 | **Home made** | 0.07 | 0 | 5 | 7 | 0.3 | 4 |
| 66 | **Matzo** | 0.06 | 0 | — | — | — | — |
| 67 | **Oatcakes** | 0.10 | 0 | 8 | — | (1.0) | (20) |
| 68 | **Sandwich** | 0.04 | 0 | — | — | — | — |
| 69 | **Semi-sweet** | 0.06 | 0 | 8 | — | — | — |
| 70 | **Short-sweet** | 0.05 | 0 | 8 | — | — | — |
| 71 | **Shortbread** | 0.07 | 0 | 5 | 7 | — | — |
| 72 | **Wafers** filled | 0.03 | 0 | — | — | — | — |
| 73 | **Water biscuits** | (0.06) | 0 | (8) | — | — | — |

Notes

[a] Also contains 2.0mg $\gamma$-tocopherol per 100g.

[b] Also contains 0.5mg $\gamma$-tocopherol per 100g.

[c] Also contains 1.4mg $\gamma$-tocopherol per 100g.

[d] Also contains 2.2mg $\gamma$-tocopherol per 100g.

[e] Also contains 1.3mg $\gamma$-tocopherol per 100g.

[f] Also contains 1.0mg $\gamma$-tocopherol per 100g.

[g] Also contains 1.4mg $\gamma$-tocopherol per 100g.

| No | Food | Description and number of samples | Water g | Sugars g | Starch and dextrins g | Dietary fibre g | Total nitrogen g |
|---|---|---|---|---|---|---|---|
| | ***Cakes*** | | | | | | |
| 74 | **Fancy iced cakes** | 10 different types | 12.7 | 54.0 | 14.8 | 2.4 | 0.66 |
| 75 | **Fruit cake** rich | eg Christmas, Dundee; recipe p334 | 20.6 | 46.7 | 11.6 | 3.5 | 0.62 |
| 76 | rich, iced | Coated with marzipan and royal icing; recipe p334 | 17.9 | 54.2 | 7.8 | 3.4 | 0.71 |
| 77 | plain | 10 cakes, 4 brands | 19.5 | 43.1 | 14.8 | 2.8 | 0.89 |
| 78 | **Gingerbread** | Recipe p335 | 19.0 | 31.8 | 30.9 | 1.3 | 1.03 |
| 79 | **Madeira cake** | 10 cakes, 4 brands | 20.2 | 36.5 | 21.9 | 1.4 | 0.94 |
| 80 | **Rock cakes** | Basic recipe, rubbing in method; recipe p335 | 15.6 | 31.3 | 28.9 | 2.4 | 0.92 |
| 81 | **Sponge cake** with fat | eg Victoria, chocolate, orange; basic recipe, creaming method; recipe p335 | 14.9 | 30.5 | 22.7 | 1.0 | 1.06 |
| 82 | without fat | Basic recipe, whisking method; recipe p335 | 30.0 | 30.9 | 22.7 | 1.0 | 1.64 |
| 83 | jam filled | 10 cakes, 3 brands; sandwich and Swiss roll | 24.5 | 47.7 | 16.5 | 1.2 | 0.74 |
| | ***Buns and pastries*** | | | | | | |
| 84 | **Currant buns** | 20 samples from 4 different shops | 28.6 | 14.0 | 40.5 | — | 1.30 |
| 85 | **Doughnuts** | 16 samples from 4 different shops | 26.4 | 15.0 | 33.8 | — | 1.03 |
| 86 | **Eclairs** | With chocolate icing and dairy cream filling; recipe p335 | 34.8 | 26.3 | 11.9 | — | 0.73 |
| 87 | **Jam tarts** | Recipe p335 | 19.2 | 37.5 | 25.3 | 1.7 | 0.61 |
| 88 | **Mince pies** | Recipe p335 | 11.5 | 30.0 | 31.7 | 2.9 | 0.74 |

| No | Food | Energy value kcal | Energy value kJ | Protein g | Fat g | Carbo-hydrate g | Na (mg) | K (mg) | Ca (mg) | Mg (mg) | P (mg) | Fe (mg) | Cu (mg) | Zn (mg) | S (mg) | Cl (mg) |
|---|---|---|---|---|---|---|---|---|---|---|---|---|---|---|---|---|
| | ***Cakes*** | | | | | | | | | | | | | | | |
| 74 | **Fancy iced cakes** | 407 | 1717 | 3.8 | 14.9 | 68.8 | 250 | 170 | 44 | 30 | 120 | 1.4 | 0.25 | 0.7 | — | 230 |
| 75 | **Fruit cake** rich | 332 | 1403 | 3.7 | 11.0 | 58.3 | 170 | 430 | 75 | 26 | 73 | 1.8 | 0.33 | — | — | 240 |
| 76 | rich, iced | 352 | 1487 | 4.1 | 11.5 | 62.0 | 120 | 360 | 71 | 37 | 86 | 1.6 | 0.24 | — | — | 170 |
| 77 | plain | 354 | 1490 | 5.1 | 12.9 | 57.9 | 250 | 390 | 60 | 25 | 110 | 1.7 | 0.25 | 0.5 | — | 320 |
| 78 | **Gingerbread** | 373 | 1573 | 6.1 | 12.6 | 62.7 | 210 | 470 | 210 | 48 | 91 | 3.8 | 0.20 | — | — | 410 |
| 79 | **Madeira cake** | 393 | 1652 | 5.4 | 16.9 | 58.4 | 380 | 120 | 42 | 12 | 120 | 1.1 | 0.10 | 0.5 | — | 500 |
| 80 | **Rock cakes** | 394 | 1658 | 5.4 | 16.3 | 60.2 | 480 | 210 | 390 | 16 | 300 | 1.4 | 0.17 | 0.4 | — | 260 |
| 81 | **Sponge cake** with fat | 464 | 1941 | 6.4 | 26.5 | 53.2 | 350 | 82 | 140 | 10 | 150 | 1.4 | 0.10 | 0.6 | — | 400 |
| 82 | without fat | 301 | 1276 | 10.0 | 6.7 | 53.6 | 82 | 120 | 74 | 13 | 160 | 1.9 | 0.11 | 1.1 | — | 110 |
| 83 | jam filled | 302 | 1280 | 4.2 | 4.9 | 64.2 | 420 | 140 | 44 | 14 | 220 | 1.6 | 0.20 | 0.5 | — | 260 |
| | ***Buns and pastries*** | | | | | | | | | | | | | | | |
| 84 | **Currant buns** | 302 | 1279 | 7.4 | 7.6 | 54.5 | 100 | 180 | 90 | 22 | 65 | 2.5 | 0.03 | — | 73 | 200 |
| 85 | **Doughnuts** | 349 | 1467 | 6.0 | 15.8 | 48.8 | 60 | 110 | 70 | 16 | 55 | 1.9 | 0.11 | — | 56 | 89 |
| 86 | **Eclairs** | 376 | 1569 | 4.1 | 24.0 | 38.2 | 160 | 92 | 48 | 16 | 68 | 1.0 | 0.15 | 0.4 | — | 250 |
| 87 | **Jam tarts** | 384 | 1616 | 3.5 | 14.9 | 62.8 | 230 | 110 | 62 | 13 | 47 | 1.6 | 0.18 | — | — | 360 |
| 88 | **Mince pies** | 435 | 1826 | 4.3 | 20.7 | 61.7 | 340 | 150 | 76 | 14 | 55 | 1.7 | 0.17 | 0.4 | — | 540 |

| No | Food | Retinol µg | Carotene µg | Vitamin D µg | Thiamin mg | Riboflavin mg | Nicotinic acid mg | Potential nicotinic acid from tryptophan mg Trp ÷ 60 | Vitamin C mg | Vitamin E mg |
|---|---|---|---|---|---|---|---|---|---|---|
| | ***Cakes*** | | | | | | | | | |
| 74 | **Fancy iced cakes** | 0 | — | 0 | 0.01 | 0.04 | 0.2 | 0.8 | 0 | — |
| 75 | **Fruit cake** rich | 120 | 10 | 1.14 | 0.08 | 0.08 | 0.5 | 0.8 | 0 | 1.4 |
| 76 | rich, iced | 80 | 7 | 0.77 | 0.12 | 0.13 | 0.5 | 0.4 | Tr | 2.4 |
| 77 | plain | — | — | — | 0.08 | 0.07 | 0.6 | 1.0 | 0 | — |
| 78 | **Gingerbread** | 130 | 2 | 1.24 | (Tr) | 0.07 | 0.7 | 1.3 | Tr | 1.2 |
| 79 | **Madeira cake** | — | — | — | 0.06 | 0.11 | 0.5 | 1.1 | 0 | — |
| 80 | **Rock cakes** | 180 | 7 | 1.59 | (Tr) | 0.07 | 0.8 | 1.1 | Tr | 1.6 |
| 81 | **Sponge cake** with fat | 300 | 0 | 2.76 | (Tr) | 0.12 | 0.6 | 1.6 | 0 | 2.7 |
| 82 | without fat | 80 | 0 | 1.02 | 0.11 | 0.24 | 0.6 | 2.7 | 0 | 0.9 |
| 83 | jam filled | — | — | — | 0.04 | 0.07 | 0.4 | 0.9 | 0 | — |
| | ***Buns and pastries*** | | | | | | | | | |
| 84 | **Currant buns** | 0 | — | 0 | (0.18) | (0.03) | (1.4) | 1.5 | 0 | — |
| 85 | **Doughnuts** | 0 | — | 0 | — | — | — | 1.2 | 0 | — |
| 86 | **Eclairs** | 200 | 70 | 0.91 | 0.05 | 0.09 | 0.3 | 1.0 | Tr | 1.2 |
| 87 | **Jam tarts** | 70 | Tr | 0.64 | 0.08 | 0.01 | 0.6 | 0.7 | 4 | 0.6 |
| 88 | **Mince pies** | 90 | 5 | 0.80 | 0.11 | 0.02 | 0.9 | 0.8 | 0 | 0.8 |

| No | Food | Vitamin $B_6$ mg | Vitamin $B_{12}$ µg | Folic acid Free µg | Folic acid Total µg | Pantothenic acid mg | Biotin µg | Notes |
|---|---|---|---|---|---|---|---|---|
| | ***Cakes*** | | | | | | | |
| 74 | **Fancy iced cakes** | — | 0 | — | — | — | — | |
| 75 | **Fruit cake** rich | 0.13 | Tr | 4 | 4 | 0.2 | 4 | |
| 76 | rich, iced | 0.10 | Tr | 5 | 10 | 0.2 | 3 | |
| 77 | plain | — | 0 | — | — | — | — | |
| 78 | **Gingerbread** | 0.06 | Tr | 5 | 6 | 0.3 | 4 | |
| 79 | **Madeira cake** | — | 0 | — | — | — | — | |
| 80 | **Rock cakes** | 0.09 | Tr | 4 | 7 | 0.3 | 3 | |
| 81 | **Sponge cake** with fat | 0.06 | Tr | 6 | 7 | 0.5 | 8 | |
| 82 | without fat | 0.08 | 1 | 10 | 10 | 0.8 | 15 | |
| 83 | jam filled | — | 0 | — | — | — | — | |
| | ***Buns and pastries*** | | | | | | | |
| 84 | **Currant buns** | — | 0 | — | — | — | — | |
| 85 | **Doughnuts** | — | 0 | — | — | — | — | |
| 86 | **Eclairs** | 0.04 | Tr | 5 | 5 | 0.3 | 4 | |
| 87 | **Jam tarts** | 0.04 | 0 | 2 | 4 | 0.1 | 1 | |
| 88 | **Mince pies** | 0.08 | 0 | 3 | 5 | 0.1 | 1 | |

| No | Food | Description and number of samples | Water g | Sugars g | Starch and dextrins g | Dietary fibre g | Total nitrogen g |
|---|---|---|---|---|---|---|---|
| | ***Buns and pastries** contd* | | | | | | |
| 89 | **Pastry, choux** raw | Recipe p 336 | 61.2 | 0.4 | 19.5 | 0.8 | 0.92 |
| 90 | cooked | Recipe p 336 | 40.4 | 0.7 | 30.0 | 1.3 | 1.42 |
| 91 | **Pastry, flaky** raw | Recipe p 336 | 29.6 | 0.8 | 35.0 | 1.5 | 0.77 |
| 92 | cooked | Recipe p 336 | 7.3 | 1.1 | 46.3 | 2.0 | 1.02 |
| 93 | **Pastry, shortcrust** raw | Recipe p 336 | 19.5 | 1.0 | 47.2 | 2.0 | 1.03 |
| 94 | cooked | Recipe p 336 | 6.9 | 1.2 | 54.6 | 2.4 | 1.20 |
| 95 | **Scones** | Recipe p 336 | 21.5 | 6.1 | 49.8 | 2.1 | 1.30 |
| 96 | **Scotch pancakes** | Drop scones; recipe p 336 | 40.7 | 8.1 | 32.5 | 1.4 | 1.13 |
| | ***Puddings*** | | | | | | |
| 97 | **Apple crumble** | Recipe p 336 | 52.3 | 23.8 | 13.2 | 2.5 | 0.32 |
| 98 | **Bread and butter pudding** | Recipe p 336 | 67.2 | 12.0 | 5.2 | 0.6 | 0.99 |
| 99 | **Cheesecake** | Recipe p 337 | 34.7 | 13.9 | 10.1 | 0.9 | 0.70 |
| 100 | **Christmas pudding** | Recipe p 337 | 39.4 | 39.1 | 8.5 | 2.0 | 0.88 |
| 101 | **Custard,** egg | Baked or sauce; recipe p 337 | 76.8 | 11.0 | 0 | 0 | 0.91 |
| 102 | made with powder | Recipe p 337 | 74.7 | 11.5 | 5.3 | — | 0.60 |
| 103 | **Custard tart** | Recipe p 337 | 48.0 | 6.0 | 23.6 | 1.0 | 0.97 |
| 104 | **Dumpling** | Recipe p 337 | 60.2 | 0.5 | 24.7 | 1.0 | 0.51 |

| No | Food | Energy value kcal | Energy value kJ | Protein g | Fat g | Carbo-hydrate g | Na mg | K mg | Ca mg | Mg mg | P mg | Fe mg | Cu mg | Zn mg | S mg | Cl mg |
|---|---|---|---|---|---|---|---|---|---|---|---|---|---|---|---|---|
| | ***Buns and pastries** contd* | | | | | | | | | | | | | | | |
| 89 | **Pastry, choux** raw | 214 | 893 | 5.5 | 13.0 | 19.9 | 260 | 70 | 51 | 9 | 84 | 1.1 | 0.07 | 0.5 | — | 390 |
| 90 | cooked | 330 | 1379 | 8.5 | 20.1 | 30.7 | 390 | 110 | 78 | 14 | 130 | 1.8 | 0.11 | 0.8 | — | 600 |
| 91 | **Pastry, flaky** raw | 427 | 1780 | 4.4 | 30.6 | 35.8 | 350 | 67 | 68 | 11 | 52 | 1.1 | 0.09 | 0.3 | — | 560 |
| 92 | cooked | 565 | 2356 | 5.8 | 40.5 | 47.4 | 470 | 88 | 90 | 15 | 68 | 1.5 | 0.12 | 0.4 | — | 740 |
| 93 | **Pastry, shortcrust** raw | 455 | 1900 | 5.9 | 27.8 | 48.2 | 410 | 85 | 92 | 15 | 69 | 1.5 | 0.11 | 0.4 | — | 660 |
| 94 | cooked | 527 | 2202 | 6.9 | 32.2 | 55.8 | 480 | 99 | 110 | 17 | 79 | 1.8 | 0.13 | 0.5 | — | 760 |
| 95 | **Scones** | 371 | 1562 | 7.5 | 14.6 | 55.9 | 800 | 140 | 620 | 19 | 470 | 1.5 | 0.12 | 0.6 | — | 480 |
| 96 | **Scotch pancakes** | 283 | 1193 | 6.7 | 11.6 | 40.6 | 400 | 320 | 120 | 16 | 110 | 1.3 | 0.10 | 0.6 | — | 510 |
| | ***Puddings*** | | | | | | | | | | | | | | | |
| 97 | **Apple crumble** | 208 | 878 | 1.8 | 6.9 | 37.0 | 68 | 100 | 28 | 5 | 30 | 0.6 | 0.09 | 0.2 | — | 110 |
| 98 | **Bread and butter pudding** | 159 | 668 | 6.1 | 7.8 | 17.2 | 150 | 200 | 130 | 18 | 140 | 0.7 | 0.08 | 0.7 | 69 | 250 |
| 99 | **Cheesecake** | 421 | 1747 | 4.2 | 34.9 | 24.0 | 260 | 120 | 67 | 11 | 87 | 0.7 | 0.10 | 0.5 | — | 360 |
| 100 | **Christmas pudding** | 304 | 1279 | 5.2 | 11.6 | 47.6 | 240 | 390 | 87 | 34 | 93 | 1.9 | 0.26 | 0.5 | 58 | 380 |
| 101 | **Custard** egg | 118 | 497 | 5.8 | 6.0 | 11.0 | 78 | 170 | 130 | 14 | 140 | 0.5 | 0.04 | 0.7 | 66 | 130 |
| 102 | made with powder | 118 | 496 | 3.8 | 4.4 | 16.8 | 76 | 170 | 140 | 14 | 110 | 0.1 | 0.03 | 0.4 | 35 | 140 |
| 103 | **Custard tart** | 287 | 1199 | 5.9 | 16.9 | 29.6 | 250 | 130 | 110 | 15 | 100 | 1.0 | 0.08 | 0.5 | — | 390 |
| 104 | **Dumpling** | 211 | 885 | 2.9 | 11.7 | 25.2 | 400 | 43 | 160 | 8 | 120 | 0.8 | 0.06 | 0.2 | — | 450 |

| No | Food | Retinol µg | Carotene µg | Vitamin D µg | Thiamin mg | Riboflavin mg | Nicotinic acid mg | Potential nicotinic acid from trytophan mg Trp ÷ 60 | Vitamin C mg | Vitamin E mg |
|---|---|---|---|---|---|---|---|---|---|---|
| | ***Buns and pastries** contd* | | | | | | | | | |
| 89 | **Pastry, choux** raw | 150 | 0 | 1.42 | 0.10 | 0.12 | 0.5 | 1.4 | 0 | 1.4 |
| 90 | cooked | 230 | 0 | 2.19 | 0.12 | 0.16 | 0.8 | 2.1 | 0 | 2.1 |
| 91 | **Pastry, flaky** raw | 150 | 0 | 1.33 | 0.15 | 0.01 | 0.9 | 0.9 | Tr | 1.4 |
| 92 | cooked | 200 | 0 | 1.76 | 0.14 | 0.01 | 1.1 | 1.2 | Tr | 1.8 |
| 93 | **Pastry, shortcrust** raw | 130 | 0 | 1.19 | 0.20 | 0.01 | 1.2 | 1.2 | 0 | 1.2 |
| 94 | cooked | 160 | 0 | 1.38 | 0.17 | 0.01 | 1.3 | 1.4 | 0 | 1.4 |
| 95 | **Scones** | 150 | 5 | 1.23 | (Tr) | 0.08 | 1.2 | 1.5 | Tr | 1.3 |
| 96 | **Scotch pancakes** | 150 | 7 | 1.26 | (Tr) | 0.12 | 0.9 | 1.5 | Tr | 1.3 |
| | ***Puddings*** | | | | | | | | | |
| 97 | **Apple crumble** | 70 | 25 | 0.66 | 0.07 | 0.02 | 0.4 | 0.3 | 6 | 0.8 |
| 98 | **Bread and butter pudding** | 70 | 30 | 0.53 | 0.05 | 0.20 | 0.3 | 1.5 | Tr | 0.4 |
| 99 | **Cheesecake** | 280 | 110 | 0.94 | 0.05 | 0.10 | 0.3 | 1.0 | 2 | — |
| 100 | **Christmas pudding** | 20 | 20 | 0.21 | 0.08 | 0.10 | 0.7 | 1.1 | 0 | 1.1 |
| 101 | **Custard** egg | 60 | 20 | 0.37 | 0.05 | 0.25 | 0.1 | 1.5 | Tr | 0.3 |
| 102 | made with powder | 40 | 20 | 0.03 | 0.05 | 0.21 | 0.1 | 0.9 | Tr | 0.1 |
| 103 | **Custard tart** | 100 | 10 | 0.78 | 0.10 | 0.11 | 0.6 | 1.4 | Tr | 0.8 |
| 104 | **Dumpling** | 10 | 10 | 0 | (Tr) | 0.01 | 0.6 | 0.6 | 0 | 0.2 |

| No | Food | Vitamin $B_6$ mg | Vitamin $B_{12}$ µg | Folic acid Free µg | Folic acid Total µg | Pantothenic acid mg | Biotin µg | Notes |
|---|---|---|---|---|---|---|---|---|
| | ***Buns and pastries** contd* | | | | | | | |
| 89 | **Pastry, choux** raw | 0.06 | Tr | 10 | 12 | 0.5 | 6 | |
| 90 | cooked | 0.08 | Tr | 8 | 9 | 0.6 | 10 | |
| 91 | **Pastry, flaky** raw | 0.07 | 0 | 6 | 10 | 0.1 | Tr | |
| 92 | cooked | 0.07 | 0 | 5 | 7 | 0.1 | Tr | |
| 93 | **Pastry, shortcrust** raw | 0.09 | 0 | 8 | 13 | 0.2 | 1 | |
| 94 | cooked | 0.08 | 0 | 5 | 8 | 0.2 | 1 | |
| 95 | **Scones** | 0.08 | Tr | 5 | 8 | 0.2 | 2 | |
| 96 | **Scotch pancakes** | 0.07 | Tr | 5 | 7 | 0.5 | 4 | |
| | ***Puddings*** | | | | | | | |
| 97 | **Apple crumble** | 0.04 | 0 | 2 | 4 | 0.1 | Tr | |
| 98 | **Bread and butter pudding** | 0.05 | Tr | 5 | 6 | 0.5 | 7 | |
| 99 | **Cheesecake** | 0.02 | Tr | 3 | 3 | — | — | |
| 100 | **Christmas pudding** | 0.11 | Tr | 4 | 8 | 0.3 | 4 | |
| 101 | **Custard** egg | 0.05 | Tr | 7 | 8 | 0.6 | 7 | |
| 102 | made with powder | 0.05 | Tr | 4 | 5 | 0.4 | 2 | |
| 103 | **Custard tart** | 0.06 | Tr | 5 | 6 | 0.4 | 4 | |
| 104 | **Dumpling** | 0.03 | 0 | 2 | 3 | 0.1 | Tr | |

| No | Food | Description and number of samples | Water g | Sugars g | Starch and dextrins g | Dietary fibre g | Total nitrogen g |
|---|---|---|---|---|---|---|---|
| | ***Puddings** contd* | | | | | | |
| 105 | **Fruit pie** individual, with pastry top and bottom | 10 pies, as purchased, 3 brands; apple, blackcurrant, blackberry, apricot | 22.9 | 30.9 | 25.8 | 2.6 | 0.75 |
| 106 | **Fruit pie** with pastry top | eg Apple, gooseberry, plum, rhubarb; recipe p 338 | 60.4 | 14.7 | 12.9 | 2.2 | 0.34 |
| 107 | **Ice cream** dairy | 10 family sized packets, 2 brands | 64.4 | 22.6 | 2.2 | — | 0.58 |
| 108 | non-dairy | 10 family sized packets, 2 brands | 65.7 | 19.7 | 1.0 | — | 0.52 |
| 109 | **Jelly** packet, cubes | 8 samples, assorted flavours | 29.9 | 62.5 | 0 | — | 1.10 |
| 110 | made with water | Recipe p 338 | 84.0 | 14.2 | 0 | — | 0.25 |
| 111 | made with milk | Recipe p 338 | 78.7 | 16.0 | 0 | — | 0.47 |
| 112 | **Lemon meringue pie** | Recipe p 338 | 35.0 | 24.8 | 21.6 | 0.7 | 0.75 |
| 113 | **Meringues** | Without cream; recipe p 338 | 2.0 | 95.6 | 0 | 0 | 0.85 |
| 114 | **Milk pudding** | eg Rice, sago, semolina, tapioca; recipe p 338 | 71.8 | 10.9 | 9.5 | — | 0.65 |
| 115 | canned, rice | 10 cans, 4 brands | 77.6 | 8.9 | 5.8 | — | 0.53 |
| 116 | **Pancakes** | Recipe p 338 | 43.4 | 16.6 | 19.6 | 0.9 | 1.00 |
| 117 | **Queen of puddings** | Recipe p 339 | 54.8 | 28.9 | 4.6 | 0.3 | 0.77 |
| 118 | **Sponge pudding** steamed | Recipe p 339 | 28.5 | 18.9 | 27.1 | 1.2 | 0.99 |
| 119 | **Suet pudding** steamed | Recipe p 339 | 36.6 | 14.0 | 26.6 | 1.1 | 0.77 |
| 120 | **Treacle tart** | Recipe p 339 | 21.0 | 33.6 | 27.7 | 1.2 | 0.65 |
| 121 | **Trifle** | Recipe p 339 | 64.5 | 18.7 | 5.6 | — | 0.57 |
| 122 | **Yorkshire pudding** | Recipe p 339 | 56.4 | 3.8 | 22.0 | 1.0 | 1.12 |

| No | Food | Energy value kcal | Energy value kJ | Protein g | Fat g | Carbo-hydrate g | Na mg | K mg | Ca mg | Mg mg | P mg | Fe mg | Cu mg | Zn mg | S mg | Cl mg |
|---|---|---|---|---|---|---|---|---|---|---|---|---|---|---|---|---|
| | ***Puddings** contd* | | | | | | | | | | | | | | | |
| 105 | **Fruit pie** individual, with pastry top and bottom | 369 | 1554 | 4.3 | 15.5 | 56.7 | 210 | 120 | 51 | 12 | 64 | 1.2 | 0.10 | 0.5 | — | 260 |
| 106 | **Fruit pie** with pastry top | 180 | 756 | 2.0 | 7.6 | 27.6 | 110 | 170 | 48 | 9 | 32 | 0.6 | 0.10 | 0.1 | — | 190 |
| 107 | **Ice cream** dairy | 167 | 704 | 3.7 | 6.6 | 24.8 | 80 | 180 | 140 | 13 | 100 | 0.2 | (0.03) | 0.4 | — | 140 |
| 108 | non-dairy | 165 | 691 | 3.3 | 8.2 | 20.7 | 70 | 150 | 120 | 11 | 90 | 0.3 | (0.03) | 0.4 | — | 140 |
| 109 | **Jelly** packet, cubes | 259 | 1104 | 6.1 | 0 | 62.5 | 25 | 25 | 32 | 4 | 7 | 1.7 | 0.16 | — | 37 | 30 |
| 110 | made with water | 59 | 251 | 1.4 | 0 | 14.2 | 6 | 6 | 7 | 1 | 2 | 0.4 | 0.04 | — | 8 | 7 |
| 111 | made with milk | 86 | 363 | 2.8 | 1.6 | 16.0 | 27 | 66 | 59 | 6 | 42 | 0.4 | 0.04 | — | 21 | 48 |
| 112 | **Lemon meringue pie** | 323 | 1359 | 4.5 | 14.6 | 46.4 | 200 | 81 | 46 | 9 | 70 | 1.0 | 0.09 | 0.4 | — | 310 |
| 113 | **Meringues** | 380 | 1620 | 5.3 | 0 | 95.6 | 110 | 91 | 4 | 6 | 20 | 0.1 | 0.05 | Tr | 110 | 100 |
| 114 | **Milk pudding** | 131 | 552 | 4.1 | 4.2 | 20.4 | 55 | 160 | 130 | 14 | 110 | 0.1 | 0.03 | — | 37 | 110 |
| 115 | canned, rice | 91 | 386 | 3.4 | 2.5 | 14.7 | 50 | 140 | 93 | 11 | 80 | 0.2 | 0.03 | 0.4 | — | 95 |
| 116 | **Pancakes** | 307 | 1286 | 6.1 | 16.3 | 36.2 | 50 | 140 | 120 | 14 | 120 | 0.9 | 0.07 | 0.6 | — | 94 |
| 117 | **Queen of puddings** | 216 | 910 | 4.8 | 7.9 | 33.5 | 150 | 110 | 80 | 12 | 100 | 0.7 | 0.07 | 0.5 | 57 | 230 |
| 118 | **Sponge pudding** steamed | 344 | 1443 | 5.9 | 16.4 | 46.0 | 310 | 88 | 210 | 11 | 190 | 1.2 | 0.09 | 0.5 | — | 260 |
| 119 | **Suet pudding** steamed | 333 | 1394 | 4.4 | 18.1 | 40.6 | 470 | 91 | 240 | 14 | 180 | 0.9 | 0.08 | 0.4 | — | 510 |
| 120 | **Treacle tart** | 371 | 1563 | 3.8 | 14.0 | 61.3 | 360 | 150 | 65 | 14 | 51 | 1.5 | 0.11 | — | — | 420 |
| 121 | **Trifle** | 160 | 674 | 3.5 | 6.1 | 24.3 | 50 | 150 | 82 | 14 | 87 | 0.7 | 0.09 | 0.4 | — | 88 |
| 122 | **Yorkshire pudding** | 215 | 902 | 6.8 | 10.1 | 25.8 | 600 | 160 | 130 | 20 | 130 | 1.0 | 0.08 | 0.7 | — | 940 |

| No | Food | Retinol µg | Carotene µg | Vitamin D µg | Thiamin mg | Riboflavin mg | Nicotinic acid mg | Potential nicotinic acid from tryptophan mg Trp ÷ 60 | Vitamin C mg | Vitamin E mg |
|---|---|---|---|---|---|---|---|---|---|---|
| | ***Puddings** contd* | | | | | | | | | |
| 105 | **Fruit pie**, individual, with pastry top and bottom | 0 | (Tr) | 0 | 0.05 | 0.02 | 0.4 | 0.9 | (Tr) | — |
| 106 | **Fruit pie** with pastry top | 40 | 75 | 0.32 | 0.05 | 0.02 | 0.5 | 0.4 | 9 *(2–20)* | 0.5 |
| 107 | **Ice cream** dairy | 14 | 0 | Tr | 0.04 | 0.18 | 0.1 | 0.9 | 0 | 0.4 |
| 108 | non-dairy | — | 0 | 0 | 0.04 | 0.15 | 0.1 | 0.8 | 0 | 1.2 |
| 109 | **Jelly** packet, cubes | 0 | 0 | 0 | 0 | 0 | 0 | 0 | 0 | 0 |
| 110 | made with water | 0 | 0 | 0 | 0 | 0 | 0 | 0 | 0 | 0 |
| 111 | made with milk | 13 | 8 | 0.01 | 0.02 | 0.07 | Tr | 0.3 | Tr | Tr |
| 112 | **Lemon meringue pie** | 100 | 0 | 0.98 | 0.07 | 0.08 | 0.5 | 1.1 | 5 | 1.0 |
| 113 | **Meringues** | 0 | 0 | 0 | 0 | 0.25 | 0.1 | 1.6 | 0 | 0 |
| 114 | **Milk pudding** | 30 | 20 | 0.02 | 0.04 | 0.14 | 0.1 | 1.0 | (Tr) | 0.1 |
| 115 | canned, rice | (30) | (20) | (0.02) | 0.03 | 0.14 | 0.2 | 0.7 | 0 | (0.1) |
| 116 | **Pancakes** | 40 | 10 | 0.23 | 0.13 | 0.19 | 0.6 | 1.4 | Tr | 0.3 |
| 117 | **Queen of puddings** | 80 | 30 | 0.38 | 0.04 | 0.15 | 0.2 | 1.2 | Tr | 0.4 |
| 118 | **Sponge pudding** steamed | 180 | Tr | 1.65 | (Tr) | 0.09 | 0.7 | 1.4 | Tr | 1.6 |
| 119 | **Suet pudding** steamed | 20 | 20 | 0.01 | (Tr) | 0.06 | 0.6 | 0.9 | Tr | Tr |
| 120 | **Treacle tart** | 70 | 0 | 0.60 | 0.09 | 0.01 | 0.7 | 0.6 | 0 | 0.6 |
| 121 | **Trifle** | 50 | 60 | 0.17 | 0.05 | 0.14 | 0.2 | 0.8 | 1 | 0.3 |
| 122 | **Yorkshire pudding** | 40 | 10 | 0.26 | 0.11 | 0.18 | 0.6 | 1.6 | Tr | 0.3 |

| No | Food | Vitamin $B_6$ mg | Vitamin $B_{12}$ µg | Folic acid Free µg | Folic acid Total µg | Panto-thenic acid mg | Biotin µg | Notes |
|---|---|---|---|---|---|---|---|---|
| | ***Puddings** contd* | | | | | | | |
| 105 | **Fruit pie** individual, with pastry top and bottom | — | 0 | — | — | — | — | |
| 106 | **Fruit pie** with pastry top | 0.03 | 0 | 3 | 4 | 0.1 | Tr | |
| 107 | **Ice cream** dairy | 0.02 | Tr | 2 | 2 | — | — | |
| 108 | non-dairy | 0.02 | Tr | 2 | 2 | — | — | |
| 109 | **Jelly** packet, cubes | 0 | 0 | 0 | 0 | 0 | 0 | |
| 110 | made with water | 0 | 0 | 0 | 0 | 0 | 0 | |
| 111 | made with milk | 0.02 | Tr | 2 | 2 | 0.2 | 1 | |
| 112 | **Lemon meringue pie** | 0.05 | Tr | 5 | 5 | 0.3 | 5 | |
| 113 | **Meringues** | Tr | Tr | Tr | Tr | 0.2 | Tr | |
| 114 | **Milk puddings** | 0.05 | Tr | 3 | 4 | 0.3 | 2 | |
| 115 | canned, rice | 0.02 | Tr | — | — | — | — | |
| 116 | **Pancakes** | 0.08 | Tr | 5 | 6 | 0.5 | 5 | |
| 117 | **Queen of puddings** | 0.03 | Tr | 3 | 5 | 0.4 | 6 | |
| 118 | **Sponge pudding** steamed | 0.05 | Tr | 5 | 7 | 0.3 | 5 | |
| 119 | **Suet pudding** steamed | 0.04 | Tr | 3 | 6 | 0.2 | 2 | |
| 120 | **Treacle tart** | 0.04 | 0 | 3 | 5 | 0.1 | 1 | |
| 121 | **Trifle** | 0.06 | Tr | 5 | 6 | 0.4 | 3 | |
| 122 | **Yorkshire pudding** | 0.07 | Tr | 5 | 6 | 0.4 | 5 | |

| No | Food | Description and number of samples | Water g | Sugars g | Starch and dextrins g | Dietary fibre g | Total nitrogen g |
|---|---|---|---|---|---|---|---|

| No | Food | Energy value kcal | Energy value kJ | Protein g | Fat g | Carbo-hydrate g | Na mg | K mg | Ca mg | Mg mg | P mg | Fe mg | Cu mg | Zn mg | S mg | Cl mg |
|---|---|---|---|---|---|---|---|---|---|---|---|---|---|---|---|---|

| No | Food | Retinol µg | Carotene µg | Vitamin D µg | Thiamin mg | Riboflavin mg | Nicotinic acid mg | Potential nicotinic acid from tryptophan mg Trp ÷ 60 | Vitamin C mg | Vitamin E mg |
|---|---|---|---|---|---|---|---|---|---|---|

| No | Food | Vitamin $B_6$ mg | Vitamin $B_{12}$ µg | Folic acid | | Pantothenic acid mg | Biotin µg | Notes |
|---|---|---|---|---|---|---|---|---|
| | | | | Free µg | Total µg | | | |

| No | Food | Description and number of samples | Water g | Lactose g | Other sugars g | Total nitrogen g |
|---|---|---|---|---|---|---|
| | ***Milk, cows'*** | | | | | |
| 124 125 | fresh, whole | Data from Milk Marketing Board and literature sources | 87.6 | 4.7 | 0 | 0.52 |
| 127 128 | fresh, whole, Channel Islands | Data from Milk Marketing Board and literature sources | 86.3 | 4.7 | 0 | 0.56 |
| 129 | sterilised | As raw milk with calculated vitamin losses | 87.6 | 4.7 | 0 | 0.52 |
| 130 | longlife (UHT treated) | As raw milk with calculated vitamin losses | 87.6 | 4.7 | 0 | 0.52 |
| 131 | fresh, skimmed | Calculated on the basis of 0.1% fat content | 90.9 | 5.0 | 0 | 0.53 |
| 132 | condensed, whole, sweetened | 8 cans of the same brand | 25.8 | 10.2 | 45.3 | 1.30 |
| 133 | condensed, skimmed, sweetened | 2 samples; vitamins calculated from condensed, whole, sweetened milk | 27.0 | (12.0) | (48.0) | 1.55 |
| 134 | evaporated, whole, unsweetened | 10 cans, 4 different brands | 68.6 | 11.3 | 0 | 1.35 |
| 135 | dried, whole | Mixed sample, 3 different types | 2.9 | 39.4 | 0 | 4.12 |
| 136 | dried, skimmed | 10 tins, 4 different brands | 4.1 | 52.8 | 0 | 5.70 |
| 137 | **Milk, goats'** | Literature sources | 87.0 | 4.6 | 0 | 0.52 |
| 138 | **Milk, human** mature | Mixed sample from 96 mothers about 1 month *post partum* | 87.1 | 7.2 | 0 | 0.20 |
| 139 | transitional | Mixed sample from 15 mothers on 10th day *post partum* | 90.2 | 6.9 | 0 | 0.31 |
| 140 | **Butter** salted | Analytical (6 samples) and literature sources | 15.4 | Tr | 0 | 0.07 |

| No | Food | Energy value kcal | Energy value kJ | Protein (N × 6.38) g | Fat g | Carbo-hydrate g | Na mg | K mg | Ca mg | Mg mg | P mg | Fe mg | Cu mg | Zn mg | S mg | Cl mg |
|---|---|---|---|---|---|---|---|---|---|---|---|---|---|---|---|---|
| 124 | ***Milk, cows'*** | | | | | | | | | | | | | | | |
| 125 | fresh, whole | 65 | 272 | 3.3 | 3.8 | 4.7 | 50 | 150 | 120 | 12 | 95 | 0.05 | 0.02 | 0.35 | 30 | 95 |
| | | | | | | | *(35–90)* | *(110–170)* | *(110–130)* | *(9–14)* | *(90–100)* | *(0.03–0.06)* | *(0.01–0.03)* | *(0.2–0.6)* | — | *(90–110)* |
| 127 | | | | | | | | | | | | | | | | |
| 128 | fresh, whole, Channel Islands | 76 | 316 | 3.6 | 4.8 | 4.7 | 50 | 140 | 120 | 12 | 95 | 0.05 | 0.02 | 0.35 | 30 | 100 |
| 129 | sterilised | 65 | 274 | 3.3 | 3.8 | 4.7 | 50 | 140 | 120 | 12 | 95 | 0.05 | 0.02 | 0.35 | 30 | 100 |
| 130 | longlife (UHT treated) | 65 | 274 | 3.3 | 3.8 | 4.7 | 50 | 140 | 120 | 12 | 95 | 0.05 | 0.02 | 0.35 | 30 | 100 |
| 131 | fresh, skimmed | 33 | 142 | 3.4 | 0.1 | 5.0 | 52 | 150 | 130 | 12 | 100 | 0.05 | 0.02 | 0.36 | 31 | 100 |
| 132 | condensed, whole, sweetened | 322 | 1362 | 8.3 | 9.0 | 55.5 | 130 | 390 | 280 | 27 | 220 | 0.20 | (0.04) | 1.0 | 81 | (260) |
| 133 | condensed, skimmed, sweetened | 267 | 1139 | 9.9 | 0.3 | 60.0 | 180 | 500 | 380 | 38 | 270 | 0.29 | 0.03 | 1.2 | 94 | 310 |
| 134 | evaporated, whole, unsweetened | 158 | 660 | 8.6 | 9.0 | 11.3 | 180 | 390 | 280 | 28 | 250 | 0.20 | (0.04) | 1.1 | 84 | (350) |
| 135 | dried, whole | 490 | 2051 | 26.3 | 26.3 | 39.4 | 440 | 1270 | 1020 | 84 | 740 | 0.40[a] | 0.14 | 3.2 | 240 | 810 |
| 136 | dried, skimmed | 355 | 1512 | 36.4 | 1.3 | 52.8 | 550 | 1650 | 1190 | 117 | 950 | 0.40 | 0.20 | 4.1 | 320 | (1100) |
| 137 | **Milk, goats'** | 71 | 296 | 3.3 | 4.5 | 4.6 | 40 | 180 | 130 | 20 | 110 | 0.04 | 0.05 | 0.30 | — | 130 |
| 138 | **Milk, human** mature | 69 | 289 | 1.3 | 4.1 | 7.2 | 14 | 58 | 34 | 3 | 14 | 0.07 | 0.04 | 0.28 | — | 42 |
| 139 | transitional | 67 | 281 | 2.0 | 3.7 | 6.9 | 48 | 68 | 25 | 2 | 16 | 0.07 | 0.04 | — | — | 86 |
| 140 | **Butter** salted | 740 | 3041 | 0.4 | 82.0 | Tr | 870[b] | 15 | 15 | 2 | 24 | 0.16 | 0.03 | 0.15 | 9 | 1340[b] |

[a] Proprietary brands for infant feeding are usually fortified to higher levels

[b] The added salt content of butter may vary between 0 and 3 g per 100 g; this is an average figure for salted butter. Unsalted butter contains 7 mg Na and 10 mg Cl per 100 g

| No | Food | Retinol µg | Carotene µg | Vitamin D µg | Thiamin mg | Riboflavin mg | Nicotinic acid mg | Potential nicotinic acid from tryptophan mg Trp ÷ 60 | Vitamin C mg | Vitamin E mg |
|---|---|---|---|---|---|---|---|---|---|---|
| | ***Milk, cows'*** | | | | | | | | | |
| 124 | fresh, whole [a], summer | 35 | 22 | 0.030 | 0.04 | 0.19 [b] | 0.08 | 0.78 | 1.5 [c] | 0.10 |
| 125 | winter | 26 | 13 | 0.013 | | | | | | 0.07 |
| | | | | | *(0.03–0.06)* | *(0.15–0.23)* | *(0.06–0.13)* | | | |
| 127 | fresh, whole, Channel Islands [a], summer | 38 | 61 | 0.038 | 0.04 | 0.19 [b] | 0.08 | 0.84 | 1.5 [c] | 0.12 |
| 128 | winter | 28 | 35 | 0.018 | | | | | | 0.09 |
| 129 | sterilised | 31 | 18 | 0.022 | 0.03 | 0.19 [b] | 0.08 | 0.78 | 0.8 [d] | 0.09 |
| 130 | longlife (UHT treated) | 31 | 18 | 0.022 | 0.04 | 0.19 | 0.08 | 0.78 | 1.5 [d] | 0.09 |
| 131 | fresh, skimmed [a] | Tr | Tr | Tr | 0.04 | 0.20 | 0.08 | 0.80 | 1.6 [c] | Tr |
| 132 | condensed, whole, sweetened | 99 | 49 | 0.088 | 0.08 | 0.48 | 0.22 | 1.95 | 2.0 | 0.42 |
| 133 | condensed, skimmed, sweetened | Tr | Tr | Tr | 0.10 | 0.58 | 0.26 | 2.33 | 2.4 | Tr |
| 134 | evaporated, whole, unsweetened | 84 | 48 | 0.088 [e] | 0.06 | 0.51 | 0.28 | 2.03 | 1.0 | 0.56 |
| 135 | dried, whole | 290 [f] | 170 | 0.24 [f] | 0.33 | 1.1 | 0.60 | 6.18 | 10.0 [f] | 0.61 |
| 136 | dried, skimmed | Tr | Tr | 0 | 0.42 | 1.6 | 1.2 | 8.55 | 6.0 | Tr |
| 137 | **Milk, goats'** | 40 | 0 | 0.060 | 0.04 | 0.15 | 0.19 | 0.78 | 1.5 | — |
| 138 | **Milk, human** mature | 60 | 0 | 0.025 | 0.02 | 0.03 | 0.22 | 0.47 | 3.7 | 0.34 |
| 139 | transitional | — | — | — | — | — | — | — | — | — |
| 140 | **Butter** salted | 750 | 470 | 0.76 | Tr | Tr | Tr | 0.11 | Tr | 2.0 |
| | | *(520–970)* | *(350–650)* | *(0.63–1.0)* | | | | | | |

| No | Food | Vitamin $B_6$ mg | Vitamin $B_{12}$ µg | Folic acid Free µg | Folic acid Total µg | Pantothenic acid mg | Biotin µg |
|---|---|---|---|---|---|---|---|
| | ***Milk, cows'*** | | | | | | |
| 124 125 | fresh, whole[a] | 0.04 | 0.3 | 4 | 5 | 0.35 | 2.0 |
| 127 128 | fresh, whole, Channel Islands[a] | 0.04 | 0.3 | 4 | 5 | 0.35 | 2.0 |
| 129 | sterilised | 0.03 | 0.2 | 3[d] | 4[d] | 0.35 | 2.0 |
| 130 | longlife (UHT treated)[b] | 0.04[g] | 0.2[h] | 4[d] | 5[d] | 0.35 | 2.0 |
| 131 | fresh, skimmed[a] | 0.04 | 0.3 | 4 | 5 | 0.36 | 2.0 |
| 132 | condensed, whole, sweetened | 0.02 | 0.5 | 4 | 8 | 0.85 | 3.0 |
| 133 | condensed, skimmed, sweetened | 0.02 | 0.5 | 5 | 10 | 1.0 | 3.6 |
| 134 | evaporated, whole, unsweetened | 0.04 | Tr | 4 | 7 | 0.85 | 3.0 |
| 135 | dried, whole | 0.23 | 2.0 | 32 | 40 | 2.7 | 10 |
| 136 | dried, skimmed | 0.25 | 3.0 | 14 | 21 | 3.5 | 16 |
| 137 | **Milk, goats'** | 0.04 | Tr | 1 | (1) | 0.34 | 2.0 |
| 138 | **Milk, human** mature | 0.01 | Tr | 3 | 5 | 0.25 | 0.7 |
| 139 | transitional | — | — | — | — | — | — |
| 140 | **Butter** salted | Tr | Tr | Tr | Tr | Tr | Tr |

Notes

[a] The small losses due to pasteurisation (see p 20) make no difference to the average composition of milk, except for vitamin C (see note c). These values are applicable to raw, pasteurised and homogenised milk.

[b] Milk that has not been exposed to light. There is a loss on exposure to sunlight of 10% per hour.

[c] As delivered to the home. This falls to 1.0 mg after 12 hours and 0.5 mg after 24 hours. Raw milk contains 2.0 mg.

[d] There may be a total loss on storage.

[e] This is an unfortified value. Most brands are fortified to a level of 2.8 µg.

[f] Proprietary brands for infant feeding are usually fortified to higher levels.

[g] There is a 35% loss on storage.

[h] There is a 20% loss on storage.

**Boiled milk**

For losses on boiling milk see p 20.

| No | Food | Description and number of samples | Water g | Lactose g | Other sugars g | Total nitrogen g |
|---|---|---|---|---|---|---|
| | ***Cream*** | | | | | |
| 142 143 | single | 3 samples; vitamins calculated | 71.9 | 3.2 | 0 | 0.38 |
| 145 146 | double | 3 samples; vitamins calculated | 48.6 | 2.0 | 0 | 0.24 |
| 148 149 | whipping | Calculated on the basis of 35% fat content | 61.5 | 2.5 | 0 | 0.30 |
| 150 | sterilised, canned | 10 cans, 6 brands; vitamins calculated | 69.8 | 2.7 | 0 | 0.40 |
| | ***Cheese*** | | | | | |
| 151 | Camembert type | Soft ripe cheese, eg Camembert, Brie | 47.5 | Tr | 0 | 3.58 |
| 152 | Cheddar type | Hard cheese, eg Cheddar, Cheshire, Gruyère, Emmental | 37.0 | Tr | 0 | 4.08 |
| 153 | Danish Blue type | Blue veined cheese, eg Danish Blue, Roquefort | 40.5 | Tr | 0 | 3.61 |
| 154 | Edam type | Semi-hard cheese, eg Edam, Gouda, St Paulin | 43.7 | Tr | 0 | 3.82 |
| 155 | Parmesan | 3 samples; vitamins from literature | 28.0 | Tr | 0 | 5.50 |
| 156 | Stilton | 3 samples; vitamins from literature | 28.2 | Tr | 0 | 4.02 |
| 157 | cottage cheese | 12 samples, 3 brands; contains added cream | 78.8 | 1.4 | 0 | 2.14 |
| 158 | cream cheese | 3 samples | 45.5 | Tr | 0 | 0.49 |
| 159 | processed cheese | 10 samples, 4 brands | 43.8 | Tr | 0 | 3.37 |
| 160 | cheese spread | 6 samples; vitamins calculated | 51.0 | 0.9 | 0 | 2.87 |
| | ***Yogurt*** low fat | | | | | |
| 161 | natural | 10 samples, 2 brands | 85.7 | 4.6 | 1.6[a] | 0.78 |
| 162 | flavoured | 10 samples; mixed banana, raspberry, strawberry | 79.0 | 4.8 | 9.2[b] | 0.79 |
| 163 | fruit | 30 samples, 2 brands; mixed strawberry, raspberry, orange, blackcurrant, pineapple | 74.9 | 3.3 | 14.6[b] | 0.76 |
| 164 | hazelnut | 6 samples, 2 brands | 73.4 | 3.2 | 13.3[b] | 0.82 |

[a] Galactose [b] Mainly sucrose

| No | Food | Energy value kcal | Energy value kJ | Protein (N × 6.38) g | Fat g | Carbo-hydrate g | Na mg | K mg | Ca mg | Mg mg | P mg | Fe mg | Cu mg | Zn mg | S mg | Cl mg |
|---|---|---|---|---|---|---|---|---|---|---|---|---|---|---|---|---|
| | ***Cream*** | | | | | | | | | | | | | | | |
| 142<br>143 | single | 212 | 876 | 2.4 | 21.2 | 3.2 | 42 | 120 | 79 | 6 | 44 | 0.31 | 0.20 | 0.26) | — | 72 |
| 145<br>146 | double | 447 | 1841 | 1.5 | 48.2 | 2.0 | 27 | 79 | 50 | 4 | 21 | 0.20 | 0.13 | (0.17) | — | 46 |
| 148<br>149 | whipping | 332 | 1367 | 1.9 | 35.0 | 2.5 | 34 | 100 | 63 | 5 | 27 | 0.25 | 0.16 | (0.21) | — | 58 |
| 150 | sterilised, canned | 230 | 950 | 2.6 | 23.3 | 2.7 | 56 | (120) | (80) | (6) | (44) | (0.30) | (0.20) | (0.26) | — | 140 |
| | ***Cheese*** | | | | | | | | | | | | | | | |
| 151 | Camembert type | 300 | 1246 | 22.8 | 23.2 | Tr | 1410 | 110 | 380 | 17 | 290 | 0.76 | 0.08 | 3.0 | — | 2320 |
| 152 | Cheddar type | 406 | 1682 | 26.0 | 33.5 | Tr | 610 | 120 | 800 | 25 | 520 | 0.40 | 0.03 | 4.0 | 230 | 1060 |
| 153 | Danish Blue type | 355 | 1471 | 23.0 | 29.2 | Tr | 1420 | 190 | 580 | 20 | 430 | 0.17 | 0.09 | — | — | 2390 |
| 154 | Edam type | 304 | 1262 | 24.4 | 22.9 | Tr | 980 | 160 | 740 | 28 | 520 | 0.21 | 0.03 | 4.0 | — | 1640 |
| 155 | Parmesan | 408 | 1696 | 35.1 | 29.7 | Tr | 760 | 150 | 1220 | 50 | 770 | 0.37 | — | 4.0 | 250 | 1110 |
| 156 | Stilton | 462 | 1915 | 25.6 | 40.0 | Tr | 1150 | 160 | 360 | 27 | 300 | 0.46 | 0.03 | — | 230 | 1720 |
| 157 | cottage cheese | 96 | 402 | 13.6 | 4.0[a] | 1.4 | 450 | 54 | 60 | 6 | 140 | 0.10 | 0.02 | 0.47 | — | 670 |
| 158 | cream cheese | 439 | 1807 | 3.1 | 47.4 | Tr | 300 | 160 | 98 | 10 | 100 | 0.12 | (0.04) | 0.48 | — | 480 |
| 159 | processed cheese | 311 | 1291 | 21.5 | 25.0 | Tr | 1360 | 82 | 700 | 24 | 490 | 0.50 | 0.50 | 3.2 | — | 1020 |
| 160 | cheese spread | 283 | 1173 | 18.3 | 22.9 | 0.9 | 1170 | 150 | 510 | 25 | 440 | 0.69 | 0.09 | — | — | 760 |
| | ***Yogurt*** low fat | | | | | | | | | | | | | | | |
| 161 | natural | 52 | 216 | 5.0 | 1.0 | 6.2 | 76 | 240 | 180 | 17 | 140 | 0.09 | 0.04 | 0.60 | — | 180 |
| 162 | flavoured | 81 | 342 | 5.0 | 0.9 | 14.0 | 64 | 220 | 170 | 17 | 140 | 0.16 | 0.10 | 0.64 | — | 160 |
| 163 | fruit | 95 | 405 | 4.8 | 1.0 | 17.9 | 64 | 220 | 160 | 17 | 140 | 0.24 | 0.07 | 0.63 | — | 150 |
| 164 | hazelnut | 106 | 449 | 5.2 | 2.6 | 16.5 | 70 | 240 | 180 | 20 | 140 | 0.23 | 0.09 | 0.69 | — | 160 |

[a] Cottage cheese made without added cream contains about 0.4 g fat per 100 g

| No | Food | Retinol µg | Carotene µg | Vitamin D µg | Thiamin mg | Riboflavin mg | Nicotinic acid mg | Potential nicotinic acid from tryptophan mgTrp ÷60 | Vitamin C mg | Vitamin E mg |
|---|---|---|---|---|---|---|---|---|---|---|
| | ***Cream*** | | | | | | | | | |
| 142 | single, summer | 200 | 125 | 0.165 | 0.03 | 0.12 | 0.07 | 0.57 | 1.2 | 0.5 |
| 143 | winter | 145 | 70 | 0.081 | | | | | | 0.4 |
| 145 | double, summer | 450 | 280 | 0.376 | 0.02 | 0.08 | 0.04 | 0.36 | 0.8 | 1.2 |
| 146 | winter | 330 | 160 | 0.183 | | | | | | 0.9 |
| 148 | whipping, summer | 325 | 205 | 0.273 | 0.02 | 0.09 | 0.05 | 0.45 | 0.9 | 0.8 |
| 149 | winter | 240 | 115 | 0.133 | | | | | | 0.7 |
| 150 | sterilised, canned | 190 | 110 | 0.135 | 0.01 | 0.10 | 0.06 | 0.60 | Tr | 0.5 |
| | ***Cheese*** | | | | | | | | | |
| 151 | Camembert type | 215 | 135 | 0.181 | 0.05 [a] | 0.60 *(0.30–0.90)* | 0.80 *(0.05–2.0)* | 5.37 | 0 | (0.6) |
| 152 | Cheddar type | 310 | 205 | 0.261 | 0.04 *(0.02–0.08)* | 0.50 *(0.30–0.80)* | 0.10 *(0.01–0.20)* | 6.12 | 0 | 0.8 |
| 153 | Danish Blue type | 270 | 170 | 0.228 | 0.03 | 0.60 *(0.40–0.80)* | 0.90 *(0.1–2.3)* | 5.42 | 0 | (0.7) |
| 154 | Edam type | 215 | 135 | 0.179 | 0.04 | 0.40 | 0.06 *(0.02–0.19)* | 5.73 | 0 | (0.8) |
| 155 | Parmesan | 325 | 195 | 0.274 | 0.02 | 0.50 | 0.30 | 8.25 | 0 | 0.9 |
| 156 | Stilton | 370 | 230 | 0.312 | 0.07 | 0.30 | — | 6.03 | 0 | (1.0) |
| 157 | cottage cheese | 32 | 18 | 0.023 | 0.02 | 0.19 | 0.08 | 3.21 | 0 | — |
| 158 | cream cheese | 385 | 220 | 0.275 | (0.02) | (0.14) | (0.08) | 0.74 | 0 | 1.0 |
| 159 | processed cheese | 240 | 120 | 0.145 | 0.02 | 0.29 | 0.07 | 5.06 | 0 | — |
| 160 | cheese spread | 180 | 105 | 0.133 | 0.02 | 0.24 | 0.06 | 4.31 | 0 | — |
| | ***Yogurt*** low fat | | | | | | | | | |
| 161 | natural | 8 [c] | 5 | Tr [c] | 0.05 | 0.26 | 0.12 | 1.04 | 0.4 | 0.03 |
| 162 | flavoured | 8 [c] | 5 | Tr [c] | 0.05 | 0.25 | 0.11 | 1.05 | 0.4 | 0.04 |
| 163 | fruit | 8 | 28 | Tr | 0.05 | 0.23 | 0.11 | 1.01 | 1.8 | 0.07 |
| 164 | hazelnut | 8 | 5 | Tr | 0.06 | 0.27 | 0.12 | 1.09 | 0.4 | 0.58 |

| No | Food | Vitamin $B_6$ mg | Vitamin $B_{12}$ µg | Folic acid Free µg | Folic acid Total µg | Pantothenic acid mg | Biotin µg |
|---|---|---|---|---|---|---|---|
| | ***Cream*** | | | | | | |
| 142, 143 | single | 0.03 | 0.2 | 3 | 4 | 0.30 | 1.4 |
| 145, 146 | double | 0.02 | 0.1 | 2 | 2 | 0.19 | 0.8 |
| 148, 149 | whipping | 0.02 | 0.2 | 2 | 3 | 0.21 | 0.9 |
| 150 | sterilised, canned | 0.01 | Tr | Tr | Tr | 0.28 | 1.3 |
| | ***Cheese*** | | | | | | |
| 151 | Camembert type | 0.20[b] | 1.2 | — | 60 *(35–95)* | 1.4 *(0.4–3.6)* | 6.0 *(1.2–17.8)* |
| 152 | Cheddar type | 0.08 *(0.05–0.14)* | 1.5 | — | 20 *(10–40)* | 0.30 *(0.1–0.7)* | 1.7 *(0.4–2.3)* |
| 153 | Danish Blue type | 0.15 *(0.06–0.24)* | 1.2 *(0.6–2.7)* | — | 50 *(20–80)* | 2.0 *(1.0–3.5)* | 1.5 *(1.0–3.6)* |
| 154 | Edam type | 0.08 *(0.05–0.12)* | 1.4 | — | 20 *(5–35)* | 0.30 *(0.1–1.3)* | 1.5 *(0.7–5.1)* |
| 155 | Parmesan | 0.10 | 1.5 | — | 20 | 0.30 | 1.7 |
| 156 | Stilton | — | — | — | — | — | — |
| 157 | cottage cheese | 0.01 | (0.5) | 2 | 9 | — | — |
| 158 | cream cheese | (0.01) | (0.3) | (4) | (5) | — | — |
| 159 | processed cheese | — | — | 1 | 2 | — | — |
| 160 | cheese spread | — | — | — | — | — | — |
| | ***Yogurt*** low fat | | | | | | |
| 161 | natural | 0.04 | Tr | 1 | 2 | — | — |
| 162 | flavoured | 0.04 | Tr | 4 | 8 | — | — |
| 163 | fruit | 0.04 | Tr | Tr | 3 | — | — |
| 164 | hazelnut | 0.04 | Tr | Tr | 5 | — | — |

Notes

[a] Rind 0.5 mg.

[b] Rind 0.40 mg.

[c] Some brands are fortified; these values apply to unfortified yogurts.

| No | Food | Description and number of samples | Water g | Lactose g | Other sugars g | Total nitrogen g |
|---|---|---|---|---|---|---|

| No | Food | Energy value | | Protein (N × 6.38) | Fat | Carbo-hydrate | mg | | | | | | | | | |
|---|---|---|---|---|---|---|---|---|---|---|---|---|---|---|---|---|
| | | kcal | kJ | g | g | g | Na | K | Ca | Mg | P | Fe | Cu | Zn | S | Cl |

| No | Food | Retinol µg | Carotene µg | Vitamin D µg | Thiamin mg | Riboflavin mg | Nicotinic acid mg | Potential nicotinic acid from tryptophan mgTrp ÷60 | Vitamin C mg | Vitamin E mg |
|---|---|---|---|---|---|---|---|---|---|---|

| No | Food | Vitamin $B_6$ mg | Vitamin $B_{12}$ µg | Folic acid Free µg | Folic acid Total µg | Panto-thenic acid mg | Biotin µg | Notes |
|---|---|---|---|---|---|---|---|---|

| No | Food | Description and number of samples | Water g | Total nitrogen g |
|---|---|---|---|---|
| | ***Eggs*** | | | |
| 165 | whole, raw[a] | 150 pooled samples of battery, deep litter and free range eggs | 74.8 | 1.97 |
| 166 | white, raw | 34 eggs, English and Danish; vitamins from literature | 88.3 | 1.44 |
| 167 | yolk, raw | 34 eggs, English and Danish; vitamins from literature | 51.0 | 2.58 |
| 168 | dried | 6 packets; vitamins from literature | 7.0 | 6.97 |
| 169 | boiled | As raw, except for vitamin losses from literature | 74.8 | 1.97 |
| 170 | fried | 6 eggs; vitamin losses from literature | 63.3 | 2.26 |
| 171 | poached | 6 eggs, poached in water; vitamin losses from literature | 74.7 | 1.99 |
| 172 | omelette | Recipe, p 340 | 68.8 | 1.70 |
| 173 | scrambled | Recipe, p 340 | 62.2 | 1.67 |
| | ***Egg and cheese dishes*** | | | |
| 174 | **Cauliflower cheese** | Recipe, p 340 | 78.4 | 0.90 |
| 175 | **Cheese pudding** | Recipe, p 340 | 68.2 | 1.63 |
| 176 | **Cheese soufflé** | Recipe, p 340 | 56.6 | 1.84 |
| 177 | **Macaroni cheese** | Recipe, p 340 | 67.4 | 1.19 |
| 178 | **Pizza,** cheese and tomato | Recipe, p 341 | 51.2 | 1.53 |
| 179 | **Quiche Lorraine** | Recipe, p 341 | 34.6 | 2.37 |
| 180 | **Scotch egg** | Recipe, p 341 | 53.1 | 1.86 |
| 181 | **Welsh rarebit** | Recipe, p 341 | 33.5 | 2.50 |

[a] An average egg is composed of 11 per cent shell, 58 per cent white and 31 per cent yolk

| No | Food | Energy value kcal | Energy value kJ | Protein g | Fat g | Carbo-hydrate g | Na mg | K mg | Ca mg | Mg mg | P mg | Fe mg | Cu mg | Zn mg | S mg | Cl mg |
|---|---|---|---|---|---|---|---|---|---|---|---|---|---|---|---|---|
| | ***Eggs*** | | | | | | | | | | | | | | | |
| 165 | whole, raw | 147 | 612 | 12.3 | 10.9 | Tr | 140 | 140 | 52 | 12 | 220 | 2.0 | 0.10 | 1.5 | 180 | 160 |
| 166 | white, raw | 36 | 153 | 9.0 | Tr | Tr | 190 | 150 | 5 | 11 | 33 | 0.1 | 0.05 | 0.03 | 180 | 170 |
| 167 | yolk, raw | 339 | 1402 | 16.1 | 30.5 | Tr | 50 | 120 | 130 | 15 | 500 | 6.1 | 0.30 | 3.6 | 170 | 140 |
| 168 | dried | 564 | 2343 | 43.6 | 43.3 | Tr | 520 | 480 | 190 | 41 | 800 | 7.9 | 0.18 | 5.0 | 630 | 590 |
| 169 | boiled | 147 | 612 | 12.3 | 10.9 | Tr | 140 | 140 | 52 | 12 | 220 | 2.0 | 0.10 | 1.5 | 180 | 160 |
| 170 | fried | 232 | 961 | 14.1 | 19.5 | Tr | 220 | 180 | 64 | 14 | 260 | 2.5 | 0.12 | 1.8 | 210 | 200 |
| 171 | poached | 155 | 644 | 12.4 | 11.7 | Tr | 110 | 120 | 52 | 11 | 240 | 2.3 | 0.10 | 1.5 | 180 | 160 |
| 172 | omelette | 190 | 787 | 10.6 | 16.4 | Tr | 1030 | 120 | 47 | 18 | 190 | 1.7 | 0.09 | 1.3 | 160 | 1540 |
| 173 | scrambled | 246 | 1018 | 10.5 | 22.7 | Tr | 1050 | 130 | 60 | 17 | 190 | 1.7 | 0.09 | 1.3 | 150 | 1580 |
| | ***Egg and cheese dishes*** | | | | | | | | | | | | | | | |
| 174 | **Cauliflower cheese** | 113 | 471 | 5.7 | 8.0 | 4.9 | 250 | 250 | 160 | 16 | 120 | 0.4 | 0.03 | 0.8 | — | 410 |
| 175 | **Cheese pudding** | 170 | 707 | 10.2 | 10.8 | 8.4 | 460 | 150 | 230 | 19 | 210 | 0.8 | 0.06 | 1.3 | — | 730 |
| 176 | **Cheese soufflé** | 252 | 1049 | 11.5 | 19.0 | 9.4 | 420 | 150 | 230 | 19 | 230 | 1.1 | 0.07 | 1.4 | — | 670 |
| 177 | **Macaroni cheese** | 174 | 726 | 7.4 | 9.7 | 15.1 | 280 | 120 | 180 | 18 | 140 | 0.4 | 0.03 | 0.9 | — | 460 |
| 178 | **Pizza,** cheese and tomato | 234 | 982 | 9.4 | 11.5 | 24.8 | 340 | 180 | 240 | 19 | 170 | 1.1 | 0.13 | 1.2 | — | 570 |
| 179 | **Quiche Lorraine** | 391 | 1627 | 14.7 | 28.1 | 21.1 | 610 | 190 | 260 | 21 | 240 | 1.3 | 0.10 | 1.8 | — | 970 |
| 180 | **Scotch egg** | 279 | 1159 | 11.6 | 20.9 | 11.8 | 480 | 150 | 56 | 13 | 190 | 1.7 | 0.20 | 1.3 | 140 | 640 |
| 181 | **Welsh rarebit** | 365 | 1523 | 15.7 | 23.6 | 23.9 | 1030 | 130 | 420 | 29 | 290 | 1.1 | 0.07 | 2.1 | 150 | 1660 |

| No | Food | Retinol µg | Carotene µg | Vitamin D µg | Thiamin mg | Riboflavin mg | Nicotinic acid mg | Potential nicotinic acid from tryptophan mg Trp ÷60 | Vitamin C mg | Vitamin E mg |
|---|---|---|---|---|---|---|---|---|---|---|
| | ***Eggs*** | | | | | | | | | |
| 165 | whole, raw | 140 | Tr | 1.75[a] | 0.09 | 0.47 | 0.07 | 3.61 | 0 | 1.6 |
| 166 | white, raw | 0 | 0 | 0 | 0 | 0.43 | 0.09 | 2.64 | 0 | 0 |
| 167 | yolk, raw | 400 | Tr | 5.0[a] | 0.30 | 0.54 | 0.02 | 4.73 | 0 | 4.6 |
| 168 | dried | 490[b] | Tr | 6.0 | 0.35[b] | 1.2 | 0.20 | 12.78 | 0 | 5.6 |
| 169 | boiled | 140 | Tr | 1.75 | 0.08 | 0.45 | 0.07 | 3.61 | 0 | 1.6 |
| 170 | fried | 140 | Tr | 1.75 | 0.07 | 0.42 | 0.07 | 4.14 | 0 | 1.6 |
| 171 | poached | 140 | Tr | 1.75 | 0.07 | 0.38 | 0.07 | 3.65 | 0 | 1.6 |
| 172 | omelette | 190 | 40 | 1.57 | 0.07 | 0.32 | 0.06 | 3.11 | 0 | 1.5 |
| 173 | scrambled | 130 | 80 | 1.54 | 0.07 | 0.33 | 0.07 | 3.05 | Tr | 1.6 |
| | ***Egg and cheese dishes*** | | | | | | | | | |
| 174 | **Cauliflower cheese** | 80 | 50 | 0.29 | 0.06 | 0.14 | 0.41 | 1.32 | 8 | 0.4 |
| 175 | **Cheese pudding** | 110 | 50 | 0.46 | 0.05 | 0.28 | 0.24 | 2.55 | Tr | 0.6 |
| 176 | **Cheese soufflé** | 200 | 40 | 1.39 | 0.07 | 0.26 | 0.26 | 2.90 | Tr | 1.3 |
| 177 | **Macaroni cheese** | 90 | 40 | 0.33 | 0.03 | 0.14 | 0.23 | 1.60 | Tr | 0.3 |
| 178 | **Pizza,** cheese and tomato | 70 | 230 | 0.06 | 0.11 | 0.14 | 1.01 | 2.06 | 3 | 0.7 |
| 179 | **Quiche Lorraine** | 160 | 50 | 0.88 | 0.14 | 0.24 | 1.05 | 3.37 | Tr | 0.9 |
| 180 | **Scotch egg** | 60 | 0 | 0.75 | 0.06 | 0.22 | 1.54 | 2.90 | 0 | 0.8 |
| 181 | **Welsh rarebit** | 210 | 130 | 0.19 | 0.07 | 0.21 | 0.67 | 3.55 | Tr | 0.4 |

| No | Food | Vitamin $B_6$ mg | Vitamin $B_{12}$ µg | Folic acid Free µg | Folic acid Total µg | Pantothenic acid mg | Biotin µg |
|---|---|---|---|---|---|---|---|
| | ***Eggs*** | | | | | | |
| 165 | whole, raw | 0.11 | 1.7[c] | 25[d] | 25 | 1.8 | 25 |
| 166 | white, raw | Tr | 0.1 | 1 | 1 | 0.3 | Tr[e] |
| 167 | yolk, raw | 0.30 | 4.9 | 48 | 52 | 4.6 | 60[e] |
| 168 | dried | 0.40 | 7.0 | — | — | 6.2 | — |
| 169 | boiled | 0.10 | 1.7 | 22 | 22 | 1.6 | 25 |
| 170 | fried | 0.09 | 1.7 | 17 | 17 | 1.4 | 25 |
| 171 | poached | 0.09 | 1.7 | 16 | 16 | 1.4 | 25 |
| 172 | omelette | 0.08 | 1.5 | 15 | 15 | 1.3 | 22 |
| 173 | scrambled | 0.09 | 1.4 | 15 | 15 | 1.3 | 20 |
| | ***Egg and cheese dishes*** | | | | | | |
| 174 | **Cauliflower cheese** | 0.11 | 0.3 | — | 13 | 0.4 | 2 |
| 175 | **Cheese pudding** | 0.06 | 0.9 | — | 8 | 0.5 | 8 |
| 176 | **Cheese soufflé** | 0.07 | 1.0 | — | 12 | 0.7 | 10 |
| 177 | **Macaroni cheese** | 0.03 | 0.3 | 2 | 3 | 0.2 | 1 |
| 178 | **Pizza,** cheese and tomato | 0.08 | 0.3 | 7 | 24 | 0.3 | 3 |
| 179 | **Quiche Lorraine** | 0.10 | 0.8 | — | 8 | 0.5 | 7 |
| 180 | **Scotch egg** | 0.07 | 1.2 | 8 | 8 | 0.8 | 12 |
| 181 | **Welsh rarebit** | 0.04 | 0.8 | — | 7 | 0.3 | 2 |

Notes

[a] If the hens have been fed a supplement, values may be considerably higher.

[b] There may be a considerable loss on storage.

[c] The value for battery eggs. Deep litter contain 2.6 µg and free range 2.9 µg.

[d] The value for battery eggs. Deep litter contain 32 µg and free range 39 µg.

[e] The natural antibiotic factor avidin, present in raw egg white, binds with the biotin in the yolk to form a complex unavailable to man. Avidin in cooked egg white is inactive.

| No | Food | Description and number of samples | Water g | Total nitrogen g |
|---|---|---|---|---|
| 140 | **Butter** salted | Analytical (6 samples) and literature sources | 15.4 | 0.07 |
| 182 | **Cod liver oil** | 3 samples | Tr | Tr |
| 183 | **Compound cooking fat** | 7 samples | Tr | Tr |
| 184 | **Dripping** beef | Analysed as purchased | 1.0 | Tr |
| 185 | **Lard** | Analysed as purchased | 1.0 | Tr |
| 186 | **Low fat spread** | One brand | 57.1 | 0 |
| 187 | **Margarine** all kinds | Hard, soft and polyunsaturated | 16.0 | 0.02 |
| 193 | **Suet** block | Analysed as purchased | Tr | 0.15 |
| 194 | shredded | 6 samples of the same brand | 1.5 | Tr |
| 195 | **Vegetable oils** | All kinds | Tr | Tr |

| No | Food | Energy value kcal | Energy value kJ | Protein g | Fat g | Carbo-hydrate g | Na (mg) | K (mg) | Ca (mg) | Mg (mg) | P (mg) | Fe (mg) | Cu (mg) | Zn (mg) | S (mg) | Cl (mg) |
|---|---|---|---|---|---|---|---|---|---|---|---|---|---|---|---|---|
| 140 | **Butter** salted | 740 | 3041 | 0.4 | 82.0 | Tr | 870 | 15 | 15 | 2 | 24 | 0.2 | 0.03 | 0.15 | 9 | 1340 |
| 182 | **Cod liver oil** | 899 | 3696 | Tr | 99.9 | 0 | Tr | Tr | Tr | Tr | Tr | Tr | Tr | Tr | Tr | Tr |
| 183 | **Compound cooking fat** | 894 | 3674 | Tr | 99.3 | 0 | Tr | Tr | Tr | Tr | Tr | Tr | Tr | Tr | Tr | Tr |
| 184 | **Dripping** beef | 891 | 3663 | Tr | 99.0 | 0 | 5 | 4 | 1 | Tr | 13 | 0.2 | — | — | 9 | 2 |
| 185 | **Lard** | 891 | 3663 | Tr | 99.0 | 0 | 2 | 1 | 1 | 1 | 3 | 0.1 | 0.02 | — | 25 | 4 |
| 186 | **Low fat spread** | 366 | 1506 | 0 | 40.7 | 0 | 690 | Tr | Tr | Tr | Tr | Tr | Tr | Tr | Tr | 1035 |
| 187 | **Margarine** all kinds | 730 | 3000 | 0.1 | 81.0 | 0.1 | 800 | 5 | 4 | 1 | 12 | 0.3 | 0.04 | — | 12 | 1200 |
| 193 | **Suet** block | 895 | 3678 | 0.9 | 99.0 | 0 | 21 | 13 | 6 | 1 | 7 | 0.4 | 0.04 | — | 20 | 18 |
| 194 | shredded | 826 | 3402 | Tr | 86.7 | 12.1 | Tr | Tr | Tr | Tr | Tr | Tr | Tr | Tr | Tr | Tr |
| 195 | **Vegetable oils** | 899 | 3696 | Tr | 99.9 | 0 | Tr | Tr | Tr | Tr | Tr | Tr | Tr | Tr | Tr | Tr |

| No | Food | Retinol µg | Carotene µg | Vitamin D µg | Thiamin mg | Riboflavin mg | Nicotinic acid mg | Potential nicotinic acid from tryptophan mgTrp ÷60 | Vitamin C mg | Vitamin E mg |
|---|---|---|---|---|---|---|---|---|---|---|
| 140 | **Butter** salted | 750 | 470 | 0.76 | Tr | Tr | Tr | 0.1 | Tr | 2.0 |
| 182 | **Cod liver oil** | 18 000 | Tr | 210 | 0 | 0 | 0 | 0 | 0 | 20.0 |
| 183 | **Compound cooking fat** | 0 | 0 | 0 | 0 | 0 | 0 | 0 | 0 | Tr |
| 184 | **Dripping** beef | — | — | Tr | Tr | Tr | Tr | Tr | 0 | (0.3) |
| 185 | **Lard** | Tr | 0 | Tr | Tr | Tr | Tr | Tr | 0 | Tr |
| 186 | **Low fat spread** | 900 *(800–1000)* | 0 | 7.94 *(7.05–8.82)* | 0 | 0 | 0 | 0 | 0 | 4.0[a] |
| 187 | **Margarine** all kinds | 900 *(800–1000)* | 0[b] | 7.94 *(7.05–8.82)* | Tr | Tr | Tr | Tr | 0 | 8.0[a] |
| 193 | **Suet** block | (52) | (73) | Tr | Tr | Tr | Tr | 0.2 | 0 | (1.5) |
| 194 | shredded | 52 | 73 | Tr | Tr | Tr | Tr | Tr | 0 | 1.5 |
| 195 | **Vegetable oils** | 0 | Tr[c] | 0 | Tr | Tr | Tr | Tr | 0 | see[d] |

| No | Food | Vitamin $B_6$ mg | Vitamin $B_{12}$ µg | Folic acid Free µg | Folic acid Total µg | Pantothenic acid mg | Biotin µg |
|---|---|---|---|---|---|---|---|
| 140 | **Butter** salted | Tr | Tr | Tr | Tr | Tr | Tr |
| 182 | **Cod liver oil** | 0 | 0 | 0 | 0 | 0 | 0 |
| 183 | **Compound cooking fat** | 0 | 0 | 0 | 0 | 0 | 0 |
| 184 | **Dripping** beef | Tr | Tr | Tr | Tr | Tr | Tr |
| 185 | **Lard** | Tr | Tr | Tr | Tr | Tr | Tr |
| 186 | **Low fat spread** | 0 | 0 | 0 | 0 | 0 | 0 |
| 187 | **Margarine** all kinds | Tr | Tr | Tr | Tr | Tr | Tr |
| 193 | **Suet** block | Tr | Tr | Tr | Tr | Tr | Tr |
| 194 | shredded | Tr | Tr | Tr | Tr | Tr | Tr |
| 195 | **Vegetable oils** | Tr | 0 | Tr | Tr | Tr | Tr |

Notes

[a] The vitamin E content will vary according to the blend of oils used. Polyunsaturated margarine contains about 25 mg $\alpha$-tocopherol per 100 g.

[b] Some margarines may be fortified with carotene.

[c] Most vegetable oils contain only a trace of carotene, with the exception of unrefined palm oil, which contains about 30 000 µg $\beta$- and 24 000 µg $\alpha$-carotene per 100 g.

[d] Active tocopherols present in vegetable oils are:

| | Tocopherols mg/100 g $\alpha$ | $\gamma$ | $\delta$ | $\alpha$T3 |
|---|---|---|---|---|
| 196 Coconut | 0.5 | 0 | 0.6 | 0.5 |
| 197 Cottonseed | 38.9 | 38.7 | 0 | 0 |
| 198 Maize | 11.2 | 60.2 | 1.8 | 0 |
| 199 Olive | 5.1 | Tr | 0 | 0 |
| 200 Palm | 25.6 | 31.6 | 7.0 | 14.3 |
| 201 Peanut | 13.0 | 21.4 | 2.1 | 0 |
| 202 Rapeseed | 18.4 | 38.0 | 1.2 | 0 |
| 203 Safflowerseed | 38.7 | 17.4 | 24.0 | 0 |
| 204 Soyabean | 10.1 | 59.3 | 26.4 | 0 |
| 205 Sunflowerseed | 48.7 | 5.1 | 0.8 | 0 |
| 206 Wheatgerm | 133.0 | 26.0 | 27.1 | 2.6 |

(from Slover, 1971)

| No | Food | Description and number of samples | Edible matter, proportion of weight purchased | Water g | Total nitrogen g |
|---|---|---|---|---|---|
| | ***Bacon*** | | | | |
| 208 | **dressed carcase** raw | Average carcase weight 68 kg, 57% lean, 32% fat in whole carcase | 0.89 | 48.8 | 2.08 |
| 210 | **lean** average, raw | Average of five different cuts | — | 67.0 | 3.23 |
| 211 | **fat** average, raw | Average of five different cuts | — | 12.8 | 0.76 |
| 212 | cooked | Average of five different cuts | — | 13.8 | 1.48 |
| 213 | **collar joint** raw, lean and fat | 12 samples, boneless; 70% lean | 0.91 | 51.3 | 2.34 |
| 214 | boiled, lean and fat | 12 samples, 73% lean; soaked for 16 hours before cooking | 0.64 | 49.0 | 3.26 |
| 215 | lean only | 12 samples; soaked for 16 hours before cooking | 0.47 | 60.8 | 4.16 |
| 216 | **gammon joint** raw, lean and fat | 12 samples, boneless, 80% lean | 0.93 | 60.8 | 2.82 |
| 217 | boiled, lean and fat | 12 samples 80% lean; soaked for 16 hours before cooking | 0.63 | 53.9 | 3.95 |
| 218 | lean only | 12 samples; soaked for 16 hours before cooking | 0.50 | 62.7 | 4.70 |
| 219 | **gammon rashers** grilled, lean and fat | 24 samples, 88% lean; rind removed before cooking | 0.60 | 52.1 | 4.72 |
| 220 | lean only | 24 samples; rind removed before cooking | 0.52 | 57.0 | 5.02 |
| 221 | **rashers, raw** back, lean and fat | 36 samples, 59% lean; rind removed | 0.93 | 40.5 | 2.27 |
| 222 | middle, lean and fat | 36 samples, 59% lean; rind removed | 0.90 | 40.8 | 2.28 |
| 223 | streaky, lean and fat | 36 samples, 61% lean; rind removed | 0.85 | 41.8 | 2.34 |
| 225 | **rashers, fried** average, lean only | Average of back, middle and streaky | — | 39.2 | 5.24 |
| 226 | back, lean and fat | 36 samples, 68% lean; rind removed before cooking | 0.55 | 29.7 | 3.99 |
| 227 | middle, lean and fat | 36 samples, 64% lean; rind removed before cooking | 0.51 | 28.7 | 3.86 |
| 228 | streaky, lean and fat | 36 samples, 60% lean; rind removed before cooking | 0.51 | 27.5 | 3.69 |
| 230 | **rashers, grilled** average, lean only | Average of back, middle and streaky | — | 46.0 | 4.88 |
| 231 | back, lean and fat | 36 samples, 72% lean; rind removed before cooking | 0.55 | 36.0 | 4.04 |
| 232 | middle, lean and fat | 36 samples, 70% lean; rind removed before cooking | 0.51 | 35.2 | 3.98 |
| 233 | streaky, lean and fat | 36 samples, 69% lean; rind removed before cooking | 0.47 | 34.6 | 3.92 |

| No | Food | Energy value kcal | Energy value kJ | Protein (N × 6.25) g | Fat g | Carbo-hydrate g | Na mg | K mg | Ca mg | Mg mg | P mg | Fe mg | Cu mg | Zn mg | S mg | Cl mg |
|---|---|---|---|---|---|---|---|---|---|---|---|---|---|---|---|---|
| | ***Bacon*** | | | | | | | | | | | | | | | |
| 208 | **dressed carcase** raw | 352 | 1453 | 13.0 | 33.3 | 0 | 1400 | 250 | 7 | 16 | 130 | 1.0 | 0.10 | 1.8 | — | 2090 |
| 210 | **lean** average, raw | 147 | 617 | 20.2 | 7.4 | 0[a] | 1870[a] | 350 | 9 | 22 | 180[a] | 1.2 | 0.12 | 2.5 | 200 | 2800[a] |
| 211 | **fat** average, raw | 747 | 3075 | 4.8 | 80.9 | 0 | 560 | 75 | 3 | 4 | 38[a] | 0.7 | 0.06 | 0.6 | — | 810 |
| 212 | cooked | 692 | 2852 | 9.3 | 72.8 | 0 | 990 | 130 | 7 | 10 | 90 | 0.8 | 0.09 | 0.8 | — | 1520 |
| 213 | **collar joint** raw, lean and fat | 319 | 1318 | 14.6 | 28.9 | 0 | 1690 | 260 | 7 | 16 | 140 | 1.2 | 0.11 | 2.4 | — | 2560 |
| 214 | boiled, lean and fat | 325 | 1346 | 20.4 | 27.0 | 0 | 1100 | 170 | 13 | 15 | 140 | 1.6 | 0.18 | 3.9 | — | 1630 |
| 215 | lean only | 191 | 801 | 26.0 | 9.7 | 0 | 1350 | 210 | 15 | 19 | 170 | 1.9 | 0.22 | 5.1 | 270 | 2000 |
| 216 | **gammon joint** raw, lean and fat | 236 | 978 | 17.6 | 18.3 | 0 | 1180 | 310 | 7 | 20 | 160 | 0.9 | 0.11 | 1.7 | — | 1800 |
| 217 | boiled, lean and fat | 269 | 1119 | 24.7 | 18.9 | 0 | 960 | 210 | 9 | 18 | 150 | 1.3 | 0.15 | 2.7 | — | 1440 |
| 218 | lean only | 167 | 703 | 29.4 | 5.5 | 0 | 1110 | 250 | 10 | 21 | 180 | 1.5 | 0.17 | 3.3 | 280 | 1670 |
| 219 | **gammon rashers** grilled, lean and fat | 228 | 953 | 29.5 | 12.2 | 0 | 2140 | 480 | 9 | 31 | 260 | 1.4 | 0.17 | 3.2 | — | 3290 |
| 220 | lean only | 172 | 726 | 31.4 | 5.2 | 0 | 2210 | 520 | 10 | 33 | 270 | 1.5 | 0.18 | 3.5 | 310 | 3410 |
| 221 | **rashers, raw** back | 428 | 1766 | 14.2 | 41.2 | 0 | 1470 | 230 | 7 | 15 | 120 | 1.0 | 0.10 | 1.6 | — | 2140 |
| 222 | middle | 425 | 1756 | 14.3 | 40.9 | 0 | 1470 | 230 | 7 | 15 | 120 | 1.0 | 0.10 | 1.6 | — | 2150 |
| 223 | streaky | 414 | 1710 | 14.6 | 39.5 | 0 | 1500 | 240 | 8 | 15 | 120 | 1.0 | 0.10 | 1.7 | — | 2190 |
| 225 | **rashers, fried** average, lean only | 332 | 1383 | 32.8 | 22.3 | 0 | 2280 | 380 | 16 | 25 | 210 | 1.5 | 0.14 | 3.6 | 310 | 3510 |
| 226 | back, lean and fat | 465 | 1926 | 24.9 | 40.6 | 0 | 1910 | 300 | 13 | 20 | 170 | 1.3 | 0.12 | 2.6 | — | 2970 |
| 227 | middle, lean and fat | 477 | 1975 | 24.1 | 42.3 | 0 | 1870 | 300 | 13 | 20 | 170 | 1.3 | 0.12 | 2.5 | — | 2910 |
| 228 | streaky, lean and fat | 496 | 2050 | 23.1 | 44.8 | 0 | 1820 | 290 | 12 | 19 | 160 | 1.2 | 0.12 | 2.4 | — | 2840 |
| 230 | **rashers, grilled** average, lean only | 292 | 1218 | 30.5 | 18.9 | 0 | 2240 | 350 | 13 | 18 | 190 | 1.6 | 0.17 | 3.7 | 290 | 3250 |
| 231 | back, lean and fat | 405 | 1681 | 25.3 | 33.8 | 0 | 2020 | 290 | 12 | 16 | 160 | 1.5 | 0.16 | 3.0 | — | 2970 |
| 232 | middle, lean and fat | 416 | 1722 | 24.9 | 35.1 | 0 | 2000 | 290 | 12 | 16 | 160 | 1.5 | 0.16 | 2.9 | — | 2940 |
| 233 | streaky, lean and fat | 422 | 1749 | 24.5 | 36.0 | 0 | 1990 | 290 | 12 | 16 | 160 | 1.5 | 0.15 | 2.9 | — | 2930 |

[a] Sweetcure bacon contains 0.5g sugars, 1200mg Na, 280mg P and 1500mg Cl per 100g lean and 140mg P per 100g fat

| No | Food | Retinol µg | Carotene µg | Vitamin D µg | Thiamin mg | Riboflavin mg | Nicotinic acid mg | Potential nicotinic acid from tryptophan mg Trp ÷ 60 | Vitamin C mg | Vitamin E mg |
|---|---|---|---|---|---|---|---|---|---|---|
| | ***Bacon*** | | | | | | | | | |
| 208 | **dressed carcase** raw | Tr | Tr | Tr | 0.40 | 0.16 | 2.9 | 2.4 | 0 | 0.08 |
| 210 | **lean** average, raw | Tr | Tr | Tr | 0.65 | 0.25 | 4.7 | 3.8 | 0 | 0.06 |
| 211 | **fat** average, raw[a] | Tr | Tr | Tr | — | — | — | 0.9 | 0 | 0.11 |
| 212 | cooked[a] | Tr | Tr | Tr | — | — | — | 1.7 | 0 | 0.36 |
| 213 | **collar joint** raw, lean and fat | Tr | Tr | Tr | 0.41 | 0.21 | 2.7 | 2.7 | 0 | 0.07 |
| 214 | boiled, lean and fat | Tr | Tr | Tr | 0.27 | 0.22 | 2.6 | 3.8 | 0 | (0.14) |
| 215 | lean only | Tr | Tr | Tr | 0.37 | 0.30 | 3.6 | 4.9 | 0 | (0.05) |
| 216 | **gammon joint** raw, lean and fat | Tr | Tr | Tr | 0.62 | 0.17 | 4.1 | 3.3 | 0 | 0.07 |
| 217 | boiled, lean and fat | Tr | Tr | Tr | 0.44 | 0.15 | 3.4 | 4.6 | 0 | (0.11) |
| 218 | lean only | Tr | Tr | Tr | 0.55 | 0.19 | 4.2 | 5.5 | 0 | (0.05) |
| 219 | **gammon rashers** grilled, lean and fat | Tr | Tr | Tr | 0.88 | 0.24 | 6.3 | 5.5 | 0 | (0.07) |
| 220 | lean only | Tr | Tr | Tr | 1.00 | 0.27 | 7.1 | 5.9 | 0 | (0.04) |
| 221 | **rashers, raw** back | Tr | Tr | Tr | 0.35 | 0.14 | 3.1 | 2.7 | 0 | 0.07 |
| 222 | middle | Tr | Tr | Tr | 0.36 | 0.14 | 3.1 | 2.7 | 0 | 0.08 |
| 223 | streaky | Tr | Tr | Tr | 0.37 | 0.15 | 3.2 | 2.7 | 0 | 0.08 |
| 225 | **rashers, fried** average, lean only | Tr | Tr | Tr | 0.61 | 0.31 | 7.7 | 6.1 | 0 | 0.06 |
| 226 | back, lean and fat | Tr | Tr | Tr | 0.41 | 0.21 | 5.2 | 4.7 | 0 | 0.18 |
| 227 | middle, lean and fat | Tr | Tr | Tr | 0.39 | 0.20 | 5.0 | 4.5 | 0 | 0.20 |
| 228 | streaky, lean and fat | Tr | Tr | Tr | 0.37 | 0.19 | 4.6 | 4.3 | 0 | 0.21 |
| 230 | **rashers, grilled** average, lean only | Tr | Tr | Tr | 0.59 | 0.23 | 6.2 | 5.7 | 0 | 0.04 |
| 231 | back, lean and fat | Tr | Tr | Tr | 0.43 | 0.17 | 4.5 | 4.7 | 0 | 0.11 |
| 232 | middle, lean and fat | Tr | Tr | Tr | 0.41 | 0.16 | 4.4 | 4.6 | 0 | 0.11 |
| 233 | streaky, lean and fat | Tr | Tr | Tr | 0.40 | 0.16 | 4.2 | 4.6 | 0 | 0.12 |

| No | Food | Vitamin $B_6$ mg | Vitamin $B_{12}$ µg | Folic acid Free µg | Folic acid Total µg | Pantothenic acid mg | Biotin µg |
|---|---|---|---|---|---|---|---|
| | ***Bacon*** | | | | | | |
| 208 | **dressed carcase** raw | 0.30 | Tr | 1 | 2 | 0.3 | 1 |
| 210 | **lean** average, raw | 0.45 | Tr | 1 | 3 | 0.6 | 2 |
| 211 | **fat** average, raw[a] | — | Tr | Tr | Tr | — | Tr |
| 212 | cooked[a] | — | Tr | Tr | Tr | — | Tr |
| 213 | **collar joint** raw, lean and fat | 0.32 | Tr | Tr | 2 | 0.4 | 1 |
| 214 | boiled, lean and fat | (0.24) | Tr | Tr | (Tr) | (0.4) | (2) |
| 215 | lean only | (0.33) | Tr | Tr | (1) | (0.5) | (3) |
| 216 | **gammon joint** raw, lean and fat | 0.36 | Tr | Tr | 3 | 0.5 | 2 |
| 217 | boiled, lean and fat | (0.26) | Tr | Tr | (Tr) | (0.4) | (2) |
| 218 | lean only | (0.33) | Tr | Tr | (1) | (0.5) | (3) |
| 219 | **gammon rashers** grilled, lean and fat | (0.33) | Tr | Tr | (2) | (0.6) | (3) |
| 220 | lean only | (0.37) | Tr | Tr | (2) | (0.7) | (3) |
| 221 | **rashers, raw** back | 0.26 | Tr | Tr | 2 | 0.4 | 1 |
| 222 | middle | 0.27 | Tr | Tr | 2 | 0.4 | 1 |
| 223 | streaky | 0.28 | Tr | Tr | 2 | 0.4 | 1 |
| 225 | **rashers, fried** average, lean only | 0.45 | Tr | Tr | 2 | 0.5 | 4 |
| 226 | back, lean and fat | 0.30 | Tr | Tr | 1 | 0.3 | 3 |
| 227 | middle, lean and fat | 0.29 | Tr | Tr | 1 | 0.3 | 2 |
| 228 | streaky, lean and fat | 0.27 | Tr | Tr | 1 | 0.3 | 2 |
| 230 | **rashers, grilled** average, lean only | 0.37 | Tr | Tr | 2 | 0.7 | 3 |
| 231 | back, lean and fat | 0.27 | Tr | Tr | 1 | 0.5 | 2 |
| 232 | middle, lean and fat | 0.26 | Tr | Tr | 1 | 0.5 | 2 |
| 233 | streaky, lean and fat | 0.25 | Tr | Tr | 1 | 0.5 | 2 |

Notes

Vitamin E, vitamin $B_6$, vitamin $B_{12}$, folic acid, pantothenic acid and biotin were analysed on pooled samples of raw lean and cooked lean, and vitamin E also on pooled samples of raw fat and cooked fat. The values for the individual cuts have been calculated from these results.

[a] Bacon fat may contain small amounts of some vitamins. It is, however, extremely difficult to obtain satisfactory analytical values for inclusion in the tables.

| No | Food | Description and number of samples | Edible matter, proportion of weight purchased | Water g | Total nitrogen g |
|---|---|---|---|---|---|
| | ***Beef*** | | | | |
| 235 | **dressed carcase** raw | Average carcase weight 224 kg, 59% lean, 23% fat in whole carcase; includes kidney knob and channel fat | 0.83 | 58.6 | 2.53 |
| 237 | **lean** average, raw | Average of six different cuts | — | 74.0 | 3.25 |
| 240 | **fat** average, raw | Average of six different cuts | — | 24.0 | 1.40 |
| 241 | cooked | Average of six different cuts | — | 25.2 | 1.91 |
| 242 | **brisket** raw, lean and fat | 18 samples, boned and rolled, 77% lean | 0.95 | 62.2 | 2.68 |
| 243 | boiled, lean and fat | 18 samples, boned and rolled, 77% lean; salt added | 0.61 | 48.4 | 4.41 |
| 244 | **forerib** raw, lean and fat | 18 samples, with bone, 72% lean | 0.75 | 57.4 | 2.56 |
| 245 | roast, lean and fat | 18 samples, 72% lean; cooked on the bone | 0.55 | 48.4 | 3.59 |
| 246 | lean only | 18 samples; cooked on the bone | 0.40 | 59.1 | 4.46 |
| 247 | **mince** raw | 18 samples | 1.00 | 64.5 | 3.01 |
| 248 | stewed | 18 samples; salt added | 0.72 | 59.1 | 3.69 |
| 249 | **rump steak** raw, lean and fat | 18 samples, 86% lean | 0.95 | 66.7 | 3.02 |
| 250 | fried, lean and fat | 18 samples, 87% lean | 0.70 | 56.2 | 4.58 |
| 251 | lean only | 18 samples | 0.60 | 61.1 | 4.92 |
| 252 | grilled, lean and fat | 18 samples, 89% lean | 0.74 | 59.3 | 4.36 |
| 253 | lean only | 18 samples | 0.66 | 63.8 | 4.58 |
| 254 | **silverside** salted, boiled, lean and fat | 17 samples, 85% lean; soaked for 18 hours before cooking | 0.56 | 54.5 | 4.58 |
| 255 | lean only | 17 samples; soaked for 18 hours before cooking. | 0.48 | 59.7 | 5.16 |
| 256 | **sirloin** raw, lean and fat | 18 samples, boneless, 72% lean | 0.92 | 59.4 | 2.65 |
| 257 | roast, lean and fat | 18 samples, boneless, 80% lean | 0.72 | 54.3 | 3.77 |
| 258 | lean only | 18 samples, boneless | 0.58 | 62.0 | 4.41 |
| 259 | **stewing steak** raw, lean and fat | 18 samples, 85% lean | 0.96 | 68.7 | 3.23 |
| 260 | stewed, lean and fat | 18 samples, 92% lean; salt added | 0.60 | 57.1 | 4.94 |
| 261 | **topside** raw, lean and fat | 18 samples, 87% lean | 0.94 | 68.4 | 3.13 |
| 262 | roast, lean and fat | 18 samples, 88% lean | 0.74 | 60.2 | 4.26 |
| 263 | lean only | 18 samples | 0.65 | 65.1 | 4.67 |

| No | Food | Energy value kcal | Energy value kJ | Protein (N × 6.25) g | Fat g | Carbo-hydrate g | Na mg | K mg | Ca mg | Mg mg | P mg | Fe mg | Cu mg | Zn mg | S mg | Cl mg |
|---|---|---|---|---|---|---|---|---|---|---|---|---|---|---|---|---|
| | ***Beef*** | | | | | | | | | | | | | | | |
| 235 | **dressed carcase** raw | 282 | 1168 | 15.8 | 24.3 | 0 | 55 | 280 | 7 | 17 | 150 | 1.9 | 0.13 | 3.3 | — | 55 |
| 237 | **lean**, average, raw | 123 | 517 | 20.3 | 4.6 | 0 | 61 | 350 | 7 | 20 | 180 | 2.1 | 0.14 | 4.3 | 190 | 59 |
| 240 | **fat**, average, raw | 637 | 2625 | 8.8 | 66.9 | 0 | 33 | 100 | 10 | 7 | 60 | 1.0 | 0.11 | 1.0 | — | 39 |
| 241 | cooked | 613 | 2526 | 11.9 | 62.8 | 0 | 50 | 160 | 14 | 11 | 90 | 1.4 | 0.14 | 1.4 | — | 56 |
| 242 | **brisket** raw, lean and fat | 252 | 1044 | 16.8 | 20.5 | 0 | 68 | 270 | 7 | 16 | 140 | 1.6 | 0.12 | 3.5 | — | 69 |
| 243 | boiled, lean and fat | 326 | 1354 | 27.6 | 23.9 | 0 | 73 | 200 | 12 | 18 | 150 | 2.8 | 0.13 | 6.3 | — | 92 |
| 244 | **forerib** raw, lean and fat | 290 | 1201 | 16.0 | 25.1 | 0 | 48 | 270 | 10 | 15 | 130 | 1.5 | 0.12 | 3.4 | — | 45 |
| 245 | roast, lean and fat | 349 | 1446 | 22.4 | 28.8 | 0 | 51 | 260 | 14 | 18 | 150 | 1.9 | 0.16 | 5.2 | — | 56 |
| 246 | lean only | 225 | 941 | 27.9 | 12.6 | 0 | 56 | 310 | 13 | 22 | 180 | 2.3 | 0.17 | 6.8 | 260 | 61 |
| 247 | **mince** raw | 221 | 919 | 18.8 | 16.2 | 0 | 86 | 290 | 15 | 17 | 160 | 2.7 | 0.15 | 4.3 | 180 | 86 |
| 248 | stewed | 229 | 955 | 23.1 | 15.2 | 0 | 320 | 290 | 18 | 20 | 170 | 3.1 | 0.24 | 5.8 | 220 | 470 |
| 249 | **rump steak** raw, lean and fat | 197 | 821 | 18.9 | 13.5 | 0 | 51 | 330 | 6 | 20 | 210 | 2.3 | 0.14 | 4.6 | — | 49 |
| 250 | fried, lean and fat | 246 | 1026 | 28.6 | 14.6 | 0 | 54 | 360 | 7 | 24 | 220 | 3.2 | 0.15 | 5.3 | — | 56 |
| 251 | lean only | 190 | 797 | 30.8 | 7.4 | 0 | 57 | 390 | 6 | 25 | 240 | 3.4 | 0.15 | 5.9 | 280 | 58 |
| 252 | grilled, lean and fat | 218 | 912 | 27.3 | 12.1 | 0 | 55 | 380 | 7 | 25 | 220 | 3.4 | 0.18 | 4.9 | — | 61 |
| 253 | lean only | 168 | 708 | 28.6 | 6.0 | 0 | 56 | 400 | 7 | 26 | 230 | 3.5 | 0.18 | 5.3 | 280 | 62 |
| 254 | **silverside** salted, boiled, lean and fat | 242 | 1012 | 28.6 | 14.2 | 0 | 910 | 200 | 11 | 18 | 140 | 2.8 | 0.25 | 5.5 | — | 1420 |
| 255 | lean only | 173 | 730 | 32.3 | 4.9 | 0 | 1000 | 230 | 10 | 20 | 150 | 3.2 | 0.27 | 6.2 | 310 | 1560 |
| 256 | **sirloin** raw, lean and fat | 272 | 1126 | 16.6 | 22.8 | 0 | 49 | 260 | 9 | 16 | 150 | 1.6 | 0.13 | 3.1 | — | 52 |
| 257 | roast, lean and fat | 284 | 1182 | 23.6 | 21.1 | 0 | 54 | 300 | 10 | 19 | 170 | 1.9 | 0.18 | 4.6 | — | 64 |
| 258 | lean only | 192 | 806 | 27.6 | 9.1 | 0 | 59 | 350 | 10 | 22 | 190 | 2.1 | 0.19 | 5.5 | 270 | 65 |
| 259 | **stewing steak** raw, lean and fat | 176 | 736 | 20.2 | 10.6 | 0 | 72 | 320 | 8 | 18 | 140 | 2.1 | 0.15 | 3.8 | — | 73 |
| 260 | stewed, lean and fat | 223 | 932 | 30.9 | 11.0 | 0 | 360 | 230 | 15 | 21 | 160 | 3.0 | 0.25 | 8.7 | — | 550 |
| 261 | **topside** raw, lean and fat | 179 | 748 | 19.6 | 11.2 | 0 | 43 | 340 | 5 | 19 | 170 | 1.9 | 0.13 | 3.3 | — | 44 |
| 262 | roast, lean and fat | 214 | 896 | 26.6 | 12.0 | 0 | 48 | 350 | 6 | 23 | 200 | 2.6 | 0.13 | 4.9 | — | 51 |
| 263 | lean only | 156 | 659 | 29.2 | 4.4 | 0 | 49 | 370 | 6 | 24 | 210 | 2.8 | 0.14 | 5.5 | 270 | 51 |

| No | Food | Retinol µg | Carotene µg | Vitamin D µg | Thiamin mg | Riboflavin mg | Nicotinic acid mg | Potential nicotinic acid from tryptophan mgTrp ÷60 | Vitamin C mg | Vitamin E mg |
|---|---|---|---|---|---|---|---|---|---|---|
| | ***Beef*** | | | | | | | | | |
| 235 | **dressed carcase** raw | (4) | Tr | Tr | 0.05 | 0.20 | 3.8 | 3.4 | 0 | 0.19 |
| 237 | **lean,** average, raw | Tr | Tr | Tr | 0.07 | 0.24 | 5.2 | 4.3 | 0 | 0.15 |
| 240 | **fat,** average, raw[a] | — | — | — | — | — | — | 1.9 | 0 | 0.32 |
| 241 | cooked[a] | — | — | — | — | — | — | 2.6 | 0 | 0.55 |
| 242 | **brisket** raw, lean and fat | Tr | Tr | Tr | 0.05 | 0.16 | 3.7 | 3.6 | 0 | 0.19 |
| 243 | boiled, lean and fat | Tr | Tr | Tr | 0.04 | 0.30 | 4.3 | 5.9 | 0 | 0.35 |
| 244 | **forerib** raw, lean and fat | Tr | Tr | Tr | 0.04 | 0.14 | 3.6 | 3.4 | 0 | 0.20 |
| 245 | roast, lean and fat | Tr | Tr | Tr | 0.04 | 0.24 | 3.9 | 4.8 | 0 | 0.36 |
| 246 | lean only | Tr | Tr | Tr | 0.05 | 0.33 | 5.5 | 6.0 | 0 | 0.29 |
| 247 | **mince** raw | Tr | Tr | Tr | 0.06 | 0.31 | 4.0 | 4.0 | 0 | (0.18) |
| 248 | stewed | Tr | Tr | Tr | 0.05 | 0.33 | 4.4 | 4.9 | 0 | (0.31) |
| 249 | **rump steak** raw, lean and fat | Tr | Tr | Tr | 0.08 | 0.26 | 4.2 | 4.0 | 0 | 0.17 |
| 250 | fried, lean and fat | Tr | Tr | Tr | 0.08 | 0.35 | 5.5 | 6.1 | 0 | 0.33 |
| 251 | lean only | Tr | Tr | Tr | 0.09 | 0.40 | 6.3 | 6.6 | 0 | 0.29 |
| 252 | grilled, lean and fat | Tr | Tr | Tr | 0.08 | 0.32 | 5.7 | 5.8 | 0 | 0.32 |
| 253 | lean only | Tr | Tr | Tr | 0.09 | 0.36 | 6.4 | 6.1 | 0 | 0.29 |
| 254 | **silverside** salted, boiled, lean and fat | Tr | Tr | Tr | 0.03 | 0.27 | 3.3 | 6.1 | 0 | 0.33 |
| 255 | lean only | Tr | Tr | Tr | 0.04 | 0.32 | 3.9 | 6.9 | 0 | 0.29 |
| 256 | **sirloin** raw, lean and fat | Tr | Tr | Tr | 0.04 | 0.17 | 4.2 | 3.5 | 0 | 0.20 |
| 257 | roast, lean and fat | Tr | Tr | Tr | 0.06 | 0.25 | 4.8 | 5.0 | 0 | 0.34 |
| 258 | lean only | Tr | Tr | Tr | 0.07 | 0.31 | 6.0 | 5.9 | 0 | 0.29 |
| 259 | **stewing steak** raw, lean and fat | Tr | Tr | Tr | 0.06 | 0.23 | 4.2 | 4.3 | 0 | 0.18 |
| 260 | stewed, lean and fat | Tr | Tr | Tr | 0.03 | 0.33 | 3.6 | 6.6 | 0 | 0.31 |
| 261 | **topside** raw, lean and fat | Tr | Tr | Tr | 0.05 | 0.21 | 4.8 | 4.2 | 0 | 0.17 |
| 262 | roast, lean and fat | Tr | Tr | Tr | 0.07 | 0.31 | 5.7 | 5.7 | 0 | 0.32 |
| 263 | lean only | Tr | Tr | Tr | 0.08 | 0.35 | 6.5 | 6.2 | 0 | 0.29 |

| No | Food | Vitamin $B_6$ mg | Vitamin $B_{12}$ µg | Folic acid Free µg | Folic acid Total µg | Pantothenic acid mg | Biotin µg |
|---|---|---|---|---|---|---|---|
| | ***Beef*** | | | | | | |
| 235 | **dressed carcase** raw | 0.23 | 1 | 4 | 10 | 0.5 | Tr |
| 237 | **lean** average, raw | 0.32 | 2 | 4 | 10 | 0.7 | Tr |
| 240 | **fat** average, raw[a] | — | Tr | — | — | — | Tr |
| 241 | cooked[a] | — | Tr | — | — | — | Tr |
| 242 | **brisket** raw, lean and fat | 0.25 | 1 | 3 | 8 | 0.5 | Tr |
| 243 | boiled, lean and fat | 0.25 | 2 | 4 | 13 | 0.7 | Tr |
| 244 | **forerib** raw, lean and fat | 0.23 | 1 | 3 | 7 | 0.5 | Tr |
| 245 | roast, lean and fat | 0.24 | 1 | 3 | 13 | 0.6 | Tr |
| 246 | lean only | 0.33 | 2 | 5 | 17 | 0.9 | Tr |
| 247 | **mince** raw | (0.27) | (2) | (3) | (9) | (0.6) | Tr |
| 248 | stewed | (0.30) | (2) | (4) | (16) | (0.8) | Tr |
| 249 | **rump steak** raw, lean and fat | 0.27 | 2 | 3 | 9 | 0.6 | Tr |
| 250 | fried, lean and fat | 0.29 | 2 | 4 | 15 | 0.8 | Tr |
| 251 | lean only | 0.33 | 2 | 5 | 17 | 0.9 | Tr |
| 252 | grilled, lean and fat | 0.29 | 2 | 4 | 15 | 0.8 | Tr |
| 253 | lean only | 0.33 | 2 | 5 | 17 | 0.9 | Tr |
| 254 | **silverside** salted boiled, lean and fat | 0.28 | 2 | 4 | 15 | 0.8 | Tr |
| 255 | lean only | 0.33 | 2 | 5 | 17 | 0.9 | Tr |
| 256 | **sirloin** raw, lean and fat | 0.23 | 1 | 3 | 7 | 0.5 | Tr |
| 257 | roast, lean and fat | 0.26 | 2 | 4 | 14 | 0.7 | Tr |
| 258 | lean only | 0.33 | 2 | 5 | 17 | 0.9 | Tr |
| 259 | **stewing steak** raw, lean and fat | 0.27 | 2 | 3 | 9 | 0.6 | Tr |
| 260 | stewed, lean and fat | 0.30 | 2 | 4 | 16 | 0.8 | Tr |
| 261 | **topside** raw, lean and fat | 0.28 | 2 | 3 | 9 | 0.6 | Tr |
| 262 | roast, lean and fat | 0.29 | 2 | 4 | 15 | 0.8 | Tr |
| 263 | lean only | 0.33 | 2 | 5 | 17 | 0.9 | Tr |

Notes

Vitamin E, vitamin $B_6$, vitamin $B_{12}$, folic acid, pantothenic acid and biotin were analysed on pooled samples of raw lean and cooked lean, and vitamin E also on pooled samples of raw fat and cooked fat. The values for the individual cuts have been calculated from these results.

[a] Beef fat may contain small amounts of some vitamins. It is, however, extremely difficult to obtain satisfactory analytical values for inclusion in the tables.

| No | Food | Description and number of samples | Edible matter, proportion of weight purchased | Water g | Total nitrogen g |
|---|---|---|---|---|---|
| | ***Lamb*** | | | | |
| 264 | **dressed carcase** raw | Average carcase weight 17 kg, 55% lean, 28% fat in whole carcase; includes kidney knob and channel fat | 0.84 | 54.4 | 2.34 |
| 266 | **lean** average, raw | Average of six different cuts | — | 70.1 | 3.33 |
| 269 | **fat** average, raw | Average of six different cuts | — | 21.2 | 0.99 |
| 270 | cooked | Average of six different cuts | — | 24.6 | 1.81 |
| 271 | **breast** raw, lean and fat | 15 samples, boneless, 59% lean | 0.96 | 48.3 | 2.67 |
| 272 | roast, lean and fat | 15 samples, boneless, 60% lean | 0.77 | 43.6 | 3.05 |
| 273 | lean only | 15 samples, boneless | 0.45 | 57.8 | 4.09 |
| 274 | **chops, loin** raw, lean and fat | 15 samples, 60% lean | 0.82 | 49.5 | 2.34 |
| 275 | grilled, lean and fat | 15 samples, 70% lean | 0.54 | 46.6 | 3.76 |
| 276 | lean and fat (weighed with bone) | Calculated from the previous item | 0.54 | 36.3 | 2.93 |
| 277 | lean only | 15 samples | 0.38 | 58.9 | 4.44 |
| 278 | lean only (weighed with fat and bone) | Calculated from the previous item | 0.38 | 32.4 | 2.44 |
| 279 | **cutlets** raw, lean and fat | 15 samples, 59% lean | 0.76 | 48.7 | 2.35 |
| 280 | grilled, lean and fat | 15 samples, 67% lean | 0.50 | 45.1 | 3.68 |
| 281 | lean and fat (weighed with bone) | Calculated from the previous item | 0.50 | 29.8 | 2.43 |
| 282 | lean only | 15 samples | 0.33 | 58.9 | 4.44 |
| 283 | lean only (weighed with fat and bone) | Calculated from the previous item | 0.33 | 25.9 | 1.95 |
| 284 | **leg** raw, lean and fat | 15 samples, 80% lean | 0.77 | 63.1 | 2.86 |
| 285 | roast, lean and fat | 15 samples, 82% lean | 0.53 | 55.3 | 4.18 |
| 286 | lean only | 15 samples | 0.43 | 61.8 | 4.71 |
| 287 | **scrag and neck** raw, lean and fat | 15 samples, 71% lean | 0.60 | 55.7 | 2.50 |
| 288 | stewed, lean and fat | 15 samples, 84% lean | 0.46 | 52.6 | 4.10 |
| 289 | lean only | 15 samples | 0.38 | 55.9 | 4.44 |
| 290 | lean only (weighed with fat and bone) | Calculated from the previous item | 0.38 | 28.5 | 2.26 |

| No | Food | Energy value kcal | Energy value kJ | Protein (N × 6.25) g | Fat g | Carbohydrate g | Na mg | K mg | Ca mg | Mg mg | P mg | Fe mg | Cu mg | Zn mg | S mg | Cl mg |
|---|---|---|---|---|---|---|---|---|---|---|---|---|---|---|---|---|
| | ***Lamb*** | | | | | | | | | | | | | | | |
| 264 | **dressed carcase** raw | 333 | 1377 | 14.6 | 30.5 | 0 | 71 | 260 | 7 | 18 | 150 | 1.4 | 0.15 | 2.9 | — | 65 |
| 266 | **lean** average, raw | 162 | 679 | 20.8 | 8.8 | 0 | 88 | 350 | 7 | 24 | 190 | 1.6 | 0.17 | 4.0 | 210 | 76 |
| 269 | **fat** average, raw | 671 | 2762 | 6.2 | 71.8 | 0 | 36 | 96 | 7 | 6 | 54 | 0.7 | 0.15 | 0.8 | — | 37 |
| 270 | cooked | 616 | 2538 | 11.3 | 63.4 | 0 | 56 | 150 | 11 | 12 | 120 | 1.4 | 0.16 | 1.4 | — | 53 |
| 271 | **breast** raw, lean and fat | 378 | 1564 | 16.7 | 34.6 | 0 | 100 | 270 | 8 | 18 | 150 | 1.3 | 0.16 | 3.2 | — | 77 |
| 272 | roast, lean and fat | 410 | 1697 | 19.1 | 37.1 | 0 | 73 | 250 | 10 | 18 | 150 | 1.5 | 0.19 | 3.6 | — | 74 |
| 273 | lean only | 252 | 1049 | 25.6 | 16.6 | 0 | 86 | 330 | 10 | 24 | 200 | 1.7 | 0.23 | 5.3 | 240 | 89 |
| 274 | **chops, loin** raw, lean and fat | 377 | 1558 | 14.6 | 35.4 | 0 | 61 | 230 | (7)[a] | 17 | 140 | 1.2 | 0.16 | 2.1 | — | 60 |
| 275 | grilled, lean and fat | 355 | 1473 | 23.5 | 29.0 | 0 | 72 | 320 | (9)[a] | 24 | 210 | 1.9 | 0.17 | 3.4 | — | 83 |
| 276 | lean and fat (weighed with bone) | 277 | 1147 | 18.3 | 22.6 | 0 | 56 | 250 | (7)[a] | 19 | 160 | 1.5 | 0.13 | 2.7 | — | 65 |
| 277 | lean only | 222 | 928 | 27.8 | 12.3 | 0 | 75 | 380 | (9)[a] | 28 | 240 | 2.1 | 0.19 | 4.1 | 270 | 90 |
| 278 | lean only (weighed with fat and bone) | 122 | 512 | 15.3 | 6.8 | 0 | 41 | 210 | (5)[a] | 15 | 130 | 1.2 | 0.10 | 2.3 | 150 | 50 |
| 279 | **cutlets** raw, lean and fat | 386 | 1593 | 14.7 | 36.3 | 0 | 60 | 230 | (7)[a] | 16 | 130 | 1.2 | 0.15 | 2.1 | — | 60 |
| 280 | grilled, lean and fat | 370 | 1534 | 23.0 | 30.9 | 0 | 71 | 320 | (9)[a] | 23 | 200 | 1.9 | 0.18 | 3.3 | — | 82 |
| 281 | lean and fat (weighed with bone) | 244 | 1013 | 15.2 | 20.4 | 0 | 47 | 210 | (6)[a] | 15 | 130 | 1.3 | 0.12 | 2.2 | — | 54 |
| 282 | lean only | 222 | 928 | 27.8 | 12.3 | 0 | 75 | 380 | (9)[a] | 28 | 240 | 2.1 | 0.19 | 4.1 | 270 | 90 |
| 283 | lean only (weighed with fat and bone) | 97 | 407 | 12.2 | 5.4 | 0 | 33 | 170 | (4)[a] | 12 | 110 | 0.9 | 0.08 | 1.8 | 120 | 40 |
| 284 | **leg** raw, lean and fat | 240 | 996 | 17.9 | 18.7 | 0 | 52 | 310 | 6 | 22 | 170 | 1.7 | 0.14 | 2.8 | — | 54 |
| 285 | roast, lean and fat | 266 | 1106 | 26.1 | 17.9 | 0 | 65 | 310 | 8 | 25 | 200 | 2.5 | 0.28 | 4.6 | — | 62 |
| 286 | lean only | 191 | 800 | 29.4 | 8.1 | 0 | 67 | 340 | 8 | 28 | 220 | 2.7 | 0.31 | 5.3 | 290 | 64 |
| 287 | **scrag and neck** raw, lean and fat | 316 | 1309 | 15.6 | 28.2 | 0 | 71 | 260 | (7)[a] | 18 | 140 | 1.2 | 0.16 | 3.6 | — | 68 |
| 288 | stewed, lean and fat | 292 | 1216 | 25.6 | 21.1 | 0 | 240 | 190 | (9)[a] | 18 | 190 | 2.2 | 0.22 | 6.1 | — | 340 |
| 289 | lean only | 253 | 1054 | 27.8 | 15.7 | 0 | 250 | 200 | (9)[a] | 19 | 190 | 2.4 | 0.33 | 6.9 | 270 | 350 |
| 290 | lean only (weighed with fat and bone) | 128 | 536 | 14.1 | 8.0 | 0 | 130 | 100 | (5)[a] | 10 | 100 | 1.2 | 0.17 | 3.5 | 140 | 180 |

[a] The calcium content is extremely variable as scrapings of bone may easily be included in the edible portion. This is a minimum value

| No | Food | Retinol µg | Carotene µg | Vitamin D µg | Thiamin mg | Riboflavin mg | Nicotinic acid mg | Potential nicotinic acid from tryptophan mgTrp ÷60 | Vitamin C mg | Vitamin E mg |
|---|---|---|---|---|---|---|---|---|---|---|
| | ***Lamb*** | | | | | | | | | |
| 264 | **dressed carcase** raw | (4) | Tr | Tr | 0.09 | 0.21 | 4.0 | 3.1 | 0 | 0.26 |
| 266 | **lean** average, raw | Tr | Tr | Tr | 0.14 | 0.28 | 6.0 | 4.4 | 0 | 0.10 |
| 269 | **fat** average, raw[a] | — | — | — | — | — | — | 1.3 | 0 | 0.30 |
| 270 | cooked[a] | — | — | — | — | — | — | 2.4 | 0 | 0.18 |
| 271 | **breast** raw, lean and fat | Tr | Tr | Tr | 0.08 | 0.17 | 3.8 | 3.6 | 0 | 0.18 |
| 272 | roast, lean and fat | Tr | Tr | Tr | 0.06 | 0.17 | 3.4 | 4.1 | 0 | 0.13 |
| 273 | lean only | Tr | Tr | Tr | 0.10 | 0.29 | 5.6 | 5.5 | 0 | 0.10 |
| 274 | **chops, loin** raw, lean and fat | Tr | Tr | Tr | 0.09 | 0.16 | 4.0 | 3.1 | 0 | 0.18 |
| 275 | grilled, lean and fat | Tr | Tr | Tr | 0.11 | 0.21 | 5.1 | 5.0 | 0 | 0.12 |
| 276 | lean and fat (weighed with bone) | Tr | Tr | Tr | 0.09 | 0.16 | 4.0 | 3.9 | 0 | 0.09 |
| 277 | lean only | Tr | Tr | Tr | 0.15 | 0.30 | 7.2 | 5.9 | 0 | 0.10 |
| 278 | lean only (weighed with fat and bone) | Tr | Tr | Tr | 0.08 | 0.17 | 4.0 | 3.3 | 0 | 0.06 |
| 279 | **cutlets** raw, lean and fat | Tr | Tr | Tr | 0.09 | 0.16 | 3.9 | 3.1 | 0 | 0.18 |
| 280 | grilled, lean and fat | Tr | Tr | Tr | 0.10 | 0.20 | 4.8 | 4.9 | 0 | 0.13 |
| 281 | lean and fat (weighed with bone) | Tr | Tr | Tr | 0.07 | 0.13 | 3.2 | 3.2 | 0 | 0.09 |
| 282 | lean only | Tr | Tr | Tr | 0.15 | 0.30 | 7.2 | 5.9 | 0 | 0.10 |
| 283 | lean only (weighed with fat and bone) | Tr | Tr | Tr | 0.07 | 0.13 | 3.2 | 2.6 | 0 | 0.04 |
| 284 | **leg** raw, lean and fat | Tr | Tr | Tr | 0.14 | 0.25 | 5.7 | 3.8 | 0 | 0.14 |
| 285 | roast, lean and fat | Tr | Tr | Tr | 0.12 | 0.31 | 5.4 | 5.6 | 0 | 0.11 |
| 286 | lean only | Tr | Tr | Tr | 0.14 | 0.38 | 6.6 | 6.3 | 0 | 0.10 |
| 287 | **scrag and neck** raw, lean and fat | Tr | Tr | Tr | 0.07 | 0.17 | 3.4 | 3.3 | 0 | 0.16 |
| 288 | stewed, lean and fat | Tr | Tr | Tr | 0.04 | 0.18 | 2.7 | 5.5 | 0 | 0.11 |
| 289 | lean only | Tr | Tr | Tr | 0.05 | 0.21 | 3.2 | 5.9 | 0 | 0.10 |
| 290 | lean only (weighed with fat and bone) | Tr | Tr | Tr | 0.03 | 0.11 | 1.6 | 3.0 | 0 | 0.05 |

| No | Food | Vitamin $B_6$ mg | Vitamin $B_{12}$ µg | Folic acid Free µg | Folic acid Total µg | Pantothenic acid mg | Biotin µg |
|---|---|---|---|---|---|---|---|
| | ***Lamb*** | | | | | | |
| 264 | **dressed carcase** raw | 0.17 | 2 | Tr | 4 | 0.5 | 1 |
| 266 | **lean** average, raw | 0.25 | 2 | Tr | 5 | 0.7 | 2 |
| 269 | **fat** average, raw[a] | — | Tr | Tr | — | — | Tr |
| 270 | cooked[a] | — | Tr | Tr | — | — | Tr |
| 271 | **breast** raw, lean and fat | 0.15 | 1 | Tr | 3 | 0.4 | 1 |
| 272 | roast, lean and fat | 0.13 | 1 | Tr | 3 | 0.4 | 1 |
| 273 | lean only | 0.22 | 2 | Tr | 4 | 0.7 | 2 |
| 274 | **chops, loin** raw, lean and fat | 0.15 | 1 | Tr | 3 | 0.4 | 1 |
| 275 | grilled, lean and fat | 0.15 | 2 | Tr | 3 | 0.5 | 1 |
| 276 | lean and fat (weighed with bone) | 0.12 | 2 | Tr | 2 | 0.4 | 1 |
| 277 | lean only | 0.22 | 2 | Tr | 4 | 0.7 | 2 |
| 278 | lean only (weighed with fat and bone) | 0.12 | 1 | Tr | 2 | 0.4 | 1 |
| 279 | **cutlets** raw, lean and fat | 0.15 | 1 | Tr | 3 | 0.4 | 1 |
| 280 | grilled, lean and fat | 0.15 | 2 | Tr | 3 | 0.5 | 1 |
| 281 | lean and fat (weighed with bone) | 0.10 | 1 | Tr | 2 | 0.3 | 1 |
| 282 | lean only | 0.22 | 2 | Tr | 4 | 0.7 | 2 |
| 283 | lean only (weighed with fat and bone) | 0.10 | 1 | Tr | 2 | 0.3 | 1 |
| 284 | **leg** raw, lean and fat | 0.20 | 2 | Tr | 4 | 0.6 | 1 |
| 285 | roast, lean and fat | 0.18 | 2 | Tr | 3 | 0.6 | 1 |
| 286 | lean only | 0.22 | 2 | Tr | 4 | 0.7 | 2 |
| 287 | **scrag and neck** raw, lean and fat | 0.18 | 2 | Tr | 4 | 0.5 | 1 |
| 288 | stewed, lean and fat | 0.19 | 2 | Tr | 4 | 0.6 | 1 |
| 289 | lean only | 0.22 | 2 | Tr | 4 | 0.7 | 2 |
| 290 | lean only (weighed with fat and bone) | 0.11 | 1 | Tr | 2 | 0.4 | 1 |

Notes

Vitamin E, vitamin $B_6$, vitamin $B_{12}$, folic acid, pantothenic acid and biotin were analysed on a pooled sample of raw lean and cooked lean, and vitamin E also on pooled samples of raw fat and cooked fat. The values for the individual cuts have been calculated from these results.

[a] Lamb fat may contain small amounts of some vitamins. It is, however, extremely difficult to obtain satisfactory analytical values for inclusion in the tables.

| No | Food | Description and number of samples | Edible matter, proportion of weight purchased | Water g | Total nitrogen g |
|---|---|---|---|---|---|
| | ***Lamb** contd* | | | | |
| 291 | **shoulder** raw, lean and fat | 15 samples, 68% lean | 0.78 | 56.1 | 2.50 |
| 292 | roast, lean and fat | 15 samples, 73% lean | 0.57 | 53.6 | 3.18 |
| 293 | lean only | 15 samples | 0.42 | 64.8 | 3.80 |
| | ***Pork*** | | | | |
| 294 | **dressed carcase** raw | Average carcase weight 52 kg, 48% lean, 25% fat in whole carcase; includes kidney knob and channel fat, head, feet and skin | 0.74 | 50.7 | 2.18 |
| 296 | **lean** average, raw | Average of three different cuts | — | 71.5 | 3.29 |
| 299 | **fat** average, raw | Average of three different cuts | — | 21.1 | 1.08 |
| 300 | cooked | Average of three different cuts | — | 20.9 | 2.37 |
| 301 | **belly, rashers** raw, lean and fat | 15 samples, 56% lean | 0.87 | 48.7 | 2.44 |
| 302 | grilled, lean and fat | 15 samples, 56% lean | 0.64 | 43.0 | 3.38 |
| 303 | **chops, loin** raw, lean and fat | 15 samples, 65% lean; without kidney | 0.83 | 54.3 | 2.55 |
| 304 | grilled, lean and fat | 15 samples, 75% lean; without kidney | 0.49 | 46.3 | 4.55 |
| 305 | lean and fat (weighed with bone) | Calculated from the previous item | 0.49 | 36.1 | 3.55 |
| 306 | lean only | 15 samples | 0.37 | 56.1 | 5.17 |
| 307 | lean only (weighed with fat and bone) | Calculated from the previous item | 0.37 | 33.1 | 3.05 |
| 308 | **leg** raw, lean and fat | 15 samples, fillet end, 73% lean | 0.85 | 59.5 | 2.66 |
| 309 | roast, lean and fat | 15 samples, fillet end, 76% lean | 0.60 | 51.9 | 4.30 |
| 310 | lean only | 15 samples, fillet end | 0.45 | 61.6 | 4.91 |
| | ***Veal*** | | | | |
| 311 | **cutlet** fried | Covered in egg and breadcrumbs | 0.74 | 54.6 | 5.02 |
| 312 | **fillet** raw | All lean | 1.00 | 74.9 | 3.37 |
| 313 | roast | All lean | 0.75 | 55.1 | 5.05 |

| No | Food | Energy value kcal | Energy value kJ | Protein (N × 6.25) g | Fat g | Carbo-hydrate g | Na mg | K mg | Ca mg | Mg mg | P mg | Fe mg | Cu mg | Zn mg | S mg | Cl mg |
|---|---|---|---|---|---|---|---|---|---|---|---|---|---|---|---|---|
| | ***Lamb** contd* | | | | | | | | | | | | | | | |
| 291 | **shoulder** raw, lean and fat | 314 | 1301 | 15.6 | 28.0 | 0 | 66 | 260 | 7 | 18 | 150 | 1.2 | 0.21 | 3.1 | — | 56 |
| 292 | roast, lean and fat | 316 | 1311 | 19.9 | 26.3 | 0 | 61 | 260 | 9 | 19 | 150 | 1.6 | 0.15 | 4.3 | — | 60 |
| 293 | lean only | 196 | 819 | 23.8 | 11.2 | 0 | 65 | 300 | 9 | 22 | 170 | 1.8 | 0.16 | 5.3 | 240 | 65 |
| | ***Pork*** | | | | | | | | | | | | | | | |
| 294 | **dressed carcase** raw | 338 | 1397 | 13.6 | 31.5 | 0 | 65 | 270 | 8 | 16 | 150 | 0.9 | 0.15 | 1.8 | — | 64 |
| 296 | **lean** average, raw | 147 | 615 | 20.7 | 7.1 | 0 | 76 | 370 | 8 | 22 | 200 | 0.9 | 0.15 | 2.4 | 200 | 71 |
| 299 | **fat** average, raw | 670 | 2757 | 6.8 | 71.4 | 0 | 38 | 87 | 7 | 5 | 49 | 0.7 | 0.10 | 0.4 | — | 44 |
| 300 | cooked | 619 | 2553 | 14.8 | 62.2 | 0 | 79 | 210 | 11 | 9 | 110 | 1.0 | 0.15 | 0.9 | — | 84 |
| 301 | **belly, rashers** raw, lean and fat | 381 | 1574 | 15.3 | 35.5 | 0 | 73 | 220 | 8 | 14 | 120 | 0.8 | 0.15 | 1.8 | — | 71 |
| 302 | grilled, lean and fat | 398 | 1646 | 21.1 | 34.8 | 0 | 95 | 310 | 11 | 19 | 170 | 1.0 | 0.16 | 2.6 | — | 92 |
| 303 | **chops, loin** raw | 329 | 1362 | 15.9 | 29.5 | 0 | 56 | 290 | (8)[a] | 17 | 160 | 0.8 | 0.13 | 1.6 | — | 54 |
| 304 | grilled, lean and fat | 332 | 1380 | 28.5 | 24.2 | 0 | 84 | 380 | (11)[a] | 26 | 230 | 1.2 | 0.17 | 2.9 | — | 79 |
| 305 | lean and fat (weighed with bone) | 258 | 1073 | 22.2 | 18.8 | 0 | 66 | 300 | (9)[a] | 20 | 180 | 0.9 | 0.13 | 2.3 | — | 62 |
| 306 | lean only | 226 | 945 | 32.3 | 10.7 | 0 | 84 | 420 | (9)[a] | 29 | 260 | 1.2 | 0.16 | 3.5 | 310 | 78 |
| 307 | lean only (weighed with fat and bone) | 133 | 558 | 19.1 | 6.3 | 0 | 50 | 250 | (5)[a] | 17 | 150 | 0.7 | 0.09 | 2.1 | 180 | 46 |
| 308 | **leg** raw, lean and fat | 269 | 1115 | 16.6 | 22.5 | 0 | 59 | 300 | 7 | 18 | 160 | 0.8 | 0.12 | 1.8 | — | 59 |
| 309 | roast, lean and fat | 286 | 1190 | 26.9 | 19.8 | 0 | 79 | 350 | 10 | 22 | 200 | 1.3 | 0.25 | 2.9 | — | 79 |
| 310 | lean only | 185 | 777 | 30.7 | 6.9 | 0 | 79 | 390 | 9 | 25 | 230 | 1.3 | 0.29 | 3.5 | 300 | 76 |
| | ***Veal*** | | | | | | | | | | | | | | | |
| 311 | **cutlet** fried | 215 | 904 | 31.4 | 8.1 | 4.4 | 110 | 420 | 10 | 33 | 280 | (1.6) | — | — | 330 | 120 |
| 312 | **fillet** raw | 109 | 459 | 21.1 | 2.7 | 0 | 110 | 360 | 8 | 25 | 260 | 1.2 | — | — | 220 | 68 |
| 313 | roast | 230 | 963 | 31.6 | 11.5 | 0 | 97 | 430 | 14 | 28 | 360 | 1.6 | — | — | 330 | 110 |

[a] The calcium content is extremely variable as scrapings of bone may easily be included in the edible portion. This is a minimum value

| No | Food | Retinol µg | Carotene µg | Vitamin D µg | Thiamin mg | Riboflavin mg | Nicotinic acid mg | Potential nicotinic acid from tryptophan mg Trp ÷ 60 | Vitamin C mg | Vitamin E mg |
|---|---|---|---|---|---|---|---|---|---|---|
| | ***Lamb** contd* | | | | | | | | | |
| 291 | **shoulder** raw, lean and fat | Tr | Tr | Tr | 0.10 | 0.18 | 3.6 | 3.3 | 0 | 0.17 |
| 292 | roast, lean and fat | Tr | Tr | Tr | 0.07 | 0.20 | 3.1 | 4.2 | 0 | 0.12 |
| 293 | lean only | Tr | Tr | Tr | 0.10 | 0.27 | 4.3 | 5.1 | 0 | 0.10 |
| | ***Pork*** | | | | | | | | | |
| 294 | **dressed carcase** raw | (4) | Tr | Tr | 0.58 | 0.19 | 4.1 | 2.5 | 0 | 0.01 |
| 296 | **lean** average, raw | Tr | Tr | Tr | 0.89 | 0.25 | 6.2 | 3.8 | 0 | 0 |
| 299 | **fat** average, raw[a] | Tr | Tr | Tr | — | — | — | 1.3 | 0 | 0.03 |
| 300 | cooked[a] | Tr | Tr | Tr | — | — | — | 2.8 | 0 | 0.12 |
| 301 | **belly, rashers** raw, lean and fat | Tr | Tr | Tr | 0.45 | 0.15 | 3.3 | 2.9 | 0 | 0.01 |
| 302 | grilled, lean and fat | Tr | Tr | Tr | 0.53 | 0.11 | 4.2 | 3.9 | 0 | 0.05 |
| 303 | **chops, loin** raw, lean and fat | Tr | Tr | Tr | 0.57 | 0.14 | 4.2 | 3.0 | 0 | 0.01 |
| 304 | grilled, lean and fat | Tr | Tr | Tr | 0.66 | 0.20 | 5.7 | 5.3 | 0 | 0.03 |
| 305 | lean and fat (weighed with bone) | Tr | Tr | Tr | 0.51 | 0.16 | 4.4 | 4.1 | 0 | 0.02 |
| 306 | lean only | Tr | Tr | Tr | 0.88 | 0.26 | 7.6 | 6.0 | 0 | 0 |
| 307 | lean only (weighed with fat and bone) | Tr | Tr | Tr | 0.52 | 0.15 | 4.5 | 3.6 | 0 | 0 |
| 308 | **leg** raw, lean and fat | Tr | Tr | Tr | 0.73 | 0.20 | 4.5 | 3.1 | 0 | 0.01 |
| 309 | roast, lean and fat | Tr | Tr | Tr | 0.65 | 0.27 | 5.0 | 5.0 | 0 | 0.03 |
| 310 | lean only | Tr | Tr | Tr | 0.85 | 0.35 | 6.6 | 5.7 | 0 | 0 |
| | ***Veal*** | | | | | | | | | |
| 311 | **cutlet** fried | Tr | Tr | Tr | — | — | — | 6.7 | 0 | — |
| 312 | **fillet** raw | Tr | Tr | Tr | 0.10 | 0.25 | 7.0 | 4.5 | 0 | — |
| 313 | roast | Tr | Tr | Tr | 0.06 | 0.27 | 7.0 | 6.7 | 0 | — |

| No | Food | Vitamin $B_6$ mg | Vitamin $B_{12}$ µg | Folic acid Free µg | Folic acid Total µg | Pantothenic acid mg | Biotin µg |
|---|---|---|---|---|---|---|---|
| | ***Lamb** contd* | | | | | | |
| 291 | **shoulder** raw, lean and fat | 0.17 | 2 | Tr | 3 | 0.5 | 1 |
| 292 | roast, lean and fat | 0.16 | 2 | Tr | 3 | 0.5 | 1 |
| 293 | lean only | 0.22 | 2 | Tr | 4 | 0.7 | 2 |
| | ***Pork*** | | | | | | |
| 294 | **dressed carcase** raw | 0.30 | 1 | Tr | 3 | 0.7 | 1 |
| 296 | **lean** average, raw | 0.45 | 3 | Tr | 5 | 1.1 | 3 |
| 299 | **fat** average, raw[a] | — | Tr | Tr | — | — | Tr |
| 300 | cooked[a] | — | Tr | Tr | — | — | Tr |
| 301 | **belly, rashers** raw, lean and fat | 0.25 | 2 | Tr | 3 | 0.6 | 2 |
| 302 | grilled, lean and fat | 0.23 | 1 | Tr | 4 | 0.7 | 2 |
| 303 | **chops, loin** raw, lean and fat | 0.29 | 2 | Tr | 3 | 0.7 | 2 |
| 304 | grilled, lean and fat | 0.31 | 1 | Tr | 6 | 1.0 | 2 |
| 305 | lean and fat (weighed with bone) | 0.24 | 1 | Tr | 5 | 0.8 | 2 |
| 306 | lean only | 0.41 | 2 | Tr | 7 | 1.3 | 3 |
| 307 | lean only (weighed with fat and bone) | 0.24 | 1 | Tr | 4 | 0.8 | 2 |
| 308 | **leg** raw, lean and fat | 0.33 | 2 | Tr | 4 | 0.8 | 2 |
| 309 | roast, lean and fat | 0.31 | 1 | Tr | 6 | 1.0 | 2 |
| 310 | lean only | 0.41 | 2 | Tr | 7 | 1.3 | 3 |
| | ***Veal*** | | | | | | |
| 311 | **cutlet** fried | — | 1 | Tr | — | — | Tr |
| 312 | **fillet** raw | 0.30 | 1 | Tr | 5 | 0.6 | Tr |
| 313 | roast | 0.32 | 1 | Tr | 4 | 0.5 | Tr |

Notes

Vitamin E, vitamin $B_6$, vitamin $B_{12}$, folic acid, pantothenic acid and biotin were analysed on a pooled sample of raw lean and cooked lean, and vitamin E also on pooled samples of raw fat and cooked fat. The values for the individual cuts have been calculated from these results.

[a] Pork fat may contain small quantities of some vitamins. It is, however, extremely difficult to obtain satisfactory analytical values for inclusion in the tables.

| No | Food | Description and number of samples | Edible matter, proportion of weight purchased | Water g | Total nitrogen g |
|---|---|---|---|---|---|
| | ***Poultry and game*** | | | | |
| 314 | **Chicken** raw, meat only | 15 samples, light and dark meat from dressed carcase | 0.44 | 74.4 | 3.28 |
| 315 | meat and skin | 15 samples, dressed carcase excluding waste | 0.64 | 64.4 | 2.82 |
| 316 | light meat | 15 samples | 0.23 | 74.4 | 3.49 |
| 317 | dark meat | 15 samples | 0.21 | 74.5 | 3.06 |
| 318 | boiled, meat only | 15 samples, light and dark meat from dressed carcase | 0.39 | 63.4 | 4.67 |
| 319 | light meat | 15 samples | 0.20 | 65.2 | 4.75 |
| 320 | dark meat | 15 samples | 0.19 | 61.5 | 4.58 |
| 321 | roast, meat only | 15 samples, light and dark meat from dressed carcase | 0.40 | 68.4 | 3.97 |
| 322 | meat and skin | 15 samples, dressed carcase excluding waste | 0.55 | 61.9 | 3.61 |
| 323 | light meat | 15 samples | 0.21 | 68.5 | 4.24 |
| 324 | dark meat | 15 samples | 0.20 | 68.2 | 3.69 |
| 325 | wing quarter (weighed with bone) | Meat only | 0.37 | 34.2 | 1.99 |
| 326 | leg quarter (weighed with bone) | Meat only | 0.42 | 42.4 | 2.46 |
| 327 | **Duck** raw, meat only | 9 samples, meat from dressed carcase | 0.28 | 75.0 | 3.15 |
| 328 | meat, fat and skin | 9 samples, dressed carcase excluding waste | 0.67 | 43.9 | 1.80 |
| 329 | roast, meat only | 11 samples, meat from dressed carcase | 0.21 | 64.2 | 4.05 |
| 330 | meat, fat and skin | 11 samples, dressed carcase excluding waste | 0.40 | 49.6 | 3.14 |
| 331 | **Goose** roast | Meat only | 0.39 | 46.7 | 4.69 |
| 332 | **Grouse** roast | Meat only | 0.51 | 61.6 | 5.00 |
| 333 | roast (weighed with bone) | Calculated from the previous item | 0.51 | 40.6 | 3.30 |
| 334 | **Partridge** roast | Meat only | 0.39 | 54.5 | 5.87 |
| 335 | roast (weighed with bone) | Calculated from the previous item | 0.39 | 32.7 | 3.52 |

| No | Food | Energy value kcal | Energy value kJ | Protein (N × 6.25) g | Fat g | Carbo-hydrate g | Na mg | K mg | Ca mg | Mg mg | P mg | Fe mg | Cu mg | Zn mg | S mg | Cl mg |
|---|---|---|---|---|---|---|---|---|---|---|---|---|---|---|---|---|
| | ***Poultry and game*** | | | | | | | | | | | | | | | |
| 314 | **Chicken** raw, meat only | 121 | 508 | 20.5 | 4.3 | 0 | 81 | 320 | 10 | 25 | 200 | 0.7 | 0.19 | 1.1 | 220 | 78 |
| 315 | meat and skin | 230 | 954 | 17.6 | 17.7 | 0 | 70 | 260 | 10 | 20 | 160 | 0.7 | 0.16 | 1.0 | — | 69 |
| 316 | light meat | 116 | 489 | 21.8 | 3.2 | 0 | 72 | 330 | 10 | 27 | 210[a] | 0.5 | 0.14 | 0.7 | 210 | 70 |
| 317 | dark meat | 126 | 528 | 19.1 | 5.5 | 0 | 89 | 300 | 11 | 22 | 180 | 0.9 | 0.25 | 1.6 | 220 | 86 |
| 318 | boiled, meat only | 183 | 767 | 29.2 | 7.3 | 0 | 82 | 300 | 11 | 25 | 190 | 1.2 | 0.20 | 2.0 | 300 | 90 |
| 319 | light meat | 163 | 686 | 29.7 | 4.9 | 0 | 70 | 370 | 9 | 26 | 200[a] | 0.6 | 0.17 | 1.0 | 290 | 82 |
| 320 | dark meat | 204 | 853 | 28.6 | 9.9 | 0 | 95 | 230 | 12 | 22 | 180 | 1.9 | 0.23 | 3.1 | 300 | 99 |
| 321 | roast, meat only | 148 | 621 | 24.8 | 5.4 | 0 | 81 | 310 | 9 | 24 | 210 | 0.8 | 0.12 | 1.5 | 260 | 87 |
| 322 | meat and skin | 216 | 902 | 22.6 | 14.0 | 0 | 72 | 270 | 9 | 21 | 170 | 0.8 | 0.12 | 1.4 | — | 77 |
| 323 | light meat | 142 | 599 | 26.5 | 4.0 | 0 | 71 | 330 | 9 | 26 | 220[a] | 0.5 | 0.11 | 1.0 | 250 | 79 |
| 324 | dark meat | 155 | 648 | 23.1 | 6.9 | 0 | 91 | 290 | 9 | 22 | 190 | 1.0 | 0.13 | 2.1 | 260 | 95 |
| 325 | wing quarter (weighed with bone) | 74 | 311 | 12.4 | 2.7 | 0 | 41 | 160 | 5 | 12 | 110 | 0.4 | 0.06 | 0.8 | 130 | 44 |
| 326 | leg quarter (weighed with bone) | 92 | 388 | 15.4 | 3.4 | 0 | 50 | 190 | 6 | 15 | 130 | 0.5 | 0.07 | 0.9 | 160 | 54 |
| 327 | **Duck** raw, meat only | 122 | 513 | 19.7 | 4.8 | 0 | 110 | 290 | 12 | 19 | 200 | 2.4 | 0.34 | 1.9 | 210 | 98 |
| 328 | meat, fat and skin | 430 | 1772 | 11.3 | 42.7 | 0 | 77 | 210 | 11 | 14 | 130 | 2.4 | 0.27 | 1.3 | — | 69 |
| 329 | roast, meat only | 189 | 789 | 25.3 | 9.7 | 0 | 96 | 270 | 13 | 20 | 200 | 2.7 | 0.31 | 2.6 | 270 | 96 |
| 330 | meat, fat and skin | 339 | 1406 | 19.6 | 29.0 | 0 | 76 | 210 | 12 | 16 | 150 | 2.7 | 0.27 | 1.8 | — | 75 |
| 331 | **Goose** roast | 319 | 1327 | 29.3 | 22.4 | 0 | 150 | 410 | 10 | 31 | 270 | 4.6 | (0.49) | — | 320 | 160 |
| 332 | **Grouse** roast | 173 | 728 | 31.3 | 5.3 | 0 | 96 | 470 | 30 | 41 | 340 | 7.6 | — | — | 340 | 130 |
| 333 | roast (weighed with bone) | 114 | 480 | 20.6 | 3.5 | 0 | 63 | 310 | 20 | 27 | 220 | 5.0 | — | — | 220 | 88 |
| 334 | **Partridge** roast | 212 | 890 | 36.7 | 7.2 | 0 | 100 | 410 | 46 | 36 | 310 | 7.7 | — | — | 400 | 99 |
| 335 | roast (weighed with bone) | 127 | 533 | 22.0 | 4.3 | 0 | 60 | 240 | 28 | 22 | 190 | 4.6 | — | — | 240 | 59 |

[a] In frozen chickens treated with polyphosphates the light meat may contain up to 250mg P per 100g

| No | Food | Retinol µg | Carotene µg | Vitamin D µg | Thiamin mg | Riboflavin mg | Nicotinic acid mg | Potential nicotinic acid from tryptophan mg Trp ÷ 60 | Vitamin C mg | Vitamin E mg |
|---|---|---|---|---|---|---|---|---|---|---|
| | ***Poultry and game*** | | | | | | | | | |
| 314 | **Chicken** raw, meat only | Tr | Tr | Tr | 0.10 | 0.16 | 7.8 | 3.8 | 0 | 0.10 |
| 315 | meat and skin | Tr | Tr | Tr | 0.08 | 0.14 | 6.0 | 3.3 | 0 | — |
| 316 | light meat | Tr | Tr | Tr | 0.10 | 0.10 | 9.9 | 4.1 | 0 | 0.08 |
| 317 | dark meat | Tr | Tr | Tr | 0.11 | 0.22 | 5.4 | 3.6 | 0 | 0.13 |
| 318 | boiled, meat only | Tr | Tr | Tr | 0.06 | 0.19 | 6.7 | 5.5 | 0 | 0.07 |
| 319 | light meat | Tr | Tr | Tr | 0.05 | 0.12 | 8.9 | 5.5 | 0 | — |
| 320 | dark meat | Tr | Tr | Tr | 0.07 | 0.28 | 4.3 | 5.3 | 0 | — |
| 321 | roast, meat only | Tr | Tr | Tr | 0.08 | 0.19 | 8.2 | 4.6 | 0 | 0.11 |
| 322 | meat and skin | Tr | Tr | Tr | — | — | — | 4.2 | 0 | — |
| 323 | light meat | Tr | Tr | Tr | 0.08 | 0.14 | 10.3 | 5.0 | 0 | 0.08 |
| 324 | dark meat | Tr | Tr | Tr | 0.09 | 0.24 | 6.1 | 4.3 | 0 | 0.15 |
| 325 | wing quarter (weighed with bone) | Tr | Tr | Tr | 0.04 | 0.10 | 4.1 | 2.3 | 0 | 0.06 |
| 326 | leg quarter (weighed with bone) | Tr | Tr | Tr | 0.05 | 0.12 | 5.1 | 2.9 | 0 | 0.07 |
| 327 | **Duck** raw, meat only | — | — | — | 0.36 | 0.45 | 5.3 | 4.2 | 0 | 0 |
| 328 | meat, fat and skin | — | — | — | — | — | — | 2.4 | 0 | — |
| 329 | roast, meat only | — | — | — | 0.26 | 0.47 | 5.1 | 5.4 | 0 | 0.02 |
| 330 | meat, fat and skin | — | — | — | — | — | — | 4.2 | — | — |
| 331 | **Goose** roast | — | — | — | — | — | — | 5.5 | — | — |
| 332 | **Grouse** roast | — | — | — | (0.32) | (0.54) | (8.8) | 5.8 | — | — |
| 333 | roast (weighed with bone) | — | — | — | (0.21) | (0.36) | (5.8) | 3.9 | — | — |
| 334 | **Partridge** roast | — | — | — | — | — | — | 6.9 | — | — |
| 335 | roast (weighed with bone) | — | — | — | — | — | — | 4.1 | — | — |

| No | Food | Vitamin $B_6$ mg | Vitamin $B_{12}$ µg | Folic acid Free µg | Folic acid Total µg | Pantothenic acid mg | Biotin µg | Notes |
|---|---|---|---|---|---|---|---|---|
| | ***Poultry and game*** | | | | | | | |
| 314 | **Chicken** raw, meat only | 0.42 | Tr | 10 | 12 | 1.2 | 2 | |
| 315 | meat and skin | 0.30 | Tr | 7 | 8 | 0.9 | 2 | |
| 316 | light meat | 0.53 | Tr | 8 | 12 | 1.2 | 2 | |
| 317 | dark meat | 0.30 | 1 | 12 | 12 | 1.3 | 3 | |
| 318 | boiled, meat only | 0.35 | Tr | 5 | 8 | 1.1 | 4 | |
| 319 | light meat | 0.33 | Tr | 4 | 4 | 1.0 | 3 | |
| 320 | dark meat | 0.37 | 1 | 7 | 13 | 1.1 | 4 | |
| 321 | roast, meat only | 0.26 | Tr | 8 | 10 | 1.2 | 3 | |
| 322 | meat and skin | — | Tr | — | — | — | — | |
| 323 | light meat | 0.35 | Tr | 6 | 7 | 1.1 | 2 | |
| 324 | dark meat | 0.16 | 1 | 10 | 13 | 1.3 | 3 | |
| 325 | wing quarter (weighed with bone) | 0.13 | Tr | 4 | 5 | 0.6 | 2 | |
| 326 | leg quarter (weighed with bone) | 0.16 | Tr | 5 | 6 | 0.7 | 2 | |
| 327 | **Duck** raw, meat only | 0.34 | 3 | 7 | 25 | 1.6 | 6 | |
| 328 | meat, fat and skin | — | — | — | — | — | — | |
| 329 | roast, meat only | 0.25 | 3 | 7 | 10 | 1.5 | 4 | |
| 330 | meat, fat and skin | — | — | — | — | — | — | |
| 331 | **Goose** roast | (0.43) | — | — | — | — | — | |
| 332 | **Grouse** roast | — | — | — | — | — | — | |
| 333 | roast (weighed with bone) | — | — | — | — | — | — | |
| 334 | **Partridge** roast | — | — | — | — | — | — | |
| 335 | roast (weighed with bone) | — | — | — | — | — | — | |

| No | Food | Description and number of samples | Edible matter, proportion of weight purchased | Water g | Total nitrogen g |
|---|---|---|---|---|---|
| | ***Poultry and game** contd* | | | | |
| 336 | **Pheasant** roast | Meat only | 0.45 | 56.9 | 5.15 |
| 337 | roast (weighed with bone) | Calculated from the previous item | 0.45 | 35.8 | 3.24 |
| 338 | **Pigeon** roast | Meat only | 0.28 | 57.2 | 4.44 |
| 339 | roast (weighed with bone) | Calculated from the previous item | 0.28 | 25.2 | 1.95 |
| 340 | **Turkey** raw, meat only | 5 samples, light and dark meat from dressed carcase | 0.57 | 75.5 | 3.51 |
| 341 | meat and skin | 5 samples, dressed carcase excluding waste | 0.70 | 72.0 | 3.29 |
| 342 | light meat | 5 samples | 0.32 | 75.2 | 3.71 |
| 343 | dark meat | 5 samples | 0.25 | 75.9 | 3.24 |
| 344 | roast, meat only | 5 samples, light and dark meat from dressed carcase | 0.46 | 68.0 | 4.61 |
| 345 | meat and skin | 5 samples, dressed carcase excluding waste | 0.57 | 65.0 | 4.48 |
| 346 | light meat | 5 samples | 0.25 | 68.4 | 4.76 |
| 347 | dark meat | 5 samples | 0.21 | 67.7 | 4.44 |
| | ***Other game*** | | | | |
| 348 | **Hare** stewed | Meat only | 0.44 | 60.7 | 4.78 |
| 349 | stewed (weighed with bone) | Calculated from the previous item | 0.44 | 44.3 | 3.48 |
| 350 | **Rabbit** raw | 9 samples, pieces of loin and leg, meat only | 0.62 | 74.6 | 3.50 |
| 351 | stewed | Meat only | 0.35 | 63.9 | 4.37 |
| 352 | stewed (weighed with bone) | Calculated from the previous item | 0.35 | 32.5 | 2.23 |
| 353 | **Venison** roast | Haunch, meat only | 0.58 | 56.8 | 5.60 |

| No | Food | Energy value kcal | Energy value kJ | Protein (N × 6.25) g | Fat g | Carbo-hydrate g | Na mg | K mg | Ca mg | Mg mg | P mg | Fe mg | Cu mg | Zn mg | S mg | Cl mg |
|---|---|---|---|---|---|---|---|---|---|---|---|---|---|---|---|---|
| | ***Poultry and game** contd* | | | | | | | | | | | | | | | |
| 336 | **Pheasant** roast | 213 | 892 | 32.2 | 9.3 | 0 | 100 | 410 | 49 | 35 | 310 | 8.4 | — | — | 310 | 110 |
| 337 | roast (weighed with bone) | 134 | 563 | 20.3 | 5.9 | 0 | 66 | 260 | 31 | 22 | 190 | 5.3 | — | — | 190 | 68 |
| 338 | **Pigeon** roast | 230 | 961 | 27.8 | 13.2 | 0 | 110 | 410 | 16 | 34 | 400 | 19.4 | — | — | 300 | 99 |
| 339 | roast (weighed with bone) | 101 | 422 | 12.2 | 5.8 | 0 | 46 | 180 | 7 | 15 | 180 | 8.5 | — | — | 130 | 44 |
| 340 | **Turkey** raw, meat only | 107 | 454 | 21.9 | 2.2 | 0 | 54 | 300 | 8 | 23 | 190 | 0.8 | 0.13 | 1.7 | 220 | 48 |
| 341 | meat and skin | 145 | 606 | 20.6 | 6.9 | 0 | 49 | 270 | 9 | 19 | 170 | 0.8 | 0.12 | 1.6 | — | 43 |
| 342 | light meat | 103 | 435 | 23.2 | 1.1 | 0 | 43 | 320 | 6 | 25 | 200 | 0.5 | 0.11 | 1.2 | 210 | 42 |
| 343 | dark meat | 114 | 478 | 20.3 | 3.6 | 0 | 68 | 270 | 11 | 21 | 180 | 1.2 | 0.16 | 2.4 | 220 | 55 |
| 344 | roast, meat only | 140 | 590 | 28.8 | 2.7 | 0 | 57 | 310 | 9 | 27 | 220 | 0.9 | 0.15 | 2.4 | 290 | 52 |
| 345 | meat and skin | 171 | 717 | 28.0 | 6.5 | 0 | 52 | 280 | 9 | 24 | 200 | 0.9 | 0.14 | 2.1 | — | 47 |
| 346 | light meat | 132 | 558 | 29.8 | 1.4 | 0 | 45 | 340 | 7 | 29 | 230 | 0.5 | 0.14 | 1.5 | 280 | 42 |
| 347 | dark meat | 148 | 624 | 27.8 | 4.1 | 0 | 71 | 270 | 12 | 23 | 210 | 1.4 | 0.16 | 3.5 | 300 | 62 |
| | ***Other game*** | | | | | | | | | | | | | | | |
| 348 | **Hare** stewed | 192 | 804 | 29.9 | 8.0 | 0 | 40 | 210 | 21 | 22 | 250 | 10.8 | — | — | 320 | 74 |
| 349 | stewed (weighed with bone) | 139 | 585 | 21.8 | 5.8 | 0 | 29 | 150 | 15 | 16 | 180 | 7.9 | — | — | 230 | 54 |
| 350 | **Rabbit** raw | 124 | 520 | 21.9 | 4.0 | 0 | 67 | 360 | 22 | 25 | 220 | 1.0 | 0.54 | 1.4 | 200 | 74 |
| 351 | stewed | 179 | 749 | 27.3 | 7.7 | 0 | 32 | 210 | 11 | 22 | 200 | 1.9 | — | — | 250 | 43 |
| 352 | stewed (weighed with bone) | 91 | 381 | 13.9 | 3.9 | 0 | 16 | 110 | 6 | 11 | 100 | 1.0 | — | — | 130 | 22 |
| 353 | **Venison** roast | 198 | 832 | 35.0 | 6.4 | 0 | 86 | 360 | 29 | 33 | 290 | 7.8 | — | — | 320 | 89 |

| No | Food | Retinol µg | Carotene µg | Vitamin D µg | Thiamin mg | Riboflavin mg | Nicotinic acid mg | Potential nicotinic acid from tryptophan mg Trp ÷ 60 | Vitamin C mg | Vitamin E mg |
|---|---|---|---|---|---|---|---|---|---|---|
| | ***Poultry and game** contd* | | | | | | | | | |
| 336 | **Pheasant** roast | — | — | — | (0.04) | (0.15) | (6.1) | 6.0 | 0 | — |
| 337 | roast (weighed with bone) | — | — | — | (0.03) | (0.09) | (3.8) | 3.8 | 0 | — |
| 338 | **Pigeon** roast | — | — | — | — | — | (8.9) | 5.2 | 0 | Tr |
| 339 | roast (weighed with bone) | — | — | — | — | — | (3.9) | 2.3 | 0 | Tr |
| 340 | **Turkey** raw, meat only | Tr | Tr | Tr | 0.09 | 0.16 | 7.9 | 4.1 | 0 | Tr |
| 341 | meat and skin | — | — | — | — | — | — | 3.8 | 0 | — |
| 342 | light meat | Tr | Tr | Tr | 0.08 | 0.11 | 9.9 | 4.3 | 0 | Tr |
| 343 | dark meat | Tr | Tr | Tr | 0.10 | 0.23 | 5.2 | 3.8 | 0 | Tr |
| 344 | roast, meat only | Tr | Tr | Tr | 0.07 | 0.21 | 8.5 | 5.4 | 0 | Tr |
| 345 | meat and skin | — | — | — | — | — | — | 5.2 | 0 | — |
| 346 | light meat | Tr | Tr | Tr | 0.07 | 0.14 | 10.0 | 5.6 | 0 | 0.02 |
| 347 | dark meat | Tr | Tr | Tr | 0.07 | 0.29 | 6.7 | 5.2 | 0 | Tr |
| | ***Other game*** | | | | | | | | | |
| 348 | **Hare** stewed | — | — | — | — | — | — | 5.6 | 0 | — |
| 349 | stewed (weighed with bone) | — | — | — | — | — | — | 4.1 | 0 | — |
| 350 | **Rabbit** raw | — | — | — | 0.10 | 0.19 | 8.4 | 4.1 | 0 | 0.13 |
| 351 | stewed | — | — | — | 0.07 | 0.28 | 8.5 | 5.1 | 0 | — |
| 352 | stewed (weighed with bone) | — | — | — | 0.04 | 0.14 | 4.3 | 2.6 | 0 | — |
| 353 | **Venison** roast | — | — | — | 0.22 | — | — | 6.5 | 0 | — |

| No | Food | Vitamin $B_6$ mg | Vitamin $B_{12}$ µg | Folic acid Free µg | Folic acid Total µg | Panto-thenic acid mg | Biotin µg | Notes |
|---|---|---|---|---|---|---|---|---|
| | ***Poultry and game** contd* | | | | | | | |
| 336 | **Pheasant** roast | — | — | — | — | — | — | |
| 337 | roast (weighed with bone) | — | — | — | — | — | — | |
| 338 | **Pigeon** roast | — | — | — | — | — | — | |
| 339 | roast (weighed with bone) | — | — | — | — | — | — | |
| 340 | **Turkey** raw, meat only | 0.46 | 2 | 11 | 15 | 0.8 | 2 | |
| 341 | meat and skin | — | — | — | — | — | — | |
| 342 | light meat | 0.59 | 1 | 7 | 8 | 0.8 | 1 | |
| 343 | dark meat | 0.30 | 3 | 17 | 25 | 0.9 | 2 | |
| 344 | roast, meat only | 0.32 | 2 | 12 | 15 | 0.8 | 2 | |
| 345 | meat and skin | — | — | — | — | — | — | |
| 346 | light meat | 0.31 | 1 | 9 | 13 | 0.7 | 1 | |
| 347 | dark meat | 0.32 | 3 | 16 | 17 | 0.9 | 2 | |
| | ***Other game*** | | | | | | | |
| 348 | **Hare** stewed | — | — | — | — | — | — | |
| 349 | stewed (weighed with bone) | — | — | — | — | — | — | |
| 350 | **Rabbit** raw | 0.50 | 10 | 4 | 5 | 0.8 | 1 | |
| 351 | stewed | 0.50 | 12 | 3 | 4 | 0.8 | 1 | |
| 352 | stewed (weighed with bone) | 0.26 | 6 | 2 | 2 | 0.4 | Tr | |
| 353 | **Venison** roast | — | — | — | — | — | — | |

| No | Food | Description and number of samples | Edible matter, proportion of weight purchased | Water g | Total nitrogen g |
|---|---|---|---|---|---|
| | ***Offal*** | | | | |
| 354 | **Brain, calf and lamb** raw | 14 samples | 1.00 | 79.4 | 1.64 |
| 355 | **calf,** boiled | 5 samples; soaked 2 hours, boiled 35 minutes | 0.80 | 73.4 | 2.03 |
| 356 | **lamb,** boiled | 11 samples; soaked 2 hours, boiled 20 minutes | 0.81 | 77.0 | 1.86 |
| 358 | **Heart, lamb** raw | 12 samples; fat and valves removed | 0.73 | 75.6 | 2.73 |
| 359 | **sheep,** roast | Ventricles only | 0.53 | 57.3 | 4.18 |
| 360 | **ox,** raw | 18 samples; fat and valves removed | 0.81 | 76.3 | 3.03 |
| 361 | stewed | 18 samples; fat and valves removed before cooking | 0.50 | 61.5 | 5.02 |
| 362 | **pig,** raw | Fat removed | — | 79.2 | 2.74 |
| 364 | **Kidney, lamb** raw | 19 samples; core removed | 0.93 | 78.9 | 2.64 |
| 365 | fried | 19 samples; core removed before cooking | 0.59 | 66.5 | 3.94 |
| 366 | **ox** raw | 18 samples; core removed | 0.82 | 79.8 | 2.51 |
| 367 | stewed | 18 samples; core removed before cooking, salt added | 0.51 | 64.1 | 4.09 |
| 368 | **pig** raw | 20 samples; core removed | 0.90 | 78.8 | 2.61 |
| 369 | stewed | 20 samples; core removed before cooking, salt added | 0.56 | 66.3 | 3.91 |
| 371 | **Liver, calf** raw | 12 samples | 1.00 | 69.7 | 3.21 |
| 372 | fried | 12 samples; coated in seasoned flour and fried | 0.84 | 52.6 | 4.31 |
| 373 | **chicken** raw | 16 samples | 1.00 | 72.9 | 3.05 |
| 374 | fried | 16 samples; coated in seasoned flour and fried | 0.84 | 64.2 | 3.31 |
| 375 | **lamb** raw | 33 samples | 1.00 | 67.3 | 3.22 |
| 376 | fried | 18 samples; coated in seasoned flour and fried | 0.88 | 58.4 | 3.67 |
| 377 | **ox** raw | 33 samples | 1.00 | 68.6 | 3.37 |
| 378 | stewed | 18 samples; coated in seasoned flour | 0.82 | 62.6 | 3.96 |

| No | Food | Energy value kcal | Energy value kJ | Protein (N × 6.25) g | Fat g | Carbo-hydrate g | Na mg | K mg | Ca mg | Mg mg | P mg | Fe mg | Cu mg | Zn mg | S mg | Cl mg |
|---|---|---|---|---|---|---|---|---|---|---|---|---|---|---|---|---|
| | ***Offal*** | | | | | | | | | | | | | | | |
| 354 | **Brain, calf and lamb** raw | 110 | 456 | 10.3 | 7.6 | 0 | 140 | 270 | (12)[a] | 15 | 340 | 1.6 | 0.30 | 1.2 | 130 | 150 |
| 355 | **calf** boiled | 152 | 630 | 12.7 | 11.2 | 0 | 210 | 190 | (16)[a] | 15 | 380 | 2.3 | 0.42 | 1.5 | — | 200 |
| 356 | **lamb** boiled | 126 | 523 | 11.6 | 8.8 | 0 | 210 | 190 | (11)[a] | 15 | 320 | 1.4 | 0.23 | 1.4 | — | 250 |
| 358 | **Heart, lamb** raw | 119 | 498 | 17.1 | 5.6 | 0 | 140 | 280 | 7 | 21 | 210 | 3.6 | 0.52 | 2.0 | 200 | 140 |
| 359 | **sheep** roast | 237 | 988 | 26.1 | 14.7 | 0 | 150 | 370 | 10 | 35 | 390 | 8.1 | — | — | 300 | 130 |
| 360 | **ox** raw | 108 | 455 | 18.9 | 3.6 | 0 | 95 | 320 | 5 | 25 | 230 | 4.9 | 0.43 | 2.0 | 190 | 95 |
| 361 | stewed | 179 | 752 | 31.4 | 5.9 | 0 | 180 | 210 | 7 | 29 | 270 | 7.7 | 0.73 | 3.5 | 310 | 210 |
| 362 | **pig** raw | 93 | 391 | 17.1 | 2.7 | 0 | 80 | 300 | 6 | 20 | 220 | 4.8 | — | — | 200 | 110 |
| 364 | **Kidney, lamb** raw | 90 | 380 | 16.5 | 2.7 | 0 | 220 | 270 | 10 | 17 | 260 | 7.4 | 0.42 | 2.4 | 180 | 270 |
| 365 | fried | 155 | 651 | 24.6 | 6.3 | 0 | 270 | 340 | 13 | 29 | 360 | 12.0 | (0.65) | 4.1 | 290 | 330 |
| 366 | **ox** raw | 86 | 363 | 15.7 | 2.6 | 0 | 180 | 230 | 10 | 15 | 230 | 5.7 | 0.42 | 1.9 | 170 | 200 |
| 367 | stewed | 172 | 720 | 25.6 | 7.7 | 0 | 400 | 180 | 16 | 19 | 300 | 8.0 | 0.66 | 3.0 | 270 | 520 |
| 368 | **pig** raw | 90 | 377 | 16.3 | 2.7 | 0 | 190 | 290 | 8 | 19 | 270 | 5.0 | 0.81 | 2.6 | 170 | 180 |
| 369 | stewed | 153 | 641 | 24.4 | 6.1 | 0 | 370 | 190 | 13 | 21 | 330 | 6.4 | 0.84 | 4.7 | — | 480 |
| 371 | **Liver, calf** raw | 153 | 642 | 20.1 | 7.3 | 1.9 | 93 | 330 | 7 | 20 | 360 | 8.0 | 11.0 | 7.8 | 240 | 89 |
| 372 | fried | 254 | 1063 | 26.9 | 13.2 | 7.3 | 170 | 410 | 15 | 26 | 470 | 7.5 | 12.0 | 6.2 | 300 | 210 |
| 373 | **chicken** raw | 135 | 567 | 19.1 | 6.3 | 0.6 | 85 | 300 | 8 | 21 | 320 | 9.5 | 0.52 | 3.4 | 220 | 100 |
| 374 | fried | 194 | 810 | 20.7 | 10.9 | 3.4 | 240 | 290 | 15 | 23 | 350 | 9.1 | 0.53 | 3.4 | 250 | 350 |
| 375 | **lamb** raw | 179 | 748 | 20.1 | 10.3 | 1.6 | 76 | 290 | 7 | 19 | 370 | 9.4 | 8.7 | 3.9 | 230 | 83 |
| 376 | fried | 232 | 970 | 22.9 | 14.0 | 3.9 | 190 | 300 | 12 | 22 | 400 | 10.0 | 9.9 | 4.4 | 270 | 250 |
| 377 | **ox** raw | 163 | 683 | 21.1 | 7.8 | 2.2 | 81 | 320 | 6 | 19 | 360 | 7.0 | 2.5 | 4.0 | 240 | 90 |
| 378 | stewed | 198 | 831 | 24.8 | 9.5 | 3.6 | 110 | 250 | 11 | 19 | 380 | 7.8 | 2.3 | 4.3 | 270 | 120 |

[a] The calcium content is extremely variable as scrapings of bone may easily be included in the edible portion. This is a minimum value

| No | Food | Retinol µg | Carotene µg | Vitamin D µg | Thiamin mg | Riboflavin mg | Nicotinic acid mg | Potential nicotinic acid from tryptophan mg Trp ÷ 60 | Vitamin C mg | Vitamin E mg |
|---|---|---|---|---|---|---|---|---|---|---|
| | ***Offal*** | | | | | | | | | |
| 354 | **Brain, calf and lamb** raw | Tr | Tr | Tr | 0.07 | 0.24 | 3.0 | 2.2 | 23 | 1.2 |
| 355 | **calf** boiled | Tr | Tr | Tr | 0.08 | 0.19 | 2.2 | 2.7 | 17 | 2.3 |
| 356 | **lamb** boiled | Tr | Tr | Tr | 0.10 | 0.24 | 2.1 | 2.5 | 17 | 1.1 |
| 358 | **Heart, lamb** raw | Tr | Tr | — | 0.48 | 0.9 | 6.9 | 3.6 | 7 | 0.37 |
| 359 | **sheep** roast | Tr | Tr | — | (0.45) | (1.5) | (9.1) | 5.6 | (11) | (0.70) |
| 360 | **ox** raw | Tr | Tr | — | 0.45 | 0.8 | 6.3 | 4.0 | 7 | 0.45 |
| 361 | stewed | Tr | Tr | — | 0.21 | 1.1 | 4.7 | 6.7 | 6 | 0.72 |
| 362 | **pig** raw | Tr | 0 | — | (0.48) | (0.9) | (6.9) | 3.7 | 5 | (0.37) |
| 364 | **Kidney, lamb** raw | 100 | — | — | 0.49 | 1.8 | 8.3 | 3.5 | 7 | 0.45 |
| 365 | fried | 160 | — | — | 0.56 | 2.3 | 9.6 | 5.3 | 9 | 0.41 |
| 366 | **ox** raw | 150 *(40–270)* | — | — | 0.37 | 2.1 | 6.0 | 3.4 | 10 | 0.18 |
| 367 | stewed | 250 | — | — | 0.25 | 2.1 | 4.8 | 5.5 | 10 | 0.42 |
| 368 | **pig** raw | 110 *(70–145)* | 0 | — | 0.32 | 1.9 | 7.5 | 3.5 | 14 | 0.38 |
| 369 | stewed | 140 | 0 | — | 0.19 | 2.1 | 6.1 | 5.2 | 11 | 0.36 |
| 371 | **Liver, calf** raw | 14 600 *(8300–31 700)* | 100 | 0.25 | 0.21 | 3.1 | 12.4 | 4.3 | 18 | 0.24 |
| 372 | fried | 17 400 | 100 | 0.25 | 0.27 | 4.2 | 15.6 | 5.8 | 13 | 0.50 |
| 373 | **chicken** raw | 9300 *(5700–12 800)* | 0 | 0.21 | 0.36 | 2.7 | 10.2 | 4.1 | 23 | 0.25 |
| 374 | fried | 11 100 | 0 | — | 0.37 | 1.7 | 10.5 | 4.4 | 13 | 0.34 |
| 375 | **lamb** raw | 18 100 *(3000–55 000)* | 60 | 0.50 | 0.27 | 3.3 | 14.2 | 4.3 | 10 | 0.46 |
| 376 | fried | 20 600 | 60 | 0.50 | 0.26 | 4.4 | 15.2 | 4.9 | 12 | 0.32 |
| 377 | **ox** raw | 16 500 *(11 600–24 000)* | 1540 | 1.13 | 0.23 | 3.1 | 13.4 | 4.5 | 23 | 0.42 |
| 378 | stewed | 20 100 | 1540 | 1.13 | 0.18 | 3.6 | 10.3 | 5.3 | 15 | 0.44 |

| No | Food | Vitamin $B_6$ mg | Vitamin $B_{12}$ µg | Folic acid Free µg | Folic acid Total µg | Pantothenic acid mg | Biotin µg | Notes |
|---|---|---|---|---|---|---|---|---|
| | ***Offal*** | | | | | | | |
| 354 | **Brain, calf and lamb** raw | 0.10 | 9 | 2 | 6 | 2.0 | 2 | |
| 355 | **calf,** boiled | 0.12 | 7 | 1 | 3 | 1.4 | 3 | |
| 356 | **lamb,** boiled | 0.08 | 8 | 1 | 6 | 1.4 | 3 | |
| 358 | **Heart, lamb,** raw | 0.29 | 8 | Tr | 2 | 2.5 | 4 | |
| 359 | **sheep** roast | (0.38) | (14) | (Tr) | (4) | (3.8) | (8) | |
| 360 | **ox** raw | 0.23 | 13 | 2 | 4 | 2.4 | 2 | |
| 361 | stewed | 0.11 | 15 | 1 | 2 | 1.6 | 4 | |
| 362 | **pig** raw | (0.29) | (8) | (Tr) | (2) | (2.5) | (4) | |
| 364 | **Kidney, lamb** raw | 0.30 | 55 | 20 | 31 | 4.3 | 37 | |
| 365 | fried | 0.30 | 79 | 39 | 79 | 5.1 | 42 | |
| 366 | **ox** raw | 0.32 | 31 | 56 | 77 | 3.1 | 24 | |
| 367 | stewed | 0.30 | 31 | 49 | 75 | 3.0 | 49 | |
| 368 | **pig** raw | 0.25 | 14 | 5 | 42 | 3.0 | 32 | |
| 369 | stewed | 0.28 | 15 | 12 | 43 | 2.4 | 53 | |
| 371 | **Liver, calf** raw | 0.54 | 100 | 190 | 240 | 8.4 | 39 | |
| 372 | fried | 0.73 | 87 | 220 | 320 | 8.8 | 53 | |
| 373 | **chicken** raw | 0.40 | 56 | 290 | 590 | 6.1 | 210 | |
| 374 | fried | 0.45 | 49 | 160 | 500 | 5.5 | 170 | |
| 375 | **lamb** raw | 0.42 | 84 | 150 | 220 | 8.2 | 41 | |
| 376 | fried | 0.49 | 81 | 140 | 240 | 7.6 | 41 | |
| 377 | **ox** raw | 0.83 | 110 | 220 | 330 | 8.1 | 33 | |
| 378 | stewed | 0.52 | 110 | 180 | 290 | 5.7 | 50 | |

| No | Food | Description and number of samples | Edible matter, proportion of weight purchased | Water g | Total nitrogen g |
|---|---|---|---|---|---|
| | ***Offal*** *contd* | | | | |
| 379 | **Liver, pig** raw | 33 samples | 1.00 | 69.5 | 3.41 |
| 380 | stewed | 18 samples; coated in seasoned flour | 0.79 | 62.1 | 4.09 |
| 381 | **Oxtail** raw | 12 samples, lean only | 0.38 | 68.6 | 3.20 |
| 382 | stewed | 12 samples, lean only; salt added | 0.27 | 53.9 | 4.88 |
| 383 | stewed (weighed with fat and bones) | Calculated from the previous item | 0.27 | 20.5 | 1.85 |
| 384 | **Sweetbread, lamb** raw | 12 samples | 1.00 | 75.5 | 2.44 |
| 385 | fried | 12 samples; soaked 2 hours, boiled for 1 hour then coated with egg and breadcrumbs and fried | 0.60 | 59.9 | 3.10 |
| 387 | **Tongue, lamb** raw | 20 samples, fat and skin removed | 0.57 | 67.9 | 2.45 |
| 388 | **sheep** stewed | Fat and skin removed | 0.33 | 56.9 | 2.91 |
| 389 | **ox** pickled, raw | 6 samples, fat and skin removed | 0.60 | 62.4 | 2.51 |
| 390 | boiled | Fat and skin removed | 0.38 | 48.6 | 3.12 |
| 391 | **Tripe** dressed | 18 samples; lime treated before purchase | 1.00 | 88.1 | 1.50 |
| 392 | stewed | 18 samples; lime treated before purchase, stewed in milk | 0.56 | 78.5 | 2.37 |

| No | Food | Energy value kcal | Energy value kJ | Protein (N × 6.25) g | Fat g | Carbo-hydrate g | Na mg | K mg | Ca mg | Mg mg | P mg | Fe mg | Cu mg | Zn mg | S mg | Cl mg |
|---|---|---|---|---|---|---|---|---|---|---|---|---|---|---|---|---|
| | ***Offal** contd* | | | | | | | | | | | | | | | |
| 379 | **Liver, pig** raw | 154 | 647 | 21.3 | 6.8 | 2.1 | 87 | 320 | 6 | 21 | 370 | 21.0 | 2.7 | 6.9 | 230 | 95 |
| 380 | stewed | 189 | 793 | 25.6 | 8.1 | 3.6 | 130 | 250 | 11 | 22 | 390 | 17.0 | 2.5 | 8.2 | 280 | 150 |
| 381 | **Oxtail** raw | 171 | 714 | 20.0 | 10.1 | 0 | 110 | 270 | 9 | 20 | 160 | 2.7 | 0.20 | 5.6 | 190 | 110 |
| 382 | stewed | 243 | 1014 | 30.5 | 13.4 | 0 | 190 | 170 | 14 | 18 | 140 | 3.8 | 0.27 | 8.8 | 290 | 270 |
| 383 | stewed (weighed with bones) | 92 | 386 | 11.6 | 5.1 | 0 | 72 | 65 | 5 | 7 | 53 | 1.4 | 0.10 | 3.3 | 110 | 100 |
| 384 | **Sweetbread, lamb** raw | 131 | 549 | 15.3 | 7.8 | 0 | 75 | 420 | 8 | 21 | 400 | 1.7 | 0.20 | 1.9 | 140 | 120 |
| 385 | fried | 230 | 960 | 19.4 | 14.6 | 5.6 | 210 | 260 | 34 | 23 | 420 | 1.8 | 0.22 | 2.1 | 160 | 260 |
| 387 | **Tongue, lamb** raw | 193 | 800 | 15.3 | 14.6 | 0 | 420 | 250 | 6 | 33 | 170 | 2.2 | 0.64 | 2.7 | 190 | 550 |
| 388 | **sheep** stewed | 289 | 1197 | 18.2 | 24.0 | 0 | 80 | 110 | 11 | 13 | 200 | 3.4 | — | — | 190 | 80 |
| 389 | **ox** pickled, raw | 220 | 914 | 15.7 | 17.5 | 0 | 1210 | 300 | 7 | 19 | 150 | 4.9 | 0.37 | 3.5 | 190 | 1750 |
| 390 | boiled | 293 | 1216 | 19.5 | 23.9 | 0 | 1000 | 150 | 31 | 16 | 230 | 3.0 | — | — | 200 | 1450 |
| 391 | **Tripe** dressed | 60 | 252 | 9.4 | 2.5 | 0 | 46 | 8 | 75 | 8 | 37 | 0.5 | 0.09 | 1.5 | 80 | 8 |
| 392 | stewed | 100 | 418 | 14.8 | 4.5 | Tr | 73 | 100 | 150 | 15 | 90 | 0.7 | 0.14 | 2.3 | 140 | 58 |

| No | Food | Retinol µg | Carotene µg | Vitamin D µg | Thiamin mg | Riboflavin mg | Nicotinic acid mg | Potential nicotinic acid from tryptophan mg Trp ÷ 60 | Vitamin C mg | Vitamin E mg |
|---|---|---|---|---|---|---|---|---|---|---|
| | ***Offal*** *contd* | | | | | | | | | |
| 379 | **Liver, pig** raw | 9200 | 0 | 1.13 | 0.31 | 3.0 | 14.8 | 4.6 | 13 | 0.17 |
| | | *(5600–14 200)* | | | | | | | | |
| 380 | stewed | 11 600 | 0 | 1.13 | 0.21 | 3.1 | 11.5 | 5.5 | 9 | 0.16 |
| 381 | **Oxtail** raw | Tr | Tr | Tr | 0.03 | 0.29 | 4.5 | 4.3 | 0 | 0.29 |
| 382 | stewed | Tr | Tr | Tr | 0.02 | 0.28 | 3.3 | 6.5 | 0 | 0.45 |
| 383 | stewed (weighed with bones) | Tr | Tr | Tr | 0.01 | 0.11 | 1.3 | 2.5 | 0 | 0.17 |
| 384 | **Sweetbread, lamb** raw | Tr | Tr | Tr | 0.03 | 0.25 | 3.7 | 3.3 | 18 | 0.44 |
| 385 | fried | Tr | Tr | Tr | 0.03 | 0.24 | 2.1 | 4.1 | 18 | 1.2 |
| 387 | **Tongue, lamb** raw | Tr | Tr | Tr | 0.17 | 0.49 | 4.9 | 3.3 | 7 | 0.21 |
| 388 | **sheep** stewed | Tr | Tr | Tr | (0.13) | (0.45) | (3.7) | 3.9 | (6) | (0.32) |
| 389 | **ox** pickled, raw | Tr | Tr | Tr | 0.10 | 0.38 | 6.4 | 3.4 | 3 | 0.28 |
| 390 | boiled | Tr | Tr | Tr | (0.06) | (0.29) | (4.1) | 4.2 | (2) | (0.35) |
| 391 | **Tripe** dressed | Tr | Tr | Tr | Tr | 0.01 | 0.06 | 2.0 | (3) | 0.08 |
| 392 | stewed | Tr | Tr | Tr | Tr | 0.08 | 0.02 | 3.2 | (3) | 0.09 |

| No | Food | Vitamin $B_6$ mg | Vitamin $B_{12}$ µg | Folic acid Free µg | Folic acid Total µg | Panto-thenic acid mg | Biotin µg | Notes |
|---|---|---|---|---|---|---|---|---|
| | ***Offal** contd* | | | | | | | |
| 379 | **Liver, pig** raw | 0.68 | 25 | 59 | 110 | 6.5 | 27 | |
| 380 | stewed | 0.64 | 26 | 33 | 110 | 4.6 | 34 | |
| 381 | **Oxtail** raw | 0.27 | 3 | 3 | 7 | 1.0 | 1 | |
| 382 | stewed | 0.14 | 2 | 3 | 9 | 0.9 | 2 | |
| 383 | stewed (weighed with bones) | 0.05 | 1 | 1 | 3 | 0.3 | 1 | |
| 384 | **Sweetbread, lamb** raw | 0.03 | 6 | 11 | 13 | 1.0 | 3 | |
| 385 | fried | 0.02 | 4 | 6 | 14 | 0.8 | 5 | |
| 387 | **Tongue, lamb** raw | 0.17 | 7 | 1 | 4 | 1.0 | 1 | |
| 388 | **sheep** stewed | (0.10) | (7) | (Tr) | (4) | (0.8) | (2) | |
| 389 | **ox** pickled, raw | 0.18 | 5 | 3 | 6 | 0.8 | 2 | |
| 390 | boiled | (0.09) | (4) | (2) | (5) | (0.5) | (3) | |
| 391 | **Tripe** dressed | Tr | Tr | Tr | 2 | Tr | Tr | |
| 392 | stewed | 0.02 | Tr | Tr | 1 | 0.2 | 2 | |

| No | Food | Description and number of samples | Edible matter, proportion of weight purchased | Water g | Total nitrogen g |
|---|---|---|---|---|---|
| | ***Meat products and dishes*** | | | | |
| | ***Canned meats*** | | | | |
| 393 | **Beef, corned** | 18 samples | 1.00 | 58.5 | 4.30 |
| 394 | **Ham** | 12 samples, 10 brands | 1.00 | 72.5 | 2.95 |
| 395 | **Ham and pork** chopped | 12 samples, 5 brands | 1.00 | 58.5 | 2.30 |
| 396 | **Luncheon meat** | 18 samples | 1.00 | 51.5 | 2.02 |
| 397 | **Stewed steak with gravy** | 12 samples, 8 brands | 1.00 | 70.0 | 2.37 |
| 398 | **Tongue** | 18 samples, lamb and ox | 1.00 | 63.9 | 2.56 |
| 400 | **Veal, jellied** | 18 samples | 1.00 | 68.8 | 4.00 |
| | ***Offal products*** | | | | |
| 401 | **Black pudding** fried | 24 samples | — | 44.0 | 2.06 |
| 402 | **Faggots** | 38 samples | 1.00 | 47.1 | 1.78 |
| 403 | **Haggis** boiled | 8 samples | 0.95 | 46.2 | 1.71 |
| 404 | **Liver sausage** | 24 samples | 1.00 | 51.8 | 2.06 |
| | ***Sausages*** | | | | |
| 405 | **Frankfurters** | 12 samples (cans and packets), 6 brands | 1.00 | 59.5 | 1.52 |
| 406 | **Polony** | 24 samples | 1.00 | 52.0 | 1.50 |
| 407 | **Salami** | 24 samples, 8 different countries of origin | 1.00 | 28.0 | 3.09 |
| 408 | **Sausages, beef** raw | 20 samples | 1.00 | 50.3 | 1.54 |
| 409 | fried | 20 samples | 0.75 | 47.7 | 2.07 |
| 410 | grilled | 20 samples | 0.75 | 47.9 | 2.08 |
| 411 | **Sausages, pork** raw | 18 samples | 1.00 | 45.4 | 1.69 |
| 412 | fried | 18 samples | 0.70 | 44.9 | 2.20 |
| 413 | grilled | 18 samples | 0.72 | 45.1 | 2.13 |
| 414 | **Saveloy** | 60 samples | 1.00 | 56.7 | 1.59 |

| No | Food | Energy value kcal | Energy value kJ | Protein (N × 6.25) g | Fat g | Carbo-hydrate g | Na mg | K mg | Ca mg | Mg mg | P mg | Fe mg | Cu mg | Zn mg | S mg | Cl mg |
|---|---|---|---|---|---|---|---|---|---|---|---|---|---|---|---|---|
| | ***Meat products and dishes*** | | | | | | | | | | | | | | | |
| | ***Canned meats*** | | | | | | | | | | | | | | | |
| 393 | **Beef, corned** | 217 | 905 | 26.9 | 12.1 | 0 | 950 | 140 | 14 | 15 | 120 | 2.9 | 0.24 | 5.6 | 240 | 1430 |
| 394 | **Ham** | 120 | 502 | 18.4 | 5.1 | 0 | 1250 | 280 | 9 | 18 | 280 | 1.2 | 0.22 | 2.3 | 180 | 1670 |
| 395 | **Ham and pork** chopped | 270 | 1118 | 14.4 | 23.6 | 0 | 1090 | 230 | 14 | 13 | 250 | 1.2 | 0.24 | 2.9 | 140 | 1210 |
| 396 | **Luncheon meat** | 313 | 1298 | 12.6 | 26.9 | 5.5 | 1050 | 140 | 15 | 8 | 200 | 1.1 | 0.33 | 2.2 | 120 | 1290 |
| 397 | **Stewed steak with gravy** | 176 | 730 | 14.8 | 12.5 | 1.0 | 380 | 240 | 14 | 14 | 98 | 2.1 | 0.19 | 3.3 | 130 | 550 |
| 398 | **Tongue** | 213 | 883 | 16.0 | 16.5 | 0 | 1050 | 97 | 32 | 14 | 140 | 2.5 | 0.29 | 2.3 | 210 | 1430 |
| 400 | **Veal, jellied** | 125 | 529 | 25.0 | 2.8 | 0 | 1190 | 240 | 15 | 19 | 180 | 1.5 | 0.34 | 3.3 | 230 | 1650 |
| | ***Offal products*** | | | | | | | | | | | | | | | |
| 401 | **Black pudding** fried | 305 | 1270 | 12.9 | 21.9 | 15.0 | 1210 | 140 | 35 | 16 | 110 | 20.0 | 0.37 | 1.3 | 110 | 1770 |
| 402 | **Faggots** | 268 | 1118 | 11.1 | 18.5 | 15.3 | 820 | 170 | 55 | 18 | 120 | 8.3 | 0.60 | 1.6 | 120 | 1160 |
| 403 | **Haggis** boiled | 310 | 1292 | 10.7 | 21.7 | 19.2 | 770 | 170 | 29 | 36 | 160 | 4.8 | 0.44 | 1.9 | 120 | 1200 |
| 404 | **Liver sausage** | 310 | 1283 | 12.9 | 26.9 | 4.3 | 860 | 170 | 26 | 12 | 230 | 6.4 | 0.63 | 2.3 | 130 | 1140 |
| | ***Sausages*** | | | | | | | | | | | | | | | |
| 405 | **Frankfurters** | 274 | 1135 | 9.5 | 25.0 | 3.0 | 980 | 98 | 34 | 9 | 130 | 1.5 | 0.24 | 1.4 | 90 | 1280 |
| 406 | **Polony** | 281 | 1168 | 9.4 | 21.1 | 14.2 | 870 | 120 | 42 | 13 | 130 | 1.3 | 0.32 | 1.2 | 90 | 1160 |
| 407 | **Salami** | 491 | 2031 | 19.3 | 45.2 | 1.9 | 1850 | 160 | 10 | 10 | 160 | 1.0 | 0.24 | 1.7 | 190 | 2460 |
| 408 | **Sausages, beef** raw | 299 | 1242 | 9.6 | 24.1 | 11.7 | 810 | 150 | 48 | 13 | 150 | 1.4 | 0.23 | 1.2 | 120 | 1100 |
| 409 | fried | 269 | 1124 | 12.9 | 18.0 | 14.9 | 1090 | 180 | 64 | 16 | 210 | 1.6 | 0.36 | 1.6 | 140 | 1470 |
| 410 | grilled | 265 | 1104 | 13.0 | 17.3 | 15.2 | 1100 | 190 | 73 | 17 | 210 | 1.7 | 0.30 | 1.7 | 140 | 1490 |
| 411 | **Sausages, pork** raw | 367 | 1520 | 10.6 | 32.1 | 9.5 | 760 | 160 | 41 | 11 | 160 | 1.1 | 0.27 | 1.2 | 120 | 1030 |
| 412 | fried | 317 | 1317 | 13.8 | 24.5 | 11.0 | 1050 | 200 | 55 | 15 | 210 | 1.5 | 0.37 | 1.7 | 160 | 1440 |
| 413 | grilled | 318 | 1320 | 13.3 | 24.6 | 11.5 | 1000 | 200 | 53 | 15 | 220 | 1.5 | 0.34 | 1.6 | 160 | 1340 |
| 414 | **Saveloy** | 262 | 1088 | 9.9 | 20.5 | 10.1 | 890 | 160 | 23 | 9 | 210 | 1.5 | 0.27 | 1.4 | 90 | 1030 |

| No | Food | Retinol µg | Carotene µg | Vitamin D µg | Thiamin mg | Riboflavin mg | Nicotinic acid mg | Potential nicotinic acid from tryptophan mg Trp ÷ 60 | Vitamin C mg | Vitamin E mg |
|---|---|---|---|---|---|---|---|---|---|---|
| | ***Meat products and dishes*** | | | | | | | | | |
| | ***Canned meats*** | | | | | | | | | |
| 393 | **Beef, corned** | Tr | Tr | Tr | Tr | 0.23 | 2.5 | 6.5 | 0 | 0.78 |
| 394 | **Ham** | Tr | Tr | Tr | 0.52 | 0.25 | 3.9 | 3.0 | 0[a] | 0.08 |
| 395 | **Ham and pork** chopped | Tr | Tr | Tr | 0.19 | 0.21 | 3.2 | 2.7 | 0[a] | 0.11 |
| 396 | **Luncheon meat** | Tr | Tr | Tr | 0.07 | 0.12 | 1.8 | 2.7 | 0[a] | 0.11 |
| 397 | **Stewed steak with gravy** | Tr | Tr | Tr | Tr | 0.13 | 2.4 | 2.8 | 0 | 0.59 |
| 398 | **Tongue** | Tr | Tr | Tr | 0.04 | 0.39 | 2.5 | 3.8 | 0 | 0.26 |
| 400 | **Veal, jellied** | Tr | Tr | Tr | 0.05 | 0.29 | 6.0 | 4.7 | 0 | 0.12 |
| | ***Offal products*** | | | | | | | | | |
| 401 | **Black pudding** fried | Tr | Tr | Tr | 0.09 | 0.07 | 1.0 | 2.8 | 0 | 0.24 |
| 402 | **Faggots** | (1500) | Tr | (0.2) | 0.14 | 0.49 | 3.0 | 2.1 | Tr | — |
| 403 | **Haggis** boiled | (1800) | Tr | (0.05) | 0.16 | 0.35 | 1.5 | 2.0 | Tr | 0.41 |
| 404 | **Liver sausage** | (8300) | Tr | (0.6) | 0.17 | 1.58 | 4.3 | 2.4 | Tr | 0.10 |
| | ***Sausages*** | | | | | | | | | |
| 405 | **Frankfurters** | Tr | Tr | Tr | 0.08 | 0.12 | 1.5 | 1.5 | 0 | 0.25 |
| 406 | **Polony** | Tr | Tr | Tr | 0.17 | 0.10 | 1.5 | 1.8 | 0 | 0.09 |
| 407 | **Salami** | Tr | Tr | Tr | 0.21 | 0.23 | 4.6 | 3.6 | 0 | 0.28 |
| 408 | **Sausages, beef** raw | Tr | Tr | Tr | 0.03 | 0.13 | 5.0 | 2.1 | 0 | 0.43 |
| 409 | fried | Tr | Tr | Tr | Tr | 0.14 | 6.9 | 2.8 | 0 | 0.28 |
| 410 | grilled | Tr | Tr | Tr | Tr | 0.14 | 5.4 | 2.8 | 0 | 0.22 |
| 411 | **Sausages, pork** raw | Tr | Tr | Tr | 0.04 | 0.12 | 3.4 | 2.3 | 0 | 0.24 |
| 412 | fried | Tr | Tr | Tr | 0.01 | 0.16 | 4.4 | 2.9 | 0 | 0.28 |
| 413 | grilled | Tr | Tr | Tr | 0.02 | 0.15 | 4.0 | 2.8 | 0 | 0.22 |
| 414 | **Saveloy** | Tr | Tr | Tr | 0.14 | 0.09 | 1.9 | 1.9 | 0 | 0.08 |

| No | Food | Vitamin $B_6$ mg | Vitamin $B_{12}$ µg | Folic acid Free µg | Folic acid Total µg | Panto-thenic acid mg | Biotin µg |
|---|---|---|---|---|---|---|---|
| | ***Meat products and dishes*** | | | | | | |
| | ***Canned meats*** | | | | | | |
| 393 | **Beef, corned** | 0.06 | 2 | 1 | 2 | 0.4 | 2 |
| 394 | **Ham** | 0.22 | Tr | Tr | Tr | 0.6 | 1 |
| 395 | **Ham and pork** chopped | 0.05 | 1 | Tr | 1 | 0.4 | 2 |
| 396 | **Luncheon meat** | 0.02 | 1 | Tr | 1 | 0.5 | Tr |
| 397 | **Stewed steak with gravy** | 0.07 | 1 | 1 | 4 | 0.3 | 1 |
| 398 | **Tongue** | 0.04 | 5 | Tr | 2 | 0.4 | 2 |
| 400 | **Veal, jellied** | 0.14 | 2 | 3 | 3 | 0.3 | 3 |
| | ***Offal products*** | | | | | | |
| 401 | **Black pudding** fried | 0.04 | 1 | 2 | 5 | 0.6 | 2 |
| 402 | **Faggots** | 0.17 | 5 | 19 | 22 | 1.1 | 4 |
| 403 | **Haggis** boiled | 0.07 | 2 | 4 | 8 | 0.5 | 12 |
| 404 | **Liver sausage** | 0.14 | 8 | 13 | 19 | 1.5 | 7 |
| | ***Sausages*** | | | | | | |
| 405 | **Frankfurters** | 0.03 | 1 | Tr | 1 | 0.4 | 2 |
| 406 | **Polony** | 0.08 | Tr | 2 | 4 | 0.5 | Tr |
| 407 | **Salami** | 0.15 | 1 | 2 | 3 | 0.8 | 3 |
| 408 | **Sausages, beef** raw | 0.06 | Tr | 2 | 2 | 0.5 | 2 |
| 409 | fried | 0.07 | 1 | 2 | 2 | 0.5 | 2 |
| 410 | grilled | 0.07 | 1 | 2 | 4 | 0.5 | 2 |
| 411 | **Sausages, pork** raw | 0.07 | 1 | Tr | 1 | 0.6 | 2 |
| 412 | fried | 0.07 | 1 | Tr | 2 | 0.6 | 3 |
| 413 | grilled | 0.06 | 1 | 1 | 3 | 0.6 | 3 |
| 414 | **Saveloy** | 0.06 | Tr | 1 | 1 | 0.4 | Tr |

Notes

[a] Some brands have ascorbic acid added, and may contain from 12 to 60mg per 100g.

| No | Food | Description and number of samples | Edible matter, proportion of weight purchased | Water g | Total nitrogen g |
|---|---|---|---|---|---|
| | ***Meat products and dishes** contd* | | | | |
| 415 | **Beefburgers** frozen, raw | 36 samples, 6 brands | 1.00 | 56.3 | 2.43 |
| 416 | fried | 36 samples, 6 brands | 0.76 | 53.0 | 3.27 |
| 417 | **Brawn** | 10 samples | 1.00 | 72.0 | 1.99 |
| 418 | **Meat paste** | 67 samples, beef, chicken, ham and tongue, liver and bacon | 1.00 | 67.1 | 2.43 |
| 419 | **White pudding** | 6 samples | 1.00 | 22.8 | 1.12 |
| | ***Meat and pastry products*** | | | | |
| 420 | **Cornish pastie** | 18 pasties, average 62% pastry, 38% filling | 1.00 | 39.2 | 1.28 |
| 421 | **Pork pie** individual | 18 pies, average 55% pastry, 42% meat filling, 3% jelly | 1.00 | 36.8 | 1.56 |
| 422 | **Sausage roll** flaky pastry | Recipe p 341 | — | 23.0 | 1.21 |
| 423 | short pastry | Recipe p 341 | — | 21.8 | 1.36 |
| 424 | **Steak and kidney pie** pastry top only | Recipe p 341 | — | 48.8 | 2.47 |
| 425 | individual | 10 pies, purchased cooked; pastry top and bottom | 1.00 | 42.6 | 1.46 |
| | ***Cooked dishes*** | | | | |
| 426 | **Beef steak pudding** | Recipe p 342 | — | 57.9 | 1.77 |
| 427 | **Beef stew** | Recipe p 342 | — | 77.7 | 1.54 |
| 428 | **Bolognese sauce** | Recipe p 342 | — | 75.0 | 1.27 |
| 429 | **Curried meat** | Recipe p 342 | — | 68.2 | 1.55 |
| 430 | **Hot pot** | Recipe p 342 | — | 72.1 | 1.48 |
| 431 | **Irish stew** | Recipe p 342 | — | 76.0 | 0.83 |
| 432 | **Irish stew** (weighed with bones) | Calculated from the previous item | — | 69.4 | 0.76 |
| 433 | **Moussaka** | Recipe p 343 | — | 65.7 | 1.49 |
| 434 | **Shepherd's pie** | Recipe p 343 | — | 76.1 | 1.24 |

| No | Food | Energy value kcal | Energy value kJ | Protein g | Fat g | Carbo-hydrate g | Na (mg) | K (mg) | Ca (mg) | Mg (mg) | P (mg) | Fe (mg) | Cu (mg) | Zn (mg) | S (mg) | Cl (mg) |
|---|---|---|---|---|---|---|---|---|---|---|---|---|---|---|---|---|
| | ***Meat products and dishes** contd* | | | | | | | | | | | | | | | |
| 415 | **Beefburgers** frozen, raw | 265 | 1102 | 15.2 | 20.5 | 5.3 | 600 | 270 | 23 | 17 | 190 | 2.5 | 0.25 | 3.2 | 160 | 800 |
| 416 | fried | 264 | 1099 | 20.4 | 17.3 | 7.0 | 880 | 340 | 33 | 23 | 250 | 3.1 | 0.28 | 4.2 | 220 | 1120 |
| 417 | **Brawn** | 153 | 636 | 12.4 | 11.5 | 0 | 750 | 85 | 38 | 7 | 59 | 1.0 | 0.19 | 1.3 | 100 | 1110 |
| 418 | **Meat paste** | 173 | 721 | 15.2 | 11.2 | 3.0 | 740 | 160 | 86 | 15 | 170 | 2.3 | 0.31 | 2.3 | 150 | 1060 |
| 419 | **White pudding** | 450 | 1876 | 7.0 | 31.8 | 36.3 | 370 | 190 | 38 | 61 | 230 | 2.1 | 0.43 | 1.6 | 110 | 600 |
| | ***Meat and pastry products*** | | | | | | | | | | | | | | | |
| 420 | **Cornish pastie** | 332 | 1388 | 8.0 | 20.4 | 31.1 | 590 | 190 | 60 | 18 | 110 | 1.5 | 0.35 | 1.0 | 100 | 860 |
| 421 | **Pork pie** individual | 376 | 1564 | 9.8 | 27.0 | 24.9 | 720 | 150 | 47 | 16 | 120 | 1.4 | 0.32 | 1.0 | 100 | 1030 |
| 422 | **Sausage roll** flaky pastry | 479 | 1991 | 7.2 | 36.2 | 33.1 | 550 | 110 | 70 | 13 | 97 | 1.3 | 0.17 | 0.7 | — | 810 |
| 423 | short pastry | 463 | 1929 | 8.1 | 31.8 | 38.4 | 580 | 120 | 82 | 15 | 110 | 1.5 | 0.18 | 0.7 | — | 850 |
| 424 | **Steak and kidney pie** pastry top only | 286 | 1195 | 15.2 | 18.3 | 16.2 | 680 | 240 | 37 | 20 | 140 | 2.8 | 0.21 | 2.4 | — | 1020 |
| 425 | individual | 323 | 1349 | 9.1 | 21.2 | 25.6 | 510 | 140 | 53 | 18 | 110 | 2.5 | 0.10 | 1.2 | — | 720 |
| | ***Cooked dishes*** | | | | | | | | | | | | | | | |
| 426 | **Beef steak pudding** | 223 | 934 | 10.8 | 12.1 | 18.9 | 360 | 180 | 110 | 15 | 140 | 1.5 | 0.11 | 1.8 | — | 430 |
| 427 | **Beef stew** | 119 | 498 | 9.6 | 7.5 | 3.6 | 400 | 200 | 19 | 14 | 73 | 1.2 | 0.10 | 1.8 | — | 590 |
| 428 | **Bolognese sauce** | 139 | 579 | 8.0 | 10.9 | 2.5 | 440 | 310 | 26 | 18 | 81 | 1.6 | 0.14 | 1.9 | 82 | 670 |
| 429 | **Curried meat** | 160 | 668 | 9.6 | 10.1 | 8.2 | 480 | 210 | 33 | 22 | 71 | 2.9 | 0.16 | 2.5 | — | 710 |
| 430 | **Hot pot** | 114 | 480 | 9.3 | 4.2 | 10.4 | 670 | 430 | 22 | 25 | 83 | 1.2 | 0.16 | 1.7 | — | 1040 |
| 431 | **Irish stew** | 124 | 520 | 5.2 | 7.3 | 10.1 | 360 | 340 | 12 | 18 | 60 | 0.6 | 0.12 | 1.1 | — | 570 |
| 432 | **Irish stew** (weighed with bones) | 114 | 475 | 4.7 | 6.7 | 9.2 | 330 | 310 | 11 | 16 | 55 | 0.5 | 0.11 | 1.0 | — | 520 |
| 433 | **Moussaka** | 195 | 811 | 9.3 | 13.4 | 9.8 | 320 | 350 | 88 | 21 | 130 | 1.3 | 0.13 | 1.8 | 99 | 510 |
| 434 | **Shepherd's pie** | 119 | 497 | 7.6 | 6.1 | 8.9 | 450 | 240 | 15 | 16 | 69 | 1.1 | 0.13 | 1.9 | 79 | 670 |

| No | Food | Retinol µg | Carotene µg | Vitamin D µg | Thiamin mg | Riboflavin mg | Nicotinic acid mg | Potential nicotinic acid from tryptophan mgTrp ÷60 | Vitamin C mg | Vitamin E mg |
|---|---|---|---|---|---|---|---|---|---|---|
| | ***Meat products and dishes** contd* | | | | | | | | | |
| 415 | **Beefburgers** frozen, raw | Tr | Tr | Tr | 0.04 | 0.21 | 3.7 | 2.8 | 0 | 0.27 |
| 416 | fried | Tr | Tr | Tr | 0.02 | 0.23 | 4.2 | 3.8 | 0 | 0.58 |
| 417 | **Brawn** | Tr | Tr | Tr | 0.05 | 0.08 | 1.0 | 2.3 | 0 | 0.06 |
| 418 | **Meat paste** | Tr | Tr | Tr | 0.03 | 0.26 | 3.8 | 2.8 | 0 | 0.17 |
| 419 | **White pudding** | Tr | Tr | Tr | 0.26 | 0.08 | 0.5 | 1.3 | 0 | 1.0 |
| | ***Meat and pastry products*** | | | | | | | | | |
| 420 | **Cornish pastie** | Tr | Tr | Tr | 0.10 | 0.06 | 1.6 | 1.7 | 0 | 1.3 |
| 421 | **Pork pie** individual | Tr | Tr | Tr | 0.16 | 0.09 | 1.8 | 2.1 | 0 | 0.43 |
| 422 | **Sausage roll** flaky pastry | 125 | Tr | 1.11 | 0.11 | 0.04 | 1.8 | 1.5 | 0 | 1.3 |
| 423 | short pastry | 100 | Tr | 0.86 | 0.12 | 0.04 | 2.0 | 1.7 | 0 | 1.0 |
| 424 | **Steak and kidney pie** pastry top only | 100 | Tr | — | 0.14 | 0.52 | 3.6 | 3.2 | 2 | 0.7 |
| 425 | individual | — | Tr | — | 0.12 | 0.15 | 1.7 | 1.7 | 0 | — |
| | ***Cooked dishes*** | | | | | | | | | |
| 426 | **Beef steak pudding** | Tr | Tr | Tr | 0.08 | 0.09 | 1.8 | 0.6 | Tr | 0.2 |
| 427 | **Beef stew** | Tr | 1600 | Tr | 0.04 | 0.10 | 1.7 | 2.1 | Tr | 0.15 |
| 428 | **Bolognese sauce** | Tr | 1940 | Tr | 0.06 | 0.12 | 1.6 | 1.7 | 5 | 1.3 |
| 429 | **Curried meat** | Tr | Tr | Tr | 0.02 | 0.09 | 0.9 | 2.0 | 2 | 0.83 |
| 430 | **Hot pot** | Tr | 1900 | Tr | 0.07 | 0.10 | 1.8 | 2.0 | 5 | 0.20 |
| 431 | **Irish stew** | Tr | Tr | Tr | 0.06 | 0.07 | 1.4 | 1.7 | 4 | 0.11 |
| 432 | **Irish stew** (weighed with bones) | Tr | Tr | Tr | 0.05 | 0.06 | 1.3 | 1.6 | 4 | 0.10 |
| 433 | **Moussaka** | 30 | 65 | 0.07 | 0.06 | 0.15 | 1.4 | 2.0 | 4 | 0.32 |
| 434 | **Shepherd's pie** | 14 | Tr | 0.14 | 0.04 | 0.12 | 1.7 | 1.5 | 2 | 0.28 |

| No | Food | Vitamin $B_6$ mg | Vitamin $B_{12}$ µg | Folic acid Free µg | Folic acid Total µg | Pantothenic acid mg | Biotin µg | Notes |
|---|---|---|---|---|---|---|---|---|
| | ***Meat products and dishes** contd* | | | | | | | |
| 415 | **Beefburgers** frozen, raw | 0.20 | 1 | 2 | 12 | 0.4 | 1 | |
| 416 | fried | 0.20 | 2 | 2 | 15 | 0.5 | 2 | |
| 417 | **Brawn** | 0.05 | Tr | Tr | 3 | 0.9 | Tr | |
| 418 | **Meat paste** | 0.08 | 3 | 7 | 9 | 0.3 | 3 | |
| 419 | **White pudding** | 0.06 | 1 | 2 | 6 | 0.8 | 18 | |
| | ***Meat and pastry products*** | | | | | | | |
| 420 | **Cornish pastie** | 0.12 | 1 | 3 | 3 | 0.6 | 1 | |
| 421 | **Pork pie** individual | 0.06 | 1 | 3 | 3 | 0.6 | 1 | |
| 422 | **Sausage roll** flaky pastry | 0.06 | Tr | 3 | 4 | 0.2 | 1 | |
| 423 | short pastry | 0.07 | Tr | 3 | 5 | 0.3 | 1 | |
| 424 | **Steak and kidney pie** pastry top only | 0.17 | 8 | 9 | 14 | 0.8 | 6 | |
| 425 | individual | 0.06 | 2 | 7 | 8 | (0.3) | (1) | |
| | ***Cooked dishes*** | | | | | | | |
| 426 | **Beef steak pudding** | 0.13 | 1 | 1 | 5 | 0.3 | Tr | |
| 427 | **Beef stew** | 0.13 | 1 | Tr | 5 | 0.3 | Tr | |
| 428 | **Bolognese sauce** | 0.16 | 1 | Tr | 10 | 0.4 | Tr | |
| 429 | **Curried meat** | 0.10 | 1 | Tr | 5 | 0.3 | Tr | |
| 430 | **Hot pot** | 0.21 | 1 | 1 | 8 | 0.4 | Tr | |
| 431 | **Irish stew** | 0.15 | 1 | 1 | 6 | 0.3 | 1 | |
| 432 | **Irish stew** (weighed with bones) | 0.14 | 1 | 1 | 5 | 0.3 | 1 | |
| 433 | **Moussaka** | 0.17 | 1 | 1 | 8 | 0.5 | 2 | |
| 434 | **Shepherd's pie** | 0.17 | 1 | 2 | 7 | 0.3 | Tr | |

| No | Food | Description and number of samples | Edible matter, proportion of weight purchased | Water g | Total nitrogen g |
|---|---|---|---|---|---|

| No | Food | Energy value | | Protein | Fat | Carbo-hydrate | mg | | | | | | | | | |
|---|---|---|---|---|---|---|---|---|---|---|---|---|---|---|---|---|
| | | kcal | kJ | g | g | g | Na | K | Ca | Mg | P | Fe | Cu | Zn | S | Cl |

| No | Food | Retinol µg | Carotene µg | Vitamin D µg | Thiamin mg | Riboflavin mg | Nicotinic acid mg | Potential nicotinic acid from tryptophan mg Trp ÷ 60 | Vitamin C mg | Vitamin E mg |
|---|---|---|---|---|---|---|---|---|---|---|

| No | Food | Vitamin $B_6$ mg | Vitamin $B_{12}$ µg | Folic acid Free µg | Folic acid Total µg | Pantothenic acid mg | Biotin µg | Notes |
|---|---|---|---|---|---|---|---|---|

| No | Food | Description and number of samples | Edible matter, proportion of weight purchased | Water g | Total nitrogen g |
|---|---|---|---|---|---|
| | ***White fish*** | | | | |
| 438 | **Cod** raw, fresh fillets | Samples from 3 different shops | 0.89 | 82.1 | 2.78 |
| 439 | frozen steaks | 12 packets, 3 brands | 1.00 | 83.9 | 2.49 |
| 440 | baked | Fillets; baked in the oven with added butter | 0.69 | 76.6 | 3.43 |
| 441 | baked (weighed with bones and skin) | Calculated from the previous item | 0.69 | 65.1 | 2.92 |
| 442 | fried in batter | Purchased cooked | 1.00 | 60.9 | 3.14 |
| 443 | grilled | Frozen steaks, 12 samples; butter and salt added | 0.63 | 78.0 | 3.32 |
| 444 | poached | Fillets; poached in milk, butter and salt added | 0.75 | 77.7 | 3.35 |
| 445 | poached (weighed with bones and skin) | Calculated from the previous item | 0.75 | 67.6 | 2.91 |
| 446 | steamed | Middle cuts | 0.66 | 79.2 | 2.98 |
| 447 | steamed (weighed with bones and skin) | Calculated from the previous item | 0.66 | 64.1 | 2.42 |
| 448 | **smoked** raw | Samples from 3 different shops | 0.99 | 78.0 | 2.93 |
| 449 | poached | Poached in milk, butter added | 0.80 | 73.7 | 3.46 |
| 450 | **dried** salt, boiled | Stockfish; soaked 24 hours and boiled | 0.99 | 64.9 | 5.20 |
| 451 | **Haddock, fresh** raw | Fillets | — | 81.3 | 2.68 |
| 452 | fried | Fish without heads, coated in crumbs; all except bones | 1.15 | 65.1 | 3.42 |
| 453 | fried (weighed with bones) | Calculated from the previous item | 1.15 | 60.0 | 3.15 |
| 454 | steamed | Middle cut | 0.59 | 75.1 | 3.65 |
| 455 | steamed (weighed with bones and skin) | Calculated from the previous item | 0.59 | 57.1 | 2.77 |
| 456 | **smoked** steamed | Flesh only | 0.55 | 71.6 | 3.73 |
| 457 | steamed (weighed with bones and skin) | Calculated from the previous item | 0.55 | 46.5 | 2.42 |

| No | Food | Energy value kcal | Energy value kJ | Protein (N × 6.25) g | Fat g | Carbo-hydrate g | Na mg | K mg | Ca mg | Mg mg | P mg | Fe mg | Cu mg | Zn mg | S mg | Cl mg |
|---|---|---|---|---|---|---|---|---|---|---|---|---|---|---|---|---|
| | ***White fish*** | | | | | | | | | | | | | | | |
| 438 | **Cod** raw, fresh fillets | 76 | 322 | 17.4 | 0.7 | 0 | 77 | 320 | 16 | 23 | 170 | 0.3 | 0.06 | 0.4 | 200 | 110 |
| 439 | frozen steaks | 68 | 287 | 15.6 | 0.6 | 0 | 68 | 310 | 11 | 22 | 160 | 0.3 | 0.06 | 0.3 | 180 | 95 |
| 440 | baked | 96 | 408 | 21.4 | 1.2 | 0 | 340 | 350 | 22 | 26 | 190 | 0.4 | 0.07 | 0.5 | 230 | 520 |
| 441 | baked (weighed with bones and skin) | 82 | 348 | 18.3 | 1.0 | 0 | 290 | 300 | 19 | 22 | 160 | 0.4 | 0.06 | 0.4 | 200 | 440 |
| 442 | fried in batter | 199 | 834 | 19.6 | 10.3 | 7.5 | 100 | 370 | 80 | 24 | 200 | 0.5 | (0.07) | — | — | 150 |
| 443 | grilled | 95 | 402 | 20.8 | 1.3 | 0 | 91 | 380 | 10 | 26 | 200 | 0.4 | 0.07 | 0.5 | 240 | 130 |
| 444 | poached | 94 | 396 | 20.9 | 1.1 | 0 | 110 | 330 | 29 | 26 | 180 | 0.3 | 0.09 | 0.5 | 250 | 150 |
| 445 | poached (weighed with bones and skin) | 82 | 346 | 18.2 | 1.0 | 0 | 96 | 290 | 25 | 23 | 160 | 0.3 | 0.08 | 0.4 | 220 | 130 |
| 446 | steamed | 83 | 350 | 18.6 | 0.9 | 0 | 100 | 360 | 15 | 21 | 240 | 0.5 | 0.10 | 0.5 | 210 | 120 |
| 447 | steamed (weighed with bones and skin | 67 | 283 | 15.1 | 0.7 | 0 | 81 | 290 | 12 | 17 | 200 | 0.4 | 0.08 | 0.4 | 170 | 97 |
| 448 | **smoked** raw | 79 | 333 | 18.3 | 0.6 | 0 | 1170 | 390 | 14 | 25 | 190 | 0.4 | 0.17 | 0.4 | 210 | 1800 |
| 449 | poached | 101 | 426 | 21.6 | 1.6 | 0 | 1200 | 360 | 25 | 25 | 190 | 0.5 | 0.23 | 0.6 | 250 | 1800 |
| 450 | **dried** salt, boiled | 138 | 586 | 32.5 | 0.9 | 0 | 400 | 31 | 22 | 35 | 160 | 1.8 | — | — | 370 | 670 |
| 451 | **Haddock, fresh** raw | 73 | 308 | 16.8 | 0.6 | 0 | 120 | 300 | 18 | 23 | 170 | 0.6 | 0.19 | 0.3 | 220 | 160 |
| 452 | fried | 174 | 729 | 21.4 | 8.3 | 3.6 | 180 | 350 | 110 | 31 | 250 | 1.2 | — | — | 290 | 180 |
| 453 | fried (weighed with bones) | 160 | 669 | 19.7 | 7.6 | 3.3 | 160 | 320 | 100 | 28 | 230 | 1.1 | — | — | 260 | 170 |
| 454 | steamed | 98 | 417 | 22.8 | 0.8 | 0 | 120 | 320 | 55 | 28 | 230 | 0.7 | 0.13 | (0.4) | 300 | (140) |
| 455 | steamed (weighed with bones and skin) | 75 | 316 | 17.3 | 0.6 | 0 | 92 | 250 | 41 | 21 | 180 | 0.5 | 0.10 | (0.3) | 230 | (110) |
| 456 | **smoked** steamed | 101 | 429 | 23.3 | 0.9 | 0 | 1220 | 290 | 58 | 25 | 250 | 1.0 | — | — | 250 | 1900 |
| 457 | steamed (weighed with bones and skin | 66 | 279 | 15.1 | 0.6 | 0 | 790 | 190 | 37 | 17 | 160 | 0.7 | — | — | 160 | 1230 |

| No | Food | Retinol µg | Carotene µg | Vitamin D µg | Thiamin mg | Riboflavin mg | Nicotinic acid mg | Potential nicotinic acid from tryptophan mg Trp ÷ 60 | Vitamin C mg | Vitamin E mg |
|---|---|---|---|---|---|---|---|---|---|---|
| | ***White fish*** | | | | | | | | | |
| 438 | **Cod** raw, fresh fillets | Tr | Tr | Tr | 0.08 *(0.05–0.18)* | 0.07 *(0.02–0.16)* | 1.7 | 3.2 | Tr | 0.44 |
| 439 | frozen steaks | Tr | Tr | Tr | 0.06 | 0.05 | 1.5 | 2.9 | Tr | — |
| 440 | baked | Tr | Tr | Tr | 0.07 | 0.07 | 1.7 | 4.0 | Tr | 0.59 |
| 441 | baked (weighed with bones and skin) | Tr | Tr | Tr | 0.06 | 0.06 | 1.3 | 3.4 | Tr | 0.50 |
| 442 | fried in batter | Tr | Tr | Tr | — | — | — | 3.7 | Tr | — |
| 443 | grilled | Tr | Tr | Tr | 0.08 | 0.06 | 1.9 | 3.9 | Tr | — |
| 444 | poached | Tr | Tr | Tr | 0.08 | 0.08 | 1.7 | 3.9 | Tr | 0.61 |
| 445 | poached (weighed with bones and skin) | Tr | Tr | Tr | 0.07 | 0.07 | 1.5 | 3.4 | Tr | 0.53 |
| 446 | steamed | Tr | Tr | Tr | (0.09) | (0.09) | (2.1) | 3.5 | Tr | (0.54) |
| 447 | steamed (weighed with bones and skin) | Tr | Tr | Tr | (0.07) | (0.07) | (1.7) | 2.8 | Tr | (0.44) |
| 448 | **smoked** raw | Tr | Tr | Tr | 0.08 | 0.07 | 1.4 | 3.4 | Tr | — |
| 449 | poached | Tr | Tr | Tr | 0.10 | 0.11 | 1.7 | 4.0 | Tr | — |
| 450 | **dried** salt, boiled | Tr | Tr | Tr | (Tr) | (Tr) | — | 6.1 | Tr | — |
| 451 | **Haddock, fresh** raw | Tr | Tr | Tr | 0.07 *(0.03–0.10)* | 0.10 *(0.02–0.16)* | 4.0 | 3.1 | Tr | — |
| 452 | fried | Tr | Tr | Tr | — | — | — | 4.0 | Tr | — |
| 453 | fried (weighed with bones) | Tr | Tr | Tr | — | — | — | 3.7 | Tr | — |
| 454 | steamed | Tr | Tr | Tr | (0.08) | (0.13) | (5.1) | 4.3 | Tr | — |
| 455 | steamed (weighed with bones and skin) | Tr | Tr | Tr | (0.06) | (0.10) | (3.9) | 3.2 | Tr | — |
| 456 | **smoked** steamed | Tr | Tr | Tr | (0.10) | (0.11) | (1.7) | 4.4 | Tr | — |
| 457 | steamed (weighed with bones and skin) | Tr | Tr | Tr | (0.07) | (0.07) | (1.1) | 2.8 | Tr | — |

| No | Food | Vitamin $B_6$ mg | Vitamin $B_{12}$ µg | Folic acid Free µg | Folic acid Total µg | Pantothenic acid mg | Biotin µg | Notes |
|---|---|---|---|---|---|---|---|---|
| | ***White fish*** | | | | | | | |
| 438 | **Cod** raw, fresh fillets | 0.33 | 2 | 8 | 12 | 0.20 | 3 | |
| 439 | frozen steaks | 0.34 | 1 | 4 | 6 | (0.20) | (3) | |
| 440 | baked | 0.38 | 2 | 7 | 12 | (0.20) | (3) | |
| 441 | baked (weighed with bones and skin) | 0.32 | 2 | 6 | 10 | (0.17) | (3) | |
| 442 | fried in batter | — | — | — | — | — | — | |
| 443 | grilled | 0.41 | 2 | 6 | 10 | (0.25) | (3) | |
| 444 | poached | 0.37 | 2 | 5 | 14 | (0.19) | (3) | |
| 445 | poached (weighed with bones and skin) | 0.32 | 2 | 4 | 12 | (0.16) | (3) | |
| 446 | steamed | (0.37) | (3) | (5) | (12) | (0.20) | (3) | |
| 447 | steamed (weighed with bones and skin) | (0.30) | (2) | (4) | (10) | (0.16) | (2) | |
| 448 | **smoked** raw | 0.32 | 2 | 3 | 5 | (0.20) | (3) | |
| 449 | poached | 0.35 | 3 | 3 | 5 | (0.20) | (3) | |
| 450 | **dried** salt, boiled | — | (Tr) | (Tr) | (Tr) | — | (Tr) | |
| 451 | **Haddock, fresh** raw | 0.20 | 1 | 5 | 13 | 0.20 | 5 | |
| 452 | fried | — | — | — | — | — | — | |
| 453 | fried (weighed with bones) | — | — | — | — | — | — | |
| 454 | steamed | (0.25) | (1) | (3) | (16) | (0.20) | (6) | |
| 455 | steamed (weighed with bones and skin) | (0.19) | (1) | (2) | (12) | (0.15) | (5) | |
| 456 | **smoked** steamed | (0.35) | (3) | (3) | (5) | (0.20) | (3) | |
| 457 | steamed (weighed with bones and skin) | (0.28) | (2) | (2) | (3) | (0.13) | (2) | |

| No | Food | Description and number of samples | Edible matter, proportion of weight purchased | Water g | Total nitrogen g |
|---|---|---|---|---|---|
| | ***White fish** contd* | | | | |
| 458 | **Halibut** raw | Literature sources | — | 78.1 | 2.83 |
| 459 | steamed | Middle cut | 0.66 | 70.9 | 3.80 |
| 460 | steamed (weighed with bones and skin) | Calculated from the previous item | 0.66 | 53.8 | 2.88 |
| 461 | **Lemon sole** raw | Literature sources | — | 81.2 | 2.74 |
| 462 | fried | Fish without head and fins, coated in crumbs; all except bones | 0.91 | 60.4 | 2.57 |
| 463 | fried (weighed with bones) | Calculated from the previous item | 0.91 | 47.7 | 2.03 |
| 464 | steamed | Flesh only from fish without head and fins | 0.62 | 77.2 | 3.29 |
| 465 | steamed (weighed with bones and skin) | Calculated from the previous item | 0.62 | 54.9 | 2.34 |
| 466 | **Plaice** raw | 8 fish, purchased whole | 0.42 | 79.5 | 2.86 |
| 467 | fried in batter | 6 samples, purchased cooked | 1.00 | 52.4 | 2.52 |
| 468 | fried in crumbs | Fillets from 8 fish, dipped in egg and breadcrumbs and fried; light skin included | 0.53 | 59.9 | 2.88 |
| 469 | steamed | Flesh only from fish without head and fins | 0.49 | 78.0 | 3.02 |
| 470 | steamed (weighed with bones and skin) | Calculated from the previous item | 0.49 | 42.1 | 1.63 |
| 471 | **Saithe** raw | Coley, coalfish; literature sources | — | 81.0 | (2.72) |
| 472 | steamed | Pieces from tail end | 0.65 | 74.8 | 3.73 |
| 473 | steamed (weighed with bones and skin) | Calculated from the previous item | 0.65 | 63.5 | 3.17 |
| 475 | **Whiting** fried | Fish without heads, coated in crumbs; all except bones | 1.02 | 63.0 | 2.90 |
| 476 | fried (weighed with bones) | Calculated from the previous item | 1.02 | 56.8 | 2.61 |
| 477 | steamed | Flesh only from fish without heads | 0.57 | 76.9 | 3.35 |
| 478 | steamed (weighed with bones) | Calculated from the previous item | 0.57 | 52.2 | 2.28 |

| No | Food | Energy value kcal | Energy value kJ | Protein (N × 6.25) g | Fat g | Carbo-hydrate g | Na mg | K mg | Ca mg | Mg mg | P mg | Fe mg | Cu mg | Zn mg | S mg | Cl mg |
|---|---|---|---|---|---|---|---|---|---|---|---|---|---|---|---|---|
| | ***White fish** contd* | | | | | | | | | | | | | | | |
| 458 | **Halibut** raw | 92 | 390 | 17.7 | 2.4 | 0 | (84) | (260) | (10) | (17) | (190) | (0.5) | (0.05) | — | (190) | (60) |
| 459 | steamed | 131 | 553 | 23.8 | 4.0 | 0 | 110 | 340 | 13 | 23 | 260 | 0.6 | 0.07 | — | 260 | 80 |
| 460 | steamed (weighed with bones and skin) | 99 | 417 | 18.0 | 3.0 | 0 | 84 | 260 | 10 | 18 | 190 | 0.5 | 0.05 | — | 190 | 61 |
| 461 | **Lemon sole** raw | 81 | 343 | 17.1 | 1.4 | 0 | (95) | (230) | (17) | (17) | (200) | (0.5) | (0.10) | — | (200) | (97) |
| 462 | fried | 216 | 904 | 16.1 | 13.0 | 9.3 | 140 | 250 | 95 | 22 | 240 | 1.1 | 0.16 | — | 190 | 120 |
| 463 | fried (weighed with bones) | 171 | 715 | 12.7 | 10.3 | 7.4 | 110 | 200 | 75 | 16 | 190 | 0.9 | 0.13 | — | 150 | 98 |
| 464 | steamed | 91 | 384 | 20.6 | 0.9 | 0 | 120 | 280 | 21 | 20 | 250 | 0.6 | 0.12 | — | 240 | 120 |
| 465 | steamed (weighed with bones and skin) | 64 | 270 | 14.6 | 0.6 | 0 | 82 | 200 | 15 | 14 | 180 | 0.4 | 0.09 | — | 170 | 83 |
| 466 | **Plaice** raw | 91 | 386 | 17.9 | 2.2 | 0 | 120 | 280 | 51 | 22 | 180 | 0.3 | 0.05 | 0.5 | 240 | 170 |
| 467 | fried in batter | 279 | 1165 | 15.8 | 18.0 | 14.4 | 220 | 230 | 93 | 21 | 170 | 1.0 | 0.17 | 1.0 | 210 | 280 |
| 468 | fried in crumbs | 228 | 951 | 18.0 | 13.7 | 8.6 | 220 | 280 | 67 | 24 | 180 | 0.8 | 0.20 | 0.7 | 240 | 310 |
| 469 | steamed | 93 | 392 | 18.9 | 1.9 | 0 | 120 | 280 | 38 | 24 | 250 | 0.6 | — | — | 250 | 110 |
| 470 | steamed (weighed with bones and skin) | 50 | 210 | 10.2 | 1.0 | 0 | 65 | 150 | 20 | 13 | 130 | 0.3 | — | — | 130 | 61 |
| 471 | **Saithe** raw | (73) | (308) | (17.0) | (0.5) | 0 | (73) | (260) | (14) | (23) | (190) | (0.5) | — | — | (190) | (200) |
| 472 | steamed | 99 | 418 | 23.3 | 0.6 | 0 | 97 | 350 | 19 | 31 | 250 | 0.6 | — | — | 270 | 83 |
| 473 | steamed (weighed with bones and skin) | 84 | 355 | 19.8 | 0.5 | 0 | 83 | 300 | 16 | 26 | 210 | 0.5 | — | — | 230 | 71 |
| 475 | **Whiting** fried | 191 | 801 | 18.1 | 10.3 | 7.0 | 200 | 320 | 48 | 33 | 260 | 0.7 | — | — | 270 | 190 |
| 476 | fried (weighed with bones) | 173 | 722 | 16.3 | 9.3 | 6.3 | 180 | 290 | 43 | 29 | 230 | 0.6 | — | — | 240 | 180 |
| 477 | steamed | 92 | 389 | 20.9 | 0.9 | 0 | 130 | 300 | 42 | 28 | 190 | 1.0 | — | — | 310 | 93 |
| 478 | steamed (weighed with bones) | 63 | 265 | 14.3 | 0.6 | 0 | 86 | 200 | 29 | 19 | 130 | 0.7 | — | — | 210 | 63 |

| No | Food | Retinol µg | Carotene µg | Vitamin D µg | Thiamin mg | Riboflavin mg | Nicotinic acid mg | Potential nicotinic acid from tryptophan mg Trp ÷ 60 | Vitamin C mg | Vitamin E mg |
|---|---|---|---|---|---|---|---|---|---|---|
| | ***White fish** contd* | | | | | | | | | |
| 458 | **Halibut** raw | Tr[a] | Tr | Tr[a] | 0.08 *(0.03–0.12)* | 0.10 *(0.04–0.18)* | 5.0 | 3.3 | Tr | 0.90 |
| 459 | steamed | Tr[a] | Tr | Tr[a] | (0.08) | (0.11) | (5.2) | 4.4 | Tr | (1.0) |
| 460 | steamed (weighed with bones and skin) | Tr[a] | Tr | Tr[a] | (0.06) | (0.08) | (4.0) | 3.4 | Tr | (0.76) |
| 461 | **Lemon sole** raw | Tr | Tr | Tr | 0.09 | 0.08 | 3.5 | 3.2 | Tr | — |
| 462 | fried | Tr | Tr | Tr | — | — | — | 3.0 | Tr | — |
| 463 | fried (weighed with bones) | Tr | Tr | Tr | — | — | — | 2.4 | Tr | — |
| 464 | steamed | Tr | Tr | Tr | (0.09) | (0.09) | (3.6) | 3.8 | Tr | — |
| 465 | steamed (weighed with bones and skin) | Tr | Tr | Tr | (0.06) | (0.06) | (2.6) | 2.7 | Tr | — |
| 466 | **Plaice** raw | Tr | Tr | Tr | 0.30 *(0.02–0.46)* | 0.10 *(0.09–0.33)* | 3.2 | 3.3 | Tr | — |
| 467 | fried in batter | Tr | Tr | Tr | 0.20 | 0.15 | 2.0 | 2.9 | Tr | — |
| 468 | fried in crumbs | Tr | Tr | Tr | 0.23 | 0.18 | 2.9 | 3.4 | Tr | — |
| 469 | steamed | Tr | Tr | Tr | (0.30) | (0.11) | (3.2) | 3.5 | Tr | — |
| 470 | steamed (weighed with bones and skin) | Tr | Tr | Tr | (0.16) | (0.06) | (1.7) | 1.9 | Tr | — |
| 471 | **Saithe** raw | Tr | Tr | Tr | 0.10 | 0.20 | 3.4 | 3.2 | Tr | 0.36 |
| 472 | steamed | Tr | Tr | Tr | (0.12) | (0.26) | (4.0) | 4.4 | Tr | (0.47) |
| 473 | steamed (weighed with bones and skin) | Tr | Tr | Tr | (0.10) | (0.22) | (3.4) | 3.7 | Tr | (0.40) |
| 475 | **Whiting** fried | Tr | Tr | Tr | — | — | — | 3.4 | Tr | — |
| 476 | fried (weighed with bones) | Tr | Tr | Tr | — | — | — | 3.1 | Tr | — |
| 477 | steamed | Tr | Tr | Tr | — | — | — | 3.9 | Tr | — |
| 478 | steamed (weighed with bones) | Tr | Tr | Tr | — | — | — | 2.7 | Tr | — |

| No | Food | Vitamin $B_6$ mg | Vitamin $B_{12}$ µg | Folic acid Free µg | Folic acid Total µg | Pantothenic acid mg | Biotin µg | Notes |
|---|---|---|---|---|---|---|---|---|
| | ***White fish** contd* | | | | | | | |
| 458 | **Halibut** raw | 0.20 | 1 | 4 | 12 | 0.30 | 5 | [a] These are values for Atlantic halibut. Pacific halibut have been reported to contain 120 µg retinol and 1 µg vitamin D per 100 g. |
| 459 | steamed | (0.23) | (1) | (2) | (14) | (0.28) | (5) | |
| 460 | steamed (weighed with bones and skin) | (0.17) | (1) | (2) | (11) | (0.21) | (4) | |
| 461 | **Lemon sole** raw | — | 1 | 5 | 11 | 0.30 | (5) | |
| 462 | fried | — | — | — | — | — | — | |
| 463 | fried (weighed with bones) | — | — | — | — | — | — | |
| 464 | steamed | — | (1) | (3) | (13) | (0.31) | (5) | |
| 465 | steamed (weighed with bones and skin) | — | (1) | (2) | (9) | (0.22) | (4) | |
| 466 | **Plaice** raw | 0.43 | 2 | 5 | 10 | 0.80 | — | |
| 467 | fried in batter | — | — | — | — | — | — | |
| 468 | fried in crumbs | 0.36 | 1 | 8 | 17 | — | — | |
| 469 | steamed | (0.47) | (2) | (3) | (11) | (0.70) | — | |
| 470 | steamed (weighed with bones and skin) | (0.25) | (1) | (2) | (6) | (0.38) | — | |
| 471 | **Saithe** raw | 0.47 | 4 | — | — | 0.38 | 7 | |
| 472 | steamed | (0.62) | (5) | — | — | (0.40) | (8) | |
| 473 | steamed (weighed with bones and skin) | (0.53) | (4) | — | — | (0.34) | (7) | |
| 475 | **Whiting** fried | — | — | — | — | — | — | |
| 476 | fried (weighed with bones) | — | — | — | — | — | — | |
| 477 | steamed | — | — | — | — | — | — | |
| 478 | steamed (weighed with bones) | — | — | — | — | — | — | |

| No | Food | Description and number of samples | Edible matter, proportion of weight purchased | Water g | Total nitrogen g |
|---|---|---|---|---|---|
| | ***Fatty fish*** | | | | |
| 480 | **Eel** raw | Yellow eels, flesh only | 0.67 | 71.3 [a] | 2.66 |
| 481 | stewed | Yellow eels, flesh only; stewed in water | — | (61.3) | (3.30) |
| 482 | **Herring** raw | 12 fish, sampled in November, flesh only | 0.55 | 63.9 [b] | 2.69 |
| 483 | fried | Flesh, skin and roes; covered in oatmeal | 0.77 | 58.7 | 3.69 |
| 484 | fried (weighed with bones) | Calculated from the previous item | 0.77 | 51.6 | 3.24 |
| 485 | grilled | 12 fish, flesh only | 0.53 | 65.5 | 3.26 |
| 486 | grilled (weighed with bones) | Calculated from the previous item | 0.53 | 44.5 | 2.22 |
| 487 | **Bloater** grilled | Flesh only from fish without heads or roes | 0.65 | 55.6 | 3.76 |
| 488 | grilled (weighed with bones) | Calculated from the previous item | 0.65 | 41.1 | 2.78 |
| 489 | **Kipper** baked | Flesh only | 0.45 | 58.7 | 4.08 |
| 490 | baked (weighed with bones) | Calculated from the previous item | 0.45 | 31.6 | 2.20 |
| 491 | **Mackerel** raw | Literature sources | — | 64.0 [b] | 3.04 |
| 492 | fried | Flesh only from fish without heads | 0.61 | 65.6 | 3.44 |
| 493 | fried (weighed with bones) | Calculated from the previous item | 0.61 | 47.8 | 2.51 |
| 494 | **Pilchards** canned in tomato sauce | 6 cans, 4 brands (South African), total contents of can | 1.00 | 70.0 | 3.01 |
| 495 | **Salmon** raw | Atlantic salmon; literature sources | — | 68.0 | (2.94) |
| 496 | steamed | Shoulder cut, flesh only | 0.73 | 65.4 | 3.21 |
| 497 | steamed (weighed with bones and skin) | Calculated from the previous item | 0.73 | 53.0 | 2.60 |

[a] The water content varies according to stage of maturity: elvers contain 81.8 g and silver eels 57.1 g water per 100 g

[b] The values for water vary throughout the year from about 75 g per 100 g in February–April to 60 g per 100 g in July–October

| No | Food | Energy value kcal | Energy value kJ | Protein (N × 6.25) g | Fat g | Carbo-hydrate g | Na mg | K mg | Ca mg | Mg mg | P mg | Fe mg | Cu mg | Zn mg | S mg | Cl mg |
|---|---|---|---|---|---|---|---|---|---|---|---|---|---|---|---|---|
| | ***Fatty fish*** | | | | | | | | | | | | | | | |
| 480 | **Eel** raw | 168 | 700 | 16.6 | 11.3 [a] | 0 | 89 | 270 | 19 | 19 | 220 | 0.7 | 0.05 | 0.5 | 190 | 57 |
| 481 | stewed | (201) | (839) | (20.6) | (13.2) | 0 | (84) | (250) | (21) | (20) | (230) | (0.9) | (0.06) | (0.6) | (230) | (53) |
| 482 | **Herring** raw | 234 | 970 | 16.8 | 18.5 [b] | 0 | 67 | 340 | 33 | 29 | 210 | 0.8 | 0.12 | 0.5 | 190 | 76 |
| 483 | fried | 234 | 975 | 23.1 | 15.1 | 1.5 | 100 | 420 | 39 | 35 | 340 | 1.0 | — | — | 260 | 130 |
| 484 | fried (weighed with bones) | 206 | 858 | 20.3 | 13.3 | 1.3 | 89 | 370 | 34 | 31 | 300 | 1.7 | — | — | 230 | 110 |
| 485 | grilled | 199 | 828 | 20.4 | 13.0 | 0 | 170 | 370 | 33 | 32 | 240 | 1.0 | 0.11 | 0.5 | 230 | 220 |
| 486 | grilled (weighed with bones) | 135 | 562 | 13.9 | 8.8 | 0 | 120 | 250 | 22 | 22 | 160 | 0.7 | 0.07 | 0.4 | 160 | 150 |
| 487 | **Bloater** grilled | 251 | 1043 | 23.5 | 17.4 | 0 | 700 | 450 | 120 | 45 | 360 | 2.2 | — | — | 310 | 1130 |
| 488 | grilled (weighed with bones) | 186 | 773 | 17.4 | 12.9 | 0 | 520 | 330 | 91 | 33 | 260 | 1.6 | — | — | 230 | 840 |
| 489 | **Kipper** baked | 205 | 855 | 25.5 | 11.4 | 0 | 990 | 520 | 65 | 48 | 430 | 1.4 | — | — | 280 | 1520 |
| 490 | baked (weighed with bones) | 111 | 464 | 13.8 | 6.2 | 0 | 540 | 280 | 35 | 26 | 230 | 0.8 | — | — | 150 | 820 |
| 491 | **Mackerel** raw | 223 | 926 | 19.0 | 16.3 [b] | 0 | (130) | (360) | (24) | (30) | (240) | (1.0) | 0.19 | 0.5 | (180) | (97) |
| 492 | fried | 188 | 784 | 21.5 | 11.3 | 0 | 150 | 420 | 28 | 35 | 280 | 1.2 | 0.20 | — | 210 | 110 |
| 493 | fried (weighed with bones) | 138 | 574 | 15.7 | 8.3 | 0 | 110 | 310 | 21 | 25 | 200 | 0.9 | 0.15 | — | 150 | 83 |
| 494 | **Pilchards** canned in tomato sauce | 126 | 531 | 18.8 | 5.4 | 0.7 | 370 | 420 | 300 | 39 | 350 | 2.7 | 0.19 | 1.6 | — | 580 |
| 495 | **Salmon** raw | (182) | (757) | (18.4) | (12.0) | 0 | (98) | (310) | (27) | (26) | (280) | (0.7) | 0.20 | 0.8 | (170) | (59) |
| 496 | steamed | 197 | 823 | 20.1 | 13.0 | 0 | 110 | 330 | 29 | 29 | 300 | 0.8 | — | — | 190 | 64 |
| 497 | steamed (weighed with bones and skin) | 160 | 666 | 16.3 | 10.5 | 0 | 87 | 270 | 23 | 23 | 250 | 0.6 | — | — | 150 | 52 |

[a] The fat content varies according to stage of maturity: elvers contain 2.2g and silver eels 27.8g fat per 100g

[b] The values for fat vary throughout the year from about 5g per 100g in February–April to 20g per 100g in July–October

| No | Food | Retinol µg | Carotene µg | Vitamin D µg | Thiamin mg | Riboflavin mg | Nicotinic acid mg | Potential nicotinic acid from tryptophan mg Trp ÷ 60 | Vitamin C mg | Vitamin E mg |
|---|---|---|---|---|---|---|---|---|---|---|
| | ***Fatty fish*** | | | | | | | | | |
| 480 | **Eel** raw | 1200 | Tr | —[b] | 0.20 | 0.35 | 3.5 | 3.1 | Tr | — |
| | | *(260–2500[a])* | | | | *(0.05–0.50)* | | | | |
| 481 | stewed | (1900) | Tr | —[b] | (0.13) | (0.40) | (2.8) | 3.9 | Tr | — |
| 482 | **Herring** raw | 45 | Tr | 22.5 | Tr | 0.18 | 4.1 | 3.1 | Tr | 0.21 |
| | | *(6–120)* | | *(7.5–42.5)* | *(Tr–0.13)* | *(0.09–0.33)* | *(2–6)* | | | |
| 483 | fried | (49) | Tr | (25.0) | Tr | (0.18) | (4.0) | 4.3 | Tr | (0.30) |
| 484 | fried (weighed with bones) | (43) | Tr | (22.0) | Tr | (0.16) | (3.5) | 3.8 | Tr | (0.26) |
| 485 | grilled | (49) | Tr | (25.0) | Tr | 0.18 | 4.0 | 3.8 | Tr | 0.30 |
| 486 | grilled (weighed with bones) | (33) | Tr | (17.0) | Tr | 0.12 | 2.7 | 2.6 | Tr | 0.20 |
| 487 | **Bloater** grilled | (49) | Tr | (25.0) | Tr | (0.18) | (4.0) | 4.4 | Tr | (0.30) |
| 488 | grilled (weighed with bones) | (36) | Tr | (18.5) | Tr | (0.13) | (3.0) | 3.2 | Tr | (0.22) |
| 489 | **Kipper** baked | (49) | Tr | (25.0) | Tr | (0.18) | (4.0) | 4.8 | Tr | (0.30) |
| 490 | baked (weighed with bones) | (26) | Tr | (13.5) | Tr | (0.10) | (2.2) | 2.6 | Tr | (0.16) |
| 491 | **Mackerel** raw | 45 | Tr | 17.5 | 0.09 | 0.35 | 8.0 | 3.6 | Tr | — |
| | | *(15–60)* | | *(2.5–25)* | *(0.02–0.20)* | *(0.16–0.66)* | | | | |
| 492 | fried | (52) | Tr | (21.1) | (0.09) | (0.38) | (8.7) | 4.0 | Tr | — |
| 493 | fried (weighed with bones) | (38) | Tr | (15.4) | (0.07) | (0.28) | (6.4) | 2.9 | Tr | — |
| 494 | **Pilchards** canned in tomato sauce | Tr[c] | Tr | 8 | 0.02 | 0.29 | 7.6 | 3.5 | Tr | 0.70 |
| 495 | **Salmon** raw | Tr[d] | Tr | Tr[d] | 0.20 | 0.15 | 7.0 | 3.4 | Tr | — |
| | | | | | | *(0.06–0.22)* | | | | |
| 496 | steamed | Tr[d] | Tr | Tr[d] | (0.20) | (0.11) | (7.0) | 3.8 | Tr | — |
| 497 | steamed (weighed with bones and skin) | Tr[d] | Tr | Tr[d] | (0.16) | (0.09) | (5.7) | 3.0 | Tr | — |

| No | Food | Vitamin $B_6$ mg | Vitamin $B_{12}$ µg | Folic acid Free µg | Folic acid Total µg | Pantothenic acid mg | Biotin µg |
|---|---|---|---|---|---|---|---|
| | ***Fatty fish*** | | | | | | |
| 480 | **Eel** raw | 0.30 | 1 | — | — | 0.15 | — |
| 481 | stewed | (0.24) | (1) | — | — | (0.17) | — |
| 482 | **Herring** raw | 0.45 | 6 | 3 | 5 | 1.0 | 10 |
| 483 | fried | (0.57) | (11) | (3) | (10) | (0.88) | (10) |
| 484 | fried (weighed with bones) | (0.50) | (10) | (3) | (9) | (0.77) | (9) |
| 485 | grilled | 0.57 | 11 | 3 | 10 | (0.88) | (10) |
| 486 | grilled (weighed with bones) | 0.39 | 8 | 2 | 7 | (0.60) | (7) |
| 487 | **Bloater** grilled | (0.57) | (11) | (3) | (10) | (0.88) | (10) |
| 488 | grilled (weighed with bones) | (0.42) | (8) | (2) | (7) | (0.65) | (7) |
| 489 | **Kipper** baked | (0.57) | (11) | (3) | (10) | (0.88) | (10) |
| 490 | baked (weighed with bones) | (0.31) | (6) | (2) | (5) | (0.48) | (5) |
| 491 | **Mackerel** raw | 0.70 | 10 | — | — | 1.0 | 7 |
| 492 | fried | (0.84) | (12) | — | — | (0.96) | (8) |
| 493 | fried (weighed with bones) | (0.61) | (9) | — | — | (0.70) | (6) |
| 494 | **Pilchards** canned in tomato sauce | — | 12 | — | — | — | — |
| 495 | **Salmon** raw | 0.75 | 5 | 4 | 26 | 2.0 | 5 |
| 496 | steamed | (0.83) | (6) | (2) | (29) | (1.8) | (4) |
| 497 | steamed (weighed with bones and skin) | (0.67) | (5) | (2) | (23) | (1.5) | (3) |

Notes

[a] The retinol content of eels increases with maturity.

[b] Whole body oil is a rich source of vitamin D, and it contains about 120µg per 100g oil.

[c] New analysis shows only a trace to be present.

[d] These are values for Atlantic salmon. Pacific salmon may contain 90 (20–150) µg retinol and 12.5 (5–20) µg vitamin D per 100g.

| No | Food | Description and number of samples | Edible matter, proportion of weight purchased | Water g | Total nitrogen g |
|---|---|---|---|---|---|
| | ***Fatty fish** contd* | | | | |
| 498 | **Salmon** canned | 10 cans, red salmon; backbone and skin removed | 0.94 | 70.4 | 3.24 |
| 499 | smoked | 4 samples | 1.00 | 64.9 | 4.06 |
| 500 | **Sardines** canned in oil, fish only | 10 cans, 6 brands; fish after draining off oil | 0.83 | 58.4 | 3.79 |
| 501 | fish plus oil | 10 cans, 6 brands; total contents of can | 1.00 | 48.5 | 3.15 |
| 502 | canned in tomato sauce | 10 cans, 4 brands; total contents of can | 1.00 | 65.0 | 2.84 |
| 504 | **Sprats** fried | Fish without heads; fried in deep fat | 0.59 | 33.7 | 3.98 |
| 505 | fried (weighed with bones) | Calculated from the previous item | 0.59 | 29.6 | 3.50 |
| 506 | **Trout, brown** steamed | Flesh only from whole fish | 0.54 | 70.6 | 3.76 |
| 507 | steamed (weighed with bones) | Calculated from the previous item | 0.54 | 46.5 | 2.48 |
| 508 | **Tuna** canned in oil | 6 cans, 2 brands, skipjack tuna | 1.00 | 54.6 | 3.65 |
| 509 | **Whitebait** fried | Whole fish; rolled in flour and fried | 0.77 | 23.5 | 3.12 |
| | ***Cartilaginous fish*** | | | | |
| 511 | **Dogfish** fried in batter | 7 samples, purchased cooked (rock salmon) | 0.92 | 54.2 | 3.42 |
| 512 | fried (weighed with waste) | Calculated from the previous item | 0.92 | 49.9 | 3.15 |
| 514 | **Skate** fried in batter | 6 samples, purchased cooked | 0.82 | 61.8 | 3.67 |
| 515 | fried (weighed with waste) | Calculated from the previous item | 0.82 | 50.7 | 3.01 |

| No | Food | Energy value kcal | Energy value kJ | Protein (N × 6.25) g | Fat g | Carbo-hydrate g | Na mg | K mg | Ca mg | Mg mg | P mg | Fe mg | Cu mg | Zn mg | S mg | Cl mg |
|---|---|---|---|---|---|---|---|---|---|---|---|---|---|---|---|---|
| | ***Fatty fish** contd* | | | | | | | | | | | | | | | |
| 498 | **Salmon** canned | 155 | 649 | 20.3 | 8.2 | 0 | 570 | 300 | 93 | 30 | 240 | 1.4 | 0.09 | 0.9 | 220 | 880 |
| 499 | smoked | 142 | 598 | 25.4 | 4.5 | 0 | 1880 | 420 | 19 | 32 | 250 | 0.6 | 0.09 | 0.4 | — | 2850 |
| 500 | **Sardines** canned in oil, fish only | 217 | 906 | 23.7 | 13.6 | 0 | 650 | 430 | 550 | 52 | 520 | 2.9 | 0.19 | 3.0 | 310 | 1000 |
| 501 | fish plus oil | 334 | 1382 | 19.7 | 28.3 | 0 | 540 | 360 | 460 | 43 | 430 | 2.4 | 0.17 | 2.5 | 260 | 830 |
| 502 | canned in tomato sauce | 177 | 740 | 17.8 | 11.6 | 0.5 | 700 | 410 | 460 | 51 | 400 | 4.6 | 0.23 | 2.7 | 230 | 1110 |
| 504 | **Sprats** fried | 441 | 1826 | 24.9 | 37.9 | 0 | 130 | 410 | 710 | 46 | 640 | 4.5 | — | — | 280 | 180 |
| 505 | fried (weighed with bones) | 388 | 1608 | 21.9 | 33.4 | 0 | 120 | 360 | 620 | 40 | 560 | 4.0 | — | — | 250 | 160 |
| 506 | **Trout, brown** steamed | 135 | 566 | 23.5 | 4.5 | 0 | 88[a] | 370 | 36 | 31 | 270 | 1.0 | — | — | 220 | 70[a] |
| 507 | steamed (weighed with bones) | 89 | 375 | 15.5 | 3.0 | 0 | 58 | 250 | 24 | 20 | 180 | 0.7 | — | — | 140 | 46 |
| 508 | **Tuna** canned in oil | 289 | 1202 | 22.8 | 22.0 | 0 | 420 | 280 | 7 | 28 | 190 | 1.1 | 0.09 | 0.8 | — | 690 |
| 509 | **Whitebait** fried | 525 | 2174 | 19.5 | 47.5 | 5.3 | 230 | 110 | 860 | 50 | 860 | 5.1 | — | — | 270 | 330 |
| | ***Cartilaginous fish*** | | | | | | | | | | | | | | | |
| 511 | **Dogfish** fried in batter | 265 | 1103 | 16.7[b] | 18.8 | 7.7 | 290 | 310 | 42 | 23 | 220 | 1.1 | 0.13 | 0.5 | 200 | 340 |
| 512 | fried (weighed with waste) | 244 | 1016 | 15.4[b] | 17.3 | 7.1 | 270 | 290 | 39 | 21 | 200 | 1.0 | 0.12 | 0.4 | 181 | 310 |
| 514 | **Skate** fried in batter | 199 | 830 | 17.9[b] | 12.1 | 4.9 | 140 | 240 | 50 | 27 | 180 | 1.0 | 0.09 | 0.9 | 250 | 170 |
| 515 | fried (weighed with waste) | 163 | 680 | 14.7[b] | 9.9 | 4.0 | 110 | 200 | 40 | 22 | 150 | 0.8 | 0.07 | 0.7 | 210 | 140 |

[a] Sea trout contains 210mg Na and 260mg Cl per 100g

[b] (Total N — non-protein N) × 6.25

| No | Food | Retinol µg | Carotene µg | Vitamin D µg | Thiamin mg | Riboflavin mg | Nicotinic acid mg | Potential nicotinic acid from tryptophan mgTrp ÷60 | Vitamin C mg | Vitamin E mg |
|---|---|---|---|---|---|---|---|---|---|---|
| | ***Fatty fish** contd* | | | | | | | | | |
| 498 | **Salmon** canned | 90 | Tr | 12.5 | 0.04 | 0.18 | 7.0 | 3.8 | Tr | 1.5 |
| | | *(20–150)* | | *(5–20)* | | | | | | |
| 499 | smoked | Tr[a] | Tr | Tr[a] | 0.16 | 0.17 | 8.8 | 4.7 | Tr | — |
| 500 | **Sardines** canned in oil, fish only | Tr[b] | Tr | 7.5 | 0.04 | 0.36 | 8.2 | 4.4 | Tr | 0.30 |
| 501 | fish plus oil | Tr[b] | Tr | 6.2 | 0.03 | 0.30 | 6.8 | 3.7 | Tr | 1.1 |
| 502 | canned in tomato sauce | Tr[b] | Tr | 7.5 | 0.02 | 0.28 | 5.5 | 3.3 | Tr | 0.51[c] |
| 504 | **Sprats** fried | — | Tr | — | — | — | — | 4.6 | Tr | — |
| 505 | fried (weighed with bones) | — | Tr | — | — | — | — | 4.1 | Tr | — |
| 506 | **Trout, brown** steamed | — | Tr | — | — | — | — | 4.4 | Tr | — |
| 507 | steamed (weighed with bones) | — | Tr | — | — | — | — | 2.9 | Tr | — |
| 508 | **Tuna** canned in oil | — | Tr | 5.8 | 0.04 | 0.11 | 12.9 | 4.3 | Tr | 6.3[d] |
| 509 | **Whitebait** fried | — | Tr | — | — | — | — | 3.6 | Tr | — |
| | ***Cartilaginous fish*** | | | | | | | | | |
| 511 | **Dogfish** fried in batter | — | Tr | — | 0.06 | 0.10 | 5.6 | — | Tr | 2.1 |
| 512 | fried (weighed with waste) | — | Tr | — | 0.06 | 0.09 | 5.2 | — | Tr | 1.9 |
| 514 | **Skate** fried in batter | — | Tr | — | 0.03 | 0.10 | 2.4 | — | Tr | 1.2 |
| 515 | fried (weighed with waste) | — | Tr | — | 0.02 | 0.08 | 2.0 | — | Tr | 1.0 |

| No | Food | Vitamin $B_6$ mg | Vitamin $B_{12}$ µg | Folic acid Free µg | Folic acid Total µg | Pantothenic acid mg | Biotin µg |
|---|---|---|---|---|---|---|---|
| | ***Fatty fish** contd* | | | | | | |
| 498 | **Salmon** canned | 0.45 | 4 | 4 | 12 | 0.50 | (5) |
| 499 | smoked | — | — | — | — | — | — |
| 500 | **Sardines** canned in oil, fish only | 0.48 | 28 | 3 | 8 | 0.50 | 5 |
| 501 | fish plus oil | 0.40 | 23 | 2 | 7 | 0.42 | 4 |
| 502 | canned in tomato sauce | 0.35 | 14 | 7 | 13 | (0.50) | (5) |
| 504 | **Sprats** fried | — | — | — | — | — | — |
| 505 | fried (weighed with bones) | — | — | — | — | — | — |
| 506 | **Trout, brown** steamed | — | — | — | — | — | — |
| 507 | steamed (weighed with bones) | — | — | — | — | — | — |
| 508 | **Tuna** canned in oil | 0.44 | 5 | 7 | 15 | 0.42 | 3 |
| 509 | **Whitebait** fried | — | — | — | — | — | — |
| | ***Cartilaginous fish*** | | | | | | |
| 511 | **Dogfish** fried in batter | — | — | — | — | — | — |
| 512 | fried (weighed with waste) | — | — | — | — | — | — |
| 514 | **Skate** fried in batter | — | — | — | — | — | — |
| 515 | fried (weighed with waste) | — | — | — | — | — | — |

Notes

[a] These are values for Atlantic salmon. Pacific salmon may contain 90µg retinol and 12.5µg vitamin D per 100g.

[b] New analysis shows only a trace to be present.

[c] Also contains 0.25 mg γ-tocopherol per 100g.

[d] Also contains 2.9 mg γ-tocopherol per 100g.

| No | Food | Description and number of samples | Edible matter, proportion of weight purchased | Water g | Total nitrogen g |
|---|---|---|---|---|---|
| | ***Crustacea*** | | | | |
| 518 | **Crab** boiled | Boiled in fresh water | 0.16 | 72.5 | 3.21 |
| 519 | boiled (weighed with shell) | Calculated from the previous item | 0.16 | 14.5 | 0.64 |
| 520 | canned | 6 cans, 2 brands | 1.00 | 79.2 | 2.90 |
| 521 | **Lobster** boiled | Boiled in fresh water | 0.29 | 72.4 | 3.54 |
| 522 | boiled (weighed with shell) | Calculated from the previous item | 0.29 | 26.1 | 1.27 |
| 523 | **Prawns** boiled | Purchased cooked, probably in sea or salt water | 0.38 | 70.0 | 3.62 |
| 524 | boiled (weighed with shell) | Calculated from the previous item | 0.38 | 26.6 | 1.38 |
| 525 | **Scampi** fried | 5 packets, frozen; prepared in breadcrumbs | 0.78 | 39.4 | 1.95 |
| 527 | **Shrimps** boiled | Purchased cooked, probably in sea or salt water | 0.33 | 62.5 | 3.80 |
| 528 | boiled (weighed with shell) | Calculated from the previous item | 0.33 | 20.6 | 1.26 |
| 529 | canned | 10 cans, 3 brands; drained shrimps | 0.65 | 74.9 | 3.33 |
| | ***Molluscs*** | | | | |
| 531 | **Cockles** boiled | Purchased cooked (in sea or salt water) without shells | 1.00 | 78.9 | 1.80 |
| 532 | **Mussels** raw | Purchased alive | 0.32 | 84.1 | 1.93 |
| 533 | boiled | Boiled in fresh water | 0.20 | 79.0 | 2.75 |
| 534 | boiled (weighed with shell) | Calculated from the previous item | 0.20 | 23.7 | 0.83 |
| 535 | **Oysters** raw | Purchased alive | 0.12 | 85.7 | 1.72 |
| 536 | raw (weighed with shell) | Calculated from the previous item | 0.12 | 10.3 | 0.21 |
| 538 | **Scallops** steamed | Purchased without shells | 0.56 | 73.1 | 3.71 |

| No | Food | Energy value kcal | Energy value kJ | Protein (N × 6.25) g | Fat g | Carbo-hydrate g | Na mg | K mg | Ca mg | Mg mg | P mg | Fe mg | Cu mg | Zn mg | S mg | Cl mg |
|---|---|---|---|---|---|---|---|---|---|---|---|---|---|---|---|---|
| | ***Crustacea*** | | | | | | | | | | | | | | | |
| 518 | **Crab** boiled | 127 | 534 | 20.1 | 5.2 | 0 | 370 | 270 | 29 | 48 | 350 | 1.3 | 4.8 | 5.5 | 470 | 570 |
| 519 | boiled (weighed with shell) | 25 | 105 | 4.0 | 1.0 | 0 | 73 | 54 | 6 | 10 | 70 | 0.3 | 1.0 | 1.1 | 93 | 110 |
| 520 | canned | 81 | 341 | 18.1 | 0.9 | 0 | 550 | 100 | 120 | 32 | 140 | 2.8 | 0.42 | 5.0 | — | 830 |
| 521 | **Lobster** boiled | 119 | 502 | 22.1 | 3.4 | 0 | 330 | 260 | 62 | 34 | 280 | 0.8 | 1.7 | 1.8 | 510 | 530 |
| 522 | boiled (weighed with shell) | 42 | 179 | 7.9 | 1.2 | 0 | 120 | 93 | 22 | 12 | 100 | 0.3 | 0.65 | 0.6 | 190 | 190 |
| 523 | **Prawns** boiled | 107 | 451 | 22.6 | 1.8 | 0 | 1590 | 260 | 150 | 42 | 350 | 1.1 | (0.70) | (1.6) | 370 | 2550 |
| 524 | boiled (weighed with shell) | 41 | 172 | 8.6 | 0.7 | 0 | 610 | 99 | 55 | 16 | 130 | 0.4 | (0.27) | (0.6) | 140 | 970 |
| 525 | **Scampi** fried | 316 | 1321 | 12.2 | 17.6 | 28.9 | 380 | 390 | 99 | 30 | 310 | 1.1 | 0.22 | 0.6 | — | 740 |
| 527 | **Shrimps** boiled | 117 | 493 | 23.8 | 2.4 | 0 | 3840 | 400 | 320 | 110 | 270 | 1.8 | 0.80 | (5.3) | 340 | 5850 |
| 528 | boiled (weighed with shell) | 39 | 164 | 7.9 | 0.8 | 0 | 1260 | 130 | 110 | 35 | 89 | 0.6 | 0.26 | (1.7) | 110 | 1930 |
| 529 | canned | 94 | 398 | 20.8 | 1.2 | 0 | 980 | 100 | 110 | 49 | 150 | 5.1 | 0.23 | 2.4 | — | 1510 |
| | ***Molluscs*** | | | | | | | | | | | | | | | |
| 531 | **Cockles** boiled | 48 | 203 | 11.3 | 0.3 | Tr | 3520 | 43 | 130 | 51 | 200 | 26.0[a] | 0.28 | 1.2 | 320 | 5220 |
| 532 | **Mussels** raw | 66 | 276 | 12.1 | 1.9 | Tr | 290 | 320 | 88 | 23 | 240 | 5.8 | 0.36 | 1.6 | 370 | 460 |
| 533 | boiled | 87 | 366 | 17.2 | 2.0 | Tr | 210 | 92 | 200 | 25 | 330 | 7.7 | 0.48 | 2.1 | 350 | 320 |
| 534 | boiled (weighed with shell) | 26 | 111 | 5.2 | 0.6 | Tr | 63 | 28 | 59 | 8 | 99 | 2.3 | 0.16 | 0.6 | 100 | 95 |
| 535 | **Oysters** raw | 51 | 217 | 10.8 | 0.9 | Tr | 510 | 260 | 190 | 42 | 270 | 6.0 | 7.6 | 45.0[b] | 250 | 820 |
| 536 | raw (weighed with shell) | 6 | 26 | 1.3 | 0.1 | Tr | 61 | 31 | 22 | 5 | 32 | 0.7 | 0.91 | 5.4 | 30 | 98 |
| 538 | **Scallops** steamed | 105 | 446 | 23.2 | 1.4 | Tr | 270 | 480 | 120 | 38 | 340 | 3.0 | — | — | 570 | 410 |

[a] The iron content of cockles can be as high as 40 mg per 100 g

[b] The zinc content of oysters may vary from 6 to 100 mg per 100 g

| No | Food | Retinol µg | Carotene µg | Vitamin D µg | Thiamin mg | Riboflavin mg | Nicotinic acid mg | Potential nicotinic acid from tryptophan mg Trp ÷ 60 | Vitamin C mg | Vitamin E mg |
|---|---|---|---|---|---|---|---|---|---|---|
| | ***Crustacea*** | | | | | | | | | |
| 518 | **Crab** boiled | Tr | Tr | Tr | 0.10 | 0.15 | 2.5 | 3.8 | Tr | — |
| 519 | boiled (weighed with shell) | Tr | Tr | Tr | 0.02 | 0.03 | 0.5 | 0.8 | Tr | — |
| 520 | canned | Tr | Tr | Tr | Tr | 0.05 | 1.1 | 3.4 | Tr | — |
| 521 | **Lobster** boiled | Tr | Tr | Tr | 0.08 | 0.05 | 1.5 | 4.1 | Tr | 1.5 |
| 522 | boiled (weighed with shell) | Tr | Tr | Tr | 0.03 | 0.02 | 0.5 | 1.5 | Tr | 0.50 |
| 523 | **Prawns** boiled | Tr | Tr | Tr | — | — | — | 4.2 | Tr | — |
| 524 | boiled (weighed with shell) | Tr | Tr | Tr | — | — | — | 1.6 | Tr | — |
| 525 | **Scampi** fried | Tr | Tr | Tr | 0.08 | 0.05 | 1.3 | 2.3 | Tr | — |
| 527 | **Shrimps** boiled | Tr | Tr | Tr | 0.03 | 0.03 | 3.0 | 4.4 | Tr | — |
| 528 | boiled (weighed with shell) | Tr | Tr | Tr | 0.01 | 0.01 | 1.0 | 1.5 | Tr | — |
| 529 | canned | Tr | Tr | Tr | 0.01 | 0.02 | 0.8 | 3.9 | Tr | — |
| | ***Molluscs*** | | | | | | | | | |
| 531 | **Cockles** boiled | — | Tr | Tr | — | — | — | 2.4 | Tr | — |
| 532 | **Mussels** raw | — | Tr | Tr | — | — | — | 2.6 | Tr | 0.90 |
| 533 | boiled | — | Tr | Tr | — | — | — | 3.7 | Tr | (1.2) |
| 534 | boiled (weighed with shell) | — | Tr | Tr | — | — | — | 1.1 | Tr | (0.36) |
| 535 | **Oysters** raw | 75 | Tr | Tr | 0.10 | 0.20 | 1.5 | 2.3 | Tr[a] | 0.85 |
| 536 | raw (weighed with shell) | 9 | Tr | Tr | 0.01 | 0.02 | 0.2 | 0.3 | Tr | 0.10 |
| 538 | **Scallops** steamed | — | Tr | Tr | — | — | — | 5.0 | Tr | — |

| No | Food | Vitamin $B_6$ mg | Vitamin $B_{12}$ µg | Folic acid Free µg | Folic acid Total µg | Pantothenic acid mg | Biotin µg |
|---|---|---|---|---|---|---|---|
| | ***Crustacea*** | | | | | | |
| 518 | **Crab** boiled | 0.35 | Tr | 3 | 20 | 0.60 | Tr |
| 519 | boiled (weighed with shell) | 0.07 | Tr | 1 | 4 | 0.12 | Tr |
| 520 | canned | — | Tr | — | — | — | Tr |
| 521 | **Lobster** boiled | — | 1 | 7 | 17 | 1.63 | 5 |
| 522 | boiled (weighed with shell) | — | Tr | 3 | 6 | 0.59 | 2 |
| 523 | **Prawns** boiled | — | — | — | — | — | — |
| 524 | boiled (weighed with shell) | — | — | — | — | — | — |
| 525 | **Scampi** fried | — | — | — | — | — | — |
| 527 | **Shrimps** boiled | 0.10 | 1 | — | — | 0.30 | 1 |
| 528 | boiled (weighed with shell) | 0.03 | Tr | — | — | 0.10 | Tr |
| 529 | canned | 0.03 | 2 | 4 | 15 | 0.35 | (1) |
| | ***Molluscs*** | | | | | | |
| 531 | **Cockles** boiled | — | Tr | — | — | — | — |
| 532 | **Mussels** raw | — | — | — | — | — | — |
| 533 | boiled | — | — | — | — | — | — |
| 534 | boiled (weighed with shell) | — | — | — | — | — | — |
| 535 | **Oysters** raw | 0.03 | 15 | 10 | — | 0.50 | 10 |
| 536 | raw (weighed with shell) | Tr | 2 | 1 | — | 0.06 | 1 |
| 538 | **Scallops** steamed | — | — | 17 | 17 | 0.14 | Tr |

Notes

[a] Some species of oysters contain vitamin C; Pacific oysters (*Ostrea gigas*) have been shown to contain 22 mg, and Olympia oysters (*Ostrea lurida*) 38 mg per 100 g.

| No | Food | Description and number of samples | Edible matter, proportion of weight purchased | Water g | Total nitrogen g |
|---|---|---|---|---|---|
| | ***Molluscs** contd* | | | | |
| 539 | **Whelks** boiled | Purchased cooked, probably boiled in sea or salt water | 0.15 | 77.5 | 2.96 |
| 540 | boiled (weighed with shell) | Calculated from the previous item | 0.15 | 11.6 | 0.44 |
| 541 | **Winkles** boiled | Purchased cooked, probably boiled in sea water | 0.19 | 79.1 | 2.45 |
| 542 | boiled (weighed with shell) | Calculated from the previous item | 0.19 | 15.1 | 0.47 |
| | ***Fish products and dishes*** | | | | |
| 543 | **Fish cakes** frozen | 14 packets, 4 brands, white fish | 1.00 | 70.2 | 1.68 |
| 544 | fried | 14 packets, 4 brands, white fish | 1.02 | 63.3 | 1.45 |
| 545 | **Fish fingers** frozen | 11 packets, 3 brands; in breadcrumbs | 1.00 | 63.9 | 2.02 |
| 546 | fried | 11 packets, 3 brands; in breadcrumbs | 0.90 | 55.6 | 2.16 |
| 547 | **Fish paste** | 30 samples, sardine, crab, lobster, salmon | 1.00 | 67.1 | 2.45 |
| 548 | **Fish pie** | Recipe p 343 | — | 74.3 | 1.13 |
| 549 | **Kedgeree** | Recipe p 343 | — | 68.4 | 2.03 |
| 550 | **Roe, cod** hard, raw | Literature sources | 1.00 | 70.0 | 3.89 |
| 551 | fried | Parboiled, sliced and fried in crumbs | 0.93 | 62.0 | 3.35 |
| 552 | **herring** soft, raw | Literature sources | 1.00 | 82.0 | 2.42 [a] |
| 553 | fried | Rolled in flour and fried | 0.80 | 52.3 | 3.85 [b] |

[a] Includes 0.29 g purine nitrogen per 100 g

[b] Includes 0.48 g purine nitrogen per 100 g

| No | Food | Energy value kcal | Energy value kJ | Protein g | Fat g | Carbo-hydrate g | mg Na | K | Ca | Mg | P | Fe | Cu | Zn | S | Cl |
|---|---|---|---|---|---|---|---|---|---|---|---|---|---|---|---|---|
| | ***Molluscs** contd* | | | | | | | | | | | | | | | |
| 539 | **Whelks** boiled | 91 | 385 | 18.5 | 1.9 | Tr | 270 | 320 | 54 | 160 | 230 | 6.2 | (7.2) | 7.2 | 450 | 590 |
| 540 | boiled (weighed with shell) | 14 | 59 | 2.8 | 0.3 | Tr | 40 | 47 | 8 | 24 | 34 | 0.9 | (1.1) | 1.1 | 67 | 88 |
| 541 | **Winkles** boiled | 74 | 312 | 15.3 | 1.4 | Tr | 1140 | 150 | 140 | 360 | 220 | 15.0 | (1.3) | (5.7) | 380 | 1800 |
| 542 | boiled (weighed with shell) | 14 | 60 | 2.9 | 0.3 | Tr | 220 | 29 | 26 | 68 | 42 | 2.9 | (0.25) | (1.1) | 72 | 340 |
| | ***Fish products and dishes*** | | | | | | | | | | | | | | | |
| 543 | **Fish cakes** frozen | 112 | 477 | 10.5 | 0.8 | 16.8 | 480 | 280 | 76 | 20 | 120 | 1.0 | 0.10 | 0.5 | — | 820 |
| 544 | fried | 188 | 785 | 9.1 | 10.5 | 15.1 | 500 | 260 | 70 | 18 | 110 | 1.0 | 0.13 | 0.4 | — | 730 |
| 545 | **Fish fingers** frozen | 178 | 749 | 12.6 | 7.5 | 16.1 | 320 | 240 | 43 | 18 | 190 | 0.7 | 0.06 | 0.4 | — | 380 |
| 546 | fried | 233 | 975 | 13.5 | 12.7 | 17.2 | 350 | 260 | 45 | 19 | 220 | 0.7 | 0.08 | 0.4 | — | 400 |
| 547 | **Fish paste** | 169 | 704 | 15.3 | 10.4 | 3.7 | 600 | 300 | 280 | 33 | 310 | 9.0 | 0.37 | 1.4 | — | 940 |
| 548 | **Fish pie** | 128 | 540 | 7.1 | 5.7 | 13.0 | 210 | 310 | 40 | 18 | 92 | 0.4 | 0.10 | 0.4 | — | 330 |
| 549 | **Kedgeree** | 151 | 633 | 13.1 | 7.1 | 9.2 | 790 | 160 | 36 | 16 | 160 | 0.9 | 0.07 | 0.6 | 150 | 1220 |
| 550 | **Roe, cod** hard, raw | 113 | 476 | 24.3 | 1.7 | 0 | — | — | — | — | — | — | — | — | — | — |
| 551 | fried | 202 | 844 | 20.9 | 11.9 | 3.0 | 130 | 260 | 17 | 11 | 500 | 1.6 | — | — | 240 | 190 |
| 552 | **herring** soft, raw | 80 | 337 | 13.3[a] | 3.0 | 0 | — | — | — | — | — | — | — | — | — | — |
| 553 | fried | 244 | 1019 | 21.1[a] | 15.8 | 4.7 | 87 | 240 | 16 | 8 | 920 | 1.5 | — | — | 240 | 120 |

[a] (Total N − purine N) × 6.25

| No | Food | Retinol µg | Carotene µg | Vitamin D µg | Thiamin mg | Riboflavin mg | Nicotinic acid mg | Potential nicotinic acid from tryptophan mg Trp ÷ 60 | Vitamin C mg | Vitamin E mg |
|---|---|---|---|---|---|---|---|---|---|---|
| | ***Molluscs** contd* | | | | | | | | | |
| 539 | **Whelks** boiled | — | Tr | Tr | — | — | — | 4.0 | Tr | 0.80 |
| 540 | boiled (weighed with shell) | — | Tr | Tr | — | — | — | 0.6 | Tr | 0.10 |
| 541 | **Winkles** boiled | — | Tr | Tr | — | — | — | 3.3 | Tr | — |
| 542 | boiled (weighed with shell) | — | Tr | Tr | — | — | — | 0.6 | Tr | — |
| | ***Fish products and dishes*** | | | | | | | | | |
| 543 | **Fish cakes** frozen | Tr | Tr | Tr | 0.06 | 0.06 | 1.3 | 2.0 | Tr | — |
| 544 | fried | Tr | Tr | Tr | 0.06 | 0.06 | 1.1 | 1.7 | Tr | — |
| 545 | **Fish fingers** frozen | Tr | Tr | Tr | 0.09 | 0.06 | 1.1 | 2.4 | Tr | — |
| 546 | fried | Tr | Tr | Tr | 0.08 | 0.07 | 1.4 | 2.5 | Tr | — |
| 547 | **Fish paste** | — | Tr | — | 0.02 | 0.20 | 4.1 | 2.9 | Tr | 0.85[a] |
| 548 | **Fish pie** | 30 | 4 | 0.17 | 0.07 | 0.09 | 1.0 | 1.4 | 2 | 0.42 |
| 549 | **Kedgeree** | 80 | 0 | 0.79 | 0.07 | 0.14 | 0.8 | 2.8 | 0 | 1.0 |
| 550 | **Roe cod** hard, raw | 140[b] | Tr | 2.0 | 1.5 | 1.0 | 1.5 | 4.5 | 30 | 6.4 |
| 551 | fried | (150)[b] | Tr | (2.2) | (1.3) | (0.9) | (1.3) | 3.9 | (26) | (6.9) |
| 552 | **herring** soft, raw | — | — | — | 0.20 | 0.50 | 2.0 | 2.5 | 5 | — |
| 553 | fried | — | — | — | (0.20) | (0.50) | (2.0) | 3.9 | (5) | — |

| No | Food | Vitamin $B_6$ mg | Vitamin $B_{12}$ µg | Folic acid Free µg | Folic acid Total µg | Pantothenic acid mg | Biotin µg |
|---|---|---|---|---|---|---|---|
| | ***Molluscs** contd* | | | | | | |
| 539 | **Whelks** boiled | — | — | — | — | — | — |
| 540 | boiled (weighed with shell) | — | — | — | — | — | — |
| 541 | **Winkles** boiled | — | — | — | — | — | — |
| 542 | boiled (weighed with shell) | — | — | — | — | — | — |
| | ***Fish products and dishes*** | | | | | | |
| 543 | **Fish cakes** frozen | — | — | — | — | — | — |
| 544 | fried | — | — | — | — | — | — |
| 545 | **Fish fingers** frozen | 0.21 | 1 | 5 | 15 | — | — |
| 546 | fried | 0.21 | 2 | 6 | 16 | — | — |
| 547 | **Fish paste** | — | — | — | — | — | — |
| 548 | **Fish pie** | 0.22 | 1 | 2 | 6 | 0.3 | 1 |
| 549 | **Kedgeree** | 0.19 | 2 | 7 | 9 | 0.5 | 7 |
| 550 | **Roe, cod** hard, raw | 0.32 | 10 | — | — | 3.0 | 13 |
| 551 | fried | (0.28) | (11) | — | — | (2.6) | (15) |
| 552 | **herring** soft, raw | — | 5 | — | — | 0.49 | — |
| 553 | fried | — | (6) | — | — | (0.49) | — |

Notes

[a] Also contains 0.17 mg γ-tocopherol per 100 g.

[b] 90 per cent is present as retinaldehyde.

| No | Food | Description and number of samples | Edible matter, proportion of weight purchased | Water g | Total nitrogen g |
|---|---|---|---|---|---|

| | | Energy value | | Protein | Fat | Carbo-hydrate | mg | | | | | | | | | |
|---|---|---|---|---|---|---|---|---|---|---|---|---|---|---|---|---|
| No | Food | kcal | kJ | g | g | g | Na | K | Ca | Mg | P | Fe | Cu | Zn | S | Cl |

| No | Food | Retinol µg | Carotene µg | Vitamin D µg | Thiamin mg | Riboflavin mg | Nicotinic acid mg | Potential nicotinic acid from tryptophan mg Trp ÷ 60 | Vitamin C mg | Vitamin E mg |
|---|---|---|---|---|---|---|---|---|---|---|

| No | Food | Vitamin $B_6$ mg | Vitamin $B_{12}$ µg | Folic acid Free µg | Folic acid Total µg | Pantothenic acid mg | Biotin µg | Notes |
|---|---|---|---|---|---|---|---|---|

| No | Food | Description and number of samples | Edible matter, proportion of weight purchased | Water g | Sugars g | Starch g | Dietary fibre g | Total nitrogen g |
|---|---|---|---|---|---|---|---|---|
| 554 | **Ackee** canned | 8 cans, drained contents only | — | 76.7 | 0.8 | Tr | 2.7 | 0.46 |
| 555 | **Artichokes, globe** boiled | Base of leaves and soft inside parts; boiled 35 minutes | 0.41 | 84.4 | — | 0 | — | 0.18 |
| 556 | boiled (weighed as served) | Calculated from the previous item | 0.41 | 36.3 | — | 0 | — | 0.08 |
| 557 | **Artichokes, Jerusalem** boiled | Flesh only; boiled 20 minutes | 0.85 | 80.2 | — | 0 | — | 0.25 |
| 558 | **Asparagus** boiled | Soft tips only; boiled 25 minutes | 0.20 | 92.4 | 1.1 | 0 | 1.5 | 0.54 |
| 559 | boiled (weighed as served) | Calculated from the previous item | 0.20 | 46.2 | 0.6 | 0 | 0.8 | 0.27 |
| 560 | **Aubergine** raw | Eggplant; flesh only | 0.77 | 93.4 | 2.9 | 0.2 | 2.5 | 0.11 |
| | **Beans** | | | | | | | |
| 561 | **French** boiled | Pods and beans; cut up and boiled 30 minutes | 1.00 | 95.5 | 0.8 | 0.3 | 3.2 | 0.12 |
| 562 | **runner** raw | Samples from 6 shops; pod ends and sides trimmed | 0.79 | 89.0 | 2.8 | 1.1 | 2.9 | 0.36 |
| 563 | boiled | Trimmed pods broken up and boiled 20 minutes | 0.99 | 90.7 | 1.3 | 1.4 | 3.4 | 0.31 |
| 564 | **broad** boiled | Whole beans without pods; boiled 30 minutes | 0.31 | 83.7 | 0.6 | 6.5 | 4.2 | 0.66 |
| 565 | **butter** raw | Whole beans | 1.00 | 11.6 | 3.6 | 46.2 | 21.6 | 3.06 |
| 566 | boiled | Soaked 24 hours, boiled 2 hours | 2.50 | 70.5 | 1.5 | 15.6 | 5.1 | 1.13 |
| 567 | **haricot** raw | Whole beans | 1.00 | 11.3 | 2.8 | 42.7 | 25.4 | 3.42 |
| 568 | boiled | Soaked 24 hours, boiled 2 hours | 2.60 | 69.6 | 0.8 | 15.8 | 7.4 | 1.06 |
| 569 | **baked** canned in tomato sauce | 11 cans, 4 brands | 1.00 | 73.6 | 5.2 | 5.1 | 7.3 | 0.82 |

| No | Food | Energy value kcal | Energy value kJ | Protein (N × 6.25) g | Fat g | Carbo-hydrate g | Na mg | K mg | Ca mg | Mg mg | P mg | Fe mg | Cu mg | Zn mg | S mg | Cl mg |
|---|---|---|---|---|---|---|---|---|---|---|---|---|---|---|---|---|
| 554 | **Ackee** canned | 151 | 625 | 2.9 | 15.2 | 0.8 | 240 | 270 | 35 | 40 | 47 | 0.7 | 0.27 | 0.6 | — | 340 |
| 555 | **Artichokes, globe** boiled | 15 | 62 | 1.1 | Tr | 2.7[a] | 15 | 330 | 44 | 27 | 40 | 0.5 | 0.09 | — | 16 | 84 |
| 556 | boiled (weighed as served) | 7 | 28 | 0.5 | Tr | 1.2[a] | 6 | 140 | 19 | 12 | 17 | 0.2 | 0.04 | — | 7 | 36 |
| 557 | **Artichokes, Jerusalem** boiled | 18 | 78 | 1.6 | Tr | 3.2[a] | 3 | 420 | 30 | 11 | 33 | 0.4 | 0.12 | 0.1 | 22 | 58 |
| 558 | **Asparagus** boiled | 18 | 75 | 3.4 | Tr | 1.1 | 2 | 240 | 26 | 10 | 85 | 0.9 | 0.20 | 0.3 | 47 | 31 |
| 559 | boiled (weighed as served) | 9 | 39 | 1.7 | Tr | 0.6 | 1 | 120 | 13 | 5 | 42 | 0.5 | 0.10 | 0.1 | 23 | 16 |
| 560 | **Aubergine** raw | 14 | 62 | 0.7 | Tr | 3.1 | 3 | 240 | 10 | 10 | 12 | 0.4 | 0.08 | — | 9 | 61 |
| | **Beans** | | | | | | | | | | | | | | | |
| 561 | **French** boiled | 7 | 31 | 0.8 | Tr | 1.1 | 3 | 100 | 39 | 10 | 15 | 0.6 | 0.10 | 0.3 | 8 | 11 |
| 562 | **runner** raw | 26 | 114 | 2.3 | 0.2 | 3.9 | 2 | 280 | 27 | 27 | 47 | 0.8 | 0.07 | 0.4 | — | 18 |
| 563 | boiled | 19 | 83 | 1.9 | 0.2 | 2.7 | 1 | 150 | 22 | 17 | 41 | 0.7 | 0.05 | 0.3 | — | 5 |
| 564 | **broad** boiled | 48 | 206 | 4.1 | 0.6 | 7.1 | 20 | 230 | 21 | 28 | 99 | 1.0 | 0.43 | — | 27 | 14 |
| 565 | **butter** raw | 273 | 1162 | 19.1 | 1.1 | 49.8 | 62 | 1700 | 85 | 164 | 320 | 5.9 | 1.22 | 2.8 | 110 | 47 |
| 566 | boiled | 95 | 405 | 7.1 | 0.3 | 17.1 | 16 | 400 | 19 | 33 | 87 | 1.7 | 0.16 | 1.0 | 47 | 2 |
| 567 | **haricot** raw | 271 | 1151 | 21.4 | 1.6 | 45.5 | 43 | 1160 | 180 | 180 | 310 | 6.7 | 0.61 | 2.8 | 170 | 2 |
| 568 | boiled | 93 | 396 | 6.6 | 0.5 | 16.6 | 15 | 320 | 65 | 45 | 120 | 2.5 | 0.14 | 1.0 | 46 | 1 |
| 569 | **baked** canned in tomato sauce | 64 | 270 | 5.1 | 0.5 | 10.3 | 480 | 300 | 45 | 31 | 91 | 1.4 | 0.21 | 0.7 | (43) | 800 |

[a] This vegetable contains inulin; 50 per cent total carbohydrate taken to be available

| No | Food | Retinol µg | Carotene µg | Vitamin D µg | Thiamin mg | Riboflavin mg | Nicotinic acid mg | Potential nicotinic acid from tryptophan mg Trp ÷ 60 | Vitamin C mg | Vitamin E mg |
|---|---|---|---|---|---|---|---|---|---|---|
| 554 | **Ackee** canned | 0 | — | 0 | 0.03 | 0.07 | 0.6 | 0.5 | 30 | — |
| 555 | **Artichokes, globe** boiled | 0 | 90 | 0 | 0.07 | 0.03 | 0.9 | 0.2 | 8 | — |
| 556 | boiled (weighed as served) | 0 | 40 | 0 | 0.03 | 0.01 | 0.4 | 0.1 | 3 | — |
| 557 | **Artichokes, Jerusalem** boiled | 0 | (Tr) | 0 | 0.10 | Tr | — | 0.3 | 2 | 0.2 |
| 558 | **Asparagus** boiled | 0 | 500 *(400–800)* | 0 | 0.10 | 0.08 | 0.8 | 0.6 | 20 *(15–30)* | 2.5 |
| 559 | boiled (weighed as served) | 0 | 250 | 0 | 0.05 | 0.04 | 0.4 | 0.3 | 10 | 1.3 |
| 560 | **Aubergine** raw | 0 | Tr | 0 | 0.05 | 0.03 | 0.8 | 0.1 | 5 | — |
| | **Beans** | | | | | | | | | |
| 561 | **French** boiled | 0 | 400 *(300–500)* | 0 | 0.04 | 0.07 | 0.3 | 0.2 | 5 | 0.2 |
| 562 | **runner** raw | 0 | 400 *(300–500)* | 0 | 0.05 | 0.10 | 0.9 | 0.4 | 20 *(15–40)* | 0.2 [a] |
| 563 | boiled | 0 | 400 | 0 | 0.03 | 0.07 | 0.5 | 0.3 | 5 [b] | 0.2 [a] |
| 564 | **broad** boiled | 0 | 250 | 0 | (0.10) | 0.04 | 3.0 | 0.7 | 15 [c] | Tr [d] |
| 565 | **butter** raw | 0 | Tr | 0 | 0.45 | 0.13 | 2.5 | 3.1 | 0 | — |
| 566 | boiled | 0 | Tr | 0 | — | — | — | 1.1 | 0 | — |
| 567 | **haricot** raw | 0 | Tr | 0 | 0.45 | 0.13 | 2.5 | 3.4 | 0 | — |
| 568 | boiled | 0 | Tr | 0 | — | — | — | 1.1 | 0 | — |
| 569 | **baked** canned in tomato sauce | 0 | — | 0 | 0.07 | 0.05 | 0.5 | 0.8 | (Tr) | 0.6 [e] |

| No | Food | Vitamin $B_6$ mg | Vitamin $B_{12}$ µg | Folic acid Free µg | Folic acid Total µg | Pantothenic acid mg | Biotin µg |
|---|---|---|---|---|---|---|---|
| 554 | **Ackee** canned | 0.06 | 0 | 8 | 41 | — | — |
| 555 | **Artichokes, globe** boiled | 0.07 | 0 | — | (30) | 0.21 | 4.1 |
| 556 | boiled (weighed as served) | 0.03 | 0 | — | (13) | 0.09 | 1.8 |
| 557 | **Artichokes, Jerusalem** boiled | — | 0 | — | — | — | — |
| 558 | **Asparagus** boiled | 0.04 | 0 | (5) | (30) | 0.13 | 0.4 |
| 559 | boiled (weighed as served) | 0.02 | 0 | (3) | (15) | 0.07 | 0.2 |
| 560 | **Aubergine** raw | 0.08 | 0 | 8 | 20 | 0.22 | — |
| | **Beans** | | | | | | |
| 561 | **French** boiled | 0.06 | 0 | 3 | 28 | 0.07 | 0.8 |
| 562 | **runner** raw | 0.07 | 0 | 57 | 60 | 0.05 | 0.7 |
| 563 | boiled | 0.04 | 0 | 3 | 28 | 0.04 | 0.5 |
| 564 | **broad** boiled | — | 0 | — | — | 3.8 | 2.1 |
| 565 | **butter** raw | 0.58 | 0 | 25 | 110 | 1.0 | — |
| 566 | boiled | — | 0 | — | — | — | — |
| 567 | **haricot** raw | 0.56 | 0 | — | — | 0.7 | — |
| 568 | boiled | — | 0 | — | — | — | — |
| 569 | **baked** canned in tomato sauce | 0.12 | 0 | 4 | 29 | — | — |

Notes

[a] Also contains 0.3 mg γ-tocopherol per 100 g.

[b] Canned green beans contain 2 mg per 100 g.

[c] Canned broad beans contain 6 mg per 100 g.

[d] Also contains 2.5 mg γ-tocopherol per 100 g.

[e] Also contains 0.8 mg γ-tocopherol per 100 g.

| No | Food | Description and number of samples | Edible matter, proportion of weight purchased | Water g | Sugars g | Starch g | Dietary fibre g | Total nitrogen g |
|---|---|---|---|---|---|---|---|---|
| | **Beans** *contd* | | | | | | | |
| 570 | **mung** green gram, raw | Literature sources | 1.00 | 12.0 | 1.2 | 34.4 | (22.0) | 3.52 |
| 571 | cooked dahl | Recipe p 343 | — | 72.5 | 0.8 | 10.6 | (6.4) | 1.02 |
| 572 | **red kidney** raw | Literature sources | 1.00 | 11.0 | (3.0) | (42.0) | (25.0) | 3.54 |
| 573 | **Beansprouts** canned | 10 cans, drained contents | 0.55 | 95.4 | 0.4 | 0.4 | 3.0 | 0.25 |
| 574 | **Beetroot** raw | Flesh only, no skin | 0.82 | 87.1 | 6.0 | 0 | 3.1 | 0.21 |
| 575 | boiled [a] | Flesh only, no skin; boiled 2 hours | 0.80 | 82.7 | 9.9 | 0 | 2.5 | 0.29 |
| 576 | **Broccoli tops** raw | 10 samples; predominantly leaves, thick stems removed | 0.70 | 89.0 | 2.5 | Tr | 3.6 | 0.52 |
| 577 | boiled | 10 samples; predominantly leaves, thick stems removed; boiled 15 minutes | 0.84 | 89.9 | 1.5 | 0.1 | 4.1 | 0.49 |
| 578 | **Brussels sprouts** raw | 10 samples; inner leaves only | 0.63 | 88.1 | 2.6 | 0.1 | 4.2 | 0.64 |
| 579 | boiled | 10 samples; inner leaves only; boiled 15 minutes | 0.72 | 91.5 | 1.6 | 0.1 | 2.9 | 0.45 |
| 580 | **Cabbage, red** raw | Inner leaves | 0.70 | 89.7 | 3.5 | Tr | 3.4 | 0.27 |
| 581 | **Savoy** raw | Inner leaves | 0.53 | 89.9 | 3.3 | Tr | 3.1 | 0.53 |
| 582 | boiled | Inner leaves; boiled 30 minutes | 0.65 | 95.7 | 1.1 | Tr | 2.5 | 0.21 |
| 583 | **spring** boiled | Inner leaves; boiled 30 minutes | 0.59 | 96.6 | 0.8 | Tr | 2.2 | 0.18 |
| 584 | **white** raw | 7 cabbages; whole cabbage as purchased | 1.00 | 90.3 | 3.7 | 0.1 | 2.7 | 0.31 |
| 585 | **winter** raw | 20 cabbages, January King; inner leaves | 0.57 | 88.3 | 2.7 | 0.1 | 3.4 | 0.45 |
| 586 | boiled | 20 cabbages, January King; inner leaves, boiled 15 minutes | 0.61 | 93.0 | 2.2 | 0.1 | 2.8 | 0.27 |

[a] Weighed cold

| No | Food | Energy value kcal | Energy value kJ | Protein (N × 6.25) g | Fat g | Carbo-hydrate g | Na mg | K mg | Ca mg | Mg mg | P mg | Fe mg | Cu mg | Zn mg | S mg | Cl mg |
|---|---|---|---|---|---|---|---|---|---|---|---|---|---|---|---|---|
| | **Beans** *contd* | | | | | | | | | | | | | | | |
| 570 | **mung** green gram, raw | 231 | 981 | 22.0 | 1.0 | 35.6 | 28 | 850 | 100 | 170 | 330 | 8.0 | 0.97 | — | 190 | 12 |
| 571 | cooked, dahl | 106 | 447 | 6.4 | 4.2 | 11.4 | 820 | 270 | 34 | 51 | 100 | 2.6 | 0.29 | — | 61 | 1260 |
| 572 | **red kidney** raw | 272 | 1159 | 22.1 | 1.7 | 45.0 | (40) | (1160) | 140 | (180) | 410 | 6.7 | (0.61) | (2.8) | (170) | (2) |
| 573 | **Beansprouts** canned | 9 | 40 | 1.6 | Tr | 0.8 | 80 | 36 | 13 | 10 | 20 | 1.0 | 0.09 | 0.8 | — | 120 |
| 574 | **Beetroot** raw | 28 | 118 | 1.3 | Tr | 6.0 | 84 | 300 | 25 | 15 | 32 | 0.4 | 0.07 | 0.4 | — | 59 |
| 575 | boiled | 44 | 189 | 1.8 | Tr | 9.9 | 64 | 350 | 30 | 17 | 36 | 0.4 | 0.08 | 0.4 | 22 | 76 |
| 576 | **Broccoli tops** raw | 23 | 96 | 3.3 | Tr | 2.5 | 12 | 340 | 100 | 18 | 67 | 1.5 | 0.07 | 0.6 | — | 55 |
| 577 | boiled | 18 | 78 | 3.1 | Tr | 1.6 | 6 | 220 | 76 | 12 | 60 | 1.0 | 0.08 | 0.4 | — | 37 |
| 578 | **Brussels sprouts** raw | 26 | 111 | 4.0 | Tr | 2.7 | 4 | 380 | 32 | 19 | 65 | 0.7 | 0.06 | 0.5 | — | 28 |
| 579 | boiled | 18 | 75 | 2.8 | Tr | 1.7 | 2 | 240 | 25 | 13 | 51 | 0.5 | 0.05 | 0.4 | 78 | 16 |
| 580 | **Cabbage, red** raw | 20 | 85 | 1.7 | Tr | 3.5 | 32 | 300 | 53 | 17 | 32 | 0.6 | 0.09 | 0.3 | 68 | 45 |
| 581 | **Savoy**, raw | 26 | 109 | 3.3 | Tr | 3.3 | 23 | 260 | 75 | 20 | 68 | 0.9 | (0.07) | 0.3 | 88 | 22 |
| 582 | boiled | 9 | 40 | 1.3 | Tr | 1.1 | 8 | 120 | 53 | 7 | 27 | 0.7 | 0.07 | 0.2 | 30 | 9 |
| 583 | **spring** boiled | 7 | 32 | 1.1 | Tr | 0.8 | 12 | 110 | 30 | 6 | 32 | 0.5 | 0.07 | 0.2 | 27 | 6 |
| 584 | **white** raw | 22 | 93 | 1.9 | Tr | 3.8 | 7 | 280 | 44 | 13 | 36 | 0.4 | (0.03) | 0.3 | — | 23 |
| 585 | **winter** raw | 22 | 92 | 2.8 | Tr | 2.8 | 7 | 390 | 57 | 17 | 54 | 0.6 | 0.06 | 0.4 | — | 31 |
| 586 | boiled | 15 | 66 | 1.7 | Tr | 2.3 | 4 | 160 | 38 | 8 | 34 | 0.4 | (0.03) | 0.2 | — | 13 |

| No | Food | Retinol µg | Carotene µg | Vitamin D µg | Thiamin mg | Riboflavin mg | Nicotinic acid mg | Potential nicotinic acid from tryptophan mg Trp ÷ 60 | Vitamin C mg | Vitamin E mg |
|---|---|---|---|---|---|---|---|---|---|---|
| | **Beans** *contd* | | | | | | | | | |
| 570 | **mung** green gram, raw | 0 | 24 | 0 | 0.45 | 0.20 | 2.0 | 3.5 | Tr | — |
| 571 | cooked, dahl | 60 | 44 | 0.06 | 0.09 | 0.04 | 0.4 | 1.0 | Tr | — |
| 572 | **red kidney** raw | 0 | Tr | 0 | 0.54 | 0.18 | 2.0 | 3.5 | Tr | — |
| 573 | **Beansprouts** canned | 0 | Tr | 0 | 0.02 | 0.03 | 0.2 | 0.3 | 1 [a] | — |
| 574 | **Beetroot** raw | 0 | Tr | 0 | 0.03 | 0.05 | 0.1 | 0.2 | 6 | 0 |
| 575 | boiled | 0 | Tr | 0 | 0.02 | 0.04 | 0.1 | 0.3 | 5 | 0 |
| 576 | **Broccoli tops** raw | 0 | 2500 *(900–7000)* | 0 | 0.10 | 0.30 | 1.0 | 0.6 | 110 *(70–160)* | 1.3 |
| 577 | boiled | 0 | 2500 *(900–7000)* | 0 | 0.06 | 0.20 | 0.6 | 0.6 | 34 *(20–70)* | 1.1 |
| 578 | **Brussels sprouts** raw | 0 | 400 *(120–550)* | 0 | 0.10 | (0.15) | 0.7 | 0.8 | 90 *(70–140)* | 1.0 |
| 579 | boiled | 0 | 400 *(120–550)* | 0 | 0.06 | (0.10) | 0.4 | 0.5 | 40 *(30–90)* | 0.9 |
| 580 | **Cabbage, red** raw | 0 | (20) | 0 | 0.06 | 0.05 | 0.3 | 0.3 | 55 | 0.2 |
| 581 | **Savoy** raw | 0 | 300 [b] | 0 | 0.06 | 0.05 | 0.3 | 0.5 | 60 *(50–80)* | 0.2 [c] |
| 582 | boiled | 0 | 300 [b] | 0 | 0.03 | 0 03 | 0.2 | 0.2 | 15 *(10–40)* | 0.2 [c] |
| 803 | **spring** boiled | 0 | 500 | 0 | 0.03 | 0.03 | 0.2 | 0.2 | 25 *(10–50)* | 0.2 |
| 584 | **white** raw | 0 | (Tr) | 0 | 0.06 | 0.05 | 0.3 | 0.3 | 40 [d] | 0.2 |
| 585 | **winter** raw | 0 | 300 [b] | 0 | 0.06 | 0.05 | 0.3 | 0.5 | 55 *(40–70)* | 0.2 [c] |
| 586 | boiled | 0 | 300 [b] | 0 | 0.03 | 0.03 | 0.2 | 0.3 | 20 *(10–40)* | 0.2 [c] |

| No | Food | Vitamin $B_6$ mg | Vitamin $B_{12}$ µg | Folic acid Free µg | Folic acid Total µg | Pantothenic acid mg | Biotin µg |
|---|---|---|---|---|---|---|---|
| | **Beans** *contd* | | | | | | |
| 570 | **mung** green gram, raw | (0.50) | 0 | 25 | 140 | — | — |
| 571 | cooked, dahl | (0.09) | 0 | 1 | 20 | — | — |
| 572 | **red kidney** raw | 0.44 | 0 | 24 | 130 | 0.50 | — |
| 573 | **Beansprouts** canned | 0.03 | 0 | 4 | 12 | — | — |
| 574 | **Beetroot** raw | 0.05 | 0 | 70 | 90 | 0.12 | Tr |
| 575 | boiled | 0.03 | 0 | 20 | (50) | 0.10 | Tr |
| 576 | **Broccoli tops** raw | 0.21 | 0 | 89 | 130 | 1.0 | (0.5) |
| 577 | boiled | 0.13 | 0 | 7 | 110 | 0.70 | (0.3) |
| 578 | **Brussels sprouts** raw | 0.28 | 0 | 84 | 110 | 0.40 | 0.4 |
| 579 | boiled | 0.17 | 0 | 7 | 87 | 0.28 | 0.3 |
| 580 | **Cabbage, red** raw | 0.21 | 0 | (60) | (90) | 0.32 | 0.1 |
| 581 | **Savoy** raw | 0.16 | 0 | (60) | (90) | 0.21 | 0.1 |
| 582 | boiled | 0.10 | 0 | (2) | (35) | 0.15 | Tr |
| 583 | **spring** boiled | 0.10 | 0 | (18) | (50) | 0.15 | Tr |
| 584 | **white** raw | 0.16 | 0 | 19 | 26 | 0.21 | 0.1 |
| 585 | **winter** raw | 0.16 | 0 | 60 | 90 | 0.21 | 0.1 |
| 586 | boiled | 0.10 | 0 | 2 | 35 | 0.15 | Tr |

Notes

[a] Fresh beansprouts contain about 30mg per 100g.

[b] This is an average figure. The amount of carotene in leafy vegetables depends on the amount of chlorophyll, and the outer green leaves may contain 50 times as much as inner white ones.

[c] The value for inner leaves. Outer leaves contain 7.0mg α-tocopherol per 100g.

[d] About 20 per cent is lost on shredding.

| No | Food | Description and number of samples | Edible matter, proportion of weight purchased | Water g | Sugars g | Starch g | Dietary fibre g | Total nitrogen g |
|---|---|---|---|---|---|---|---|---|
| 587 | **Carrots, old** raw | Flesh only | 0.96 | 89.9 | 5.4 | 0 | 2.9 | 0.11 |
| 588 | boiled | Flesh only; cut up and boiled 45 minutes | 0.87 | 91.5 | 4.2 | 0.1 | 3.1 | 0.10 |
| 589 | **young** boiled | Purchased with leaves; flesh only, boiled 25 minutes | 0.50 | 91.1 | 4.4 | 0.1 | 3.0 | 0.14 |
| 590 | canned | 6 samples; drained contents | 0.63 | 91.2 | 4.4 | Tr | 3.7 | 0.11 |
| 591 | **Cauliflower** raw | 16 cauliflowers; flower and stalk | 0.62 | 92.7 | 1.5 | Tr | 2.1 | 0.30 |
| 592 | boiled | 16 cauliflowers; flower and stalk, boiled 20 minutes | 0.60 | 94.5 | 0.8 | Tr | 1.8 | 0.26 |
| 593 | **Celeriac** boiled | Flesh only; boiled 30 minutes | 0.79 | 90.2 | 1.5 | 0.5 | 4.9 | 0.26 |
| 594 | **Celery** raw | Stem only | 0.73 | 93.5 | 1.2 | 0.1 | 1.8 | 0.15 |
| 595 | boiled | Stem only; boiled 30 minutes | 0.72 | 95.7 | 0.7 | 0 | 2.2 | 0.10 |
| 596 | **Chicory** raw | Stem and young leaves | 0.79 | 96.2 | — | 0 | — | 0.12 |
| 597 | **Cucumber** raw | Flesh only | 0.77 | 96.4 | 1.8 | 0 | 0.4 | 0.10 |
| 598 | **Endive** raw | Leaves only | 0.63 | 93.7 | 1.0 | 0 | 2.2 | 0.28 |
| 599 | **Horseradish** raw | Flesh of root | 0.45 | 74.7 | 7.3 | 3.7 | 8.3 | 0.72 |
| 600 | **Laverbread** | 6 samples; cooked puréed seaweed coated in oatmeal | 1.00 | 87.7 | Tr | 1.6 | 3.1 | 0.51 |
| 601 | **Leeks** raw | Bulb only | 0.36 | 86.0 | 6.0 | 0 | 3.1 | 0.31 |
| 602 | boiled | Bulb only; boiled 30 minutes | 0.44 | 90.8 | 4.6 | 0 | 3.9 | 0.28 |
| 603 | **Lentils** raw | As purchased | 1.00 | 12.2 | 2.4 | 50.8 | 11.7 | 3.80 |
| 604 | split, boiled | As purchased; boiled 20 minutes | 3.27 | 72.1 | 0.8 | 16.2 | 3.7 | 1.22 |
| 605 | masur dahl, cooked | Recipe p 344 | — | 78.4 | 0.7 | 10.7 | 2.4 | 0.78 |

| | | Energy value | | Protein (N × 6.25) | Fat | Carbo-hydrate | mg | | | | | | | | | |
|---|---|---|---|---|---|---|---|---|---|---|---|---|---|---|---|---|
| No | Food | kcal | kJ | g | g | g | Na | K | Ca | Mg | P | Fe | Cu | Zn | S | Cl |
| 587 | **Carrots, old** raw | 23 | 98 | 0.7 | Tr | 5.4 | 95 | 220 | 48 | 12 | 21 | 0.6 | 0.08 | 0.4 | 7 | 69 |
| 588 | boiled | 19 | 79 | 0.6 | Tr | 4.3 | 50 | 87 | 37 | 6 | 17 | 0.4 | 0.08 | 0.3 | 5 | 31 |
| 589 | **young** boiled | 20 | 87 | 0.9 | Tr | 4.5 | 23 | 240 | 29 | 8 | 30 | 0.4 | 0.08 | 0.3 | 9 | 28 |
| 590 | canned | 19 | 82 | 0.7 | Tr | 4.4 | 280 | 84 | 27 | 5 | 15 | 1.3 | 0.04 | 0.3 | — | 450 |
| 591 | **Cauliflower** raw | 13 | 56 | 1.9 | Tr | 1.5 | 8 | 350 | 21 | 14 | 45 | 0.5 | (0.03) | 0.3 | — | 31 |
| 592 | boiled | 9 | 40 | 1.6 | Tr | 0.8 | 4 | 180 | 18 | 8 | 32 | 0.4 | (0.03) | 0.2 | — | 14 |
| 593 | **Celeriac** boiled | 14 | 59 | 1.6 | Tr | 2.0 | 28 | 400 | 47 | 12 | 71 | 0.8 | 0.13 | — | 13 | 23 |
| 594 | **Celery** raw | 8 | 36 | 0.9 | Tr | 1.3 | 140 | 280 | 52 | 10 | 32 | 0.6 | 0.11 | 0.1 | 15 | 180 |
| 595 | boiled | 5 | 21 | 0.6 | Tr | 0.7 | 67 | 130 | 52 | 9 | 19 | 0.4 | 0.11 | 0.1 | 8 | 100 |
| 596 | **Chicory** raw | 9 | 38 | 0.8 | Tr | 1.5 [a] | 7 | 180 | 18 | 13 | 21 | 0.7 | 0.14 | 0.2 | 13 | 25 |
| 597 | **Cucumber** raw | 10 | 43 | 0.6 | 0.1 | 1.8 | 13 | 140 | 23 | 9 | 24 | 0.3 | 0.09 | 0.1 | 11 | 25 |
| 598 | **Endive** raw | 11 | 47 | 1.8 | Tr | 1.0 | 10 | 380 | 44 | 10 | 67 | 2.8 | 0.09 | — | 26 | 71 |
| 599 | **Horseradish** raw | 59 | 253 | 4.5 | Tr | 11.0 | 8 | 580 | 120 | 36 | 70 | 2.0 | 0.14 | — | 210 | 19 |
| 600 | **Laverbread** | 52 | 217 | 3.2 | 3.7 | 1.6 | 560 | 220 | 20 | 31 | 51 | 3.5 | 0.12 | 0.8 | — | 820 |
| 601 | **Leeks** raw | 31 | 128 | 1.9 | Tr | 6.0 | 9 | 310 | 63 | 10 | 43 | 1.1 | 0.10 | (0.1) | — | 43 |
| 602 | boiled | 24 | 104 | 1.8 | Tr | 4.6 | 6 | 280 | 61 | 13 | 28 | 2.0 | 0.09 | (0.1) | 49 | 43 |
| 603 | **Lentils** raw | 304 | 1293 | 23.8 | 1.0 | 53.2 | 36 | 670 | 39 | 77 | 240 | 7.6 | 0.58 | 3.1 | 120 | 64 |
| 604 | split, boiled | 99 | 420 | 7.6 | 0.5 | 17.0 | 12 | 210 | 13 | 25 | 77 | 2.4 | 0.19 | 1.0 | 39 | 20 |
| 605 | masur dahl, cooked | 90 | 380 | 4.9 | 3.1 | 11.4 | 320 | 150 | 11 | 17 | 52 | 1.7 | 0.12 | 0.6 | 28 | 490 |

[a] This vegetable contains inulin; 50 per cent total carbohydrate taken to be available

| No | Food | Retinol µg | Carotene µg | Vitamin D µg | Thiamin mg | Riboflavin mg | Nicotinic acid mg | Potential nicotinic acid from tryptophan mg Trp ÷ 60 | Vitamin C mg | Vitamin E mg |
|---|---|---|---|---|---|---|---|---|---|---|
| 587 | **Carrots, old** raw | 0 | 12 000 *(10 000–14 000)* | 0 | 0.06 | 0.05 | 0.6 | 0.1 | 6 *(4–10)* | 0.5 |
| 588 | boiled | 0 | 12 000 *(10 000–14 000)* | 0 | 0.05 | 0.04 | 0.4 | 0.1 | 4 *(2–6)* | 0.5 |
| 589 | **young** boiled | 0 | 6000 *(5000–7000)* | 0 | 0.05 | 0.04 | 0.4 | 0.1 | 4 *(2–6)* | 0.5 |
| 590 | canned | 0 | 7000 | 0 | 0.04 | 0.02 | 0.3 | 0.1 | 3 | (0.5) |
| 591 | **Cauliflower** raw | 0 | 30 *(6–50)* | 0 | 0.10 | 0.10 | 0.6 | 0.5 | 60 *(50–90)* | 0.2 [a] |
| 592 | boiled | 0 | 30 *(6–50)* | 0 | 0.06 | 0.06 | 0.4 | 0.4 | 20 *(15–40)* | 0.1 [b] |
| 593 | **Celeriac** boiled | 0 | 0 | 0 | 0.04 | 0.04 | 0.5 | 0.3 | 4 | — |
| 594 | **Celery** raw | 0 | Tr | 0 | 0.03 | 0.03 | 0.3 | 0.2 | 7 | 0.2 |
| 595 | boiled | 0 | Tr | 0 | 0.02 | 0.02 | 0.2 | 0.1 | 5 | 0.2 |
| 596 | **Chicory** raw | 0 | Tr | 0 | 0.05 | 0.05 | 0.5 | 0.1 | 4 | — |
| 597 | **Cucumber** raw | 0 | Tr | 0 | 0.04 | 0.04 | 0.2 | 0.1 | 8 | Tr |
| 598 | **Endive** raw | 0 | 2000 *(1000–6000)* | 0 | 0.06 | 0.10 | 0.4 | 0.3 | 12 | — |
| 599 | **Horseradish** raw | 0 | 0 | 0 | 0.05 | 0.03 | 0.5 | 0.7 | 120 | — |
| 600 | **Laverbread** | 0 | — | 0 | 0.03 | 0.10 | 0.6 | 0.5 | 5 | 1.1 |
| 601 | **Leeks** raw | 0 | 40 [c] | 0 | 0.10 | 0.05 | 0.6 | 0.3 | 18 *(15–30)* | 0.8 |
| 602 | boiled | 0 | 40 [c] | 0 | 0.07 | 0.03 | 0.4 | 0.3 | 15 *(10–25)* | 0.8 |
| 603 | **Lentils** raw | 0 | 60 | 0 | 0.50 | 0.20 | 2.0 | 3.8 | Tr | — |
| 604 | split, boiled | 0 | 20 | 0 | 0.11 | 0.04 | 0.4 | 1.2 | Tr | — |
| 605 | masur dahl, cooked | 27 | 30 | 0.03 | 0.07 | 0.03 | 0.3 | 0.8 | Tr | — |

| No | Food | Vitamin $B_6$ mg | Vitamin $B_{12}$ µg | Folic acid Free µg | Folic acid Total µg | Panto-thenic acid mg | Biotin µg |
|---|---|---|---|---|---|---|---|
| 587 | **Carrots, old** raw | 0.15 | 0 | 12 | 15 | 0.25 | 0.6 |
| 588 | boiled | 0.09 | 0 | 1 | 8 | 0.18 | 0.4 |
| 589 | **young** boiled | 0.09 | 0 | 1 | 8 | 0.18 | 0.4 |
| 590 | canned | 0.02 | 0 | 1 | 7 | 0.10 | 0.4 |
| 591 | **Cauliflower** raw | 0.20 | 0 | 30 | 39 | 0.60 | 1.5 |
| 592 | boiled | 0.12 | 0 | 2 | 49 | 0.42 | 1.0 |
| 593 | **Celeriac** boiled | 0.10 | 0 | — | — | — | — |
| 594 | **Celery** raw | 0.10 | 0 | 6 | 12 | 0.40 | 0.1 |
| 595 | boiled | 0.06 | 0 | (1) | (6) | 0.28 | Tr |
| 596 | **Chicory** raw | 0.05 | 0 | 33 | 52 | — | — |
| 597 | **Cucumber** raw | 0.04 | 0 | 14 | 16 | 0.30 | (0.4) |
| 598 | **Endive** raw | — | 0 | 62 | 330 | — | — |
| 599 | **Horseradish** raw | 0.15 | 0 | — | — | — | — |
| 600 | **Laverbread** | — | 0 | 8 | 47 | — | — |
| 601 | **Leeks** raw | 0.25 | 0 | — | — | 0.12 | 1.4 |
| 602 | boiled | 0.15 | 0 | 7 | — | 0.10 | 1.0 |
| 603 | **Lentils** raw | 0.60 | 0 | 25 | 35 | 1.36 | — |
| 604 | split, boiled | 0.11 | 0 | 1 | 5 | 0.31 | — |
| 605 | masur dahl, cooked | 0.07 | 0 | 1 | 4 | 0.20 | — |

Notes

[a] Also contains 0.2mg γ-tocopherol per 100g.

[b] Also contains 0.1mg γ-tocopherol per 100g.

[c] Bulb only. The leaves contain about 2000 µg.

| No | Food | Description and number of samples | Edible matter, proportion of weight purchased | Water g | Sugars g | Starch and dextrins g | Dietary fibre g | Total nitrogen g |
|---|---|---|---|---|---|---|---|---|
| 606 | **Lettuce** raw | 29 lettuces; inner leaves of long and headed forms | 0.70 | 95.9 | 1.2 | Tr | 1.5 | 0.16 |
| 607 | **Marrow** raw | 10 marrows; flesh only | 0.50 | 93.5 | 3.0 | 0.7 | (1.8) | 0.10 |
| 608 | boiled | Flesh only; boiled 25 minutes | 0.64 | 97.8 | 1.3 | 0.1 | 0.6 | 0.06 |
| 609 | **Mushrooms** raw | Flesh and stem | 0.75 | 91.5 | 0 | 0 | 2.5 | 0.64[a] |
| 610 | fried | Flesh and stem; fried in dripping | 0.61 | 64.2 | 0 | 0 | (4.0) | 0.90[a] |
| 611 | **Mustard and cress** raw | Leaves and stems | 1.00 | 92.5 | 0.9 | 0 | 3.7 | 0.26 |
| 612 | **Okra** raw | Literature sources (ladies' fingers) | 0.88 | 90.0 | 2.3 | Tr | (3.2) | 0.32 |
| 613 | **Onions** raw | Flesh only | 0.97 | 92.8 | 5.2 | 0 | 1.3 | 0.15 |
| 614 | boiled | Flesh only; boiled 30 minutes | 0.85 | 96.6 | 2.7 | 0 | 1.3 | 0.09 |
| 615 | fried | Flesh only; cut up and fried in dripping | 0.49 | 42.0 | 10.1 | 0 | (4.5) | 0.29 |
| 616 | spring, raw | Flesh of bulb | 0.31 | 86.8 | 8.5 | 0 | 3.1 | 0.15 |
| 617 | **Parsley** raw | Leaves | 0.53 | 78.7 | Tr | 0 | 9.1 | 0.83 |
| 618 | **Parsnips** raw | Flesh only | 0.74 | 82.5 | 8.8 | 2.5 | 4.0 | 0.27 |
| 619 | boiled | Flesh only; boiled 30 minutes | 0.78 | 83.2 | 2.7 | 10.8 | 2.5 | 0.20 |
| 620 | **Peas, fresh** raw | Whole peas, no pods | 0.37 | 78.5 | 4.0 | 6.6 | 5.2 | 0.92 |
| 621 | boiled | Whole peas, no pods; boiled 20 minutes | 0.37 | 80.0 | 1.8 | 5.9 | 5.2 | 0.80 |
| 622 | **frozen** raw | 15 packets | 1.00 | 79.1 | 4.1 | 3.4 | 7.8 | 0.91 |
| 623 | boiled | 15 packets; boiled 5 minutes | — | 80.7 | 1.0 | 3.3 | 12.0 | 0.87 |
| 624 | **canned** garden | 10 cans; drained contents | 0.63 | 81.6 | 3.6 | 3.4 | 6.3 | 0.74 |
| 625 | processed | 10 cans; drained contents | 0.54 | 71.5 | 1.3 | 12.4 | 7.9 | 0.99 |

[a] 60 per cent of this nitrogen is present as urea

| No | Food | Energy value kcal | Energy value kJ | Protein (N × 6.25) g | Fat g | Carbo-hydrate g | Na mg | K mg | Ca mg | Mg mg | P mg | Fe mg | Cu mg | Zn mg | S mg | Cl mg |
|---|---|---|---|---|---|---|---|---|---|---|---|---|---|---|---|---|
| 606 | **Lettuce** raw | 12 | 51 | 1.0 | 0.4 | 1.2 | 9 | 240 | 23 | 8 | 27 | 0.9 | (0.03) | 0.2 | — | 53 |
| 607 | **Marrow** raw | 16 | 69 | 0.6 | Tr | 3.7 | 1 | 210 | 17 | 12 | 20 | 0.2 | (0.03) | 0.2 | — | 30 |
| 608 | boiled | 7 | 29 | 0.4 | Tr | 1.4 | 1 | 84 | 14 | 7 | 13 | 0.2 | 0.03 | 0.2 | 6 | 14 |
| 609 | **Mushrooms** raw | 13 | 53 | 1.8[a] | 0.6 | 0 | 9 | 470 | 3 | 13 | 140 | 1.0 | 0.64 | 0.1 | 34 | 85 |
| 610 | fried | 210 | 863 | 2.2[a] | 22.3 | 0 | 11 | 570 | 4 | 16 | 170 | 1.3 | 0.78 | 0.1 | 74 | 100 |
| 611 | **Mustard and cress** raw | 10 | 47 | 1.6 | Tr | 0.9 | 19 | 340 | 66 | 27 | 66 | (1.0) | 0.12 | — | 170 | 89 |
| 612 | **Okra** raw | 17 | 71 | 2.0 | Tr | 2.3 | 7 | 190 | 70 | 60 | 60 | 1.0 | 0.19 | — | 30 | 41 |
| 613 | **Onions** raw | 23 | 99 | 0.9 | Tr | 5.2 | 10 | 140 | 31 | 8 | 30 | 0.3 | 0.08 | 0.1 | 51 | 20 |
| 614 | boiled | 13 | 53 | 0.6 | Tr | 2.7 | 7 | 78 | 24 | 5 | 16 | 0.3 | 0.07 | 0.1 | 24 | 5 |
| 615 | fried | 345 | 1424 | 1.8 | 33.3 | 10.1 | 20 | 270 | 61 | 15 | 59 | 0.6 | 0.16 | 0.1 | 88 | 38 |
| 616 | spring, raw | 35 | 151 | 0.9 | Tr | 8.5 | 13 | 230 | 140 | 11 | 24 | 1.2 | 0.13 | — | 50 | 36 |
| 617 | **Parsley** raw | 21 | 88 | 5.2 | Tr | Tr | 33 | 1080 | 330 | 52 | 130 | 8.0 | 0.52 | 0.9 | — | 160 |
| 618 | **Parsnips** raw | 49 | 210 | 1.7 | Tr | 11.3 | 17 | 340 | 55 | 22 | 69 | 0.6 | 0.10 | 0.1 | 17 | 41 |
| 619 | boiled | 56 | 238 | 1.3 | Tr[b] | 13.5 | 4 | 290 | 36 | 13 | 32 | 0.5 | 0.10 | 0.1 | 15 | 33 |
| 620 | **Peas, fresh** raw | 67 | 283 | 5.8 | 0.4 | 10.6 | 1 | 340 | 15 | 30 | 100 | 1.9 | 0.23 | 0.7 | 50 | 38 |
| 621 | boiled | 52 | 223 | 5.0 | 0.4 | 7.7 | Tr | 170 | 13 | 21 | 83 | 1.2 | 0.15 | 0.5 | 44 | 8 |
| 622 | **frozen** raw | 53 | 227 | 5.7 | 0.4 | 7.2 | 3 | 190 | 33 | 27 | 90 | 1.5 | 0.22 | 0.9 | — | 20 |
| 623 | boiled | 41 | 175 | 5.4 | 0.4 | 4.3 | 2 | 130 | 31 | 23 | 84 | 1.4 | 0.19 | 0.7 | — | 12 |
| 624 | **canned** garden | 47 | 201 | 4.6 | 0.3 | 7.0 | 230 | 130 | 24 | 17 | 73 | 1.6 | 0.16 | 0.7 | — | 350 |
| 625 | processed | 80 | 339 | 6.2 | 0.4 | 13.7 | 330 | 170 | 27 | 24 | 91 | 1.5 | 0.22 | 0.8 | — | 510 |

[a] (Total N − urea N) × 6.25

[b] Roast parsnips contain 6.5 g fat per 100 g

| No | Food | Retinol µg | Carotene µg | Vitamin D µg | Thiamin mg | Riboflavin mg | Nicotinic acid mg | Potential nicotinic acid from tryptophan mg Trp 60 ÷ | Vitamin C mg | Vitamin E mg |
|---|---|---|---|---|---|---|---|---|---|---|
| 606 | **Lettuce** raw | 0 | 1000 [a] | 0 | 0.07 | 0.08 | 0.3 | 0.1 | 15 *(10–30)* | 0.5 [b] |
| 607 | **Marrow** raw | 0 | 30 | 0 | Tr | (Tr) | 0.3 | 0.1 | 5 | Tr |
| 608 | boiled | 0 | 30 | 0 | Tr | (Tr) | 0.2 | 0.1 | 2 | Tr |
| 609 | **Mushrooms** raw | 0 | 0 | 0 | 0.10 | 0.40 | 4.0 | 0.6 | 3 | Tr |
| 610 | fried | 0 | 0 | 0 | (0.07) | 0.35 | 3.5 | 0.9 | 1 | Tr |
| 611 | **Mustard and cress** raw | 0 | (500) | 0 | — | — | — | 0.3 | 40 | 0.7 |
| 612 | **Okra** raw | 0 | 90 | 0 | 0.10 | 0.10 | 1.0 | 0.3 | 25 | — |
| 613 | **Onions** raw | 0 | 0 | 0 | 0.03 | 0.05 | 0.2 | 0.2 | 10 *(3–15)* | Tr |
| 614 | boiled | 0 | 0 | 0 | 0.02 | 0.04 | 0.1 | 0.1 | 6 | Tr |
| 615 | fried | 0 | 0 | 0 | — | — | — | 0.4 | — | — |
| 616 | spring, raw | 0 | Tr | 0 | (0.03) | (0.05) | (0.2) | 0.2 | 25 *(20–30)* | Tr |
| 617 | **Parsley** raw | 0 | 7000 *(3000–10 000)* | 0 | 0.15 | 0.30 | 1.0 | 0.8 | 150 *(100–200)* | 1.8 |
| 618 | **Parsnips** raw | 0 | Tr | 0 | 0.10 | 0.08 | 1.0 | 0.3 | 15 *(5–30)* | 1.0 |
| 619 | boiled | 0 | Tr | 0 | 0.07 | 0.06 | 0.7 | 0.2 | 10 *(5–20)* | 1.0 |
| 620 | **Peas, fresh** raw | 0 | 300 *(250–400)* | 0 | 0.32 | 0.15 | 2.5 | 0.9 | 25 *(15–35)* | Tr [d] |
| 621 | boiled | 0 | 300 | 0 | 0.25 | 0.11 | 1.5 | 0.8 | 15 [c] | Tr [d] |
| 622 | **frozen** raw | 0 | 300 | 0 | 0.32 | 0.10 | 2.1 | 0.9 | 17 | Tr [e] |
| 623 | boiled | 0 | 300 | 0 | 0.24 | 0.07 | 1.5 | 0.9 | 13 | Tr [f] |
| 624 | **canned** garden | 0 | 300 | 0 | 0.13 | 0.10 | 2.1 | 0.7 | 8 | Tr [d] |
| 625 | processed | 0 | 300 | 0 | 0.10 | 0.04 | 0.5 | 1.0 | Tr | Tr [g] |

| No | Food | Vitamin $B_6$ mg | Vitamin $B_{12}$ µg | Folic acid Free µg | Folic acid Total µg | Panto-thenic acid mg | Biotin µg |
|---|---|---|---|---|---|---|---|
| 606 | **Lettuce** raw | 0.07 | 0 | 19 | 34 | 0.20 | 0.7 |
| 607 | **Marrow** raw | 0.06 | 0 | 13 | 13 | 0.10 | 0.4 |
| 608 | boiled | 0.03 | 0 | (1) | (6) | 0.07 | — |
| 609 | **Mushrooms** raw | 0.10 | 0 | 20 | 23 | 2.0 | — |
| 610 | fried | (0.06) | 0 | 17 | (20) | (1.4) | — |
| 611 | **Mustard and cress** raw | — | 0 | — | — | — | — |
| 612 | **Okra** raw | 0.08 | 0 | 25 | 100 | 0.26 | — |
| 613 | **Onions** raw | 0.10 | 0 | 15 | 16 | 0.14 | 0.9 |
| 614 | boiled | 0.06 | 0 | Tr | 8 | 0.10 | 0.6 |
| 615 | fried | — | 0 | — | — | — | — |
| 616 | spring, raw | (0.10) | 0 | 40 | 40 | (0.14) | (0.9) |
| 617 | **Parsley** raw | 0.20 | 0 | — | — | 0.30 | 0.4 |
| 618 | **Parsnips** raw | 0.10 | 0 | 57 | 67 | 0.50 | 0.1 |
| 619 | boiled | 0.06 | 0 | (6) | (30) | 0.35 | Tr |
| 620 | **Peas, fresh** raw | 0.16 | 0 | — | — | 0.75 | 0.5 |
| 621 | boiled | 0.10 | 0 | — | — | 0.32 | 0.4 |
| 622 | **frozen** raw | 0.10 | 0 | 2 | 78 | (0.75) | 0.5 |
| 623 | boiled | 0.07 | 0 | 5 | 78 | (0.32) | 0.4 |
| 624 | **canned** garden | 0.06 | 0 | 8 | 52 | 0.15 | (0.4) |
| 625 | processed | 0.03 | 0 | 1 | 3 | (0.08) | (Tr) |

Notes

[a] This is an average figure. The outer green leaves may contain 50 times as much carotene as the inner white ones.

[b] Also contains 0.7 mg γ-tocopherol per 100g.

[c] Cooked air-dried peas contain 11 mg per 100g and cooked accelerated-freeze-dried peas 16 mg per 100g.

[d] Also contains 0.8 mg γ-tocopherol per 100g.

[e] Also contains 1.0 mg γ-tocopherol per 100g.

[f] Also contains 0.9 mg γ-tocopherol per 100g.

[g] Also contains 1.2 mg γ-tocopherol per 100g.

| No | Food | Description and number of samples | Edible matter, proportion of weight purchased | Water g | Sugars g | Starch g | Dietary fibre g | Total nitrogen g |
|---|---|---|---|---|---|---|---|---|
| | **Peas** *contd* | | | | | | | |
| 626 | **dried** raw | Whole peas | 1.00 | 13.3 | 2.4 | 47.6 | 16.7 | 3.45 |
| 627 | boiled | Whole peas; soaked 24 hours, boiled 2 hours | 2.70 | 70.3 | 0.9 | 18.2 | 4.8 | 1.11 |
| 628 | **split** dried, raw | Peas as purchased | 1.00 | 12.1 | 1.9 | 54.7 | 11.9 | 3.54 |
| 629 | boiled | Soaked 24 hours, boiled 2 hours | 2.50 | 67.3 | 0.9 | 21.0 | 5.1 | 1.33 |
| 630 | **chick** Bengal gram, raw | Literature sources | 1.00 | 9.9 | (10.0) | (40.0) | (15.0) | 3.23 |
| 631 | cooked, dahl | Whole peas; recipe p 344 | — | 65.8 | (5.2) | (16.8) | (6.0) | 1.28 |
| 632 | channa dahl | 10 samples; made from split peas | — | 74.2 | 1.5 | 8.9 | 5.2 | 0.85 |
| 633 | **red** pigeon, raw | Literature sources | 1.00 | 10.0 | (9.0) | (45.0) | (15.0) | 3.20 |
| 634 | **Peppers, green** raw | 30 peppers; flesh only | 0.86 | 93.5 | 2.2 | Tr | 0.9 | 0.15 |
| 635 | boiled | 30 peppers; flesh only, boiled 15 minutes | 0.72 | 93.7 | 1.7 | 0.1 | 0.9 | 0.15 |
| 636 | **Plantain** green, raw | Literature sources | 0.61 | 67.0 | 0.8 | 27.5 | (5.8) | 0.16 |
| 637 | boiled | 10 samples; boiled 30 minutes | 0.71 | 63.9 | 0.9 | 30.2 | 6.4 | 0.16 |
| 638 | ripe, fried | 8 samples; fried in oil | 0.43 | 34.7 | 11.5 | 36.0 | 5.8 | 0.24 |
| 639 | **Potatoes, old** raw | Flesh only | 0.86 | 75.8 | 0.5 | 20.3 | 2.1 | 0.34 |
| 640 | boiled | Flesh only, boiled 30 minutes | 0.86 | 80.5 | 0.4 | 19.3 | 1.0 | 0.23 |
| 641 | mashed | Boiled and mashed with margarine and milk | 0.94 | 76.9 | 0.6 | 17.4 | 0.9 | 0.24 |
| 642 | baked | Baked in skins; flesh only | 0.68 | 71.0 | 0.6 | 24.4 | 2.5 | 0.41 |
| 643 | baked (weighed with skins) | Calculated from the previous item | 0.68 | 57.5 | 0.5 | 19.8 | 2.0 | 0.33 |
| 644 | roast | Flesh only; roasted in shallow fat | 0.66 | 64.3 | — | — | — | 0.45 |
| 645 | chips | Fried in deep fat | 0.49 | 47.0 | — | — | — | 0.61 |

| No | Food | Energy value kcal | Energy value kJ | Protein (N × 6.25) g | Fat g | Carbo-hydrate g | Na mg | K mg | Ca mg | Mg mg | P mg | Fe mg | Cu mg | Zn mg | S mg | Cl mg |
|---|---|---|---|---|---|---|---|---|---|---|---|---|---|---|---|---|
| | **Peas** *contd* | | | | | | | | | | | | | | | |
| 626 | **dried** raw | 286 | 1215 | 21.6 | 1.3 | 50.0 | 38 | 990 | 61 | 116 | 300 | 4.7 | 0.49 | 3.5 | 130 | 60 |
| 627 | boiled | 103 | 438 | 6.9 | 0.4 | 19.1 | 13 | 270 | 24 | 30 | 110 | 1.4 | 0.17 | 1.0 | 39 | 9 |
| 628 | **split** dried, raw | 310 | 1318 | 22.1 | 1.0 | 56.6 | 38 | 910 | 33 | 130 | 270 | 5.4 | 0.58 | (4.0) | 170 | 56 |
| 629 | boiled | 118 | 503 | 8.3 | 0.3 | 21.9 | 14 | 270 | 11 | 30 | 120 | 1.7 | 0.25 | (1.2) | 46 | 10 |
| 630 | **chick** Bengal gram, raw | 320 | 1362 | 20.2 | 5.7 | 50.0 | 40 | 800 | 140 | 160 | 300 | 6.4 | 0.76 | — | 180 | 60 |
| 631 | cooked, dahl | 144 | 610 | 8.0 | 3.3 | 22.0 | 850 | 400 | 64 | 67 | 130 | 3.1 | 0.33 | — | 84 | 1310 |
| 632 | channa dahl | 97 | 407 | 5.3 | 4.5 | 9.5 | 480 | 260 | 30 | 31 | 92 | 1.8 | 0.20 | 0.8 | — | 700 |
| 633 | **red** pigeon, raw | 301 | 1278 | 20.0 | 2.0 | 54.0 | 29 | 1100 | 100 | 130 | 300 | 5.0 | 1.25 | — | 180 | 5 |
| 634 | **Peppers green** raw | 15 | 65 | 0.9 | 0.4 | 2.2 | 2 | 210 | 9 | 11 | 25 | 0.4 | 0.07 | 0.2 | — | 18 |
| 635 | boiled | 14 | 59 | 0.9 | 0.4 | 1.8 | 2 | 170 | 9 | 10 | 22 | 0.4 | 0.06 | 0.2 | — | 15 |
| 636 | **Plantain** green, raw | 112 | 477 | 1.0 | 0.2 | 28.3 | (1) | (350) | 7 | 33 | 35 | 0.5 | 0.16 | 0.1 | 15 | (80) |
| 637 | boiled | 122 | 518 | 1.0 | 0.1 | 31.1 | 4 | 330 | 9 | 34 | 34 | 0.4 | 0.10 | 0.2 | — | 50 |
| 638 | ripe, fried | 267 | 1126 | 1.5 | 9.2 | 47.5 | 3 | 610 | 6 | 54 | 66 | 0.8 | 0.20 | 0.4 | — | 110 |
| 639 | **Potatoes, old** raw | 87 | 372 | 2.1 | 0.1 | 20.8 | 7 | 570 | 8 | 24 | 40 | 0.5 | 0.15 | 0.3 | 35 | 79 |
| 640 | boiled | 80 | 343 | 1.4 | 0.1 | 19.7 | 3 | 330 | 4 | 15 | 29 | 0.3 | 0.11 | 0.2 | 22 | 41 |
| 641 | mashed | 119 | 499 | 1.5 | 5.0 | 18.0 | 24 | 300 | 12 | 14 | 32 | 0.3 | 0.10 | 0.3 | 24 | 71 |
| 642 | baked | 105 | 448 | 2.6 | 0.1 | 25.0 | 8 | 680 | 9 | 29 | 48 | 0.8 | 0.18 | 0.3 | 42 | 94 |
| 643 | baked (weighed with skins) | 85 | 364 | 2.1 | 0.1 | 20.3 | 6 | 550 | 8 | 24 | 39 | 0.6 | 0.15 | 0.2 | 34 | 76 |
| 644 | roast | 157 | 662 | 2.8 | 4.8 | 27.3 | 9 | 750 | 10 | 32 | 53 | 0.7 | 0.20 | 0.4 | 56 | 100 |
| 645 | chips | 253 | 1065 | 3.8 | 10.9 [a] | 37.3 | 12 | 1020 | 14 | 43 | 72 | 0.9 | 0.27 | 0.6 | 45 | 140 |

[a] The fat content may vary from 7 to 15g per 100g

| No | Food | Retinol µg | Carotene µg | Vitamin D µg | Thiamin mg | Riboflavin mg | Nicotinic acid mg | Potential nicotinic acid from tryptophan mgTrp ÷ 60 | Vitamin C mg | Vitamin E mg |
|---|---|---|---|---|---|---|---|---|---|---|
| | **Peas** *contd* | | | | | | | | | |
| 626 | **dried** raw | 0 | 250 | 0 | 0.60 | 0.30 | 3.0 | 3.5 | Tr | Tr |
| 627 | boiled | 0 | 80 | 0 | 0.11 | 0.07 | 1.0 | 1.1 | Tr | Tr |
| 628 | **split** dried, raw | 0 | 150 | 0 | 0.70 | 0.20 | 3.2 | 3.5 | Tr | Tr |
| 629 | boiled | 0 | (50) | 0 | 0.11 | 0.06 | 1.0 | 1.3 | Tr | Tr |
| 630 | **chick** Bengal gram, raw | 0 | 190 | 0 | 0.50 | 0.15 | 1.5 | 2.7 | 3 | — |
| 631 | cooked, dahl | 52 | 210 | 0.05 | 0.14 | 0.05 | 0.5 | 1.1 | 3 | — |
| 632 | channa dahl | — | — | — | 0.08 | 0.03 | 0.4 | 0.7 | Tr | — |
| 633 | **red** pigeon, raw | 0 | 30 | 0 | 0.50 | 0.15 | 2.3 | 1.6 | Tr | — |
| 634 | **Peppers, green** raw | 0 | 200 *(60–1000)* | 0 | Tr | 0.03 | 0.7 | 0.2 | 100 *(60–170)* | 0.8 |
| 635 | boiled | 0 | 200 *(60–1000)* | 0 | 0.01 | 0.02 | 0.6 | 0.2 | 60 | 0.8 |
| 636 | **Plantain** green, raw | 0 | 60 | 0 | 0.05 | 0.05 | 0.7 | 0.2 | 20 | — |
| 637 | boiled | 0 | 60 | 0 | Tr | 0.01 | 0.3 | 0.2 | 3 | — |
| 638 | ripe, fried | 0 | (120) | 0 | 0.11 | 0.02 | 0.6 | 0.2 | 12 | — |
| 639 | **Potatoes, old** raw | 0 | Tr | 0 | 0.11 | 0.04 | 1.2 | 0.5 | *(8–20[a])* | 0.1 |
| 640 | boiled | 0 | Tr | 0 | 0.08 | 0.03 | 0.8 | 0.3 | *(4–14[b])* | 0.1 |
| 641 | mashed | Tr | Tr | Tr | 0.08 | 0.04 | 0.8 | 0.4 | *(4–12[b])* | 0.1 |
| 642 | baked | 0 | Tr | 0 | 0.10 | 0.04 | 1.2 | 0.6 | *(5–16[b])* | 0.1 |
| 643 | baked (weighed with skins) | 0 | Tr | 0 | 0.08 | 0.03 | 1.0 | 0.5 | *(4–13[b])* | 0.1 |
| 644 | roast | 0 | Tr | 0 | 0.10 | 0.04 | 1.2 | 0.7 | *(5–16[b])* | 0.1 |
| 645 | chips | 0 | Tr | 0 | 0.10 | 0.04 | 1.2 | 0.9 | *(5–16[b])* | 0.1 |

| No | Food | Vitamin $B_6$ mg | Vitamin $B_{12}$ µg | Folic acid Free µg | Folic acid Total µg | Pantothenic acid mg | Biotin µg |
|---|---|---|---|---|---|---|---|
| | **Peas** *contd* | | | | | | |
| 626 | **dried** raw | 0.13 | 0 | 21 | 33 | 2.0 | — |
| 627 | boiled | — | 0 | Tr | — | — | — |
| 628 | **split** dried, raw | 0.13 | 0 | 21 | 33 | 2.0 | — |
| 629 | boiled | — | 0 | Tr | — | — | — |
| 630 | **chick** Bengal gram, raw | — | 0 | 30 | 180 | — | — |
| 631 | cooked, dahl | — | 0 | 2 | 37 | — | — |
| 632 | channa dahl | — | 0 | 4 | 30 | — | — |
| 633 | **red** pigeon, raw | — | 0 | 19 | 100 | — | — |
| 634 | **Peppers, green** raw | 0.17 | 0 | 5 | 11 | 0.23 | — |
| 635 | boiled | 0.14 | 0 | 1 | 11 | 0.16 | — |
| 636 | **Plantain** green, raw | (0.50) | 0 | 2 | 16 | 0.37 | — |
| 637 | boiled | (0.30) | 0 | 5 | 18 | 0.26 | — |
| 638 | ripe, fried | (1.0) | 0 | 16 | 37 | 0.73 | — |
| 639 | **Potatoes, old** raw | 0.25 | 0 | 10 | 14 | 0.30 | 0.1 |
| 640 | boiled | 0.18 | 0 | 3 | 10 | 0.20 | Tr |
| 641 | mashed | 0.18 | 0 | (3) | (10) | 0.20 | Tr |
| 642 | baked | 0.18 | 0 | 3 | 10 | 0.20 | Tr |
| 643 | baked (weighed with skins) | 0.14 | 0 | 2 | 8 | 0.16 | Tr |
| 644 | roast | 0.18 | 0 | 3 | 7 | 0.20 | Tr |
| 645 | chips | 0.18 | 0 | (3) | (10) | 0.20 | Tr |

Notes

| [a] Raw potatoes | Vitamin C mg per 100g |
|---|---|
| Maincrop, freshly dug | 30 |
| stored 1–3 months | 20 |
| stored 4–5 months | 15 |
| stored 6–7 months | 10 |
| stored 8–9 months | 8 |

| [b] Method of cooking | Vitamin C % of value in raw potato |
|---|---|
| Boiled, peeled<br>Mashed | 50–70 |
| Boiled, unpeeled<br>Baked<br>Roast<br>Steamed | 60–80 |
| Fried in deep fat (chips) | 65–75 |

| No | Food | Description and number of samples | Edible matter, proportion of weight purchased | Water g | Sugars g | Starch g | Dietary fibre g | Total nitrogen g |
|---|---|---|---|---|---|---|---|---|
| | **Potatoes** *contd* | | | | | | | |
| 646 | **old** chips, frozen | 11 packets, as purchased | 1.00 | 73.1 | 0.4 | 19.2 | 1.9 | 0.35 |
| 647 | frozen, fried | 11 packets; fried in shallow oil | 0.74 | 48.3 | 0.5 | 28.5 | 3.2 | 0.48 |
| 648 | **new** boiled | Flesh only; boiled 15 minutes | 0.96 | 78.8 | 0.7 | 17.6 | 2.0 | 0.25 |
| 649 | canned | 10 cans; drained contents | 0.63 | 84.2 | 0.4 | 12.2 | 2.5 | 0.19 |
| 650 | **instant** powder | 20 packets | 1.00 | 7.2 | 2.2 | 71.0 | 16.5 | 1.45 |
| 651 | made up | Calculated from the powder | 4.50 | 79.4 | 0.5 | 15.6 | 3.6 | 0.32 |
| 652 | **crisps** | 26 packets, mixed plain and flavoured | 1.00 | 2.7 | 0.7 | 48.6 | 11.9 | 1.00 |
| 653 | **Pumpkin** raw | Flesh only | 0.81 | 94.7 | 2.7 | 0.7 | 0.5 | 0.10 |
| 654 | **Radishes** raw | Flesh and skin; purchased with leaves | 0.50 | 93.3 | 2.8 | 0 | 1.0 | 0.16 |
| 655 | **Salsify** boiled | Flesh only; boiled 45 minutes | 0.63 | 81.2 | — | 0 | — | 0.30 |
| 656 | **Seakale** boiled | Stem only; boiled 20 minutes | 0.74 | 95.6 | 0.6 | 0 | 1.2 | 0.23 |
| 657 | **Spinach** boiled | Leaves; boiled 15 minutes without added water | 0.42 | 85.1 | 1.2 | 0.2 | 6.3 | 0.81 |
| 658 | **Spring greens** boiled | Leaves; boiled 30 minutes | 1.00 | 93.6 | 0.9 | 0 | 3.8 | 0.27 |
| 659 | **Swedes** raw | Flesh only | 0.86 | 91.4 | 4.2 | 0.1 | 2.7 | 0.18 |
| 660 | boiled | Flesh only; boiled 45 minutes | 0.82 | 91.6 | 3.7 | 0.1 | 2.8 | 0.14 |
| 661 | **Sweetcorn, on-the-cob** raw | 16 cobs; kernels only | 0.66 | 65.2 | 1.7 | 22.0 | 3.7 | 0.66 |
| 662 | boiled | 16 cobs; boiled 15 minutes; kernels only | 0.64 | 65.1 | 1.7 | 21.1 | 4.7 | 0.65 |
| 663 | **canned** kernels | 10 cans; whole contents | 1.00 | 73.4 | 8.9 | 7.2 | 5.7 | 0.47 |

| No | Food | Energy value kcal | Energy value kJ | Protein (N × 6.25) g | Fat g | Carbo-hydrate g | Na (mg) | K (mg) | Ca (mg) | Mg (mg) | P (mg) | Fe (mg) | Cu (mg) | Zn (mg) | S (mg) | Cl (mg) |
|---|---|---|---|---|---|---|---|---|---|---|---|---|---|---|---|---|
| | **Potatoes** *contd* | | | | | | | | | | | | | | | |
| 646 | **old** chips, frozen | 109 | 462 | 2.2 | 3.0 | 19.6 | 25 | 420 | 8 | 21 | 61 | 0.7 | 0.11 | 0.3 | — | 45 |
| 647 | frozen, fried | 291 | 1214 | 3.0 | 18.9 | 29.0 | 34 | 540 | 11 | 27 | 77 | 1.0 | 0.15 | 0.4 | — | 71 |
| 648 | **new** boiled | 76 | 324 | 1.6 | 0.1 | 18.3 | 41 | 330 | 5 | 20 | 33 | 0.4 | 0.15 | 0.3 | 24 | 46 |
| 649 | canned | 53 | 226 | 1.2 | 0.1 | 12.6 | 260 | 230 | 11 | 10 | 31 | 0.7 | 0.08 | 0.3 | — | 440 |
| 650 | **instant** powder | 318 | 1356 | 9.1 | 0.8 | 73.2 | 1190 | 1550 | 89 | 69 | 220 | 2.4 | 0.37 | 1.1 | — | 1750 |
| 651 | made up | 70 | 299 | 2.0 | 0.2 | 16.1 | 260 | 340 | 20 | 15 | 48 | 0.5 | 0.08 | 0.2 | — | 380 |
| 652 | **crisps** | 533 | 2224 | 6.3 | 35.9 | 49.3 | 550 | 1190 | 37 | 56 | 130 | 2.1 | 0.22 | 0.8 | — | 890 |
| 653 | **Pumpkin** raw | 15 | 65 | 0.6 | Tr | 3.4 | 1 | 310 | 39 | 8 | 19 | 0.4 | 0.08 | (0.2) | 10 | 37 |
| 654 | **Radishes** raw | 15 | 62 | 1.0 | Tr | 2.8 | 59 | 240 | 44 | 11 | 27 | 1.9 | 0.13 | 0.1 | 38 | 19 |
| 655 | **Salsify** boiled | 18 | 77 | 1.9 | Tr | 2.8[a] | 8 | 180 | 60 | 14 | 53 | 1.2 | 0.12 | — | 25 | 46 |
| 656 | **Seakale** boiled | 8 | 33 | 1.4 | Tr | 0.6 | 4 | 50 | 48 | 11 | 34 | 0.6 | 0.07 | — | 52 | 12 |
| 657 | **Spinach** boiled | 30 | 128 | 5.1 | 0.5 | 1.4 | 120 | 490 | 600 | 59 | 93 | 4.0 | 0.26 | 0.4 | 86 | 56 |
| 658 | **Spring greens** boiled | 10 | 43 | 1.7 | Tr | 0.9 | 10 | 120 | 86 | 9 | 31 | 1.3 | 0.08 | 0.4 | 29 | 16 |
| 659 | **Swedes** raw | 21 | 88 | 1.1 | Tr | 4.3 | 52 | 140 | 56 | 11 | 19 | 0.4 | 0.05 | — | 39 | 31 |
| 660 | boiled | 18 | 76 | 0.9 | Tr | 3.8 | 14 | 100 | 42 | 7 | 18 | 0.3 | 0.04 | — | 31 | 9 |
| 661 | **Sweetcorn, on-the-cob** raw | 127 | 538 | 4.1 | 2.4 | 23.7 | 1 | 300 | 4 | 46 | 130 | 1.1 | 0.16 | 1.2 | — | 11 |
| 662 | boiled | 123 | 520 | 4.1 | 2.3 | 22.8 | 1 | 280 | 4 | 45 | 120 | 0.9 | 0.15 | 1.0 | — | 14 |
| 663 | **canned** kernels | 76 | 325 | 2.9 | (0.5) | 16.1 | 310 | 200 | 3 | 23 | 67 | 0.6 | 0.05 | 0.6 | — | 460 |

[a] This vegetable contains inulin; 50 per cent total carbohydrate taken to be available

| No | Food | Retinol µg | Carotene µg | Vitamin D µg | Thiamin mg | Riboflavin mg | Nicotinic acid mg | Potential nicotinic acid from tryptophan mgTrp ÷ 60 | Vitamin C mg | Vitamin E mg |
|---|---|---|---|---|---|---|---|---|---|---|
| | **Potatoes** *contd* | | | | | | | | | |
| 646 | **old** chips, frozen | 0 | Tr | 0 | 0.08 | 0.01 | 1.6 | 0.5 | 6 | — |
| 647 | frozen, fried | 0 | Tr | 0 | 0.09 | 0.02 | 2.1 | 0.7 | 4 | — |
| 648 | **new** boiled | 0 | Tr | 0 | 0.11 | 0.03 | 1.2 | 0.4 | 18[a] | 0.1 |
| 649 | canned | 0 | Tr | 0 | 0.02 | 0.03 | 0.7 | 0.3 | 17 | 0.1 |
| 650 | **instant** powder | 0 | Tr | 0 | 0.04 | 0.14 | 5.6 | 2.2 | 12[b] | — |
| 651 | made up | 0 | Tr | 0 | 0.01 | 0.03 | 1.2 | 0.5 | 3[b] | — |
| 652 | **crisps** | 0 | Tr | 0 | 0.19 | 0.07 | 4.6 | 1.5 | 17 | 6.1 |
| 653 | **Pumpkin** raw | 0 | 1500 *(700–2000)* | 0 | 0.04 | 0.04 | 0.4 | 0.1 | 5 | Tr |
| 654 | **Radishes** raw | 0 | Tr | 0 | 0.04 | 0.02 | 0.2 | 0.2 | 25 *(10–35)* | 0 |
| 655 | **Salsify** boiled | 0 | — | 0 | 0.03 | — | — | 0.3 | 4 | — |
| 656 | **Seakale** boiled | 0 | — | 0 | 0.06 | — | — | 0.2 | 18 | — |
| 657 | **Spinach** boiled | 0 | 6000 *(4000–10 000)* | 0 | 0.07 | 0.15 | 0.4 | 1.4 | 25 *(10–60)* | 2.0 |
| 658 | **Spring greens** boiled | 0 | 4000 *(1000–10 000)* | 0 | 0.06 | 0.20 | 0.5 | 0.3 | 30 *(20–70)* | (1.1) |
| 659 | **Swedes** raw | 0 | Tr | 0 | 0.06 | 0.04 | 1.2 | 0.2 | 25 *(15–40)* | 0 |
| 660 | boiled | 0 | Tr | 0 | 0.04 | 0.03 | 0.8 | 0.2 | 17 *(8–25)* | 0 |
| 661 | **Sweetcorn, on-the-cob** raw | 0 | (240) | 0 | 0.15 | 0.08 | 1.8 | 0.4 | 12 | 0.8[c] |
| 662 | boiled | 0 | (240) | 0 | 0.20 | 0.08 | 1.7 | 0.4 | 9 | 0.5[d] |
| 663 | **canned** kernels | 0 | (210) | 0 | 0.05 | 0.08 | 1.2 | 0.3 | 5 | (0.5)[d] |

| No | Food | Vitamin $B_6$ mg | Vitamin $B_{12}$ µg | Folic acid Free µg | Folic acid Total µg | Panto-thenic acid mg | Biotin µg |
|---|---|---|---|---|---|---|---|
| | **Potatoes** *contd* | | | | | | |
| 646 | **old** chips, frozen | 0.28 | 0 | 3 | 12 | — | Tr |
| 647 | frozen, fried | 0.39 | 0 | 5 | 11 | — | Tr |
| 648 | **new** boiled | 0.20 | 0 | 3 | 10 | 0.20 | Tr |
| 649 | canned | 0.16 | 0 | 3 | 11 | — | Tr |
| 650 | **instant** powder | (0.82) | 0 | 10 | 24 | (0.91) | (0.5) |
| 651 | made up | (0.18) | 0 | 2 | 5 | (0.20) | (0.1) |
| 652 | **crisps** | 0.89 | 0 | 4 | 20 | — | — |
| 653 | **Pumpkin** raw | 0.06 | 0 | (13) | (13) | 0.40 | (0.4) |
| 654 | **Radishes** raw | 0.10 | 0 | 18 | 24 | 0.18 | — |
| 655 | **Salsify** boiled | — | 0 | — | — | — | — |
| 656 | **Seakale** boiled | — | 0 | — | — | — | — |
| 657 | **Spinach** boiled | 0.18 | 0 | 30 | (140) | 0.21 | 0.1 |
| 658 | **Spring greens** boiled | (0.16) | 0 | (7) | (110) | 0.30 | (0.4) |
| 659 | **Swedes** raw | 0.20 | 0 | 23 | 27 | 0.11 | 0.1 |
| 660 | boiled | 0.12 | 0 | 9 | 21 | 0.07 | Tr |
| 661 | **Sweetcorn, on-the-cob** raw | 0.19 | 0 | 43 | 52 | 0.54 | — |
| 662 | boiled | 0.16 | 0 | 18 | 33 | 0.38 | — |
| 663 | **canned** kernels | (0.16) | 0 | 9 | 32 | 0.22 | — |

Notes

[a] Raw new potatoes contain 30mg per 100g.

[b] Some brands are fortified and may contain up to 10 times these values.

[c] Also contains 1.6mg γ-tocopherol per 100g.

[d] Also contains 1.0mg γ-tocopherol per 100g.

| No | Food | Description and number of samples | Edible matter, proportion of weight purchased | Water g | Sugars g | Starch g | Dietary fibre g | Total nitrogen g |
|---|---|---|---|---|---|---|---|---|
| 664 | **Sweet potatoes** raw | Literature sources | 0.86 | 70.0 | (9.7) | (11.8) | (2.5) | 0.19 |
| 665 | boiled | Flesh only; boiled 30 minutes | 0.88 | 72.0 | 9.1 | 11.0 | 2.3 | 0.17 |
| 666 | **Tomatoes** raw | Flesh, skin and seeds | 1.00 | 93.4 | 2.8 | Tr | 1.5 | 0.14 |
| 667 | fried | Flesh, skin and seeds; fried in dripping | 0.87 | 86.5 | 3.3 | Tr | 3.0 | 0.16 |
| 668 | canned | 10 cans; drained contents [a] | 0.60 | 94.0 | 2.0 | Tr | 0.9 | 0.17 |
| 669 | **Turnips** raw | Flesh only | 0.84 | 93.3 | 3.8 | 0 | 2.8 | 0.12 |
| 670 | boiled | Flesh only; boiled 30 minutes | 0.80 | 94.5 | 2.3 | 0 | 2.2 | 0.11 |
| 671 | **Turnip tops** boiled | Leaves; boiled 20 minutes | 0.45 | 92.8 | 0 | 0.1 | 3.9 | 0.43 |
| 672 | **Watercress** raw | Leaves and part of stem | 0.77 | 91.1 | 0.6 | 0.1 | 3.3 | 0.46 |
| 673 | **Yam** raw | Literature sources | 0.86 | 73.0 | 1.0 | 31.4 | (4.1) | 0.32 |
| 674 | boiled | 6 samples; flesh only, boiled 30 minutes | 0.91 | 65.8 | 0.2 | 29.6 | 3.9 | 0.25 |

[a] The values given are also applicable to the total contents of the can

| No | Food | Energy value kcal | Energy value kJ | Protein (N × 6.25) g | Fat g | Carbo-hydrate g | Na mg | K mg | Ca mg | Mg mg | P mg | Fe mg | Cu mg | Zn mg | S mg | Cl mg |
|---|---|---|---|---|---|---|---|---|---|---|---|---|---|---|---|---|
| 664 | **Sweet potatoes** raw | 91 | 387 | 1.2 | 0.6 | 21.5 | (19) | (320) | (22) | (13) | (47) | (0.7) | (0.16) | — | (16) | (64) |
| 665 | boiled | 85 | 363 | 1.1 | 0.6 | 20.1 | 18 | 300 | 21 | 12 | 44 | 0.6 | 0.15 | — | 15 | 60 |
| 666 | **Tomatoes** raw | 14 | 60 | 0.9 | Tr | 2.8 | 3 | 290 | 13 | 11 | 21 | 0.4 | 0.10 | 0.2 | 11 | 51 |
| 667 | fried | 69 | 288 | 1.0 | 5.9 | 3.3 | 3 | 340 | 15 | 13 | 25 | 0.5 | 0.12 | 0.2 | 9 | 59 |
| 668 | canned | 12 | 51 | 1.1 | Tr | 2.0 | 29 | 270 | 9 | 11 | 22 | 0.9 | 0.11 | 0.3 | — | 78 |
| 669 | **Turnips** raw | 20 | 86 | 0.8 | 0.3 | 3.8 | 58 | 240 | 59 | 7 | 28 | 0.4 | 0.07 | — | 22 | 70 |
| 670 | boiled | 14 | 60 | 0.7 | 0.3 | 2.3 | 28 | 160 | 55 | 7 | 19 | 0.4 | 0.04 | — | 21 | 31 |
| 671 | **Turnip tops** boiled | 11 | 48 | 2.7 | Tr | 0.1 | 7 | 78 | 98 | 10 | 45 | 3.1 | 0.09 | 0.4 | 39 | 15 |
| 672 | **Watercress** raw | 14 | 61 | 2.9 | Tr | 0.7 | 60 | 310 | 220 | 17 | 52 | 1.6 | 0.14 | 0.2 | 130 | 160 |
| 673 | **Yam** raw | 131 | 560 | 2.0 | 0.2 | 32.4 | — | (500) | 10 | (40) | (40) | 0.3 | 0.16 | 0.4 | — | — |
| 674 | boiled | 119 | 508 | 1.6 | 0.1 | 29.8 | 17 | 300 | 9 | 14 | 33 | 0.3 | 0.15 | 0.4 | — | 40 |

| No | Food | Retinol µg | Carotene µg | Vitamin D µg | Thiamin mg | Riboflavin mg | Nicotinic acid mg | Potential nicotinic acid from tryptophan mg Trp ÷ 60 | Vitamin C mg | Vitamin E mg |
|---|---|---|---|---|---|---|---|---|---|---|
| 664 | **Sweet potatoes** raw | 0 | 4000 [a] | 0 | 0.10 | 0.06 | 0.8 | 0.4 | 25 | (4.0) |
| 665 | boiled | 0 | 4000 [a] | 0 | 0.08 | 0.04 | 0.6 | 0.3 | 15 | (4.0) |
| 666 | **Tomatoes** raw | 0 | 600 *(200–1000)* | 0 | 0.06 | 0.04 | 0.7 | 0.1 | 20 *(10–30)* | 1.2 [b] |
| 667 | fried | 0 | — | 0 | — | — | — | 0.1 | (10) | — |
| 668 | canned | 0 | 500 *(300–600)* | 0 | 0.06 | 0.03 | 0.7 | 0.1 | 18 | 1.2 [b] |
| 669 | **Turnips** raw | 0 | 0 | 0 | 0.04 | 0.05 | 0.6 | 0.2 | 25 *(15–40)* | 0 |
| 670 | boiled | 0 | 0 | 0 | 0.03 | 0.04 | 0.4 | 0.2 | 17 *(8–25)* | 0 |
| 671 | **Turnip tops** boiled | 0 | 6000 *(4000–12 000)* | 0 | 0.06 | 0.20 | 0.5 | 0.4 | 40 *(20–70)* | (1.0) |
| 672 | **Watercress** raw | 0 | 3000 *(1500–3500)* | 0 | 0.10 | 0.10 | 0.6 | 0.5 | 60 *(40–80)* | 1.0 |
| 673 | **Yam** raw | 0 | 12 | 0 | 0.10 | 0.03 | 0.4 | 0.4 | 10 | — |
| 674 | boiled | 0 | 12 | 0 | 0.05 | 0.01 | 0.5 | 0.3 | 2 | — |

| No | Food | Vitamin $B_6$ mg | Vitamin $B_{12}$ µg | Folic acid Free µg | Folic acid Total µg | Pantothenic acid mg | Biotin µg |
|---|---|---|---|---|---|---|---|
| 664 | **Sweet potatoes** raw | 0.22 | 0 | 35 | 52 | 0.94 | — |
| 665 | boiled | 0.13 | 0 | 4 | 25 | 0.66 | — |
| 666 | **Tomatoes** raw | 0.11 | 0 | 15 | 28 | 0.33 | 1.5 |
| 667 | fried | — | 0 | — | — | — | — |
| 668 | canned | 0.11 | 0 | 11 | 25 | 0.20 | 1.5 |
| 669 | **Turnips** raw | 0.11 | 0 | 17 | 20 | 0.20 | 0.1 |
| 670 | boiled | 0.06 | 0 | (1) | (10) | 0.14 | Tr |
| 671 | **Turnip tops** boiled | 0.16 | 0 | (7) | (110) | 0.30 | (0.4) |
| 672 | **Watercress** raw | 0.13 | 0 | (200) | — | 0.10 | 0.4 |
| 673 | **Yam** raw | — | 0 | — | — | 0.63 | — |
| 674 | boiled | — | 0 | 2 | 6 | 0.44 | — |

Notes

[a] There is considerable variation according to variety; some yellow sweet potatoes contain 12 000µg but the white varieties contain only a trace.

[b] Also contains 0.2 mg γ-tocopherol per 100 g.

| No | Food | Description and number of samples | Edible matter, proportion of weight purchased | Water g | Sugars g | Starch g | Dietary fibre g | Total nitrogen g |
|---|---|---|---|---|---|---|---|---|

| | | Energy value | | Protein | | Carbo- | mg | | | | | | | | | |
|---|---|---|---|---|---|---|---|---|---|---|---|---|---|---|---|---|
| No | Food | kcal | kJ | (N × 6.25) g | Fat g | hydrate g | Na | K | Ca | Mg | P | Fe | Cu | Zn | S | Cl |

| No | Food | Reitnol µg | Carotene µg | Vitamin D µg | Thiamin mg | Riboflavin mg | Nicotinic acid mg | Potential nicotinic acid from tryptophan mg Trp ÷60 | Vitamin C mg | Vitamin E mg |
|---|---|---|---|---|---|---|---|---|---|---|

| No | Food | Vitamin $B_6$ mg | Vitamin $B_{12}$ µg | Folic acid Free µg | Folic acid Total µg | Pantothenic acid mg | Biotin µg | Notes |
|---|---|---|---|---|---|---|---|---|

| No | Food | Description and number of samples | Edible matter, proportion of weight purchased | Water g | Sugars g | Starch g | Dietary fibre g | Total nitrogen g |
|---|---|---|---|---|---|---|---|---|
| 675 | **Apples, eating** | Flesh only, no skin or core | 0.77 | 84.3 | 11.8 | 0.1 | 2.0[a] | 0.04 |
| 676 | eating (weighed with skin and core) | Calculated from the previous item | 0.77 | 64.9 | 9.1 | 0.1 | 1.5 | 0.03 |
| 677 | **cooking** raw | Flesh only, no skin or core | 0.81 | 85.6 | 9.2 | 0.4 | 2.4 | 0.05 |
| 678 | baked without sugar | Flesh only, no skin, cored before cooking | 0.70 | 85.0 | 9.6 | 0.4 | 2.5 | 0.05 |
| 679 | baked (weighed with skin) | Calculated from the previous item | 0.70 | 68.0 | 7.7 | 0.3 | 2.0 | 0.04 |
| 680 | stewed without sugar | Flesh and juice, peeled and cored before cooking | 1.00 | 87.7 | 7.9 | 0.3 | 2.1 | 0.04 |
| 681 | stewed with sugar | Flesh and juice, peeled and cored before cooking | 1.11 | 79.3 | 17.0 | 0.3 | 1.9 | 0.04 |
| 682 | **Apricots, fresh** raw | Flesh and skin, no stones | 0.92 | 86.6 | 6.7 | 0 | 2.1 | 0.09 |
| 683 | raw (weighed with stones) | Calculated from the previous item | 0.92 | 79.6 | 6.2 | 0 | 1.9 | 0.08 |
| 684 | stewed without sugar | Fruit and juice, no stones | 1.10 | 87.9 | 5.6 | 0 | 1.7 | 0.07 |
| 685 | stewed without sugar (weighed with stones) | Calculated from the previous item | 1.10 | 82.6 | 5.3 | 0 | 1.6 | 0.07 |
| 686 | stewed with sugar | Fruit and juice, no stones | 1.21 | 79.4 | 15.6 | 0 | 1.6 | 0.06 |
| 687 | stewed with sugar (weighed with stones) | Calculated from the previous item | 1.21 | 74.6 | 14.7 | 0 | 1.5 | 0.06 |

[a] Apple peel contains 3.7g per 100g

| No | Food | Energy value kcal | Energy value kJ | Protein (N × 6.25) g | Fat g | Carbo-hydrate g | Na mg | K mg | Ca mg | Mg mg | P mg | Fe mg | Cu mg | Zn mg | S mg | Cl mg |
|---|---|---|---|---|---|---|---|---|---|---|---|---|---|---|---|---|
| 675 | **Apples, eating** | 46 | 196 | 0.3 | Tr | 11.9 | 2 | 120 | 4 | 5 | 8 | 0.3 | 0.04 | 0.1 | 6 | 1 |
| 676 | eating (weighed with skin and core) | 35 | 151 | 0.2 | Tr | 9.2 | 2 | 92 | 3 | 4 | 6 | 0.2 | 0.03 | 0.1 | 5 | 1 |
| 677 | **cooking** raw | 37 | 159 | 0.3 | Tr | 9.6 | 2 | 120 | 4 | 3 | 16 | 0.3 | 0.09 | 0.1 | 3 | 5 |
| 678 | baked without sugar | 39 | 165 | 0.3 | Tr | 10.0 | 2 | 130 | 4 | 3 | 17 | 0.3 | 0.09 | 0.1 | 3 | 5 |
| 679 | baked (weighed with skin) | 31 | 133 | 0.3 | Tr | 8.0 | 2 | 100 | 3 | 2 | 13 | 0.2 | 0.07 | 0.1 | 2 | 4 |
| 680 | stewed without sugar | 32 | 136 | 0.3 | Tr | 8.2 | 2 | 100 | 3 | 3 | 14 | 0.3 | 0.08 | 0.1 | 3 | 4 |
| 681 | stewed with sugar | 66 | 282 | 0.3 | Tr | 17.3 | 2 | 94 | 3 | 2 | 13 | 0.2 | 0.07 | 0.1 | 2 | 4 |
| 682 | **Apricots** fresh raw | 28 | 117 | 0.6 | Tr | 6.7 | Tr | 320 | 17 | 12 | 21 | 0.4 | 0.12 | 0.1 | 6 | Tr |
| 683 | raw (weighed with stones) | 25 | 108 | 0.5 | Tr | 6.2 | Tr | 290 | 16 | 11 | 20 | 0.3 | 0.11 | 0.1 | 6 | Tr |
| 684 | stewed without sugar | 23 | 98 | 0.4 | Tr | 5.7 | Tr | 270 | 15 | 10 | 18 | 0.3 | 0.10 | 0.1 | 5 | Tr |
| 685 | stewed without sugar (weighed with stones) | 21 | 92 | 0.4 | Tr | 5.3 | Tr | 250 | 14 | 9 | 17 | 0.3 | 0.09 | 0.1 | 5 | Tr |
| 686 | stewed with sugar | 60 | 256 | 0.4 | Tr | 15.6 | Tr | 240 | 14 | 10 | 17 | 0.2 | 0.10 | 0.1 | 5 | Tr |
| 687 | stewed with sugar (weighed with stones) | 57 | 242 | 0.4 | Tr | 14.7 | Tr | 230 | 13 | 9 | 16 | 0.2 | 0.09 | 0.1 | 5 | Tr |

| No | Food | Retinol µg | Carotene µg | Vitamin D µg | Thiamin mg | Riboflavin mg | Nicotinic acid mg | Potential nicotinic acid from tryptophan mg Trp ÷ 60 | Vitamin C mg | Vitamin E mg |
|---|---|---|---|---|---|---|---|---|---|---|
| 675 | **Apples, eating** | 0 | 30 | 0 | 0.04 | 0.02 | 0.1 | Tr | 3 [a] | 0.2 |
| 676 | eating (weighed with skin and core) | 0 | 23 | 0 | 0.03 | 0.02 | 0.1 | Tr | 2 | 0.2 |
| 677 | **cooking** raw | 0 | 30 | 0 | 0.04 | 0.02 | 0.1 | Tr | 15 [b] | 0.2 |
| 678 | baked without sugar | 0 | 30 | 0 | 0.03 | 0.02 | 0.1 | Tr | 14 | 0.2 |
| 679 | baked (weighed with skin) | 0 | 20 | 0 | 0.03 | 0.01 | 0.1 | Tr | 10 | 0.1 |
| 680 | stewed without sugar | 0 | 25 | 0 | 0.03 | 0.02 | 0.1 | Tr | 12 | 0.2 |
| 681 | stewed with sugar | 0 | 25 | 0 | 0.03 | 0.02 | 0.1 | Tr | 11 | 0.2 |
| 682 | **Apricots** fresh, raw | 0 | 1500 *(1000–2400)* | 0 | 0.04 | 0.05 | 0.6 | Tr | 7 | — |
| 683 | raw (weighed with stones) | 0 | 1380 | 0 | 0.04 | 0.05 | 0.5 | Tr | 6 | — |
| 684 | stewed without sugar | 0 | 1260 | 0 | 0.03 | 0.04 | 0.4 | Tr | 5 | — |
| 685 | stewed without sugar (weighed with stones) | 0 | 1180 | 0 | 0.03 | 0.04 | 0.4 | Tr | 5 | — |
| 686 | stewed with sugar | 0 | 1150 | 0 | 0.03 | 0.04 | 0.4 | Tr | 5 | — |
| 687 | stewed with sugar (weighed with stones) | 0 | 1080 | 0 | 0.03 | 0.04 | 0.4 | Tr | 5 | — |

| No | Food | Vitamin $B_6$ mg | Vitamin $B_{12}$ µg | Folic acid Free µg | Folic acid Total µg | Pantothenic acid mg | Biotin µg |
|---|---|---|---|---|---|---|---|
| 675 | **Apples, eating** | 0.03 | 0 | 2 | 5 | 0.10 | 0.3 |
| 676 | eating (weighed with skin and core) | 0.02 | 0 | 2 | 4 | 0.08 | 0.2 |
| 677 | **cooking** raw | 0.03 | 0 | 2 | 5 | 0.10 | 0.3 |
| 678 | baked without sugar | 0.02 | 0 | Tr | 3 | 0.09 | 0.3 |
| 679 | baked (weighed with skin) | 0.01 | 0 | Tr | 2 | 0.06 | 0.2 |
| 680 | stewed without sugar | 0.02 | 0 | Tr | 2 | 0.08 | 0.3 |
| 681 | stewed with sugar | 0.02 | 0 | Tr | 2 | 0.07 | 0.2 |
| 682 | **Apricots** fresh, raw | 0.07 | 0 | (4) | (5) | 0.30 | — |
| 683 | raw (weighed with stones) | 0.06 | 0 | (4) | (5) | 0.28 | — |
| 684 | stewed without sugar | 0.04 | 0 | Tr | (2) | 0.23 | — |
| 685 | stewed without sugar (weighed with stones) | 0.04 | 0 | Tr | (2) | 0.22 | — |
| 686 | stewed with sugar | 0.04 | 0 | Tr | (2) | 0.21 | — |
| 687 | stewed with sugar (weighed with stones) | 0.04 | 0 | Tr | (2) | 0.20 | — |

Notes

[a] Value for Cox's Orange Pippin. The vitamin C content varies according to variety, and there is more in the peel than in the flesh. Some values for different varieties are:

| | Vitamin C mg/100g Peeled | Vitamin C mg/100g Unpeeled |
|---|---|---|
| Cox's Orange Pippin | 3 | 5 |
| Granny Smith | 2 | 8 |
| Laxton Superb, Golden Delicious, Newton Wonder | 3 | 10 |
| Worcester Pearmain, Lord Lambourne | 10 | 16 |
| Sturmer Pippin | 20 | 30 |

[b] Value for peeled Bramley's Seedlings. Unpeeled Bramley's Seedlings contain 20mg per 100g

| No | Food | Description and number of samples | Edible matter, proportion of weight purchased | Water g | Sugars g | Starch g | Dietary fibre g | Total nitrogen g |
|---|---|---|---|---|---|---|---|---|
| 688 | **Apricots** dried, raw | Whole fruit | 1.00 | 14.7 | 43.4 | 0 | 24.0 | 0.76 |
| 689 | stewed without sugar | Fruit and juice | 2.70 | 68.4 | 16.1 | 0 | 8.9 | 0.28 |
| 690 | stewed with sugar | Fruit and juice | 2.81 | 76.4 | 19.9 | 0 | 8.5 | 0.27 |
| 691 | canned | Fruit and syrup | 1.00 | 67.8 | 27.7 | 0 | 1.3 | 0.08 |
| 692 | **Avocado pears** | 10 pears, flesh only; Fuerte variety | 0.71 | 68.7 [a] | 1.8 | Tr | 2.0 | 0.67 |
| 693 | **Bananas** raw | Flesh only, no skin | 0.59 | 70.7 | 16.2 | 3.0 | 3.4 | 0.18 |
| 694 | raw (weighed with skin) | Calculated from the previous item | 0.59 | 41.6 | 9.6 | 1.8 | 2.0 | 0.11 |
| 695 | **Bilberries** raw | Whole fruit; literature sources | 0.98 | 84.9 | 14.3 | 0 | — | 0.10 |
| 696 | **Blackberries** raw | Whole fruit | 1.00 | 82.0 | 6.4 | 0 | 7.3 | 0.20 |
| 697 | stewed without sugar | Fruit and juice | 1.17 | 84.6 | 5.5 | 0 | 6.3 | 0.17 |
| 698 | stewed with sugar | Fruit and juice | 1.28 | 76.5 | 14.8 | 0 | 5.7 | 0.16 |
| 699 | **Cherries, eating** raw | Flesh and skin, no stalks or stones | 0.87 | 81.5 | 11.9 | 0 | 1.7 | 0.09 |
| 700 | raw (weighed with stones) | Calculated from the previous item | 0.87 | 71.0 | 10.4 | 0 | 1.5 | 0.08 |
| 701 | **cooking** raw | Flesh and skin, no stalks or stones | 0.84 | 79.8 | 11.6 | 0 | 1.7 | 0.09 |
| 702 | raw (weighed with stones) | Calculated from the previous item | 0.84 | 67.0 | 9.8 | 0 | 1.4 | 0.08 |
| 703 | stewed without sugar | Fruit and juice, no stones | 1.03 | 83.4 | 9.7 | 0 | 1.4 | 0.08 |
| 704 | stewed without sugar (weighed with stones) | Calculated from the previous item | 1.03 | 72.6 | 8.4 | 0 | 1.2 | 0.07 |

[a] The water content varies from 52 to 79 g per 100 g according to season (Pearson 1975)

| No | Food | Energy value kcal | Energy value kJ | Protein (N × 6.25) g | Fat g | Carbo-hydrate g | Na mg | K mg | Ca mg | Mg mg | P mg | Fe mg | Cu mg | Zn mg | S mg | Cl mg |
|---|---|---|---|---|---|---|---|---|---|---|---|---|---|---|---|---|
| 688 | **Apricots** dried, raw | 182 | 776 | 4.8 | Tr | 43.4 | 56 | 1880 | 92 | 65 | 120 | 4.1 | 0.27 | 0.2 | 160 | 35 |
| 689 | stewed without sugar | 66 | 288 | 1.8 | Tr | 16.1 | 21 | 700 | 34 | 24 | 44 | 1.5 | 0.10 | 0.1 | 59 | 13 |
| 690 | stewed with sugar | 81 | 347 | 1.7 | Tr | 19.9 | 20 | 670 | 33 | 23 | 43 | 1.5 | 0.10 | 0.1 | 57 | 12 |
| 691 | canned | 106 | 452 | 0.5 | Tr | 27.7 | 1 | 260 | 12 | 7 | 13 | 0.7 | 0.05 | 0.1 | 1 | 2 |
| 692 | **Avocado pears** | 223 | 922 | 4.2 | 22.2[a] | 1.8 | 2 | 400 | 15 | 29 | 31 | 1.5 | 0.21 | — | 19 | 6 |
| 693 | **Bananas** raw | 79 | 337 | 1.1 | 0.3 | 19.2 | 1 | 350 | 7 | 42 | 28 | 0.4 | 0.16 | 0.2 | 13 | 79 |
| 694 | raw (weighed with skin) | 47 | 202 | 0.7 | 0.2 | 11.4 | 1 | 210 | 4 | 25 | 17 | 0.2 | 0.09 | 0.2 | 8 | 46 |
| 695 | **Bilberries** raw | 56 | 240 | 0.6 | Tr | 14.3 | 1 | 65 | 10 | 2 | 9 | 0.7 | 0.11 | 0.1 | — | 5 |
| 696 | **Blackberries** raw | 29 | 125 | 1.3 | Tr | 6.4 | 4 | 210 | 63 | 30 | 24 | 0.9 | 0.12 | — | 9 | 22 |
| 697 | stewed without sugar | 25 | 107 | 1.1 | Tr | 5.5 | 3 | 180 | 54 | 26 | 21 | 0.8 | 0.10 | — | 8 | 19 |
| 698 | stewed with sugar | 60 | 254 | 1.0 | Tr | 14.8 | 3 | 160 | 49 | 23 | 19 | 0.7 | 0.09 | — | 7 | 17 |
| 699 | **Cherries, eating** raw | 47 | 201 | 0.6 | Tr | 11.9 | 3 | 280 | 16 | 10 | 17 | 0.4 | 0.07 | 0.1 | 7 | Tr |
| 700 | raw (weighed with stones) | 41 | 175 | 0.5 | Tr | 10.4 | 2 | 240 | 14 | 8 | 15 | 0.3 | 0.06 | 0.1 | 6 | Tr |
| 701 | **cooking** raw | 46 | 196 | 0.6 | Tr | 11.6 | 4 | 310 | 20 | 12 | 21 | 0.3 | 0.10 | 0.1 | 8 | Tr |
| 702 | raw (weighed with stones) | 39 | 165 | 0.5 | Tr | 9.8 | 3 | 260 | 17 | 10 | 18 | 0.3 | 0.08 | 0.1 | 7 | Tr |
| 703 | stewed without sugar | 39 | 165 | 0.5 | Tr | 9.8 | 3 | 250 | 18 | 10 | 17 | 0.3 | 0.08 | 0.1 | 7 | Tr |
| 704 | stewed without sugar (weighed with stones) | 33 | 141 | 0.4 | Tr | 8.4 | 3 | 220 | 16 | 9 | 15 | 0.3 | 0.07 | 0.1 | 6 | Tr |

[a] The fat content varies from 11 to 39g per 100g according to season (Pearson 1975)

| No | Food | Retinol µg | Carotene µg | Vitamin D µg | Thiamin mg | Riboflavin mg | Nicotinic acid mg | Potential nicotinic acid from tryptophan mg Trp ÷ 60 | Vitamin C mg | Vitamin E mg |
|---|---|---|---|---|---|---|---|---|---|---|
| 688 | **Apricots** dried, raw | 0 | 3600 *(2400–4400)* | 0 | Tr | 0.20 | 3.0 | 0.8 | Tr | — |
| 689 | stewed without sugar | 0 | 1330 | 0 | Tr | 0.06 | 1.1 | 0.3 | Tr | — |
| 690 | stewed with sugar | 0 | 1280 | 0 | Tr | 0.06 | 1.1 | 0.3 | Tr | — |
| 691 | canned | 0 | 1000 | 0 | 0.02 | 0.01 | 0.3 | 0.1 | 2 | — |
| 692 | **Avocado pears** | 0 | 100 | —[a] | 0.10 | 0.10 | 1.0 | 0.8 | 15 *(5–30)* | 3.2 |
| 693 | **Bananas** raw | 0 | 200 | 0 | 0.04 | 0.07 | 0.6 | 0.2 | 10 | 0.2 |
| 694 | raw (weighed with skin) | 0 | 120 | 0 | 0.02 | 0.04 | 0.4 | 0.1 | 6 | 0.1 |
| 695 | **Bilberries,** raw | 0 | 130 | 0 | 0.02 | 0.02 | 0.4 | 0.1 | 22 *(10–44)* | — |
| 696 | **Blackberries** raw | 0 | 100 | 0 | 0.03 | 0.04 | 0.4 | 0.2 | 20 | 3.5[b] |
| 697 | stewed without sugar | 0 | 85 | 0 | 0.03 | 0.03 | 0.3 | 0.2 | 15 | 3.0[c] |
| 698 | stewed with sugar | 0 | 80 | 0 | 0.02 | 0.03 | 0.3 | 0.2 | 14 | 2.7[c] |
| 699 | **Cherries, eating** raw | 0 | 120 | 0 | 0.05 | 0.07 | 0.3 | 0.1 | 5 | 0.1 |
| 700 | raw (weighed with stones) | 0 | 100 | 0 | 0.04 | 0.06 | 0.3 | 0.1 | 4 | 0.1 |
| 701 | **cooking** raw | 0 | 120 | 0 | 0.05 | 0.07 | 0.3 | 0.1 | 5 | 0.1 |
| 702 | raw (weighed with stones) | 0 | 100 | 0 | 0.04 | 0.06 | 0.3 | 0.1 | 4 | 0.1 |
| 703 | stewed without sugar | 0 | 100 | 0 | 0.03 | 0.06 | 0.3 | 0.1 | 3 | 0.1 |
| 704 | stewed without sugar (weighed with stones) | 0 | 85 | 0 | 0.03 | 0.05 | 0.3 | 0.1 | 3 | 0.1 |

| No | Food | Vitamin $B_6$ mg | Vitamin $B_{12}$ µg | Folic acid Free µg | Folic acid Total µg | Pantothenic acid mg | Biotin µg |
|---|---|---|---|---|---|---|---|
| 688 | **Apricots** dried, raw | 0.17 | 0 | 10 | 14 | 0.70 | — |
| 689 | stewed without sugar | 0.05 | 0 | Tr | 2 | 0.23 | — |
| 690 | stewed with sugar | 0.05 | 0 | Tr | 2 | 0.23 | — |
| 691 | canned | 0.05 | 0 | 4 | (5) | 0.10 | — |
| 692 | **Avocado pears** | 0.42 | 0 | 55 | 66 | 1.07 | 3.2 |
| 693 | **Bananas** raw | 0.51 | 0 | 14 | 22 | 0.26 | — |
| 694 | raw (weighed with skin) | 0.30 | 0 | 8 | 13 | 0.15 | — |
| 695 | **Bilberries** raw | 0.06 | 0 | 2 | 6 | 0.16 | — |
| 696 | **Blackberries** raw | 0.05 | 0 | — | — | 0.25 | 0.4 |
| 697 | stewed without sugar | 0.03 | 0 | — | — | 0.19 | 0.3 |
| 698 | stewed with sugar | 0.03 | 0 | — | — | 0.18 | 0.3 |
| 699 | **Cherries, eating** raw | 0.05 | 0 | 6 | 8 | 0.26 | 0.4 |
| 700 | raw (weighed with stones) | 0.04 | 0 | 5 | 7 | 0.23 | 0.3 |
| 701 | **cooking** raw | 0.05 | 0 | 6 | 8 | 0.26 | 0.4 |
| 702 | raw (weighed with stones) | 0.04 | 0 | 5 | 7 | 0.22 | 0.3 |
| 703 | stewed without sugar | 0.02 | 0 | Tr | 3 | 0.20 | 0.3 |
| 704 | stewed without sugar (weighed with stones) | 0.02 | 0 | Tr | 3 | 0.17 | 0.3 |

Notes

[a] Avocado pears have been reported to contain vitamin D (Zanobini, Firenzuoli and Bianchi 1974).

[b] Value for wild blackberries, which also contain 4.7 mg γ-tocopherol and 4.5 mg δ-tocopherol. Cultivated blackberries contain 0.6 mg α-tocopherol, 1.1 mg γ-tocopherol and 1.0 mg δ-tocopherol per 100 g (Booth and Bradford 1963a).

[c] Value for wild blackberries.

| No | Food | Description and number of samples | Edible matter, proportion of weight purchased | Water g | Sugars g | Starch g | Dietary fibre g | Total nitrogen g |
|---|---|---|---|---|---|---|---|---|
| 705 | **Cherries, cooking** stewed with sugar | Fruit and juice, no stones | 1.13 | 72.8 | 19.7 | 0 | 1.2 | 0.07 |
| 706 | stewed with sugar (weighed with stones) | Calculated from the previous item | 1.13 | 64.8 | 17.5 | 0 | 1.1 | 0.06 |
| 707 | **Cranberries** raw | Whole fruit | 1.00 | 87.0 | 3.5 | 0 | 4.2 | 0.06 |
| 708 | **Currants, black** raw | Whole fruit, no stalks | 0.98 | 77.4 | 6.6 | 0 | 8.7 | 0.15 |
| 709 | stewed without sugar | Fruit and juice | 1.15 | 80.7 | 5.6 | 0 | 7.4 | 0.13 |
| 710 | stewed with sugar | Fruit and juice | 1.26 | 72.9 | 15.0 | 0 | 6.8 | 0.12 |
| 711 | **red** raw | Whole fruit, no stalks | 0.97 | 82.8 | 4.4 | 0 | 8.2 | 0.18 |
| 712 | stewed without sugar | Fruit and juice | 1.14 | 85.3 | 3.8 | 0 | 7.0 | 0.15 |
| 713 | stewed with sugar | Fruit and juice | 1.25 | 88.2 | 13.3 | 0 | 6.4 | 0.14 |
| 714 | **white** raw | Whole fruit, no stalks | 0.96 | 83.3 | 5.6 | 0 | 6.8 | 0.20 |
| 715 | stewed without sugar | Fruit and juice | 1.13 | 85.7 | 4.8 | 0 | 5.8 | 0.17 |
| 716 | stewed with sugar | Fruit and juice | 1.24 | 77.5 | 14.2 | 0 | 5.3 | 0.16 |
| 717 | **dried** | Whole fruit | 1.00 | 22.0 | 63.1 | 0 | 6.5 | 0.27 |
| 718 | **Damsons** raw | Flesh and skin, no stalks or stones | 0.90 | 77.5 | 9.6 | 0 | 4.1 | 0.08 |
| 719 | raw (weighed with stones) | Calculated from the previous item | 0.90 | 69.8 | 8.6 | 0 | 3.7 | 0.07 |
| 720 | stewed without sugar | Fruit and juice, no stones | 1.08 | 80.7 | 8.1 | 0 | 3.5 | 0.07 |
| 721 | stewed without sugar (weighed with stones) | Calculated from the previous item | 1.08 | 74.2 | 7.4 | 0 | 3.2 | 0.06 |

| No | Food | Energy value kcal | Energy value kJ | Protein (N × 6.25) g | Fat g | Carbo-hydrate g | Na mg | K mg | Ca mg | Mg mg | P mg | Fe mg | Cu mg | Zn mg | S mg | Cl mg |
|---|---|---|---|---|---|---|---|---|---|---|---|---|---|---|---|---|
| 705 | **Cherries, cooking** stewed with sugar | 77 | 328 | 0.4 | Tr | 20.1 | 2 | 230 | 15 | 9 | 16 | 0.2 | 0.07 | 0.1 | 6 | Tr |
| 706 | stewed with sugar (weighed with stones) | 67 | 287 | 0.4 | Tr | 17.5 | 2 | 200 | 13 | 8 | 14 | 0.2 | 0.06 | 0.1 | 5 | Tr |
| 707 | **Cranberries** raw | 15 | 63 | 0.4 | Tr | 3.5 | 2 | 120 | 15 | 8 | 11 | 1.1 | 0.14 | — | 11 | Tr |
| 708 | **Currants, black** raw | 28 | 121 | 0.9 | Tr | 6.6 | 3 | 370 | 60 | 17 | 43 | 1.3 | 0.14 | — | 33 | 15 |
| 709 | stewed without sugar | 24 | 103 | 0.8 | Tr | 5.6 | 3 | 320 | 51 | 16 | 37 | 1.1 | 0.12 | — | 28 | 13 |
| 710 | stewed with sugar | 59 | 254 | 0.8 | Tr | 15.0 | 2 | 290 | 47 | 13 | 34 | 1.0 | 0.11 | — | 26 | 12 |
| 711 | **red** raw | 21 | 89 | 1.1 | Tr | 4.4 | 2 | 280 | 36 | 13 | 30 | 1.2 | 0.12 | — | 29 | 14 |
| 712 | stewed without sugar | 18 | 76 | 0.9 | Tr | 3.8 | 2 | 240 | 31 | 11 | 26 | 1.0 | 0.10 | — | 25 | 12 |
| 713 | stewed with sugar | 53 | 228 | 0.9 | Tr | 13.3 | 2 | 220 | 28 | 10 | 23 | 0.9 | 0.09 | — | 23 | 11 |
| 714 | **white** raw | 26 | 112 | 1.3 | Tr | 5.6 | 2 | 290 | 22 | 13 | 28 | 0.9 | 0.14 | — | 24 | 11 |
| 715 | stewed without sugar | 22 | 96 | 1.1 | Tr | 4.8 | 2 | 250 | 19 | 11 | 24 | 0.8 | 0.12 | — | 21 | 9 |
| 716 | stewed with sugar | 57 | 244 | 1.0 | Tr | 14.2 | 2 | 230 | 17 | 10 | 22 | 0.7 | 0.11 | — | 19 | 9 |
| 717 | **dried** | 243 | 1039 | 1.7 | Tr | 63.1 | 20 | 710 | 95 | 36 | 40 | 1.8 | 0.48 | (0.1) | 31 | 16 |
| 718 | **Damsons** raw | 38 | 162 | 0.5 | Tr | 9.6 | 2 | 290 | 24 | 11 | 16 | 0.4 | 0.08 | (0.1) | 6 | Tr |
| 719 | raw (weighed with stones) | 34 | 144 | 0.4 | Tr | 8.6 | 2 | 260 | 21 | 10 | 15 | 0.4 | 0.07 | (0.1) | 6 | Tr |
| 720 | stewed without sugar | 32 | 136 | 0.4 | Tr | 8.1 | 2 | 240 | 20 | 10 | 14 | 0.3 | 0.07 | (0.1) | 5 | Tr |
| 721 | stewed without sugar (weighed with stones) | 29 | 125 | 0.4 | Tr | 7.4 | 2 | 220 | 18 | 9 | 13 | 0.3 | 0.06 | (0.1) | 5 | Tr |

| No | Food | Retinol µg | Carotene µg | Vitamin D µg | Thiamin mg | Riboflavin mg | Nicotinic acid mg | Potential nicotinic acid from tryptophan mgTrp ÷ 60 | Vitamin C mg | Vitamin E mg |
|---|---|---|---|---|---|---|---|---|---|---|
| 705 | **Cherries, cooking** stewed with sugar | 0 | 90 | 0 | 0.03 | 0.06 | 0.2 | 0.1 | 3 | 0.1 |
| 706 | stewed with sugar (weighed with stones) | 0 | 80 | 0 | 0.03 | 0.05 | 0.2 | 0.1 | 3 | 0.1 |
| 707 | **Cranberries** raw | 0 | 20 | 0 | 0.03 | 0.02 | 0.1 | 0.1 | 12 | — |
| 708 | **Currants, black** raw | 0 | 200 | 0 | 0.03 | 0.06 | 0.3 | 0.1 | 200 *(150–230)* | 1.0 |
| 709 | stewed without sugar | 0 | 170 | 0 | 0.03 | 0.05 | 0.3 | 0.1 | 150 | 0.9 |
| 710 | stewed with sugar | 0 | 160 | 0 | 0.02 | 0.05 | 0.2 | 0.1 | 140[a] | 0.8 |
| 711 | **red** raw | 0 | 70 | 0 | 0.04 | (0.06) | 0.1 | 0.2 | 40 | 0.1 |
| 712 | stewed without sugar | 0 | 60 | 0 | 0.03 | (0.05) | 0.1 | 0.1 | 31 | 0.1 |
| 713 | stewed with sugar | 0 | 55 | 0 | 0.03 | (0.05) | 0.1 | 0.1 | 28 | 0.1 |
| 714 | **white** raw | 0 | Tr | 0 | (0.04) | (0.06) | (0.1) | 0.2 | (40) | (0.1) |
| 715 | stewed without sugar | 0 | Tr | 0 | (0.03) | (0.05) | (0.1) | 0.2 | (31) | (0.1) |
| 716 | stewed with sugar | 0 | Tr | 0 | (0.03) | (0.05) | (0.1) | 0.2 | (28) | (0.1) |
| 717 | **dried** | 0 | 30 | 0 | 0.03 | (0.08) | (0.5) | 0.1 | 0 | — |
| 718 | **Damsons** raw | 0 | (220) | 0 | 0.10 | 0.03 | 0.3 | 0.1 | (3) | 0.7 |
| 719 | raw (weighed with stones) | 0 | (200) | 0 | 0.09 | 0.03 | 0.3 | 0.1 | (3) | 0.6 |
| 720 | stewed without sugar | 0 | (180) | 0 | 0.08 | 0.03 | 0.3 | 0.1 | (3) | 0.5 |
| 721 | stewed without sugar (weighed with stones) | 0 | (170) | 0 | 0.07 | 0.03 | 0.3 | 0.1 | (3) | 0.5 |

| No | Food | Vitamin $B_6$ mg | Vitamin $B_{12}$ µg | Folic acid Free µg | Folic acid Total µg | Pantothenic acid mg | Biotin µg | Notes |
|---|---|---|---|---|---|---|---|---|
| 705 | **Cherries, cooking** stewed with sugar | 0.02 | 0 | Tr | 3 | 0.13 | 0.2 | [a] Canned blackcurrants contain 100 mg per 100 g. |
| 706 | stewed with sugar (weighed with stones) | 0.02 | 0 | Tr | 3 | 0.12 | 0.2 | |
| 707 | **Cranberries** raw | 0.04 | 0 | 1 | 2 | 0.22 | — | |
| 708 | **Currants, black** raw | 0.08 | 0 | — | — | 0.40 | 2.4 | |
| 709 | stewed without sugar | 0.06 | 0 | — | — | 0.31 | 2.1 | |
| 710 | stewed with sugar | 0.05 | 0 | — | — | 0.28 | 1.9 | |
| 711 | **red** raw | 0.05 | 0 | — | — | 0.06 | 2.6 | |
| 712 | stewed without sugar | 0.03 | 0 | — | — | 0.05 | 2.2 | |
| 713 | stewed with sugar | 0.03 | 0 | — | — | 0.05 | 2.0 | |
| 714 | **white** raw | (0.05) | 0 | — | — | (0.06) | (2.6) | |
| 715 | stewed without sugar | (0.03) | 0 | — | — | (0.05) | (2.2) | |
| 716 | stewed with sugar | (0.03) | 0 | — | — | (0.05) | (2.0) | |
| 717 | **dried** | (0.30) | 0 | 4 | 11 | (0.10) | — | |
| 718 | **Damsons** raw | (0.05) | 0 | (1) | (3) | 0.27 | 0.1 | |
| 719 | raw (weighed with stones) | (0.05) | 0 | (1) | (3) | 0.24 | 0.1 | |
| 720 | stewed without sugar | (0.03) | 0 | Tr | (1) | 0.21 | 0.1 | |
| 721 | stewed without sugar (weighed with stones) | (0.03) | 0 | Tr | (1) | 0.19 | 0.1 | |

| No | Food | Description and number of samples | Edible matter, proportion of weight purchased | Water g | Sugars g | Starch g | Dietary fibre g | Total nitrogen g |
|---|---|---|---|---|---|---|---|---|
| 722 | **Damsons** stewed with sugar | Fruit and juice, no stones | 1.19 | 72.0 | 17.8 | 0 | 3.1 | 0.05 |
| 723 | stewed with sugar (weighed with stones) | Calculated from the previous item | 1.19 | 67.0 | 16.6 | 0 | 2.9 | 0.05 |
| 724 | **Dates** dried | Flesh and skin, no stones | 0.86 | 14.6 | 63.9 | 0 | 8.7 | 0.32 |
| 725 | dried (weighed with stones) | Calculated from the previous item | 0.86 | 12.6 | 54.9 | 0 | 7.5 | 0.28 |
| 726 | **Figs, green** raw | Whole fruit, no stalks | 0.98 | 84.6 | 9.5 | 0 | 2.5 | 0.21 |
| 727 | **dried** raw | Whole fruit | 1.00 | 16.8 | 52.9 | 0 | 18.5 | 0.57 |
| 728 | stewed without sugar | Fruit and juice | 1.80 | 53.8 | 29.4 | 0 | 10.3 | 0.32 |
| 729 | stewed with sugar | Fruit and juice | 1.91 | 50.7 | 34.3 | 0 | 9.7 | 0.30 |
| 730 | **Fruit pie filling** canned | 10 cans, blackcurrant, blackberry and apple, gooseberry, apple, cherry | 1.00 | 72.6 | 23.2 | 1.9 | (1.8) | 0.04 |
| 731 | **Fruit salad** canned | Fruit and syrup | 1.00 | 71.1 | 25.0 | 0 | 1.1 | 0.04 |
| 732 | **Gooseberries, green** raw | Flesh, skin and pips, no 'tops' or 'tails' | 0.99 | 89.9 | 3.4 | 0 | 3.2 | 0.18 |
| 733 | stewed without sugar | Fruit and juice | 1.16 | 91.4 | 2.9 | 0 | 2.7 | 0.15 |
| 734 | stewed with sugar | Fruit and juice | 1.27 | 82.7 | 12.5 | 0 | 2.5 | 0.14 |
| 735 | **ripe** raw | Flesh, skin and pips, no 'tops' or 'tails' | 0.99 | 83.7 | 9.2 | 0 | 3.5 | 0.09 |
| 736 | **Grapes, black** raw | Flesh only, no skin, pips or stalks | 0.81 | 80.7 | 15.5 | 0 | 0.4 | 0.09 |
| 737 | raw (whole grapes weighed) | Calculated from the previous item | 0.81 | 65.2 | 13.0 | 0 | 0.3 | 0.08 |

| No | Food | Energy value kcal | Energy value kJ | Protein (N × 6.25) g | Fat g | Carbo-hydrate g | mg Na | K | Ca | Mg | P | Fe | Cu | Zn | S | Cl |
|---|---|---|---|---|---|---|---|---|---|---|---|---|---|---|---|---|
| 722 | **Damsons** stewed with sugar | 69 | 293 | 0.3 | Tr | 18.0 | 2 | 220 | 17 | 9 | 13 | 0.3 | 0.05 | (0.1) | 5 | Tr |
| 723 | stewed with sugar (weighed with stones) | 63 | 271 | 0.3 | Tr | 16.6 | 2 | 200 | 16 | 8 | 12 | 0.3 | 0.05 | (0.1) | 5 | Tr |
| 724 | **Dates** dried | 248 | 1056 | 2.0 | Tr | 63.9 | 5 | 750 | 68 | 59 | 64 | 1.6 | 0.21 | 0.3 | 51 | 290 |
| 725 | dried (weighed with stones) | 213 | 909 | 1.7 | Tr | 54.9 | 4 | 650 | 58 | 50 | 55 | 1.4 | 0.18 | 0.3 | 44 | 250 |
| 726 | **Figs, green** raw | 41 | 174 | 1.3 | Tr | 9.5 | 2 | 270 | 34 | 20 | 32 | 0.4 | 0.06 | 0.3 | 13 | 18 |
| 727 | **dried** raw | 213 | 908 | 3.6 | Tr | 52.9 | 87 | 1010 | 280 | 92 | 92 | 4.2 | 0.24 | 0.9 | 81 | 170 |
| 728 | stewed without sugar | 118 | 504 | 2.0 | Tr | 29.4 | 48 | 560 | 160 | 51 | 51 | 2.3 | 0.13 | 0.5 | 45 | 94 |
| 729 | stewed with sugar | 136 | 581 | 1.9 | Tr | 34.3 | 46 | 530 | 140 | 48 | 48 | 2.2 | 0.13 | 0.5 | 42 | 89 |
| 730 | **Fruit pie filling** canned | 95 | 407 | 0.3 | Tr | 25.1 | 30 | 79 | 18 | 4 | 9 | 0.5 | (0.03) | 0.1 | — | 45 |
| 731 | **Fruit salad** canned | 95 | 405 | 0.3 | Tr | 25.0 | 2 | 120 | 8 | 8 | 10 | 1.0 | 0.03 | — | 2 | 3 |
| 732 | **Gooseberries, green** raw | 17 | 73 | 1.1 | Tr | 3.4 | 2 | 210 | 28 | 7 | 34 | 0.3 | 0.13 | 0.1 | 16 | 7 |
| 733 | stewed without sugar | 14 | 62 | 0.9 | Tr | 2.9 | 2 | 180 | 24 | 6 | 29 | 0.3 | 0.11 | 0.1 | 14 | 6 |
| 734 | stewed with sugar | 50 | 215 | 0.9 | Tr | 12.5 | 2 | 160 | 22 | 5 | 27 | 0.2 | 0.10 | 0.1 | 13 | 5 |
| 735 | **ripe** raw | 37 | 157 | 0.6 | Tr | 9.2 | 1 | 170 | 19 | 9 | 19 | 0.6 | 0.15 | 0.1 | 14 | 11 |
| 736 | **Grapes, black** raw | 61 | 258 | 0.6 | Tr | 15.5 | 2 | 320 | 4 | 4 | 16 | 0.3 | 0.08 | 0.1 | 7 | Tr |
| 737 | raw (whole grapes weighed) | 51 | 217 | 0.5 | Tr | 13.0 | 1 | 270 | 4 | 3 | 14 | 0.3 | 0.07 | 0.1 | 6 | Tr |

| No | Food | Retinol µg | Carotene µg | Vitamin D µg | Thiamin mg | Riboflavin mg | Nicotinic acid mg | Potential nicotinic acid from tryptophan mg Trp ÷ 60 | Vitamin C mg | Vitamin E mg |
|---|---|---|---|---|---|---|---|---|---|---|
| 722 | **Damsons** stewed with sugar | 0 | (170) | 0 | 0.06 | 0.02 | 0.2 | 0.1 | (2) | 0.5 |
| 723 | stewed with sugar (weighed with stones) | 0 | (160) | 0 | 0.06 | 0.02 | 0.2 | 0.1 | (2) | 0.5 |
| 724 | **Dates** dried | 0 | 50 | 0 | 0.07 | 0.04 | 2.0 | 0.9 | 0 | — |
| 725 | dried (weighed with stones) | 0 | 43 | 0 | 0.06 | 0.03 | 1.7 | 0.8 | 0 | — |
| 726 | **Figs, green** raw | 0 | (500) | 0 | 0.06 | 0.05 | 0.4 | 0.2 | 2 | — |
| 727 | **dried** raw | 0 | 50 | 0 | 0.10 | 0.08 | 1.7 | 0.5 | 0 | — |
| 728 | stewed without sugar | 0 | 30 | 0 | 0.05 | 0.04 | 0.9 | 0.3 | 0 | — |
| 729 | stewed with sugar | 0 | 30 | 0 | 0.05 | 0.04 | 0.9 | 0.3 | 0 | — |
| 730 | **Fruit pie filling** canned | 0 | — | 0 | Tr | 0.01 | 0.1 | Tr | (Tr) | — |
| 731 | **Fruit salad** canned[a] | 0 | 300 | 0 | 0.02 | 0.01 | 0.3 | Tr | 3 | — |
| 732 | **Gooseberries, green** raw | 0 | 180 | 0 | (0.04) | 0.03 | 0.3 | 0.2 | 40 *(25–50)* | 0.4 |
| 733 | stewed without sugar | 0 | 150 | 0 | 0.03 | 0.03 | 0.3 | 0.2 | 31 | 0.3 |
| 734 | stewed with sugar | 0 | 140 | 0 | 0.03 | 0.02 | 0.2 | 0.1 | 28[b] | 0.3 |
| 735 | **ripe** raw | 0 | 180 | 0 | (0.04) | 0.03 | 0.3 | 0.1 | 40 *(25–50)* | 0.4 |
| 736 | **Grapes, black** raw | 0 | (Tr) | 0 | 0.04 | 0.02 | 0.3 | Tr | 4 | — |
| 737 | raw (whole grapes weighed) | 0 | (Tr) | 0 | 0.03 | 0.02 | 0.2 | Tr | 3 | — |

| No | Food | Vitamin $B_6$ mg | Vitamin $B_{12}$ µg | Folic acid Free µg | Folic acid Total µg | Pantothenic acid mg | Biotin µg |
|---|---|---|---|---|---|---|---|
| 722 | **Damsons** stewed with sugar | 0.03 | 0 | Tr | (1) | 0.18 | 0.1 |
| 723 | stewed with sugar (weighed with stones) | 0.03 | 0 | Tr | (1) | 0.17 | 0.1 |
| 724 | **Dates** dried | 0.15 | 0 | 14 | 21 | 0.80 | — |
| 725 | dried (weighed with stones) | 0.13 | 0 | 12 | 18 | 0.69 | — |
| 726 | **Figs, green** raw | 0.11 | 0 | — | — | 0.30 | — |
| 727 | **dried** raw | 0.18 | 0 | 3 | 9 | 0.44 | — |
| 728 | stewed without sugar | 0.08 | 0 | Tr | 2 | 0.22 | — |
| 729 | stewed with sugar | 0.07 | 0 | Tr | 2 | 0.21 | — |
| 730 | **Fruit pie filling** canned | (Tr) | 0 | 1 | 1 | (Tr) | (Tr) |
| 731 | **Fruit salad** canned [a] | 0.01 | 0 | (1) | (4) | 0.04 | 0.1 |
| 732 | **Gooseberries, green** raw | 0.02 | 0 | — | — | 0.15 | 0.5 |
| 733 | stewed without sugar | 0.02 | 0 | — | — | 0.12 | 0.4 |
| 734 | stewed with sugar | 0.02 | 0 | — | — | 0.11 | 0.4 |
| 735 | **ripe** raw | 0.02 | 0 | — | — | 0.30 | 0.1 |
| 736 | **Grapes, black** raw | 0.10 | 0 | 3 | 6 | 0.05 | 0.3 |
| 737 | raw (whole grapes weighed) | 0.08 | 0 | 2 | 5 | 0.04 | 0.2 |

**Notes**

[a] Calculated assuming that canned fruit salad contains canned fruit in the following proportions:

| | % |
|---|---|
| Apricots or peaches | 35 |
| Pears | 35 |
| Cherries | 10 |
| Grapes | 10 |
| Pineapple | 10 |

[b] Canned gooseberries contain 24 mg per 100 g.

| No | Food | Description and number of samples | Edible matter, proportion of weight purchased | Water g | Sugars g | Starch g | Dietary fibre g | Total nitrogen g |
|---|---|---|---|---|---|---|---|---|
| 738 | **Grapes, white** raw | Flesh and skin, no pips or stalks | 0.95 | 79.3 | 16.1 | 0 | 0.9 | 0.10 |
| 739 | raw (whole grapes weighed) | Calculated from the previous item | 0.95 | 75.5 | 15.3 | 0 | 0.9 | 0.10 |
| 740 | **Grapefruit** raw | Flesh only, no skin, pith or pips | 0.48 | 90.7 | 5.3 | 0 | 0.6 | 0.10 |
| 741 | raw (whole fruit weighed) | Calculated from the previous item | 0.48 | 43.5 | 2.5 | 0 | 0.3 | 0.05 |
| 742 | canned | 10 cans, fruit and syrup | 1.00 | 81.8 | 15.5 | 0 | 0.4 | 0.08 |
| 743 | **Greengages** raw | Flesh and skin, no stalks or stones | 0.95 | 78.2 | 11.8 | 0 | 2.6 | 0.12 |
| 744 | raw (weighed with stones) | Calculated from the previous item | 0.95 | 74.4 | 11.2 | 0 | 2.5 | 0.11 |
| 745 | stewed without sugar | Fruit and juice, no stones | 1.13 | 81.4 | 10.0 | 0 | 2.2 | 0.09 |
| 746 | stewed without sugar (weighed with stones) | Calculated from the previous item | 1.13 | 78.1 | 9.6 | 0 | 2.1 | 0.09 |
| 747 | stewed with sugar | Fruit and juice, no stones | 1.23 | 72.8 | 19.2 | 0 | 2.1 | 0.09 |
| 748 | stewed with sugar (weighed with stones) | Calculated from the previous item | 1.23 | 70.6 | 18.6 | 0 | 2.0 | 0.09 |
| 749 | **Guavas** canned | 10 cans, fruit and syrup | 1.00 | 77.6 | 15.7 | Tr | 3.6 | 0.06 |
| 750 | **Lemons** whole | Whole fruit including skin, no pips | 0.99 | 85.2 | 3.2 | 0 | 5.2 | 0.12 |
| 751 | juice, fresh | Strained juice from fresh lemons | 0.36 | 91.3 | 1.6 | 0 | 0 | 0.05 |
| 752 | **Loganberries** raw | Whole fruit | 1.00 | 85.0 | 3.4 | 0 | 6.2 | 0.17 |
| 753 | stewed without sugar | Fruit and juice | 1.08 | 86.1 | 3.1 | 0 | 5.7 | 0.16 |

| No | Food | Energy value kcal | Energy value kJ | Protein (N × 6.25) g | Fat g | Carbo-hydrate g | Na mg | K mg | Ca mg | Mg mg | P mg | Fe mg | Cu mg | Zn mg | S mg | Cl mg |
|---|---|---|---|---|---|---|---|---|---|---|---|---|---|---|---|---|
| 738 | **Grapes, white** raw | 63 | 268 | 0.6 | Tr | 16.1 | 2 | 250 | 19 | 7 | 22 | 0.3 | 0.10 | 0.1 | 9 | Tr |
| 739 | raw (whole grapes weighed) | 60 | 255 | 0.6 | Tr | 15.3 | 2 | 240 | 18 | 6 | 21 | 0.3 | 0.10 | 0.1 | 9 | Tr |
| 740 | **Grapefruit** raw | 22 | 95 | 0.6 | Tr | 5.3 | 1 | 230 | 17 | 10 | 16 | 0.3 | 0.06 | 0.1 | 5 | 1 |
| 741 | raw (whole fruit weighed) | 11 | 45 | 0.3 | Tr | 2.5 | 1 | 110 | 8 | 5 | 8 | 0.1 | 0.03 | 0.1 | 3 | 1 |
| 742 | canned | 60 | 257 | 0.5 | Tr | 15.5 | 10 | 79 | 17 | 7 | 13 | 0.7 | (0.03) | 0.4 | — | (5) |
| 743 | **Greengages** raw | 47 | 202 | 0.8 | Tr | 11.8 | 1 | 310 | 17 | 8 | 23 | 0.4 | 0.08 | (0.1) | 3 | 1 |
| 744 | raw (weighed with stones) | 45 | 191 | 0.7 | Tr | 11.2 | 1 | 290 | 16 | 7 | 22 | 0.4 | 0.08 | (0.1) | 3 | 1 |
| 745 | stewed without sugar | 40 | 170 | 0.6 | Tr | 10.0 | 1 | 260 | 15 | 6 | 20 | 0.3 | 0.07 | (0.1) | 3 | 1 |
| 746 | stewed without sugar (weighed with stones) | 38 | 164 | 0.6 | Tr | 9.6 | 1 | 250 | 14 | 6 | 19 | 0.3 | 0.07 | (0.1) | 3 | 1 |
| 747 | stewed with sugar | 75 | 321 | 0.6 | Tr | 19.4 | 1 | 240 | 13 | 5 | 18 | 0.3 | 0.06 | (0.1) | 2 | 1 |
| 748 | stewed with sugar (weighed with stones) | 72 | 308 | 0.6 | Tr | 18.6 | 1 | 230 | 13 | 5 | 17 | 0.3 | 0.06 | (0.1) | 2 | 1 |
| 749 | **Guavas** canned | 60 | 258 | 0.4 | Tr | 15.7 | 7 | 120 | 8 | 6 | 11 | 0.5 | 0.10 | 0.4 | — | 10 |
| 750 | **Lemons** whole | 15 | 65 | 0.8 | Tr | 3.2 | 6 | 160 | 110 | 12 | 21 | 0.4 | 0.26 | 0.1 | 12 | 5 |
| 751 | juice, fresh | 7 | 31 | 0.3 | Tr | 1.6 | 2 | 140 | 8 | 7 | 10 | 0.1 | 0.13 | Tr | 2 | 3 |
| 752 | **Loganberries** raw | 17 | 73 | 1.1 | Tr | 3.4 | 3 | 260 | 35 | 25 | 24 | 1.4 | 0.14 | — | 18 | 16 |
| 753 | stewed without sugar | 16 | 67 | 1.0 | Tr | 3.1 | 3 | 240 | 32 | 23 | 22 | 1.3 | 0.13 | — | 17 | 15 |

| No | Food | Retinol µg | Carotene µg | Vitamin D µg | Thiamin mg | Riboflavin mg | Nicotinic acid mg | Potential nicotinic acid from tryptophan mg Trp ÷ 60 | Vitamin C mg | Vitamin E mg |
|---|---|---|---|---|---|---|---|---|---|---|
| 738 | **Grapes, white** raw | 0 | Tr | 0 | 0.04 | 0.02 | 0.3 | Tr | 4 | — |
| 739 | raw (whole grapes weighed) | 0 | Tr | 0 | 0.04 | 0.02 | 0.3 | Tr | 4 | — |
| 740 | **Grapefruit** raw | 0 | Tr | 0 | 0.05 | 0.02 | 0.2 | 0.1 | 40 *(35–45)* | 0.3 |
| 741 | raw (whole fruit weighed) | 0 | Tr | 0 | 0.02 | 0.01 | 0.1 | Tr | 19 | 0.1 |
| 742 | canned | 0 | Tr | 0 | 0.04 | 0.01 | 0.2 | 0.1 | 30 | Tr |
| 743 | **Greengages** raw | 0 | — | 0 | (0.05) | (0.03) | (0.4) | 0.1 | (3) | (0.7) |
| 744 | raw (weighed with stones) | 0 | — | 0 | (0.05) | (0.03) | (0.4) | 0.1 | (3) | (0.7) |
| 745 | stewed without sugar | 0 | — | 0 | (0.04) | (0.03) | (0.3) | 0.1 | (3) | (0.6) |
| 746 | stewed without sugar (weighed with stones) | 0 | — | 0 | (0.04) | (0.03) | (0.3) | 0.1 | (3) | (0.6) |
| 747 | stewed with sugar | 0 | — | 0 | (0.04) | (0.02) | (0.3) | 0.1 | (2) | (0.5) |
| 748 | stewed with sugar (weighed with stones) | 0 | — | 0 | (0.04) | (0.02) | (0.3) | 0.1 | (2) | (0.5) |
| 749 | **Guavas** canned | 0 | (100) | 0 | (0.04) | (0.03) | (0.9) | 0.1 | 180[a] | — |
| 750 | **Lemons** whole | 0 | Tr | 0 | 0.05 | 0.04 | 0.2 | 0.1 | 80 | — |
| 751 | juice, fresh | 0 | Tr | 0 | 0.02 | 0.01 | 0.1 | Tr | 50[b] *(40–60)* | — |
| 752 | **Loganberries** raw | 0 | (80) | 0 | (0.02) | 0.03 | (0.4) | 0.2 | 35 | (0.3) |
| 753 | stewed without sugar | 0 | (75) | 0 | (0.02) | 0.03 | (0.4) | 0.2 | 29 | (0.3) |

| No | Food | Vitamin $B_6$ mg | Vitamin $B_{12}$ µg | Folic acid Free µg | Folic acid Total µg | Pantothenic acid mg | Biotin µg |
|---|---|---|---|---|---|---|---|
| 738 | **Grapes, white** raw | 0.10 | 0 | 3 | 6 | 0.05 | 0.3 |
| 739 | raw (whole grapes weighed) | 0.10 | 0 | 3 | 6 | 0.05 | 0.3 |
| 740 | **Grapefruit** raw | 0.03 | 0 | 9 | 12 | 0.28 | (1.0) |
| 741 | raw (whole fruit weighed) | 0.01 | 0 | 4 | 6 | 0.13 | (0.5) |
| 742 | canned | 0.02 | 0 | 3 | 4 | 0.12 | 1.0 |
| 743 | **Greengages** raw | (0.05) | 0 | (1) | (3) | (0.20) | (Tr) |
| 744 | raw (weighed with stones) | (0.05) | 0 | (1) | (3) | (0.20) | (Tr) |
| 745 | stewed without sugar | (0.03) | 0 | (Tr) | (1) | (0.16) | (Tr) |
| 746 | stewed without sugar (weighed with stones) | (0.03) | 0 | (Tr) | (1) | (0.15) | (Tr) |
| 747 | stewed with sugar | (0.03) | 0 | (Tr) | (1) | (0.14) | (Tr) |
| 748 | stewed with sugar (weighed with stones) | (0.03) | 0 | (Tr) | (1) | (0.14) | (Tr) |
| 749 | **Guavas** canned | — | 0 | — | — | — | — |
| 750 | **Lemons** whole | 0.11 | 0 | — | — | 0.23 | 0.5 |
| 751 | juice, fresh | 0.05 | 0 | 7 | 7 | 0.10 | 0.3 |
| 752 | **Loganberries** raw | (0.06) | 0 | — | — | (0.24) | — |
| 753 | stewed without sugar | (0.05) | 0 | — | — | (0.20) | — |

Notes

[a] Raw guavas contain about 200 mg per 100 g; the value may range from 20 to 600 mg per 100 g.

[b] Limes contain 25 mg vitamin C per 100 g.

| No | Food | Description and number of samples | Edible matter, proportion of weight purchased | Water g | Sugars g | Starch g | Dietary fibre g | Total nitrogen g |
|---|---|---|---|---|---|---|---|---|
| 754 | **Loganberries** stewed with sugar | Fruit and juice | 1.19 | 77.3 | 13.4 | 0 | 5.2 | 0.14 |
| 755 | canned | Fruit and juice | 1.00 | 66.3 | 26.2 | 0 | 3.3 | 0.10 |
| 756 | **Lychees** raw | Flesh only; literature sources | 0.60 | 82.0 | 16.0 | 0 | (0.5) | 0.14 |
| 757 | canned | 10 cans ; fruit and syrup | 1.00 | 79.3 | 17.7 | 0 | 0.4 | 0.06 |
| 758 | **Mandarin oranges** canned | 10 cans; fruit and syrup | 1.00 | 84.3 | 14.2 | 0 | 0.3 | 0.10 |
| 759 | **Mangoes** raw | Flesh only; literature sources | 0.66 | 83.0 | 15.3 | Tr | (1.5) | 0.08 |
| 760 | canned | 10 cans; fruit and syrup | 1.00 | 74.8 | 20.2 | 0.1 | 1.0 | 0.05 |
| 761 | **Medlars** raw | Flesh only, no skin or stones | 0.81 | 74.5 | 10.6 | 0 | 10.2 | 0.08 |
| 762 | **Melons, Canteloupe** raw | Flesh only, no skin or seeds | 0.59 | 93.6 | 5.3 | 0 | 1.0 | 0.16 |
| 763 | raw (weighed with skin) | Calculated from the previous item | 0.59 | 58.6 | 3.3 | 0 | 0.6 | 0.10 |
| 764 | **yellow, Honeydew** raw | Flesh only, no skin or seeds | 0.59 | 94.2 | 5.0 | 0 | 0.9 | 0.10 |
| 765 | raw (weighed with skin) | Calculated from the previous item | 0.59 | 59.0 | 3.1 | 0 | 0.6 | 0.06 |
| 766 | **watermelon** raw | Flesh only; literature sources | 0.50 | 94.0 | 5.3 | 0 | — | 0.06 |
| 767 | raw (weighed with skin) | Calculted from the previous item | 0.50 | 47.0 | 2.7 | 0 | — | 0.03 |
| 768 | **Mulberries** raw | Whole fruit | 1.00 | 85.0 | 8.1 | 0 | 1.7 | 0.21 |
| 769 | **Nectarines** raw | Flesh and skin, no stones | 0.92 | 80.2 | 12.4 | 0 | 2.4 | 0.15 |
| 770 | raw (weighed with stones) | Calculated from the previous item | 0.92 | 74.0 | 11.4 | 0 | 2.2 | 0.14 |

| No | Food | Energy value kcal | Energy value kJ | Protein (N× 6.25) g | Fat g | Carbo-hydrate g | Na mg | K mg | Ca mg | Mg mg | P mg | Fe mg | Cu mg | Zn mg | S mg | Cl mg |
|---|---|---|---|---|---|---|---|---|---|---|---|---|---|---|---|---|
| 754 | **Loganberries** stewed with sugar | 54 | 230 | 0.9 | Tr | 13.4 | 3 | 220 | 29 | 21 | 20 | 1.2 | 0.12 | — | 15 | 13 |
| 755 | canned | 101 | 429 | 0.6 | Tr | 26.2 | 1 | 97 | 18 | 11 | 23 | 1.4 | 0.04 | — | 3 | 5 |
| 756 | **Lychees** raw | 64 | 271 | 0.9 | Tr | 16.0 | 3 | 170 | 8 | 10 | 35 | 0.5 | — | — | 19 | 3 |
| 757 | canned | 68 | 290 | 0.4 | Tr | 17.7 | 2 | 75 | 4 | 6 | 12 | 0.7 | 0.11 | 0.2 | — | (5) |
| 758 | **Mandarin oranges** canned | 56 | 237 | 0.6 | Tr | 14.2 | 9 | 88 | 18 | 9 | 12 | 0.4 | 0.05 | 0.4 | — | 2 |
| 759 | **Mangoes** raw | 59 | 253 | 0.5 | Tr | 15.3 | 7 | 190 | 10 | 18 | 13 | 0.5 | 0.12 | — | — | — |
| 760 | canned | 77 | 330 | 0.3 | Tr | 20.3 | 3 | 100 | 10 | 7 | 10 | 0.4 | 0.09 | 0.3 | — | (5) |
| 761 | **Medlars** raw | 42 | 178 | 0.5 | Tr | 10.6 | 6 | 250 | 30 | 11 | 28 | 0.5 | 0.17 | — | 17 | 3 |
| 762 | **Melons, Canteloupe** raw | 24 | 102 | 1.0 | Tr | 5.3 | 14 | 320 | 19 | 20 | 30 | 0.8 | 0.04 | 0.1 | 12 | 44 |
| 753 | raw (weighed with skin) | 15 | 63 | 0.6 | Tr | 3.3 | 9 | 200 | 12 | 13 | 19 | 0.5 | 0.03 | 0.1 | 7 | 27 |
| 764 | **yellow, Honeydew** raw | 21 | 90 | 0.6 | Tr | 5.0 | 20 | 220 | 14 | 13 | 9 | 0.2 | 0.04 | 0.1 | 6 | 45 |
| 765 | raw (weighed with skin) | 13 | 56 | 0.4 | Tr | 3.1 | 12 | 140 | 9 | 8 | 5 | 0.2 | 0.03 | 0.1 | 4 | 28 |
| 766 | **watermelon** raw | 21 | 92 | 0.4 | Tr | 5.3 | 4 | 120 | 5 | 11 | 8 | 0.3 | 0.03 | (0.1) | — | — |
| 767 | raw (weighed with skin) | 11 | 47 | 0.2 | Tr | 2.7 | 2 | 60 | 3 | 6 | 4 | 0.2 | 0.02 | (Tr) | — | — |
| 768 | **Mulberries** raw | 36 | 152 | 1.3 | Tr | 8.1 | 2 | 260 | 36 | 15 | 48 | 1.6 | 0.06 | — | 9 | 4 |
| 769 | **Nectarines** raw | 50 | 214 | 0.9 | Tr | 12.4 | 9 | 270 | 4 | 13 | 24 | 0.5 | 0.06 | 0.1 | 10 | 5 |
| 770 | raw (weighed with stones) | 46 | 198 | 0.9 | Tr | 11.4 | 8 | 250 | 4 | 12 | 22 | 0.4 | 0.06 | 0.1 | 9 | 4 |

| No | Food | Retinol µg | Carotene µg | Vitamin D µg | Thiamin mg | Riboflavin mg | Nicotinic acid mg | Potential nicotinic acid from tryptophan mg Trp ÷ 60 | Vitamin C mg | Vitamin E mg |
|---|---|---|---|---|---|---|---|---|---|---|
| 754 | **Loganberries** stewed with sugar | 0 | (70) | 0 | (0.02) | 0.03 | (0.3) | 0.1 | 26 | (0.3) |
| 755 | canned | 0 | (70) | 0 | (0.01) | 0.02 | (0.3) | 0.1 | 25 | — |
| 756 | **Lychees** raw | 0 | (Tr) | 0 | 0.04 | 0.04 | 0.3 | 0.1 | 40 | — |
| 757 | canned | 0 | (Tr) | 0 | (0.03) | (0.03) | (0.2) | 0.1 | 8 | — |
| 758 | **Mandarin oranges** canned | 0 | 50 | 0 | 0.07 | 0.02 | 0.2 | 0.1 | 14 | (Tr) |
| 759 | **Mangoes** raw | 0 | 1200[a] | 0 | 0.03 | 0.04 | 0.3 | 0.1 | 30 *(10–180)* | — |
| 760 | canned | 0 | (1200) | 0 | (0.02) | (0.03) | (0.2) | Tr | 10 | — |
| 761 | **Medlars** raw | 0 | — | 0 | — | — | — | 0.1 | 2 | — |
| 762 | **Melons, Canteloupe** raw | 0 | 2000[b] | 0 | 0.05 | 0.03 | 0.5 | Tr | 25 | 0.1 |
| 763 | raw (weighed with skin) | 0 | 1180[b] | 0 | 0.03 | 0.02 | 0.3 | Tr | 15 | 0.1 |
| 764 | **yellow, Honeydew** raw | 0 | 100[c] | 0 | 0.05 | 0.03 | 0.5 | Tr | 25 | 0.1 |
| 765 | raw (weighed with skin) | 0 | 60[c] | 0 | 0.03 | 0.02 | 0.3 | Tr | 15 | 0.1 |
| 766 | **watermelon** raw | 0 | 20 | 0 | 0.02 | 0.02 | 0.2 | 0.1 | 5 | (0.1) |
| 767 | raw (weighed with skin) | 0 | 10 | 0 | 0.01 | 0.01 | 0.1 | Tr | 3 | (Tr) |
| 768 | **Mulberries** raw | 0 | Tr | 0 | 0.05 | (0.04) | (0.4) | 0.2 | 10 | — |
| 769 | **Nectarines** raw | 0 | (500) | 0 | (0.02) | (0.05) | (1.0) | 0.1 | (8) | — |
| 770 | raw (weighed with stones) | 0 | (460) | 0 | (0.02) | (0.05) | (0.9) | 0.1 | (7) | — |

| No | Food | Vitamin $B_6$ mg | Vitamin $B_{12}$ µg | Folic acid Free µg | Folic acid Total µg | Pantothenic acid mg | Biotin µg |
|---|---|---|---|---|---|---|---|
| 754 | **Loganberries** stewed with sugar | (0.05) | 0 | — | — | (0.18) | — |
| 755 | canned | (0.04) | 0 | — | — | (0.17) | — |
| 756 | **Lychees** raw | — | 0 | — | — | — | — |
| 757 | canned | — | 0 | — | — | — | — |
| 758 | **Mandarin oranges** canned | 0.03 | 0 | 5 | 8 | (0.15) | (0.8) |
| 759 | **Mangoes** raw | — | 0 | — | — | 0.16 | — |
| 760 | canned | — | 0 | — | — | — | — |
| 761 | **Medlars** raw | — | 0 | — | — | — | — |
| 762 | **Melons, Canteloupe** raw | 0.07 | 0 | 30 | 30 | 0.23 | — |
| 763 | raw (weighed with skin) | 0.04 | 0 | 18 | 18 | 0.14 | — |
| 764 | **yellow, Honeydew** raw | 0.07 | 0 | (30) | (30) | 0.23 | — |
| 765 | raw (weighed with skin) | 0.04 | 0 | (18) | (18) | 0.14 | — |
| 766 | **watermelon** raw | (0.07) | 0 | 2 | 3 | 1.55 | — |
| 767 | raw (weighed with skin) | (0.04) | 0 | 1 | 2 | 0.78 | — |
| 768 | **Mulberries** raw | (0.05) | 0 | — | — | (0.25) | (0.4) |
| 769 | **Nectarines** raw | (0.02) | 0 | 5 | 5 | (0.15) | — |
| 770 | raw (weighed with stones) | (0.02) | 0 | 5 | 5 | (0.14) | — |

Notes

[a] Value for ripe, orange coloured mangoes. The carotene content varies according to the colour, and unripe, green mangoes contain about one-tenth of this amount.

[b] Value for orange coloured flesh.

[c] Value for green coloured flesh.

| No | Food | Description and number of samples | Edible matter, proportion of weight purchased | Water g | Sugars g | Starch g | Dietary fibre g | Total nitrogen g |
|---|---|---|---|---|---|---|---|---|
| 771 | **Olives** in brine | Bottled in brine; flesh and skin, no stones | 0.80 | 76.5 | Tr | 0 | 4.4 | 0.14 |
| 772 | in brine (weighed with stones) | Calculated from the previous item | 0.80 | 61.1 | Tr | 0 | 3.5 | 0.11 |
| 773 | **Oranges** raw | Flesh only, no peel or pips | 0.75 | 86.1 | 8.5 | 0 | 2.0 | 0.13 |
| 774 | raw (weighed with peel and pips) | Calculated from the previous item | 0.75 | 64.8 | 6.4 | 0 | 1.5 | 0.10 |
| 775 | juice, fresh | Strained juice from fresh oranges | 0.46 | 87.7 | 9.4 | 0 | 0 | 0.10 |
| 776 | **Passion fruit** raw | Granadilla; flesh and seeds, no skin | 0.42 | 73.3 | 6.2 | 0 | 15.9 | 0.44 |
| 777 | raw (weighed with skin) | Calculated from the previous item | 0.42 | 30.8 | 2.6 | 0 | 6.7 | 0.18 |
| 778 | **Paw paw** canned | Papaya; 10 cans, fruit and juice | 1.00 | 80.4 | 17.0 | 0 | 0.5 | 0.03 |
| 779 | **Peaches** fresh, raw | Flesh and skin, no stones | 0.87 | 86.2 | 9.1 | 0 | 1.4 | 0.10 |
| 780 | raw (weighed with stones) | Calculated from the previous item | 0.87 | 75.1 | 7.9 | 0 | 1.2 | 0.09 |
| 781 | dried, raw | Whole fruit | 1.00 | 15.5 | 53.0 | 0 | 14.3 | 0.55 |
| 782 | stewed without sugar | Fruit and juice | 2.70 | 68.7 | 19.6 | 0 | 5.3 | 0.20 |
| 783 | stewed with sugar | Fruit and juice | 2.81 | 66.0 | 23.3 | 0 | 5.1 | 0.20 |
| 784 | canned | Fruit and syrup | 1.00 | 74.3 | 22.9 | 0 | 1.0 | 0.06 |
| 785 | **Pears, eating** | Flesh only, no skin or core | 0.72 | 83.2 | 10.6 | 0 | 2.3 | 0.04 |
| 786 | eating (weighed with skin and core) | Calculated from the previous item | 0.72 | 59.9 | 7.6 | 0 | 1.7 | 0.03 |

| No | Food | Energy value kcal | Energy value kJ | Protein (N × 6.25) g | Fat g | Carbo-hydrate g | Na mg | K mg | Ca mg | Mg mg | P mg | Fe mg | Cu mg | Zn mg | S mg | Cl mg |
|---|---|---|---|---|---|---|---|---|---|---|---|---|---|---|---|---|
| 771 | **Olives** in brine | 103 | 422 | 0.9 | 11.0 | Tr | 2250 | 91 | 61 | 22 | 17 | 1.0 | 0.23 | — | 36 | 3750 |
| 772 | in brine (weighed with stones) | 82 | 338 | 0.7 | 8.8 | Tr | 1800 | 73 | 49 | 18 | 13 | 0.8 | 0.18 | — | 29 | 3000 |
| 773 | **Oranges** raw | 35 | 150 | 0.8 | Tr | 8.5 | 3 | 200 | 41 | 13 | 24 | 0.3 | 0.07 | 0.2 | 9 | 3 |
| 774 | raw (weighed with peel and pips) | 26 | 113 | 0.6 | Tr | 6.4 | 2 | 150 | 31 | 10 | 18 | 0.3 | 0.05 | 0.2 | 7 | 2 |
| 775 | juice, fresh | 38 | 161 | 0.6 | Tr | 9.4 | 2 | 180 | 12 | 12 | 22 | 0.3 | 0.05 | 0.2 | 5 | 1 |
| 776 | **Passion fruit** raw | 34 | 147 | 2.8 | Tr | 6.2 | 28 | 350 | 16 | 39 | 54 | 1.1 | 0.12 | — | 19 | 37 |
| 777 | raw (weighed with skin) | 14 | 60 | 1.1 | Tr | 2.6 | 12 | 150 | 7 | 16 | 23 | 0.5 | 0.05 | — | 8 | 15 |
| 778 | **Paw paw** canned | 65 | 275 | 0.2 | Tr | 17.0 | 8 | 110 | 23 | 8 | 6 | 0.4 | 0.10 | 0.3 | — | 40 |
| 779 | **Peaches** fresh, raw | 37 | 156 | 0.6 | Tr | 9.1 | 3 | 260 | 5 | 8 | 19 | 0.4 | 0.05 | 0.1 | 6 | Tr |
| 780 | raw (weighed with stones) | 32 | 137 | 0.6 | Tr | 7.9 | 2 | 230 | 4 | 7 | 16 | 0.3 | 0.04 | 0.1 | 5 | Tr |
| 781 | dried, raw | 212 | 906 | 3.4 | Tr | 53.0 | 6 | 1100 | 36 | 54 | 120 | 6.8 | 0.63 | — | 240 | 11 |
| 782 | stewed without sugar | 79 | 336 | 1.3 | Tr | 19.6 | 2 | 410 | 13 | 20 | 44 | 2.5 | 0.23 | — | 89 | 4 |
| 783 | stewed with sugar | 93 | 395 | 1.3 | Tr | 23.3 | 2 | 390 | 13 | 19 | 43 | 2.4 | 0.22 | — | 85 | 4 |
| 784 | canned | 87 | 373 | 0.4 | Tr | 22.9 | 1 | 150 | 4 | 6 | 10 | 0.4 | 0.06 | — | 1 | 4 |
| 785 | **Pears, eating** | 41 | 175 | 0.3 | Tr | 10.6 | 2 | 130 | 8 | 7 | 10 | 0.2 | 0.15 | 0.1 | 5 | Tr |
| 786 | eating (weighed with skin and core) | 29 | 125 | 0.2 | Tr | 7.6 | 1 | 94 | 6 | 5 | 7 | 0.1 | 0.11 | 0.1 | 4 | Tr |

| No | Food | Retinol µg | Carotene µg | Vitamin D µg | Thiamin mg | Riboflavin mg | Nicotinic acid mg | Potential nicotinic acid from tryptophan mg Trp ÷ 60 | Vitamin C mg | Vitamin E mg |
|---|---|---|---|---|---|---|---|---|---|---|
| 771 | **Olives** in brine | 0 | 180[a] | 0 | Tr | Tr | (Tr) | 0.1 | 0 | — |
| 772 | in brine (weighed with stones) | 0 | 140 | 0 | Tr | Tr | (Tr) | 0.1 | 0 | — |
| 773 | **Oranges** raw | 0 | 50 | 0 | 0.10 | 0.03 | 0.2 | 0.1 | 50 *(40–60)* | 0.2 |
| 774 | raw (weighed with peel and pips) | 0 | 38 | 0 | 0.08 | 0.02 | 0.2 | 0.1 | 38 | 0.2 |
| 775 | juice, fresh | 0 | 50 | 0 | 0.08 | 0.02 | 0.2 | 0.1 | 50[b] *(40–60)* | Tr |
| 776 | **Passion fruit** raw | 0 | 10 | 0 | Tr | 0.10 | 1.5 | 0.4 | 20 | — |
| 777 | raw (weighed with skin) | 0 | 4 | 0 | Tr | 0.04 | 0.6 | 0.2 | 8 | — |
| 778 | **Paw paw** canned | 0 | (500) | 0 | 0.02 | 0.02 | 0.2 | Tr | 15 | — |
| 779 | **Peaches** fresh, raw | 0 | 500 *(250–1000)* | 0 | 0.02 | 0.05 | 1.0 | Tr | 8 | — |
| 780 | raw (weighed with stones) | 0 | 440 | 0 | 0.02 | 0.04 | 0.9 | Tr | 7 | — |
| 781 | dried, raw | 0 | 2000 *(1200–2600)* | 0 | Tr | 0.19 | 5.3 | 0.3 | Tr | — |
| 782 | stewed without sugar | 0 | 740 | 0 | Tr | 0.06 | 2.0 | 0.1 | Tr | — |
| 783 | stewed with sugar | 0 | 710 | 0 | Tr | 0.06 | 1.9 | 0.1 | Tr | — |
| 784 | canned | 0 | 250 | 0 | 0.01 | 0.02 | 0.6 | Tr | 4 | — |
| 785 | **Pears, eating** | 0 | 10 | 0 | 0.03 | 0.03 | 0.2 | Tr | 3 | Tr |
| 786 | eating (weighed with skin and core) | 0 | 7 | 0 | 0.02 | 0.02 | 0.1 | Tr | 2 | Tr |

| No | Food | Vitamin $B_6$ mg | Vitamin $B_{12}$ µg | Folic acid Free µg | Folic acid Total µg | Panto-thenic acid mg | Biotin µg |
|---|---|---|---|---|---|---|---|
| 771 | **Olives** in brine | 0.02 | 0 | — | — | 0.02 | (Tr) |
| 772 | in brine (weighed with stones) | 0.02 | 0 | — | — | 0.02 | (Tr) |
| 773 | **Oranges** raw | 0.06 | 0 | 30 | 37 | 0.25 | 1.0 |
| 774 | raw (weighed with peel and pips) | 0.05 | 0 | 23 | 28 | 0.18 | 0.8 |
| 775 | juice, fresh | 0.04 | 0 | 30 [b] | 37 [b] | 0.19 | 0.8 |
| 776 | **Passion fruit** raw | — | 0 | — | — | — | — |
| 777 | raw (weighed with skin) | — | 0 | — | — | — | — |
| 778 | **Paw paw** canned | — | 0 | — | — | (0.20) | — |
| 779 | **Peaches** fresh, raw | 0.02 | 0 | 2 | 3 | 0.15 | (0.2) |
| 780 | raw (weighed with stones) | 0.02 | 0 | 2 | 3 | 0.13 | (0.2) |
| 781 | dried, raw | 0.10 | 0 | (10) | (14) | (0.30) | — |
| 782 | stewed without sugar | 0.03 | 0 | Tr | (2) | (0.10) | — |
| 783 | stewed with sugar | 0.03 | 0 | Tr | (2) | (0.10) | — |
| 784 | canned | 0.02 | 0 | (2) | (3) | 0.05 | 0.2 |
| 785 | **Pears, eating** | 0.02 | 0 | 4 | 11 | 0.07 | 0.1 |
| 786 | eating (weighed with skin and core) | 0.01 | 0 | 3 | 8 | 0.05 | 0.1 |

Notes

[a] Value for green olives. Ripe, black olives contain 40µg per 100g.

[b] These values also apply to frozen reconstituted orange juice.

| No | Food | Description and number of samples | Edible matter, proportion of weight purchased | Water g | Sugars g | Starch g | Dietary fibre g | Total nitrogen g |
|---|---|---|---|---|---|---|---|---|
| 787 | **Pears, cooking** raw | Flesh only, no skin or core | 0.77 | 83.0 | 9.3 | Tr | 2.9 | 0.04 |
| 788 | stewed without sugar | Flesh and juice, peeled and cored before cooking | 0.96 | 85.5 | 7.9 | Tr | 2.5 | 0.03 |
| 789 | stewed with sugar | Flesh and juice, peeled and cored before cooking | 1.07 | 77.3 | 17.1 | Tr | 2.3 | 0.03 |
| 790 | canned | Fruit and syrup | 1.00 | 76.2 | 20.0 | 0 | 1.7 | 0.06 |
| 791 | **Pineapple** fresh | Flesh only, no skin or core | 0.53 | 84.3 | 11.6 | 0 | 1.2 | 0.08 |
| 792 | canned | Fruit and syrup | 1.00 | 77.1 | 20.2 | 0 | 0.9 | 0.04 |
| 793 | **Plums, Victoria dessert** raw | Flesh and skin, no stalks or stones | 0.94 | 84.1 | 9.6 | 0 | 2.1 | 0.09 |
| 794 | raw (weighed with stones) | Calculated from the previous item | 0.94 | 79.1 | 9.0 | 0 | 2.0 | 0.08 |
| 795 | **cooking** raw | Flesh and skin, no stalks or stones | 0.91 | 85.1 | 6.2 | 0 | 2.5 | 0.09 |
| 796 | raw (weighed with stones) | Calculated from the previous item | 0.91 | 77.5 | 5.6 | 0 | 2.3 | 0.08 |
| 797 | stewed without sugar | Fruit and juice, no stones | 1.09 | 86.3 | 5.2 | 0 | 2.2 | 0.08 |
| 798 | stewed without sugar (weighed with stones) | Calculated from the previous item | 1.09 | 80.3 | 4.8 | 0 | 2.0 | 0.07 |
| 799 | stewed with sugar | Fruit and juice, no stones | 1.20 | 77.7 | 15.1 | 0 | 1.9 | 0.06 |
| 800 | stewed with sugar (weighed with stones) | Calculated from the previous item | 1.20 | 73.0 | 14.2 | 0 | 1.8 | 0.06 |
| 801 | **Pomegranate** juice | Juice from fresh fruit | 0.56 | 85.4 | 11.6 | 0 | 0 | 0.03 |

| No | Food | Energy value kcal | Energy value kJ | Protein (N × 6.25) g | Fat g | Carbo-hydrate g | Na mg | K mg | Ca mg | Mg mg | P mg | Fe mg | Cu mg | Zn mg | S mg | Cl mg |
|---|---|---|---|---|---|---|---|---|---|---|---|---|---|---|---|---|
| 787 | **Pears, cooking** | 36 | 154 | 0.3 | Tr | 9.3 | 3 | 100 | 7 | 4 | 15 | 0.2 | 0.11 | 0.1 | 3 | 2 |
| 788 | stewed without sugar | 30 | 130 | 0.2 | Tr | 7.9 | 3 | 85 | 6 | 3 | 13 | 0.2 | 0.09 | 0.1 | 3 | 2 |
| 789 | stewed with sugar | 65 | 277 | 0.2 | Tr | 17.1 | 2 | 78 | 5 | 3 | 12 | 0.2 | 0.09 | 0.1 | 2 | 2 |
| 790 | canned | 77 | 327 | 0.4 | Tr | 20.0 | 1 | 90 | 5 | 6 | 5 | 0.3 | 0.04 | — | 1 | 3 |
| 791 | **Pineapple** fresh | 46 | 194 | 0.5 | Tr | 11.6 | 2 | 250 | 12 | 17 | 8 | 0.4 | 0.08 | 0.1 | 3 | 29 |
| 792 | canned | 77 | 328 | 0.3 | Tr | 20.2 | 1 | 94 | 13 | 8 | 5 | 0.4 | 0.05 | — | 3 | 4 |
| 793 | **Plums, Victoria dessert** raw | 38 | 164 | 0.6 | Tr | 9.6 | 2 | 190 | 11 | 7 | 16 | 0.4 | 0.10 | Tr | 4 | Tr |
| 794 | raw (weighed with stones) | 36 | 153 | 0.5 | Tr | 9.0 | 2 | 180 | 10 | 7 | 15 | 0.3 | 0.09 | Tr | 3 | Tr |
| 795 | **cooking** raw | 26 | 109 | 0.6 | Tr | 6.2 | 2 | 200 | 14 | 8 | 15 | 0.3 | 0.09 | Tr | 5 | Tr |
| 796 | raw (weighed with stones) | 23 | 98 | 0.5 | Tr | 5.6 | 2 | 180 | 13 | 7 | 13 | 0.3 | 0.08 | Tr | 4 | Tr |
| 797 | stewed without sugar | 22 | 92 | 0.5 | Tr | 5.2 | 2 | 160 | 12 | 6 | 12 | 0.3 | 0.08 | Tr | 3 | Tr |
| 798 | stewed without sugar (weighed with stones) | 20 | 84 | 0.4 | Tr | 4.8 | 2 | 150 | 11 | 6 | 11 | 0.3 | 0.07 | Tr | 3 | Tr |
| 799 | stewed with sugar | 59 | 252 | 0.4 | Tr | 15.3 | 2 | 150 | 11 | 5 | 11 | 0.2 | 0.06 | Tr | 3 | Tr |
| 800 | stewed with sugar (weighed with stones) | 55 | 234 | 0.4 | Tr | 14.2 | 2 | 140 | 10 | 5 | 10 | 0.2 | 0.06 | Tr | 3 | Tr |
| 801 | **Pomegranate** juice | 44 | 189 | 0.2 | Tr | 11.6 | 1 | 200 | 3 | 3 | 8 | 0.2 | 0.07 | — | 4 | 53 |

| No | Food | Retinol µg | Carotene µg | Vitamin D µg | Thiamin mg | Riboflavin mg | Nicotinic acid mg | Potential nicotinic acid from tryptophan mg Trp ÷ 60 | Vitamin C mg | Vitamin E mg |
|---|---|---|---|---|---|---|---|---|---|---|
| 787 | **Pears, cooking** raw | 0 | 10 | 0 | 0.03 | 0.03 | 0.2 | Tr | 3 | Tr |
| 788 | stewed without sugar | 0 | 9 | 0 | 0.03 | 0.03 | 0.2 | Tr | 3 | Tr |
| 789 | stewed with sugar | 0 | 8 | 0 | 0.02 | 0.02 | 0.2 | Tr | 2 | Tr |
| 790 | canned | 0 | 10 | 0 | 0.01 | 0.01 | 0.2 | 0.1 | 1 | Tr |
| 791 | **Pineapple** fresh | 0 | 60 | 0 | 0.08 | 0.02 | 0.2 | 0.1 | 25 *(20–40)* | — |
| 792 | canned | 0 | 40 | 0 | 0.05 | 0.02 | 0.2 | Tr | 12 | — |
| 793 | **Plums, Victoria dessert** raw | 0 | 220 | 0 | 0.05 | 0.03 | 0.5 | 0.1 | 3 | (0.7) |
| 794 | raw (weighed with stones) | 0 | 210 | 0 | 0.05 | 0.03 | 0.5 | 0.1 | 3 | (0.7) |
| 795 | **cooking** raw | 0 | 220 | 0 | 0.05 | 0.03 | 0.5 | 0.1 | 3 | (0.7) |
| 796 | raw (weighed with stones) | 0 | 200 | 0 | 0.05 | 0.03 | 0.5 | 0.1 | 3 | (0.6) |
| 797 | stewed without sugar | 0 | 180 | 0 | 0.04 | 0.03 | 0.5 | 0.1 | 3 | (0.5) |
| 798 | stewed without sugar (weighed with stones) | 0 | 170 | 0 | 0.04 | 0.03 | 0.5 | 0.1 | 3 | (0.5) |
| 799 | stewed with sugar | 0 | 170 | 0 | 0.04 | 0.02 | 0.4 | 0.1 | 2 | (0.4) |
| 800 | stewed with sugar (weighed with stones) | 0 | 160 | 0 | 0.04 | 0.02 | 0.4 | 0.1 | 2 | (0.4) |
| 801 | **Pomegranate** juice | 0 | 0 | 0 | 0.02 | 0.03 | 0.2 | Tr | 8 | — |

| No | Food | Vitamin $B_6$ mg | Vitamin $B_{12}$ µg | Folic acid Free µg | Folic acid Total µg | Pantothenic acid mg | Biotin µg | Notes |
|---|---|---|---|---|---|---|---|---|
| 787 | **Pears, cooking** raw | 0.02 | 0 | 4 | 11 | 0.07 | 0.1 | |
| 788 | stewed without sugar | 0.02 | 0 | Tr | 5 | 0.05 | 0.1 | |
| 789 | stewed with sugar | 0.02 | 0 | Tr | 5 | 0.05 | 0.1 | |
| 790 | canned | 0.01 | 0 | Tr | (5) | 0.02 | Tr | |
| 791 | **Pineapple** fresh | 0.09 | 0 | 9 | 11 | 0.16 | Tr | |
| 792 | canned | 0.07 | 0 | 2 | — | 0.10 | Tr | |
| 793 | **Plums, Victoria dessert** raw | 0.05 | 0 | 1 | 3 | 0.15 | Tr | |
| 794 | raw (weighed with stones) | 0.05 | 0 | 1 | 3 | 0.14 | Tr | |
| 795 | **cooking** raw | 0.05 | 0 | 1 | 3 | 0.15 | Tr | |
| 796 | raw (weighed with stones) | 0.05 | 0 | 1 | 3 | 0.14 | Tr | |
| 797 | stewed without sugar | 0.03 | 0 | Tr | 1 | 0.12 | Tr | |
| 798 | stewed without sugar (weighed with stones) | 0.03 | 0 | Tr | 1 | 0.11 | Tr | |
| 799 | stewed with sugar | 0.03 | 0 | Tr | 1 | 0.11 | Tr | |
| 800 | stewed with sugar (weighed with stones) | 0.03 | 0 | Tr | 1 | 0.10 | Tr | |
| 801 | **Pomegranate** juice | — | 0 | — | — | — | — | |

| No | Food | Description and number of samples | Edible matter, proportion of weight purchased | Water g | Sugars g | Starch g | Dietary fibre g | Total nitrogen g |
|---|---|---|---|---|---|---|---|---|
| 802 | **Prunes** dried, raw | Flesh and skin, no stones | 0.83 | 23.3 | 40.3 | 0 | 16.1 | 0.39 |
| 803 | raw (weighed with stones) | Calculated from the previous item | 0.83 | 19.3 | 33.5 | 0 | 13.4 | 0.32 |
| 804 | stewed without sugar | Fruit and juice, no stones | 1.65 | 60.5 | 20.4 | 0 | 8.1 | 0.20 |
| 805 | stewed without sugar (weighed with stones) | Calculated from the previous item | 1.65 | 55.1 | 18.6 | 0 | 7.4 | 0.18 |
| 806 | stewed with sugar | Fruit and juice, no stones | 1.76 | 57.1 | 26.5 | 0 | 7.7 | 0.19 |
| 807 | stewed with sugar (weighed with stones) | Calculated from the previous item | 1.76 | 52.0 | 24.1 | 0 | 7.0 | 0.17 |
| 808 | **Quinces** raw | Flesh only, no skin or core | 0.69 | 84.2 | 6.3 | Tr | 6.4 | 0.05 |
| 809 | **Raisins** dried | Flesh and skin, no stones | 0.92 | 21.5 | 64.4 | 0 | 6.8 | 0.17 |
| 810 | **Raspberries** raw | Whole fruit | 1.00 | 83.2 | 5.6 | 0 | 7.4 | 0.14 |
| 811 | stewed without sugar | Fruit and juice | 0.95 | 82.2 | 5.9 | 0 | 7.8 | 0.15 |
| 812 | stewed with sugar | Fruit and juice | 1.05 | 72.6 | 17.3 | 0 | 7.0 | 0.13 |
| 813 | canned | Fruit and syrup | 1.00 | 74.0 | 22.5 | 0 | (5.0) | 0.10 |
| 814 | **Rhubarb** raw | Stems only | 0.67 | 94.2 | 1.0 | 0 | 2.6 | 0.10 |
| 815 | stewed without sugar | Stems and juice | 0.78 | 94.6 | 0.9 | 0 | 2.4 | 0.09 |
| 816 | stewed with sugar | Stems and juice | 0.94 | 85.0 | 11.4 | 0 | 2.2 | 0.08 |
| 817 | **Strawberries** raw | Flesh and pips, no stalks | 0.97 | 88.9 | 6.2 | 0 | 2.2 | 0.10 |
| 818 | canned | 10 cans; fruit and syrup | 1.00 | 79.4 | 21.1 | 0 | 1.0 | 0.07 |
| 819 | **Sultanas** dried | Whole fruit | 1.00 | 18.3 | 64.7 | 0 | 7.0 | 0.28 |
| 820 | **Tangerines** raw | Flesh only, no peel or pips | 0.70 | 86.7 | 8.0 | 0 | 1.9 | 0.14 |
| 821 | raw (weighed with peel and pips) | Calculated from the previous item | 0.70 | 60.6 | 5.6 | 0 | 1.3 | 0.10 |

| No | Food | Energy value kcal | Energy value kJ | Protein (N × 6.25) g | Fat g | Carbo-hydrate g | Na mg | K mg | Ca mg | Mg mg | P mg | Fe mg | Cu mg | Zn mg | S mg | Cl mg |
|---|---|---|---|---|---|---|---|---|---|---|---|---|---|---|---|---|
| 802 | **Prunes** dried, raw | 161 | 686 | 2.4 | Tr | 40.3 | 12 | 860 | 38 | 27 | 83 | 2.9 | 0.16 | — | 19 | 3 |
| 803 | raw (weighed with stones) | 134 | 570 | 2.0 | Tr | 33.5 | 10 | 720 | 31 | 22 | 69 | 2.4 | 0.13 | — | 15 | 2 |
| 804 | stewed without sugar | 82 | 349 | 1.3 | Tr | 20.4 | 7 | 440 | 19 | 13 | 42 | 1.4 | 0.08 | — | 9 | 1 |
| 805 | stewed without sugar (weighed with stones) | 74 | 316 | 1.1 | Tr | 18.6 | 6 | 400 | 17 | 12 | 38 | 1.3 | 0.07 | — | 8 | 1 |
| 806 | stewed with sugar | 104 | 444 | 1.2 | Tr | 26.5 | 5 | 420 | 18 | 13 | 40 | 1.4 | 0.08 | — | 9 | 1 |
| 807 | stewed with sugar (weighed with stones) | 95 | 404 | 1.1 | Tr | 24.1 | 5 | 380 | 16 | 12 | 36 | 1.3 | 0.07 | — | 8 | 1 |
| 808 | **Quinces** raw | 25 | 106 | 0.3 | Tr | 6.3 | 3 | 200 | 14 | 6 | 19 | 0.3 | 0.13 | — | 5 | 2 |
| 809 | **Raisins** dried | 246 | 1049 | 1.1 | Tr | 64.4 | 52 | 860 | 61 | 42 | 33 | 1.6 | 0.24 | 0.1 | 23 | 9 |
| 810 | **Raspberries** raw | 25 | 105 | 0.9 | Tr | 5.6 | 3 | 220 | 41 | 22 | 29 | 1.2 | 0.21 | — | 17 | 22 |
| 811 | stewed without sugar | 26 | 110 | 0.9 | Tr | 5.9 | 3 | 230 | 43 | 23 | 31 | 1.3 | 0.22 | — | 18 | 23 |
| 812 | stewed with sugar | 68 | 290 | 0.8 | Tr | 17.3 | 3 | 210 | 39 | 21 | 28 | 1.1 | 0.20 | — | 16 | 21 |
| 813 | canned | 87 | 370 | 0.6 | Tr | 22.5 | 4 | 100 | 14 | 11 | 14 | 1.7 | 0.10 | — | — | 5 |
| 814 | **Rhubarb** raw | 6 | 26 | 0.6 | Tr | 1.0 | 2 | 430 | 100 | 14 | 21 | 0.4 | 0.13 | — | 8 | 87 |
| 815 | stewed without sugar | 6 | 25 | 0.6 | Tr | 0.9 | 2 | 400 | 93 | 13 | 19 | 0.4 | 0.12 | — | 7 | 81 |
| 816 | stewed with sugar | 45 | 191 | 0.5 | Tr | 11.4 | 2 | 360 | 84 | 12 | 18 | 0.3 | 0.11 | — | 7 | 73 |
| 817 | **Strawberries** raw | 26 | 109 | 0.6 | Tr | 6.2 | 2 | 160 | 22 | 12 | 23 | 0.7 | 0.13 | 0.1 | 13 | 18 |
| 818 | canned | 81 | 344 | 0.4 | Tr | 21.1 | 7 | 97 | 14 | 7 | 15 | 0.9 | (0.03) | 0.2 | — | (5) |
| 819 | **Sultanas** dried | 250 | 1066 | 1.8 | Tr | 64.7 | 53 | 860 | 52 | 35 | 95 | 1.8 | 0.35 | (0.1) | 44 | 16 |
| 820 | **Tangerines** raw | 34 | 143 | 0.9 | Tr | 8.0 | 2 | 160 | 42 | 11 | 17 | 0.3 | 0.09 | 0.1 | 10 | 2 |
| 821 | raw (weighed with peel and pips) | 23 | 100 | 0.6 | Tr | 5.6 | 2 | 110 | 29 | 8 | 12 | 0.2 | 0.06 | 0.1 | 7 | 2 |

| No | Food | Retinol µg | Carotene µg | Vitamin D µg | Thiamin mg | Riboflavin mg | Nicotinic acid mg | Potential nicotinic acid from tryptophan mg Trp ÷ 60 | Vitamin C mg | Vitamin E mg |
|---|---|---|---|---|---|---|---|---|---|---|
| 802 | **Prunes** dried, raw | 0 | 1000 | 0 | 0.10 | 0.20 | 1.5 | 0.4 | Tr | — |
| 803 | raw (weighed with stones) | 0 | 830 | 0 | 0.08 | 0.17 | 1.2 | 0.3 | Tr | — |
| 804 | stewed without sugar | 0 | 510 | 0 | 0.04 | 0.09 | 0.8 | 0.2 | Tr | — |
| 805 | stewed without sugar (weighed with stones) | 0 | 460 | 0 | 0.04 | 0.08 | 0.7 | 0.2 | Tr | — |
| 806 | stewed with sugar | 0 | 470 | 0 | 0.04 | 0.09 | 0.7 | 0.2 | Tr | — |
| 807 | stewed with sugar (weighed with stones) | 0 | 430 | 0 | 0.04 | 0.08 | 0.6 | 0.2 | Tr | — |
| 808 | **Quinces** raw | 0 | Tr | 0 | 0.02 | 0.02 | 0.2 | Tr | 15 | — |
| 809 | **Raisins** dried | 0 | 30 | 0 | 0.10 | 0.08 | 0.5 | 0.1 | 0 | — |
| 810 | **Raspberries** raw | 0 | 80 | 0 | 0.02 | 0.03 | 0.4 | 0.1 | 25 [a] *(14–35)* | 0.3 [b] |
| 811 | stewed without sugar | 0 | 85 | 0 | 0.02 | 0.03 | 0.4 | 0.1 | 23 | 0.3 [b] |
| 812 | stewed with sugar | 0 | 75 | 0 | 0.02 | 0.03 | 0.4 | 0.1 | 22 | 0.3 [b] |
| 813 | canned | 0 | (75) | 0 | 0.01 | 0.03 | 0.3 | 0.1 | 7 | — |
| 814 | **Rhubarb** raw | 0 | 60 | 0 | 0.01 | 0.03 | 0.3 | 0.1 | 10 | 0.2 |
| 815 | stewed without sugar | 0 | 55 | 0 | Tr | 0.03 | 0.3 | 0.1 | 8 | 0.2 |
| 816 | stewed with sugar | 0 | 50 | 0 | Tr | 0.03 | 0.3 | 0.1 | 7 [c] | 0.2 |
| 817 | **Strawberries** raw | 0 | 30 | 0 | 0.02 | 0.03 | 0.4 | 0.1 | 60 [d] *(40–90)* | 0.2 |
| 818 | canned | 0 | (Tr) | 0 | 0.01 | (0.02) | (0.3) | 0.1 | 21 | — |
| 819 | **Sultanas** dried | 0 | 30 | 0 | 0.10 | (0.08) | (0.5) | 0.1 | 0 | 0.7 |
| 820 | **Tangerines** raw | 0 | 100 | 0 | 0.07 | 0.02 | 0.2 | 0.1 | 30 | — |
| 821 | raw (weighed with peel and pips) | 0 | 70 | 0 | 0.05 | 0.01 | 0.1 | 0.1 | 21 | — |

| No | Food | Vitamin $B_6$ mg | Vitamin $B_{12}$ µg | Folic acid Free µg | Folic acid Total µg | Pantothenic acid mg | Biotin µg |
|---|---|---|---|---|---|---|---|
| 802 | **Prunes** dried, raw | 0.24 | 0 | 1 | 4 | 0.46 | (Tr) |
| 803 | raw (weighed with stones) | 0.20 | 0 | 1 | 3 | 0.38 | (Tr) |
| 804 | stewed without sugar | 0.10 | 0 | Tr | Tr | 0.21 | (Tr) |
| 805 | stewed without sugar (weighed with stones) | 0.09 | 0 | Tr | Tr | 0.19 | (Tr) |
| 806 | stewed with sugar | 0.10 | 0 | Tr | Tr | 0.20 | (Tr) |
| 807 | stewed with sugar (weighed with stones) | 0.09 | 0 | Tr | Tr | 0.18 | (Tr) |
| 808 | **Quinces** raw | — | 0 | — | — | — | — |
| 809 | **Raisins** dried | 0.30 | 0 | 4 | 4 | 0.10 | — |
| 810 | **Raspberries** raw | 0.06 | 0 | — | — | 0.24 | 1.9 |
| 811 | stewed without sugar | 0.05 | 0 | — | — | 0.23 | 2.0 |
| 812 | stewed with sugar | 0.05 | 0 | — | — | 0.21 | 1.8 |
| 813 | canned | 0.04 | 0 | — | — | 0.17 | — |
| 814 | **Rhubarb** raw | 0.03 | 0 | 8 | 8 | 0.08 | — |
| 815 | stewed without sugar | 0.02 | 0 | 1 | 4 | 0.06 | — |
| 816 | stewed with sugar | 0.02 | 0 | 1 | 4 | 0.05 | — |
| 817 | **Strawberries** raw | 0.06 | 0 | 15 | 20 | 0.34 | 1.1 |
| 818 | canned | 0.03 | 0 | 8 | 20 | 0.21 | (1.0) |
| 819 | **Sultanas** dried | (0.30) | 0 | (4) | (4) | (0.10) | — |
| 820 | **Tangerines** raw | 0.07 | 0 | 19 | 21 | 0.20 | — |
| 821 | raw (weighed with peel and pips) | 0.05 | 0 | 13 | 15 | 0.14 | — |

Notes

[a] Frozen raspberries contain 20mg per 100g.

[b] Also contains 1.5mg $\gamma$-tocopherol and 2.7mg $\delta$-tocopherol per 100g.

[c] Canned rhubarb contains 1mg per 100g.

[d] Frozen strawberries contain 50mg per 100g.

| No | Food | Description and number of samples | Edible matter, proportion of weight purchased | Water g | Sugars g | Starch g | Dietary fibre g | Total nitrogen g |
|---|---|---|---|---|---|---|---|---|

| No | Food | Energy value | | Protein ($N \times 6.25$) | Fat | Carbo-hydrate | mg | | | | | | | | | |
|---|---|---|---|---|---|---|---|---|---|---|---|---|---|---|---|---|
| | | kcal | kJ | g | g | g | Na | K | Ca | Mg | P | Fe | Cu | Zn | S | Cl |

| No | Food | Retinol µg | Carotene µg | Vitamin D µg | Thiamin mg | Riboflavin mg | Nicotinic acid mg | Potential nicotinic acid from tryptophan mg Trp ÷60 | Vitamin C mg | Vitamin E mg |
|---|---|---|---|---|---|---|---|---|---|---|

| No | Food | Vitamin $B_6$ mg | Vitamin $B_{12}$ µg | Folic acid Free µg | Folic acid Total µg | Pantothenic acid mg | Biotin µg | Notes |
|---|---|---|---|---|---|---|---|---|

| No | Food | Description and number of samples | Edible matter, proportion of weight purchased | Water g | Sugars g | Starch g | Dietary fibre g | Total nitrogen g |
|---|---|---|---|---|---|---|---|---|
| 822 | **Almonds** | Kernel only, no shell | 0.37 | 4.7 | 4.3 | 0 | 14.3 | 3.27 |
| 823 | (weighed with shells) | Calculated from the previous item | 0.37 | 1.7 | 1.6 | 0 | 5.3 | 1.21 |
| 824 | **Barcelona nuts** | Kernel only, no shell | 0.62 | 5.7 | 3.4 | 1.8 | 10.3 | 2.06 |
| 825 | (weighed with shells) | Calculated from the previous item | 0.62 | 3.5 | 2.1 | 1.1 | 6.4 | 1.28 |
| 826 | **Brazil nuts** | Kernel only, no shell | 0.45 | 8.5 | 1.7 | 2.4 | 9.0 | 2.21 |
| 827 | (weighed with shells) | Calculated from the previous item | 0.45 | 3.8 | 0.8 | 1.1 | 4.1 | 0.99 |
| 828 | **Chestnuts** | Kernel only, no shell | 0.83 | 51.7 | 7.0 | 29.6 | 6.8 | 0.37 |
| 829 | (weighed with shells) | Calculated from the previous item | 0.83 | 42.8 | 5.8 | 24.6 | 5.7 | 0.31 |
| 830 | **Cob** or **hazel nuts** | Kernel only, no shell | 0.36 | 41.1 | 4.7 | 2.1 | 6.1 | 1.44 |
| 831 | (weighed with shells) | Calculated from the previous item | 0.36 | 14.8 | 1.7 | 0.8 | 2.2 | 0.52 |
| 832 | **Coconut** fresh | Kernel only, no shell | 0.70 | 42.0 | 3.7 | 0 | 13.6 | 0.61 |
| 833 | milk | Drained fluid from fresh coconut | 0.15 | 92.2 | 4.9 | 0 | (Tr) | 0.06 |
| 834 | desiccated | As purchased | 1.00 | 2.3 | 6.4 | 0 | 23.5 | 1.05 |
| 835 | **Peanuts** fresh | Kernel only, no shell | 0.69 | 4.5 | 3.1 | 5.5 | 8.1 | 4.50 |
| 836 | (weighed with shells) | Calculated from the previous item | 0.69 | 3.1 | 2.1 | 3.8 | 5.6 | 3.10 |
| 837 | roasted and salted | As purchased | 1.00 | 4.5 | 3.1 | 5.5 | 8.1 | 4.50 |
| 838 | **Peanut butter** smooth | 10 samples, 3 brands | 1.00 | 1.1 | 6.7 | 6.4 | 7.6 | 4.17 |
| 839 | **Walnuts** | Kernel only, no shell | 0.64 | 23.5 | 3.2 | 1.8 | 5.2 | 2.00 |
| 840 | (weighed with shells) | Calculated from the previous item | 0.64 | 15.0 | 2.0 | 1.2 | 3.3 | 1.28 |

| | | Energy value | | Protein (see p7) | Fat | Carbo-hydrate | mg | | | | | | | | | |
|---|---|---|---|---|---|---|---|---|---|---|---|---|---|---|---|---|
| No | Food | kcal | kJ | g | g | g | Na | K | Ca | Mg | P | Fe | Cu | Zn | S | Cl |
| 822 | **Almonds** | 565 | 2336 | 16.9 | 53.5 | 4.3 | 6 | 860 | 250 | 260 | 440 | 4.2 | 0.14 | 3.1 | 150 | 2 |
| 823 | (weighed with shells) | 210 | 865 | 6.3 | 19.8 | 1.6 | 2 | 320 | 92 | 95 | 160 | 1.6 | 0.05 | 1.1 | 54 | 1 |
| 824 | **Barcelona nuts** | 639 | 2637 | 10.9 | 64.0 | 5.2 | 3 | 940 | 170 | 200 | 300 | 3.0 | 0.96 | — | 180 | 34 |
| 825 | (weighed with shells) | 396 | 1632 | 6.8 | 39.6 | 3.2 | 2 | 580 | 110 | 130 | 190 | 1.8 | 0.60 | — | 110 | 21 |
| 826 | **Brazil nuts** | 619 | 2545 | 12.0 | 61.5 | 4.1 | 2 | 760 | 180 | 410 | 590 | 2.8 | 1.10 | 4.2 | 290 | 61 |
| 827 | (weighed with shells) | 277 | 1142 | 5.4 | 27.6 | 1.8 | 1 | 340 | 79 | 190 | 270 | 1.3 | 0.50 | 1.9 | 130 | 27 |
| 828 | **Chestnuts** | 170 | 720 | 2.0 | 2.7 | 36.6 | 11 | 500 | 46 | 33 | 74 | 0.9 | 0.23 | — | 29 | 15 |
| 829 | (weighed with shells) | 140 | 595 | 1.6 | 2.2 | 30.4 | 9 | 410 | 38 | 27 | 61 | 0.7 | 0.19 | — | 24 | 12 |
| 830 | **Cob** or **hazel nuts** | 380 | 1570 | 7.6 | 36.0 | 6.8 | 1 | 350 | 44 | 56 | 230 | 1.1 | 0.21 | 2.4 | 75 | 6 |
| 831 | (weighed with shells) | 137 | 567 | 2.8 | 13.0 | 2.4 | 1 | 120 | 16 | 20 | 82 | 0.4 | 0.08 | 0.9 | 27 | 2 |
| 832 | **Coconut** fresh | 351 | 1446 | 3.2 | 36.0 | 3.7 | 17 | 440 | 13 | 52 | 94 | 2.1 | 0.32 | 0.5 | 44 | 110 |
| 833 | milk | 21 | 91 | 0.3 | (0.2) | 4.9 | 110 | 310 | 29 | 30 | 37 | 0.1 | 0.04 | — | 24 | 180 |
| 834 | desiccated | 604 | 2492 | 5.6 | 62.0 | 6.4 | 28 | 750 | 22 | 90 | 160 | 3.6 | 0.55 | — | 76 | 200 |
| 835 | **Peanuts** fresh | 570 | 2364 | 24.3 | 49.0 | 8.6 | 6 | 680 | 61 | 180 | 370 | 2.0 | 0.27 | 3.0 | 380 | 7 |
| 836 | (weighed with shells) | 394 | 1631 | 16.8 | 33.8 | 5.9 | 4 | 470 | 42 | 130 | 250 | 1.4 | 0.19 | 2.1 | 260 | 5 |
| 837 | roasted and salted | 570 | 2364 | 24.3 | 49.0 | 8.6 | 440 | 680 | 61 | 180 | 370 | 2.0 | 0.27 | 3.0 | 380 | 660 |
| 838 | **Peanut butter** smooth | 623 | 2581 | 22.6 | 53.7 | 13.1 | 350 | 700 | 37 | 180 | 330 | 2.1 | 0.70 | 3.0 | — | 500 |
| 839 | **Walnuts** | 525 | 2166 | 10.6 | 51.5 | 5.0 | 3 | 690 | 61 | 130 | 510 | 2.4 | 0.31 | 3.0 | 100 | 23 |
| 840 | (weighed with shells) | 336 | 1388 | 6.8 | 33.0 | 3.2 | 2 | 440 | 39 | 84 | 330 | 1.5 | 0.20 | 1.9 | 67 | 15 |

| No | Food | Retinol µg | Carotene µg | Vitamin D µg | Thiamin mg | Riboflavin mg | Nicotinic acid mg | Potential nicotinic acid from tryptophan mgTrp ÷60 | Vitamin C mg | Vitamin E mg |
|---|---|---|---|---|---|---|---|---|---|---|
| 822 | **Almonds** | 0 | 0 | 0 | 0.24 [a] | 0.92 | 2.0 | 2.7 | Tr | 20.0 [b] |
| 823 | (weighed with shells) | 0 | 0 | 0 | 0.09 | 0.34 | 0.7 | 1.0 | Tr | 7.4 |
| 824 | **Barcelona nuts** | 0 | 0 | 0 | 0.11 | — | — | 3.1 | Tr | — |
| 825 | (weighed with shells) | 0 | 0 | 0 | 0.07 | — | — | 1.9 | Tr | — |
| 826 | **Brazil nuts** | 0 | 0 | 0 | 1.00 | 0.12 | 1.6 | 2.6 | Tr | 6.5 [b] |
| 827 | (weighed with shells) | 0 | 0 | 0 | 0.45 | 0.05 | 0.7 | 1.2 | Tr | 2.9 |
| 828 | **Chestnuts** | 0 | 0 | 0 | 0.20 | 0.22 | 0.2 | 0.4 | Tr | 0.5 [b] |
| 829 | (weighed with shells) | 0 | 0 | 0 | 0.17 | 0.18 | 0.2 | 0.4 | Tr | 0.4 |
| 830 | **Cob** or **hazel nuts** | 0 | 0 | 0 | 0.40 | — | 0.9 | 2.2 | Tr | 21.0 [b] |
| 831 | (weighed with shells) | 0 | 0 | 0 | 0.14 | — | 0.3 | 0.8 | Tr | 7.6 |
| 832 | **Coconut**, fresh | 0 | 0 | 0 | 0.03 | 0.02 | 0.3 | 0.7 | 2 | 0.7 [b] |
| 833 | milk | 0 | 0 | 0 | Tr | Tr | 0.1 | 0.1 | 2 | Tr |
| 834 | desiccated | 0 | 0 | 0 | 0.06 | 0.04 | 0.6 | 1.2 | 0 | — |
| 835 | **Peanuts** fresh | 0 | 0 | 0 | 0.90 | 0.10 | 16 | 5.3 | Tr | 8.1 [b] |
| 836 | (weighed with shells) | 0 | 0 | 0 | 0.62 | 0.07 | 11 | 3.6 | Tr | 5.6 |
| 837 | roasted and salted | 0 | 0 | 0 | 0.23 | 0.10 | 16 | 5.3 | Tr | (8.1) [b] |
| 838 | **Peanut butter** smooth | 0 | 0 | 0 | 0.17 | 0.10 | 15 | 4.9 | Tr | 4.7 [b] |
| 839 | **Walnuts** | 0 | 0 | 0 | 0.30 | 0.13 | 1.0 | 2.0 | Tr [c] | 0.8 [b] |
| 840 | (weighed with shells) | 0 | 0 | 0 | 0.19 | 0.08 | 0.6 | 1.3 | Tr | 0.5 |

| No | Food | Vitamin $B_6$ mg | Vitamin $B_{12}$ µg | Folic acid Free µg | Folic acid Total µg | Pantothenic acid mg | Biotin µg |
|---|---|---|---|---|---|---|---|
| 822 | **Almonds** | 0.10 | 0 | 33 | 96 | 0.47[a] | 0.4 |
| 823 | (weighed with shells) | 0.04 | 0 | 12 | 36 | 0.17 | 0.1 |
| 824 | **Barcelona nuts** | — | 0 | — | — | — | — |
| 825 | (weighed with shells) | — | 0 | — | — | — | — |
| 826 | **Brazil nuts** | 0.17 | 0 | — | — | 0.23 | — |
| 827 | (weighed with shells) | 0.08 | 0 | — | — | 0.10 | — |
| 828 | **Chestnuts** | 0.33 | 0 | — | — | 0.47 | 1.3 |
| 829 | (weighed with shells) | 0.27 | 0 | — | — | 0.39 | 1.1 |
| 830 | **Cob** or **hazel nuts** | 0.55 | 0 | 23 | 72 | 1.15 | — |
| 831 | (weighed with shells) | 0.20 | 0 | 8 | 26 | 0.41 | — |
| 832 | **Coconut** fresh | 0.04 | 0 | 9 | 26 | 0.20 | — |
| 833 | milk | 0.03 | 0 | — | — | 0.05 | — |
| 834 | desiccated | — | 0 | — | — | — | — |
| 835 | **Peanuts** fresh | (0.50) | 0 | 28 | 110 | 2.7 | — |
| 836 | (weighed with shells) | (0.35) | 0 | 19 | 76 | 1.9 | — |
| 837 | **Peanuts** roasted and salted | 0.40 | 0 | — | — | 2.1 | — |
| 838 | **Peanut butter** smooth | 0.50 | 0 | 16 | 53 | (2.1) | — |
| 839 | **Walnuts** | 0.73 | 0 | 48 | 66 | 0.90 | 2.0 |
| 840 | (weighed with shells) | 0.47 | 0 | 31 | 42 | 0.58 | 1.3 |

Notes

[a] The thiamin content is reduced to 0.05 mg per 100 g on roasting, and the pantothenic acid to 0.25 mg.

[b] Most nuts contain only γ-tocopherol in addition to α-tocopherol. Values for γ-tocopherol are:

| | γ-tocopherol mg/100 g |
|---|---|
| Almonds | 3.0 |
| Brazil nuts | 11.0 |
| Chestnuts | 7.0 |
| Cob nuts | 1.5 |
| Coconut, fresh | 0.3 |
| Peanuts | 8.8 |
| Peanut butter | 2.9 |
| Walnuts | 18.0 |

[c] Value for ripe walnuts. Unripe walnuts contain 1300–3000 mg per 100 g.

| No | Food | Description and number of samples | Water g | Sugars g | Starch and dextrins g | Dietary fibre g | Total nitrogen g |
|---|---|---|---|---|---|---|---|
| | ***Sugars*** | | | | | | |
| 841 | **Glucose** liquid, BP | 1 sample | 20.4 | 40.2 | 44.5 | 0 | Tr |
| 842 | **Sugar** Demerara | 5 samples | Tr | 104.5[a] | 0 | 0 | 0.08 |
| 843 | white | Granulated and loaf | Tr | 105.0[b] | 0 | 0 | Tr |
| 844 | **Syrup** golden | 3 samples of the same brand | 20.0 | 79.0 | 0 | 0 | 0.05 |
| 845 | **Treacle** black | 3 samples | 28.5 | 67.2 | 0 | 0 | 0.19 |
| | ***Preserves*** | | | | | | |
| 846 | **Cherries** glacé | 3 samples | — | 55.8 | 0 | — | 0.10 |
| 847 | **Honey** comb | 2 samples | 20.2 | 74.4 | 0 | — | 0.09 |
| 848 | in jars | 2 samples | 23.0 | 76.4 | 0 | — | 0.06 |
| 849 | **Jam** fruit with edible seeds | Blackberry, blackcurrant, gooseberry, raspberry, strawberry; 2 samples of each, different brands | 29.8 | 69.0 | 0 | 1.1 | 0.10 |
| 850 | stone fruit | Apricot, damson, greengage, plum; 2 samples of each, different brands | 29.6 | 69.3 | 0 | 1.0 | 0.06 |
| 851 | **Lemon curd** starch base | 10 jars, 4 brands | 30.1 | 40.4 | 22.3 | 0.2 | 0.09 |
| 852 | home made | Recipe p 344 | 42.1 | 41.3 | 0 | 0 | 0.53 |
| 853 | **Marmalade** | 4 brands | 28.0 | 69.5 | 0 | 0.7 | 0.01 |
| 854 | **Marzipan** almond paste | Recipe p 344 | 10.5 | 49.2 | 0 | 6.4 | 1.62 |
| 855 | **Mincemeat** | 10 samples of the same brand | 27.5 | 62.1 | Tr | 3.3 | 0.10 |

[a] 99.3 g per 100 g expressed as sucrose

[b] 99.9 g per 100 g expressed as sucrose

| No | Food | Energy value kcal | Energy value kJ | Protein (N × 6.25) g | Fat g | Carbo-hydrate g | Na mg | K mg | Ca mg | Mg mg | P mg | Fe mg | Cu mg | Zn mg | S mg | Cl mg |
|---|---|---|---|---|---|---|---|---|---|---|---|---|---|---|---|---|
| | ***Sugars*** | | | | | | | | | | | | | | | |
| 841 | **Glucose** liquid, BP | 318 | 1355 | Tr | 0 | 84.7 | 150 | 3 | 8 | 2 | 11 | 0.5 | 0.09 | — | — | 190 |
| 842 | **Sugar** Demerara | 394 | 1681 | 0.5 | 0 | 104.5[a] | 6 | 89 | 53 | 15 | 20 | 0.9 | 0.06 | — | 14 | 35 |
| 843 | white | 394 | 1680 | Tr | 0 | 105.0[b] | Tr | 2 | 2 | Tr | Tr | Tr | 0.02 | — | Tr | Tr |
| 844 | **Syrup** golden | 298 | 1269 | 0.3 | 0 | 79.0 | 270 | 240 | 26 | 10 | 20 | 1.5 | 0.09 | — | 54 | 42 |
| 845 | **Treacle** black | 257 | 1096 | 1.2 | 0 | 67.2 | 96 | 1470 | 500 | 140 | 31 | 9.2 | 0.43 | — | 69 | 820 |
| | ***Preserves*** | | | | | | | | | | | | | | | |
| 846 | **Cherries** glacé | 212 | 903 | 0.6 | 0 | 55.8 | 65 | 18 | 44 | 8 | 18 | 2.9 | 1.28 | — | 21 | 71 |
| 847 | **Honey** comb | 281 | 1201 | 0.6 | 4.6[c] | 74.4 | 7 | 35 | 8 | 2 | 32 | 0.2 | 0.04 | — | 1 | 26 |
| 848 | in jars | 288 | 1229 | 0.4 | Tr | 76.4 | 11 | 51 | 5 | 2 | 17 | 0.4 | 0.05 | — | 1 | 18 |
| 849 | **Jam** fruit with edible seeds | 261 | 1114 | 0.6 | 0 | 69.0 | 16 | 110 | 24 | 10 | 18 | 1.5 | 0.23 | — | 7 | 9 |
| 850 | stone fruit | 261 | 1116 | 0.4 | 0 | 69.3 | 12 | 100 | 12 | 5 | 18 | 1.0 | 0.12 | — | 3 | 4 |
| 851 | **Lemon curd** starch base | 283 | 1202 | 0.6 | 5.1 | 62.7 | 65 | 11 | 9 | 2 | 15 | 0.5 | (0.03) | 1.3 | — | 150 |
| 852 | home made | 290 | 1216 | 3.3 | 13.5 | 41.3 | 150 | 66 | 18 | 5 | 62 | 0.6 | 0.06 | 0.4 | 48 | 220 |
| 853 | **Marmalade** | 261 | 1114 | 0.1 | 0 | 69.5 | 18 | 44 | 35 | 4 | 13 | 0.6 | 0.12 | — | 2 | 7 |
| 854 | **Marzipan** almond paste | 443 | 1856 | 8.7 | 24.9 | 49.2 | 13 | 400 | 120 | 120 | 220 | 2.0 | 0.08 | 1.5 | 81 | 13 |
| 855 | **Mincemeat** | 235 | 1163 | 0.6 | 4.3 | 62.1 | 140 | 190 | 30 | 10 | 17 | 1.5 | 0.20 | 0.2 | — | 200 |

[a] 99.3g per 100g expressed as sucrose [b] 99.9g per 100g expressed as sucrose

[c] Waxy material, probably not available as fat; disregarded in calculating energy values

| No | Food | Retinol µg | Carotene µg | Vitamin D µg | Thiamin mg | Riboflavin mg | Nicotinic acid mg | Potential nicotinic acid from tryptophan mg Trp ÷ 60 | Vitamin C mg | Vitamin E mg |
|---|---|---|---|---|---|---|---|---|---|---|
| | ***Sugars*** | | | | | | | | | |
| 841 | **Glucose** liquid, BP | 0 | 0 | 0 | 0 | 0 | 0 | 0 | 0 | 0 |
| 842 | **Sugar** Demerara | 0 | 0 | 0 | Tr | Tr | Tr | Tr | 0 | 0 |
| 843 | white | 0 | 0 | 0 | 0 | 0 | 0 | 0 | 0 | 0 |
| 844 | **Syrup** golden | 0 | 0 | 0 | Tr | Tr | Tr | Tr | 0 | 0 |
| 845 | **Treacle** black | 0 | 0 | 0 | Tr | Tr | Tr | Tr | 0 | 0 |
| | ***Preserves*** | | | | | | | | | |
| 846 | **Cherries** glacé | 0 | — | 0 | Tr | Tr | Tr | Tr | Tr | Tr |
| 847 | **Honey** comb | 0 | 0 | 0 | Tr | 0.05 | 0.2 | Tr | Tr | — |
| 848 | in jars | 0 | 0 | 0 | Tr | 0.05 | 0.2 | Tr | Tr | — |
| 849 | **Jam** fruit with edible seeds | 0 | Tr | 0 | Tr | Tr | Tr | Tr | 10[a] | Tr |
| 850 | stone fruit | 0 | Tr | 0 | Tr | Tr | Tr | Tr | Tr | Tr |
| 851 | **Lemon curd** starch base | (10) | 0 | (0.10) | Tr | (0.02) | Tr | 0.1 | (Tr) | — |
| 852 | home made | 130 | 60 | 0.55 | 0.02 | 0.12 | Tr | 1.0 | 8 | 0.4 |
| 853 | **Marmalade** | 0 | 50 | 0 | Tr | Tr | Tr | Tr | 10 | Tr |
| 854 | **Marzipan** almond paste | 10 | 0 | 0.13 | 0.12 | 0.45 | 0.9 | 1.5 | 2 | 9.1 |
| 855 | **Mincemeat** | 0 | (10) | 0 | (0.03) | (0.02) | (0.2) | 0.1 | Tr | — |

| No | Food | Vitamin $B_6$ mg | Vitamin $B_{12}$ µg | Folic acid Free µg | Folic acid Total µg | Panto-thenic acid mg | Biotin µg | Notes |
|---|---|---|---|---|---|---|---|---|
| | ***Sugars*** | | | | | | | |
| 841 | **Glucose** liquid, BP | 0 | 0 | 0 | 0 | 0 | 0 | |
| 842 | **Sugar** Demerara | Tr | 0 | Tr | Tr | Tr | Tr | |
| 843 | white | 0 | 0 | 0 | 0 | 0 | 0 | |
| 844 | **Syrup** golden | Tr | 0 | Tr | Tr | Tr | Tr | |
| 845 | **Treacle** black | Tr | 0 | Tr | Tr | Tr | Tr | |
| | ***Preserves*** | | | | | | | |
| 846 | **Cherries** glacé | Tr | 0 | Tr | Tr | Tr | Tr | |
| 847 | **Honey** comb | — | 0 | — | — | — | — | |
| 848 | in jars | — | 0 | — | — | — | — | |
| 849 | **Jam** fruit with edible seeds | Tr | 0 | Tr | Tr | Tr | Tr | |
| 850 | stone fruit | Tr | 0 | Tr | Tr | Tr | Tr | |
| 851 | **Lemon curd** starch base | Tr | Tr | Tr | Tr | (0.10) | 1 | |
| 852 | home made | 0.03 | Tr | 4 | 4 | 0.49 | 7 | |
| 853 | **Marmalade** | Tr | 0 | 5 | 5 | Tr | Tr | |
| 854 | **Marzipan** almond paste | 0.06 | Tr | 17 | 45 | 0.35 | 2 | |
| 855 | **Mincemeat** | (0.10) | 0 | (Tr) | (Tr) | 0.03 | (Tr) | |

[a] Blackcurrant jam contains 24mg per 100g.

| No | Food | Description and number of samples | Water g | Sugars g | Starch and dextrins g | Dietary fibre g | Total nitrogen g |
|---|---|---|---|---|---|---|---|
| 856 | **Boiled sweets** | 6 samples | — | 86.9 | 0.4 | 0 | 0.01 |
| | **Chocolate** | | | | | | |
| 857 | milk | 10 samples of the same brand | 2.2 | 56.5 | 2.9 | — | 1.35 |
| 858 | plain | 10 samples of the same brand | 0.6 | 59.5 | 5.3 | — | 0.75 |
| 859 | fancy and filled | 8 samples of different brands, mixed, milk and plain | 5.7 | 65.8 | 7.5 | — | 0.66 |
| 860 | Bounty Bar | 8 samples | 7.6 | 53.7 | 4.6 | — | 0.77 |
| 861 | Mars Bar | 8 samples | 6.9 | 65.8 | 0.7 | — | 0.84 |
| 862 | **Fruit gums** | 8 samples of the same brand | 12.0 | 42.6 | 2.2 | — | 0.16 |
| 863 | **Liquorice allsorts** | 6 samples | 6.6 | 67.2 | 6.9 | — | 0.63 |
| 864 | **Pastilles** | 6 samples of different brands | 10.2 | 61.9 | — | — | 0.84 |
| 865 | **Peppermints** | Several samples of 6 different brands | 0.2 | 102.2 | 0 | 0 | 0.08 |
| 866 | **Toffees** mixed | 8 samples of different brands | 4.8 | 70.1 | 1.0 | — | 0.34 |

| No | Food | Energy value kcal | Energy value kJ | Protein (N × 6.25) g | Fat g | Carbo-hydrate g | Na mg | K mg | Ca mg | Mg mg | P mg | Fe mg | Cu mg | Zn mg | S mg | Cl mg |
|---|---|---|---|---|---|---|---|---|---|---|---|---|---|---|---|---|
| 856 | **Boiled sweets** | 327 | 1397 | Tr | Tr | 87.3 | 25 | 8 | 5 | 2 | 12 | 0.4 | 0.09 | — | — | 68 |
| | **Chocolate** | | | | | | | | | | | | | | | |
| 857 | milk | 529 | 2214 | 8.4 | 30.3 | 59.4 | 120 | 420 | 220 | 55 | 240 | 1.6 | 0.30 | 0.2 | — | 270 |
| 858 | plain | 525 | 2197 | 4.7 | 29.2 | 64.8 | 11 | 300 | 38 | 100 | 140 | 2.4 | 0.70 | 0.2 | — | 100 |
| 859 | fancy and filled | 460 | 1938 | 4.1 | 18.8 | 73.3 | 60 | 240 | 92 | 51 | 120 | 1.8 | 0.45 | — | — | 180 |
| 860 | Bounty Bar | 473 | 1980 | 4.8 | 26.1 | 58.3 | 180 | 320 | 110 | 43 | 140 | 1.3 | 0.47 | — | — | 400 |
| 861 | Mars Bar | 441 | 1853 | 5.3 | 18.9 | 66.5 | 150 | 250 | 160 | 35 | 150 | 1.1 | 0.31 | — | — | 300 |
| 862 | **Fruit gums** | 172 | 734 | 1.0 | 0 | 44.8 | 64 | 360 | 360 | 110 | 4 | 4.2 | 1.43 | — | — | 160 |
| 863 | **Liquorice allsorts** | 313 | 1333 | 3.9 | 2.2 | 74.1 | 75 | 220 | 63 | 38 | 29 | 8.1 | 0.39 | — | — | 120 |
| 864 | **Pastilles** | 253 | 1079 | 5.2 | 0 | 61.9 | 77 | 40 | 40 | 12 | Tr | 1.4 | 0.32 | — | — | 120 |
| 865 | **Peppermints** | 392 | 1670 | 0.5 | 0.7 | 102.2 | 9 | Tr | 7 | 3 | Tr | 0.2 | 0.04 | — | — | 22 |
| 866 | **Toffees** mixed | 430 | 1810 | 2.1 | 17.2 | 71.1 | 320 | 210 | 95 | 25 | 64 | 1.5 | 0.40 | — | — | 480 |

| No | Food | Retinol µg | Carotene µg | Vitamin D µg | Thiamin mg | Riboflavin mg | Nicotinic acid mg | Potential nicotinic acid from tryptophan mgTrp ÷ 60 | Vitamin C mg | Vitamin E mg |
|---|---|---|---|---|---|---|---|---|---|---|
| 856 | **Boiled sweets** | 0 | 0 | 0 | 0 | 0 | 0 | 0 | 0 | 0 |
| | **Chocolate** | | | | | | | | | |
| 857 | milk | Tr | (40) | Tr | 0.10 | 0.23 | 0.2 | 1.4 | 0 | 0.5 [a] |
| 858 | plain | 0 | (40) | 0 | 0.07 | 0.08 | 0.4 | 0.8 | 0 | 0.5 [b] |
| 859 | fancy and filled | 0 | (40) | Tr | (0.10) | (0.10) | (0.3) | 0.7 | 0 | — |
| 860 | Bounty Bar | 0 | (40) | Tr | (0.04) | (0.10) | (0.3) | 0.8 | 0 | — |
| 861 | Mars Bar | 0 | (40) | Tr | (0.05) | (0.20) | (0.3) | 0.9 | 0 | — |
| 862 | **Fruit gums** | 0 | 0 | 0 | 0 | 0 | 0 | 0 | 0 | 0 |
| 863 | **Liquorice allsorts** | 0 | 0 | 0 | 0 | 0 | 0 | 0.7 | 0 | 0 |
| 864 | **Pastilles** | 0 | 0 | 0 | 0 | 0 | 0 | 0 | 0 | 0 |
| 865 | **Peppermints** | 0 | 0 | 0 | 0 | 0 | 0 | 0 | 0 | 0 |
| 866 | **Toffees** mixed | 0 | — | 0 | 0 | 0 | 0 | 0.4 | 0 | — |

| No | Food | Vitamin $B_6$ mg | Vitamin $B_{12}$ µg | Folic acid Free µg | Folic acid Total µg | Pantothenic acid mg | Biotin µg |
|---|---|---|---|---|---|---|---|
| 856 | **Boiled sweets** | 0 | 0 | 0 | 0 | 0 | 0 |
| | **Chocolate** | | | | | | |
| 857 | milk | (0.02) | Tr | (9) | (10) | (0.6) | (3) |
| 858 | plain | (0.02) | 0 | (9) | (10) | (0.6) | (3) |
| 859 | fancy and filled | (0.02) | Tr | (9) | (10) | (0.6) | (3) |
| 860 | Bounty Bar | (0.02) | Tr | — | — | (0.6) | (3) |
| 861 | Mars Bar | (0.02) | Tr | — | — | (0.6) | (3) |
| 862 | **Fruit gums** | 0 | 0 | 0 | 0 | 0 | 0 |
| 863 | **Liquorice allsorts** | 0 | 0 | 0 | 0 | 0 | 0 |
| 864 | **Pastilles** | 0 | 0 | 0 | 0 | 0 | 0 |
| 865 | **Peppermints** | 0 | 0 | 0 | 0 | 0 | 0 |
| 866 | **Toffees** mixed | 0 | 0 | 0 | 0 | 0 | 0 |

Notes

[a] Also contains 2.4 mg γ-tocopherol per 100 g.

[b] Also contains 3.5 mg γ-tocopherol per 100 g.

| No | Food | Description and number of samples | Water g | Sugars g | Starch and dextrins g | Dietary fibre g | Total nitrogen g |
|---|---|---|---|---|---|---|---|
| 867 | **Bournvita** | 6 samples | 1.5 | 52.0 | 27.0 [a] | — | 1.39 |
| 868 | **Cocoa powder** | 10 samples, 2 brands | 3.4 | Tr | 11.5 | — [b] | 3.70 [c] |
| 869 | **Coffee and chicory essence** | 7 bottles of the same brand | 36.9 | 53.8 | 2.2 | — [b] | 0.33 [d] |
| 870 | **Coffee** ground, roasted | 5 samples | 4.1 | Tr | 28.5 | — [b] | 2.04 [e] |
| 871 | infusion, 5 minutes | 60g coffee from mixed sample; boiled in percolater with 900ml water and strained | — | Tr | 0.3 | — | 0.04 |
| 872 | instant | 10 jars, 2 brands | 3.4 | 6.5 | 4.5 [a] | — [b] | 3.26 [f] |
| 873 | **Drinking chocolate** | 10 tins, 3 brands | 2.1 | 73.8 | 3.6 | — [b] | 1.04 [g] |
| 874 | **Horlicks malted milk** | Mixed sample | 2.5 | 49.4 | 23.5 [a] | — | 2.21 |
| 875 | **Ovaltine** | Mixed sample | 2.3 | 73.0 | 8.2 [a] | — | 1.57 |
| 876 | **Tea** Indian | 5 samples | 9.3 | (3.0) | Tr | — | 4.08 [h] |
| 877 | Indian, infusion | 10g from mixed sample; infused with 1000ml boiling water 2–10 minutes and strained | — | Tr | 0 | — | Tr |

[a] Dextrins only
[b] Complex polysaccharides, which are probably unavailable, are present in these foods
[c] Includes 0.74g purine nitrogen
[d] Includes 0.08g purine nitrogen
[e] Includes 0.38g purine nitrogen
[f] Includes 0.93g purine nitrogen
[g] Includes 0.16g purine nitrogen
[h] Includes 0.95g purine nitrogen

| No | Food | Energy value kcal | Energy value kJ | Protein (N × 6.25) g | Fat g | Carbo-hydrate g | Na mg | K mg | Ca mg | Mg mg | P mg | Fe mg | Cu mg | Zn mg | S mg | Cl mg |
|---|---|---|---|---|---|---|---|---|---|---|---|---|---|---|---|---|
| 867 | **Bournvita** | 377 | 1601 | 8.7 | 5.1 | 79.0 | 460 | 380 | 93 | 110 | 350 | 1.9 | 0.5 | 1.1 | — | — |
| 868 | **Cocoa powder** | 312 | 1301 | 18.5 [a] | 21.7 | 11.5 | 950 | 1500 | 130 | 520 | 660 | 10.5 | 3.9 | 6.9 | — | 460 |
| 869 | **Coffee and chicory essence** | 218 | 931 | 1.6 [a] | 0.2 | 56.0 | 65 | 750 | 30 | 39 | 90 | 0.7 | 0.6 | — | — | 85 |
| 870 | **Coffee** ground, roasted | 287 | 1203 | 10.4 [a] | 15.4 | 28.5 | 74 | 2020 | 130 | 240 | 160 | 4.1 | 0.82 | — | 110 | 24 |
| 871 | infusion, 5 minutes | 2 | 8 | 0.2 | Tr | 0.3 | Tr | 66 | 2 | 6 | 2 | Tr | Tr | — | — | Tr |
| 872 | instant | 100 | 424 | 14.6 [a] | 0 | 11.0 | 41 | 4000 | 160 | 390 | 350 | 4.4 | 0.05 | 0.5 | — | 50 |
| 873 | **Drinking chocolate** | 366 | 1554 | 5.5 [a] | 6.0 | 77.4 | 250 | 410 | 33 | 150 | 190 | 2.4 | 1.1 | 1.9 | — | 130 |
| 874 | **Horlicks malted milk** | 396 | 1679 | 13.8 | 7.5 | 72.9 | 350 | 750 | 230 | 46 | 300 | 1.8 | 0.8 | — | 68 | 610 |
| 875 | **Ovaltine** | 378 | 1606 | 9.8 | 3.8 | 81.2 | 150 | 850 | 36 | 150 | 400 | 2.6 | 1.2 | — | — | — |
| 876 | **Tea** Indian | 108 | 455 | 19.6 [a] | (2.0) | (3.0) | 45 | 2160 | 430 | 250 | 630 | 15.2 | 1.6 | (3.0) | 180 | 52 |
| 877 | Indian, infusion | <1 | 2 | 0.1 | Tr | Tr | Tr | 17 | Tr | 1 | 1 | Tr | Tr | Tr | — | Tr |

[a] (Total N − purine N) × 6.25

| No | Food | Retinol µg | Carotene µg | Vitamin D µg | Thiamin mg | Riboflavin mg | Nicotinic acid mg | Potential nicotinic acid from tryptophan mg Trp ÷ 60 | Vitamin C mg | Vitamin E mg |
|---|---|---|---|---|---|---|---|---|---|---|
| 867 | **Bournvita** | 0 | 0 | 0 | — | — | — | 1.9 | 0 | — |
| 868 | **Cocoa powder** | 0 | (40) | 0 | 0.16 | 0.06 | 1.7 | 5.6 | 0 | 0.4 [a] |
| 869 | **Coffee and chicory essence** | 0 | — | 0 | 0 | 0.03 | 2.8 | — | 0 | — |
| 870 | **Coffee** ground, roasted | 0 | — | 0 | — | 0.20 | 10 [b] | — | 0 | — |
| 871 | infusion, 5 minutes | 0 | — | 0 | — | 0.01 | 0.7 | Tr | 0 | — |
| 872 | instant | 0 | — | 0 | 0 | 0.11 | 22 [c] | 2.9 | 0 | — |
| 873 | **Drinking chocolate** | 0 | — | 0 | 0.06 | 0.04 | 0.5 | 1.6 | 0 | 0.1 [d] |
| 874 | **Horlicks malted milk** | 465 | — | 1.55 | 0.84 | 1.06 | 11.2 | 2.9 | 0 | — |
| 875 | **Ovaltine** | — | — | (30.6) | (1.76) | — | — | 2.1 | — | — |
| 876 | **Tea** Indian | 0 | Tr | 0 | 0.14 | 1.2 | 7.5 | — | Tr | — |
| 877 | Indian, infusion | 0 | 0 | 0 | Tr | 0.01 | 0.1 | 0 | 0 | — |

| No | Food | Vitamin $B_6$ mg | Vitamin $B_{12}$ µg | Folic acid Free µg | Folic acid Total µg | Pantothenic acid mg | Biotin µg |
|---|---|---|---|---|---|---|---|
| 867 | **Bournvita** | — | 0 | — | — | — | — |
| 868 | **Cocoa powder** | 0.07 | 0 | 31 | 38 | — | — |
| 869 | **Coffee and chicory essence** | — | 0 | — | — | — | — |
| 870 | **Coffee** ground, roasted | — | 0 | — | — | — | — |
| 871 | infusion, 5 minutes | — | 0 | — | — | — | — |
| 872 | instant | 0.03 | 0 | — | — | 0.4 | — |
| 873 | **Drinking chocolate** | 0.02 | 0 | 9 | 10 | — | — |
| 874 | **Horlicks malted milk** | — | — | — | — | — | — |
| 875 | **Ovaltine** | — | — | — | — | — | — |
| 876 | **Tea** Indian | — | 0 | — | — | 1.3 | — |
| 877 | Indian, infusion | — | 0 | — | — | Tr | — |

Notes

[a] Also contains 2.8 mg γ-tocopherol per 100g.

[b] Increases during roasting of coffee beans; a dark roasted variety may contain 3 or 4 times as much.

[c] Can be as high as 39 mg per 100g. Decaffeinated instant coffee contains about the same amount.

[d] Also contains 0.8 mg γ-tocopherol per 100g.

| No | Food | Description and number of samples | Specific gravity | Water g | Sugars g | Starch and dextrins g | Dietary fibre g | Total nitrogen g |
|---|---|---|---|---|---|---|---|---|
| 878 | **Coca-cola** | 8 cans and 5 bottles | 1.039 | 89.8 | 10.5 | Tr | 0 | Tr |
| 879 | **Grapefruit juice** canned unsweetened | 10 cans, 7 brands | — | 89.8 | 7.9 | Tr | 0 | 0.05 |
| 880 | sweetened | 5 cans of different brands | — | 87.3 | 9.7 | Tr | 0 | 0.08 |
| 881 | **Lemonade** bottled | 7 bottles of the same brand | 1.015 | 94.6 | 5.6 | 0 | 0 | Tr |
| 882 | **Lime juice cordial** undiluted | 6 bottles of the same brand | 1.102 | 70.5 | 24.8 | Tr | 0 | 0.01 |
| 883 | **Lucozade** | Mixed sample | 1.074 | 81.7 | 9.0 | 9.0[a] | 0 | Tr |
| 884 | **Orange drink** undiluted | Mixed sample | 1.116 | 71.2 | 28.5 | 0 | 0 | Tr |
| 885 | **Orange juice** canned, unsweetened | 9 cans, 6 brands | — | 88.7 | 8.5 | Tr | 0 | 0.07 |
| 886 | sweetened | 5 cans, 4 brands | — | 85.8 | 12.8 | Tr | 0 | 0.11 |
| 887 | **Pineapple juice** canned | 6 cans of different brands | 1.054 | 86.1 | 13.4 | Tr | 0 | 0.05 |
| 888 | **Ribena** undiluted | Mixed sample | 1.283 | 39.8 | 60.9 | 0 | 0 | 0.02 |
| 889 | **Rosehip syrup** undiluted | 9 bottles, 4 brands | — | 32.5 | 61.8 | 0.1 | 0 | — |
| 890 | **Tomato juice** canned | 10 cans, 6 brands | — | 93.3 | 3.2 | 0.2 | — | 0.12 |

[a] Dextrins only

| No | Food | Energy value kcal | Energy value kJ | Protein (N × 6.25) g | Fat g | Carbo-hydrate g | Na mg | K mg | Ca mg | Mg mg | P mg | Fe mg | Cu mg | Zn mg | S mg | Cl mg |
|---|---|---|---|---|---|---|---|---|---|---|---|---|---|---|---|---|
| 878 | **Coca-cola** | 39 | 168 | Tr | 0 | 10.5 | 8 | 1 | 4 | 1 | 15 | Tr | (0.03) | Tr | — | (10) |
| 879 | **Grapefruit juice** canned | | | | | | | | | | | | | | | |
| | unsweetened | 31 | 132 | 0.3 | Tr | 7.9 | 3 | 110 | 9 | 8 | 12 | 0.3 | (0.03) | 0.4 | — | (10) |
| 880 | sweetened | 38 | 164 | 0.5 | Tr | 9.7 | 2 | 110 | 9 | 9 | 12 | 0.3 | (0.03) | 0.3 | — | (10) |
| 881 | **Lemonade** bottled | 21 | 90 | Tr | 0 | 5.6 | 7 | 1 | 5 | Tr | Tr | Tr | 0.01 | — | — | Tr |
| 882 | **Lime juice cordial** undiluted | 112 | 479 | 0.1 | 0 | 29.8 | 8 | 49 | 9 | 4 | 5 | 0.3 | 0.07 | — | — | 4 |
| 883 | **Lucozade** | 68 | 288 | Tr | 0 | 18.0 | 29 | 1 | 5 | 1 | 4 | 0.1 | 0.04 | — | — | 35 |
| 884 | **Orange drink** undiluted | 107 | 456 | Tr | 0 | 28.5 | 21 | 17 | 8 | 3 | 2 | 0.1 | 0.01 | — | — | 4 |
| 885 | **Orange juice** canned | | | | | | | | | | | | | | | |
| | unsweetened | 33 | 143 | 0.4 | Tr | 8.5 | 4 | 130 | 9 | 9 | 15 | 0.5 | (0.03) | 0.3 | — | (10) |
| 886 | sweetened | 51 | 217 | 0.7 | Tr | 12.8 | 3 | 120 | 9 | 8 | 14 | 0.3 | (0.03) | 0.3 | — | (10) |
| 887 | **Pineapple juice** canned | 53 | 225 | 0.4 | 0.1 | 13.4 | 1 | 140 | 12 | 12 | 10 | 0.7 | 0.09 | — | — | 38 |
| 888 | **Ribena** undiluted | 229 | 976 | 0.1 | 0 | 60.9 | 20 | 86 | 9 | 5 | 10 | 0.5 | 0.02 | — | — | 7 |
| 889 | **Rosehip syrup** undiluted | 232 | 990 | (Tr) | 0 | 61.9 | 280 | 26 | — | — | — | — | — | — | — | — |
| 890 | **Tomato juice** canned | 16 | 66 | 0.7 | Tr | 3.4 | 230 | 260 | 10 | 10 | 20 | 0.5 | 0.05 | 0.4 | — | 370 |

| No | Food | Retinol µg | Carotene µg | Vitamin D µg | Thiamin mg | Riboflavin mg | Nicotinic acid mg | Potential nicotinic acid from tryptophan mg Trp ÷ 60 | Vitamin C mg | Vitamin E mg |
|---|---|---|---|---|---|---|---|---|---|---|
| 878 | **Coca-cola** | 0 | 0 | 0 | 0 | 0 | 0 | 0 | 0 | 0 |
| 879 | **Grapefruit juice** canned unsweetened | 0 | Tr | 0 | (0.04) | (0.01) | (0.2) | 0.1 | 28 | Tr |
| 880 | sweetened | 0 | Tr | 0 | (0.04) | (0.01) | (0.2) | 0.1 | 29 | Tr |
| 881 | **Lemonade** bottled | 0 | Tr | 0 | Tr | Tr | Tr | Tr | Tr [a] | Tr |
| 882 | **Lime juice cordial** undiluted | 0 | Tr | 0 | Tr | Tr | Tr | Tr | Tr | Tr |
| 883 | **Lucozade** | 0 | 0 | 0 | Tr | Tr | Tr | Tr | 3 | 0 |
| 884 | **Orange drink** undiluted | 0 | — | 0 | Tr | Tr | Tr | Tr | Tr [b] | Tr |
| 885 | **Orange juice** canned, unsweetened | 0 | (50) | 0 | (0.07) | (0.02) | (0.2) | 0.1 | 35 | Tr |
| 886 | sweetened | 0 | (50) | 0 | (0.07) | (0.02) | (0.2) | 0.1 | 31 | Tr |
| 887 | **Pineapple juice** canned | 0 | (40) | 0 | 0.05 | 0.02 | 0.2 | 0.1 | 8 | — |
| 888 | **Ribena** undiluted | 0 | — | 0 | — | — | — | Tr | 210 | — |
| 889 | **Rosehip syrup** undiluted | 0 | — | 0 | 0 | Tr | Tr | Tr | 295 | Tr |
| 890 | **Tomato juice** canned | 0 | (500) | 0 | (0.06) | (0.03) | (0.7) | 0.1 | 20 | (0.2) |

| No | Food | Vitamin $B_6$ mg | Vitamin $B_{12}$ µg | Folic acid Free µg | Folic acid Total µg | Panto-thenic acid mg | Biotin µg |
|---|---|---|---|---|---|---|---|
| 878 | **Coca-cola** | 0 | 0 | 0 | 0 | 0 | 0 |
| 879 | **Grapefruit juice** canned | | | | | | |
| | unsweetened | (0.01) | 0 | 4 | 6 | (0.12) | (1) |
| 880 | sweetened | (0.01) | 0 | 4 | 6 | (0.12) | (1) |
| 881 | **Lemonade** bottled | Tr | 0 | Tr | Tr | Tr | Tr |
| 882 | **Lime juice cordial** undiluted | Tr | 0 | Tr | Tr | Tr | Tr |
| 883 | **Lucozade** | Tr | 0 | Tr | Tr | Tr | Tr |
| 884 | **Orange drink** undiluted | Tr | 0 | Tr | Tr | Tr | Tr |
| 885 | **Orange juice** canned | | | | | | |
| | unsweetened | (0.04) | 0 | 7 | 7 | (0.15) | (1) |
| 886 | sweetened | (0.04) | 0 | 7 | 7 | (0.15) | (1) |
| 887 | **Pineapple juice** canned | 0.10 | 0 | 2 | — | 0.10 | — |
| 888 | **Ribena** undiluted | — | 0 | — | — | — | — |
| 889 | **Rosehip syrup** undiluted | Tr | 0 | Tr | Tr | Tr | Tr |
| 890 | **Tomato juice** canned | (0.11) | 0 | 4 | 13 | (0.20) | (1) |

Notes

[a] Vitamin C may be added to some brands, and the content may range from 5 to 15 mg per 100 g.

[b] Vitamin C is added to some brands, and the content may range from 20 to 60 mg per 100 g. There is a loss on storage of opened bottles, particularly when exposed to light.

| No | Food | Description and number of samples | Specific gravity | Alcohol g | Solids g | Sugars g | Total nitrogen g |
|---|---|---|---|---|---|---|---|
| | ***Beers*** | | | | | | |
| 891 | **Brown ale** bottled | 6 samples from different brewers | 1.008 | 2.2 | 4.2 | 3.0 | 0.04 |
| 892 | **Canned beer** bitter | 6 samples | 1.008 | 3.1 | 3.3 | 2.3 | 0.04 |
| 893 | **Draught** bitter | 5 samples from different brewers | 1.004 | 3.1 | 3.3 | 2.3 | 0.04 |
| 894 | mild | 5 samples from different brewers | 1.001 | 2.6 | 2.5 | 1.6 | 0.03 |
| 895 | **Keg** bitter | 6 samples from different brewers | 1.009 | 3.0 | 3.6 | 2.3 | 0.04 |
| 896 | **Lager** bottled | 6 samples | 1.005 | 3.2 | 2.4 | 1.5 | 0.03 |
| 897 | **Pale ale** bottled | 6 samples from diffeent brewers | 1.003 | 3.3 | 3.3 | 2.0 | 0.05 |
| 898 | **Stout** bottled | 4 samples from different brewers | 1.014 | 2.9 | 5.8 | 4.2 | 0.05 |
| 899 | **Stout** extra | 6 samples of the same brand | 1.002 | 4.3 | 3.6 | 2.1 | 0.05 |
| 900 | **Strong ale** | 6 samples from different brewers, barley wine type | 1.018 | 6.6 | 8.0 | 6.1 | 0.11 |
| | ***Ciders*** | | | | | | |
| 901 | **Cider** dry | 3 samples of different brands | 1.007 | 3.8 | 3.7 | 2.6 | Tr |
| 902 | sweet | 3 samples of different brands | 1.012 | 3.7 | 5.1 | 4.3 | Tr |
| 903 | vintage | 3 samples of the same brand | 1.017 | 10.5 | 8.9 | 7.3 | Tr |
| | ***Wines*** | | | | | | |
| 904 | **Red wine** | 3 samples, Beaujolais, Burgundy, claret | 0.998 | 9.5 | 2.3 | 0.3 | 0.03 |
| 905 | **Rosé** medium | 5 samples from different vintners | 1.003 | 8.7 | 4.0 | 2.5 | 0.01 |
| 906 | **White wine** dry | 5 samples from different vintners | 0.995 | 9.1 | 1.8 | 0.6 | 0.02 |
| 907 | medium | 1 sample, Graves | 1.005 | 8.8 | 5.4 | 3.4 | 0.02 |
| 908 | sweet | 1 sample, Sauternes | 1.016 | 10.2 | 9.2 | 5.9 | 0.03 |
| 909 | sparkling | 1 sample, Champagne | 0.995 | 9.9 | 3.3 | 1.4 | 0.04 |

| No | Food | Energy value kcal | Energy value kJ | Protein (N × 6.25) g | Fat g | Carbo-hydrate g | Na mg | K mg | Ca mg | Mg mg | P mg | Fe mg | Cu mg | Zn mg | S mg | Cl mg |
|---|---|---|---|---|---|---|---|---|---|---|---|---|---|---|---|---|
| | ***Beers*** | | | | | | | | | | | | | | | |
| 891 | **Brown ale** bottled | 28 | 117 | 0.3 | Tr | 3.0 | 16 | 33 | 7 | 6 | 11 | 0.03 | 0.07 | — | — | 37 |
| 892 | **Canned beer** bitter | 32 | 132 | 0.3 | Tr | 2.3 | 9 | 37 | 8 | 7 | 11 | 0.01 | Tr | Tr | — | — |
| 893 | **Draught** bitter | 32 | 132 | 0.3 | Tr | 2.3 | 12 | 38 | 11 | 9 | 13 | 0.01 | 0.08 | — | — | 32 |
| 894 | mild | 25 | 104 | 0.2 | Tr | 1.6 | 11 | 33 | 10 | 8 | 12 | 0.02 | 0.05 | — | — | 34 |
| 895 | **Keg** bitter | 31 | 129 | 0.3 | Tr | 2.3 | 8 | 35 | 8 | 7 | 9 | 0.01 | 0.01 | 0.02 | — | 30 |
| 896 | **Lager** bottled | 29 | 120 | 0.2 | Tr | 1.5 | 4 | 34 | 4 | 6 | 12 | Tr | Tr | — | — | 19 |
| 897 | **Pale ale** bottled | 32 | 133 | 0.3 | Tr | 2.0 | 10 | 49 | 9 | 10 | 15 | 0.02 | 0.04 | — | — | 31 |
| 898 | **Stout** bottled | 37 | 156 | 0.3 | Tr | 4.2 | 23 | 45 | 8 | 8 | 17 | 0.05 | 0.08 | — | — | 48 |
| 899 | **Stout** extra | 39 | 163 | 0.3 | Tr | 2.1 | 4 | 86 | 5 | 9 | 28 | 0.02 | 0.03 | — | — | 24 |
| 900 | **Strong ale** | 72 | 301 | 0.7 | Tr | 6.1 | 15 | 110 | 14 | 20 | 40 | 0.03 | 0.08 | — | — | 57 |
| | ***Ciders*** | | | | | | | | | | | | | | | |
| 901 | **Cider** dry | 36 | 152 | Tr | 0 | 2.6 | 7 | 72 | 8 | 3 | 3 | 0.49 | 0.04 | — | — | 6 |
| 902 | sweet | 42 | 176 | Tr | 0 | 4.3 | 7 | 72 | 8 | 3 | 3 | 0.49 | 0.04 | — | — | 6 |
| 903 | vintage | 101 | 421 | Tr | 0 | 7.3 | 2 | 97 | 5 | 4 | 9 | 0.31 | 0.02 | — | — | 5 |
| | ***Wines*** | | | | | | | | | | | | | | | |
| 904 | **Red wine** | 68 | 284 | 0.2 | 0 | 0.3 | 10 | 130 | 7 | 11 | 14 | 0.90 | 0.12 | — | — | 18 |
| 905 | **Rosé** medium | 71 | 294 | 0.1 | 0 | 2.5 | 4 | 75 | 12 | 7 | 6 | 0.95 | 0.02 | 0.04 | — | 7 |
| 906 | **White wine** dry | 66 | 275 | 0.1 | 0 | 0.6 | 4 | 61 | 9 | 8 | 6 | 0.50 | 0.01 | 0.01 | — | 10 |
| 907 | medium | 75 | 311 | 0.1 | 0 | 3.4 | 21 | 88 | 14 | 9 | 8 | 1.21 | 0.01 | — | — | 4 |
| 908 | sweet | 94 | 394 | 0.2 | 0 | 5.9 | 13 | 110 | 14 | 11 | 13 | 0.58 | 0.05 | — | — | 7 |
| 909 | sparkling | 76 | 315 | 0.3 | 0 | 1.4 | 4 | 57 | 3 | 6 | 7 | 0.50 | 0.01 | — | — | 7 |

| No | Food | Retinol µg | Carotene µg | Vitamin D µg | Thiamin mg | Riboflavin mg | Nicotinic acid mg | Potential nicotinic acid from tryptophan mg Trp ÷ 60 | Vitamin C mg | Vitamin E mg |
|---|---|---|---|---|---|---|---|---|---|---|
| | ***Beers*** | | | | | | | | | |
| 891 | **Brown ale** bottled | 0 | Tr | 0 | Tr | 0.02 | 0.26 | 0.13 | 0 | — |
| 892 | **Canned beer** bitter | 0 | Tr | 0 | Tr | (0.03) | (0.30) | 0.13 | 0 | — |
| 893 | **Draught** bitter | 0 | Tr | 0 | Tr | 0.04 | 0.47 | 0.13 | 0 | — |
| 894 | mild | 0 | Tr | 0 | Tr | (0.03) | (0.30) | 0.10 | 0 | — |
| 895 | **Keg** bitter | 0 | Tr | 0 | Tr | 0.03 | 0.32 | 0.13 | 0 | — |
| 896 | **Lager** bottled | 0 | Tr | 0 | Tr | 0.02 | 0.33 | 0.21 | 0 | — |
| 897 | **Pale ale** bottled | 0 | Tr | 0 | Tr | 0.02 | 0.35 | 0.17 | 0 | — |
| 898 | **Stout** bottled | 0 | Tr | 0 | Tr | 0.03 | 0.26 | 0.17 | 0 | — |
| 899 | **Stout** extra | 0 | Tr | 0 | Tr | 0.04 | 0.51 | 0.17 | 0 | — |
| 900 | **Strong ale** | 0 | Tr | 0 | Tr | 0.06 | 0.83 | 0.37 | 0 | — |
| | ***Ciders*** | | | | | | | | | |
| 901 | **Cider** dry | 0 | Tr | 0 | Tr | Tr | 0.01 | Tr | 0 | — |
| 902 | sweet | 0 | Tr | 0 | Tr | Tr | 0.01 | Tr | 0 | — |
| 903 | vintage | 0 | Tr | 0 | Tr | Tr | (0.01) | Tr | 0 | — |
| | ***Wines*** | | | | | | | | | |
| 904 | **Red wine** | 0 | Tr | 0 | Tr | 0.02 | 0.09 | Tr | 0 | — |
| 905 | **Rosé** medium | 0 | Tr | 0 | Tr | 0.01 | 0.07 | Tr | 0 | — |
| 906 | **White wine** dry | 0 | Tr | 0 | Tr | 0.01 | 0.06 | Tr | 0 | — |
| 907 | medium | 0 | Tr | 0 | Tr | 0.01 | 0.08 | Tr | 0 | — |
| 908 | sweet | 0 | Tr | 0 | Tr | 0.01 | 0.08 | Tr | 0 | — |
| 909 | sparkling | 0 | Tr | 0 | Tr | 0.01 | 0.07 | Tr | 0 | — |

| No | Food | Vitamin $B_6$ mg | Vitamin $B_{12}$ µg | Folic acid Free µg | Folic acid Total µg | Pantothenic acid mg | Biotin µg | Notes |
|---|---|---|---|---|---|---|---|---|
| | ***Beers*** | | | | | | | |
| 891 | **Brown ale** bottled | 0.012 | 0.11 | 2.3 | 4.0 | (0.10) | (0.5) | |
| 892 | **Canned beer** bitter | (0.020) | (0.15) | (3.5) | (4.0) | (0.10) | (0.5) | |
| 893 | **Draught** bitter | 0.023 | 0.17 | 4.1 | 8.8 | (0.10) | (0.5) | |
| 894 | mild | (0.020) | (0.15) | (4.0) | (4.5) | (0.10) | (0.5) | |
| 895 | **Keg** bitter | 0.019 | 0.15 | 3.9 | 4.6 | (0.10) | (0.5) | |
| 896 | **Lager** bottled | 0.021 | 0.14 | 4.3 | 4.3 | (0.10) | (0.5) | |
| 897 | **Pale ale** bottled | 0.014 | 0.14 | 3.5 | 4.1 | (0.10) | (0.5) | |
| 898 | **Stout** bottled | 0.014 | 0.11 | 3.8 | 4.4 | (0.10) | (0.5) | |
| 899 | **Stout** extra | 0.016 | 0.17 | 5.5 | 5.9 | — | — | |
| 900 | **Strong ale** | 0.042 | 0.37 | 5.9 | 8.8 | — | — | |
| | ***Ciders*** | | | | | | | |
| 901 | **Cider** dry | 0.005 | — | — | — | 0.04 | 0.6 | |
| 902 | sweet | 0.005 | — | — | — | 0.03 | 0.6 | |
| 903 | vintage | (0.005) | — | — | — | (0.03) | (0.6) | |
| | ***Wines*** | | | | | | | |
| 904 | **Red wine** | 0.015 | Tr | 0.2 | 0.2 | (0.04) | — | |
| 905 | **Rosé** medium | 0.023 | Tr | 0.2 | 0.2 | (0.04) | — | |
| 906 | **White wine** dry | 0.020 | Tr | 0.2 | 0.2 | (0.03) | — | |
| 907 | medium | 0.014 | Tr | 0.2 | 0.2 | (0.03) | — | |
| 908 | sweet | 0.012 | Tr | 0.1 | 0.1 | (0.03) | — | |
| 909 | sparkling | 0.017 | Tr | 0.1 | 0.1 | (0.03) | — | |

| No | Food | Description and number of samples | Specific gravity | Alcohol g | Solids g | Sugars g | Total nitrogen g |
|---|---|---|---|---|---|---|---|
| | ***Wines, liqueur (fortified)*** | | | | | | |
| 910 | **Port** | 2 samples | 1.026 | 15.9 | 13.0 | 12.0 | 0.02 |
| 911 | **Sherry** dry | 1 sample | 0.988 | 15.7 | 3.3 | 1.4 | 0.03 |
| 912 | medium | 5 samples from different importers | 0.998 | 14.8 | 4.7 | 3.6 | 0.02 |
| 913 | sweet | 1 sample | 1.009 | 15.6 | 9.6 | 6.9 | 0.05 |
| | ***Vermouths*** | | | | | | |
| 914 | **Vermouth** dry | 5 samples of different brands | 1.005 | 13.9 | 6.6 | 5.5 | 0.01 |
| 915 | sweet | 5 samples of different brands | 1.046 | 13.0 | 16.4 | 15.9 | Tr |
| | ***Liqueurs*** | | | | | | |
| 916 | **Advocaat** | 4 samples of different brands | 1.093 | 12.8 | 39.6 | 28.4 | 0.75 |
| 917 | **Cherry brandy** | 6 samples of different brands | 1.093 | 19.0 | 33.3 | 32.6 | Tr |
| 918 | **Curaçao** | 4 samples of different brands | 1.052 | 29.3 | 27.8 | 28.3 | Tr |
| | ***Spirits*** | | | | | | |
| 919 | **70% proof** | Mean of brandy, gin, rum, whisky | 0.950 | 31.7 | Tr | Tr | Tr |

| No | Food | Energy value | | Protein (N × 6.25) | Fat | Carbo-hydrate | mg | | | | | | | | | |
|---|---|---|---|---|---|---|---|---|---|---|---|---|---|---|---|---|
| | | kcal | kJ | g | g | g | Na | K | Ca | Mg | P | Fe | Cu | Zn | S | Cl |
| | ***Wines, liqueur (fortified)*** | | | | | | | | | | | | | | | |
| 910 | **Port** | 157 | 655 | 0.1 | 0 | 12.0 | 4 | 97 | 4 | 11 | 12 | 0.40 | 0.10 | — | — | 8 |
| 911 | **Sherry** dry | 116 | 481 | 0.2 | 0 | 1.4 | 10 | 57 | 7 | 13 | 11 | 0.39 | 0.03 | — | — | 12 |
| 912 | medium | 118 | 489 | 0.1 | 0 | 3.6 | 6 | 89 | 9 | 8 | 7 | 0.53 | 0.10 | 0.27 | — | 7 |
| 913 | sweet | 136 | 568 | 0.3 | 0 | 6.9 | 13 | 110 | 7 | 11 | 10 | 0.37 | 0.11 | — | — | 14 |
| | ***Vermouths*** | | | | | | | | | | | | | | | |
| 914 | **Vermouth** dry | 118 | 493 | 0.1 | 0 | 5.5 | 17 | 40 | 7 | 5 | 7 | 0.34 | 0.06 | 0.04 | — | 9 |
| 915 | sweet | 151 | 631 | Tr | 0 | 15.9 | 28 | 30 | 6 | 4 | 6 | 0.36 | 0.04 | 0.03 | — | 16 |
| | ***Liqueurs*** | | | | | | | | | | | | | | | |
| 916 | **Advocaat** | 272 | 1139 | 4.7 | 6.3 | 28.4 | — | — | — | — | — | — | — | — | — | — |
| 917 | **Cherry brandy** | 255 | 1073 | Tr | 0 | 32.6 | — | — | — | — | — | — | — | — | — | — |
| 918 | **Curaçao** | 311 | 1303 | Tr | 0 | 28.3 | — | — | — | — | — | — | — | — | — | — |
| | ***Spirits*** | | | | | | | | | | | | | | | |
| 919 | **70% proof** | 222 | 919 | Tr | 0 | Tr | Tr | Tr | Tr | Tr | Tr | Tr | Tr | Tr | Tr | Tr |

| No | Food | Retinol µg | Carotene µg | Vitamin D µg | Thiamin mg | Riboflavin mg | Nicotinic acid mg | Potential nicotinic acid from tryptophan mg Trp ÷ 60 | Vitamin C mg | Vitamin E mg |
|---|---|---|---|---|---|---|---|---|---|---|
| | ***Wines, liqueur (fortified)*** | | | | | | | | | |
| 910 | **Port** | 0 | Tr | 0 | Tr | 0.01 | 0.06 | Tr | 0 | 0 |
| 911 | **Sherry** dry | 0 | Tr | 0 | Tr | 0.01 | 0.10 | Tr | 0 | 0 |
| 912 | medium | 0 | Tr | 0 | Tr | 0.01 | 0.08 | Tr | 0 | 0 |
| 913 | sweet | 0 | Tr | 0 | Tr | 0.01 | 0.07 | Tr | 0 | 0 |
| | ***Vermouths*** | | | | | | | | | |
| 914 | **Vermouth** dry | 0 | 0 | 0 | Tr | Tr | 0.04 | 0 | 0 | 0 |
| 915 | sweet | 0 | 0 | 0 | Tr | Tr | 0.04 | 0 | 0 | 0 |
| | ***Liqueurs*** | | | | | | | | | |
| 916 | **Advocaat** | — | — | Tr | — | — | — | 1.4 | 0 | — |
| 917 | **Cherry brandy** | 0 | Tr | 0 | Tr | Tr | Tr | 0 | 0 | 0 |
| 918 | **Curaçao** | 0 | 0 | 0 | Tr | Tr | Tr | 0 | 0 | 0 |
| | ***Spirits*** | | | | | | | | | |
| 919 | **70% proof** | 0 | 0 | 0 | 0 | 0 | 0 | 0 | 0 | 0 |

| No | Food | Vitamin $B_6$ mg | Vitamin $B_{12}$ µg | Folic acid Free µg | Folic acid Total µg | Panto-thenic acid mg | Biotin µg | Notes |
|---|---|---|---|---|---|---|---|---|
| | ***Wines, liqueur (fortified)*** | | | | | | | |
| 910 | **Port** | 0.010 | Tr | 0.1 | 0.1 | — | — | |
| 911 | **Sherry** dry | 0.008 | Tr | 0.1 | 0.1 | — | — | |
| 912 | medium | 0.009 | Tr | 0.1 | 0.1 | — | — | |
| 913 | sweet | 0.008 | Tr | 0.1 | 0.1 | — | — | |
| | ***Vermouths*** | | | | | | | |
| 914 | **Vermouth** dry | 0.008 | Tr | Tr | Tr | — | — | |
| 915 | sweet | 0.004 | Tr | Tr | Tr | — | — | |
| | ***Liqueurs*** | | | | | | | |
| 916 | **Advocaat** | — | — | — | — | — | — | |
| 917 | **Cherry brandy** | Tr | Tr | Tr | Tr | — | — | |
| 918 | **Curacao** | Tr | Tr | Tr | Tr | — | — | |
| | ***Spirits*** | | | | | | | |
| 919 | **70% proof** | 0 | 0 | 0 | 0 | 0 | 0 | |

| No | Food | Description and number of samples | Water g | Sugars g | Starch and dextrins g | Dietary fibre g | Total nitrogen g |
|---|---|---|---|---|---|---|---|
| 920 | **Bread sauce** | Recipe p 344 | 76.0 | 4.4 | 8.4 | 0.5 | 0.70 |
| 921 | **Brown sauce** bottled | 6 bottles of different brands | 64.0 | 23.1 | 2.1 | — | 0.18 |
| 922 | **Cheese sauce** | Recipe p 344 | 66.5 | 4.2 | 4.8 | 0.2 | 1.31 |
| 923 | **Chutney** apple | Recipe p 345 | 45.0 | 50.1 | 0.4 | 1.8 | 0.12 |
| 924 | tomato | Recipe p 345 | 58.2 | 39.5 | 0.2 | 1.9 | 0.18 |
| 925 | **French dressing** | Recipe p 345 | 23.5 | 0.2 | 0 | 0 | 0.02 |
| 926 | **Mayonnaise** | Recipe p 345 | 28.0 | 0.1 | 0 | 0 | 0.29 |
| 927 | **Onion sauce** | Recipe p 345 | 81.5 | 4.2 | 3.7 | 0.7 | 0.46 |
| 928 | **Piccalilli** | 12 jars, 5 brands | 86.4 | 2.6 | 3.4 | 1.9 | 0.18 |
| 929 | **Pickle** sweet | 10 jars, 3 brands, including Branston, Pan Yan | 58.9 | 32.6 | 1.8 | 1.7 | 0.09 |
| 930 | **Salad cream** | 6 bottles of the same brand | 52.7 | 13.4 | 1.7 | — | 0.30 |
| 931 | **Tomato ketchup** | 6 bottles of different brands | 64.8 | 22.9 | 1.1 | — | 0.34 |
| 932 | **Tomato purée** | Purée or paste in tubes; calculated values | 65.7 | 11.4 | 0 | — | 0.97 |
| 933 | **Tomato sauce** | Recipe p 346 | 81.5 | 3.6 | 4.5 | 1.9 | 0.39 |
| 934 | **White sauce** savoury | Recipe p 346 | 73.2 | 5.1 | 5.9 | 0.3 | 0.68 |
| 935 | sweet | Recipe p 346 | 67.6 | 13.5 | 5.5 | 0.3 | 0.63 |

| No | Food | Energy value kcal | Energy value kJ | Protein g | Fat g | Carbo-hydrate g | Na mg | K mg | Ca mg | Mg mg | P mg | Fe mg | Cu mg | Zn mg | S mg | Cl mg |
|---|---|---|---|---|---|---|---|---|---|---|---|---|---|---|---|---|
| 920 | **Bread sauce** | 110 | 463 | 4.3 | 5.0 | 12.8 | 490 | 140 | 120 | 17 | 100 | 0.4 | 0.05 | 0.5 | 40 | 780 |
| 921 | **Brown sauce** bottled | 99 | 422 | 1.1 | Tr | 25.2 | 980 | 390 | 43 | 29 | 36 | 3.1 | 0.33 | — | — | 1550 |
| 922 | **Cheese sauce** | 198 | 825 | 8.3 | 14.6 | 9.0 | 450 | 150 | 260 | 18 | 190 | 0.3 | 0.03 | 1.1 | — | 730 |
| 923 | **Chutney** apple | 193 | 824 | 0.7 | 0.1 | 50.5 | 180 | 200 | 26 | 18 | 30 | 0.9 | 0.10 | 0.1 | 29 | 280 |
| 924 | tomato | 154 | 658 | 1.1 | 0.1 | 39.7 | 130 | 310 | 30 | 20 | 39 | 1.1 | 0.14 | 0.2 | 32 | 230 |
| 925 | **French dressing** | 658 | 2706 | 0.1 | 73.0 | 0.2 | 960 | 22 | 5 | 13 | 8 | 0.1 | 0.01 | — | 6 | 1480 |
| 926 | **Mayonnaise** | 718 | 2952 | 1.8 | 78.9 | 0.1 | 360 | 24 | 16 | 7 | 59 | 0.7 | 0.03 | 0.4 | 21 | 570 |
| 927 | **Onion sauce** | 99 | 413 | 2.9 | 6.4 | 7.9 | 440 | 130 | 96 | 14 | 75 | 0.3 | 0.05 | 0.3 | — | 690 |
| 928 | **Piccalilli** | 33 | 141 | 1.1 | 0.7 | 6.0 | 1200 | 55 | 24 | 10 | 23 | 0.9 | 0.10 | 0.2 | — | 1700 |
| 929 | **Pickle** sweet | 134 | 572 | 0.6 | 0.3 | 34.4 | 1700 | 110 | 19 | 10 | 11 | 2.0 | 0.10 | 1.4 | — | 2600 |
| 930 | **Salad cream** | 311 | 1288 | 1.9 | 27.4 | 15.1 | 840 | 80 | 34 | 21 | 90 | 0.8 | 0.08 | — | — | 1300 |
| 931 | **Tomato ketchup** | 98 | 420 | 2.1 | Tr | 24.0 | 1120 | 590 | 25 | 19 | 43 | 1.2 | 0.40 | — | — | 1810 |
| 932 | **Tomato purée** | 67 | 286 | 6.1 | Tr | 11.4 | 20[a] | 1540 | 51 | 66 | 130 | 5.1 | 0.63 | 1.7 | — | 290[a] |
| 933 | **Tomato sauce** | 86 | 359 | 2.4 | 5.1 | 8.1 | 340 | 320 | 28 | 14 | 37 | 0.7 | 0.12 | 0.4 | — | 560 |
| 934 | **White sauce** savoury | 151 | 630 | 4.3 | 10.3 | 11.0 | 410 | 160 | 140 | 16 | 110 | 0.3 | 0.04 | 0.4 | — | 650 |
| 935 | sweet | 172 | 722 | 3.9 | 9.5 | 19.0 | 110 | 150 | 130 | 13 | 100 | 0.2 | 0.04 | 0.4 | — | 180 |

[a] Values for a brand without added salt. If salt is added at a level of 1 per cent, the purée contains about 420 mg sodium and 890 mg chloride per 100 g

| No | Food | Retinol µg | Carotene µg | Vitamin D µg | Thiamin mg | Riboflavin mg | Nicotinic acid mg | Potential nicotinic acid from tryptophan mg Trp ÷ 60 | Vitamin C mg | Vitamin E mg |
|---|---|---|---|---|---|---|---|---|---|---|
| 920 | **Bread sauce** | 40 | 15 | 0.16 | 0.05 | 0.12 | 0.3 | 1.0 | Tr | 0.2 |
| 921 | **Brown sauce** bottled | 0 | — | 0 | — | — | — | 0.2 | — | — |
| 922 | **Cheese sauce** | 140 | 50 | 0.56 | 0.05 | 0.23 | 0.2 | 1.9 | Tr | 0.6 |
| 923 | **Chutney** apple | 0 | 10 | 0 | 0.02 | 0.03 | 0.1 | 0.1 | 4 | 0.1 |
| 924 | tomato | 0 | 360 | 0 | 0.04 | 0.05 | 0.5 | 0.1 | 8 | 0.8 |
| 925 | **French dressing** | 0 | 0 | 0 | 0 | 0 | 0 | 0 | 0 | 3.9 |
| 926 | **Mayonnaise** | 80 | Tr | 1.0 | 0.06 | 0.11 | Tr | 1.0 | 0 | 4.9 |
| 927 | **Onion sauce** | 60 | 10 | 0.39 | 0.04 | 0.12 | 0.2 | 0.7 | 2 | 1.0 |
| 928 | **Piccalilli** | 0 | — | 0 | 0.16 | 0.01 | 0.2 | 0.2 | Tr | — |
| 929 | **Pickle** sweet | 0 | — | 0 | 0.03 | 0.01 | 0.2 | 0.1 | — | — |
| 930 | **Salad cream** | — | — | — | — | — | — | 0.4 | 0 | — |
| 931 | **Tomato ketchup** | 0 | — | 0 | — | — | — | 0.3 | — | — |
| 932 | **Tomato purée** | 0 | 2860 | 0 | 0.34 | 0.17 | 4.0 | 0.8 | (100) | 6.9 |
| 933 | **Tomato sauce** | 30 | 1230 | 0.27 | 0.08 | 0.05 | 1.0 | 0.4 | 10 | 1.4 |
| 934 | **White sauce** savoury | 100 | 20 | 0.63 | 0.06 | 0.16 | 0.2 | 1.0 | Tr | 0.7 |
| 935 | sweet | 90 | 20 | 0.58 | 0.05 | 0.15 | 0.2 | 0.9 | Tr | 0.6 |

| No | Food | Vitamin $B_6$ mg | Vitamin $B_{12}$ µg | Folic acid Free µg | Folic acid Total µg | Panto-thenic acid mg | Biotin µg | Notes |
|---|---|---|---|---|---|---|---|---|
| 920 | **Bread sauce** | 0.03 | Tr | 3 | 5 | 0.3 | 2 | |
| 921 | **Brown sauce** bottled | — | 0 | Tr | Tr | — | — | |
| 922 | **Cheese sauce** | 0.05 | Tr | 3 | 5 | 0.3 | 2 | |
| 923 | **Chutney** apple | 0.05 | 0 | 3 | 4 | 0.1 | Tr | |
| 924 | tomato | 0.09 | 0 | 7 | 11 | 0.2 | 1 | |
| 925 | **French dressing** | 0 | 0 | 0 | 0 | 0 | 0 | |
| 926 | **Mayonnaise** | 0.10 | 1 | 14 | (14) | 1.0 | 12 | |
| 927 | **Onion sauce** | 0.05 | Tr | 2 | 4 | 0.3 | 1 | |
| 928 | **Piccalilli** | — | 0 | — | — | — | Tr | |
| 929 | **Pickle** sweet | — | 0 | — | — | — | Tr | |
| 930 | **Salad cream** | — | — | — | — | — | — | |
| 931 | **Tomato ketchup** | — | 0 | — | — | — | — | |
| 932 | **Tomato purée** | 0.63 | 0 | (63) | (140) | 1.1 | 8 | |
| 933 | **Tomato sauce** | 0.11 | 0 | 2 | 15 | 0.3 | 2 | |
| 934 | **White sauce** savoury | 0.04 | Tr | 3 | 4 | 0.3 | 2 | |
| 935 | sweet | 0.04 | Tr | 3 | 4 | 0.3 | 2 | |

| No | Food | Description and number of samples | Water g | Sugars g | Starch and dextrins g | Dietary fibre g | Total nitrogen g |
|---|---|---|---|---|---|---|---|
| 937 | **Bone and vegetable broth**[a] | Mean of 6 samples, analysed as served in hospital | 90.3 | 1.0 | 0.1 | — | 0.59 |
| | ***Soup*** | | | | | | |
| 938 | **Chicken, cream of** canned, ready to serve | 10 cans, 3 brands | 87.9 | 1.1 | 3.4 | — | 0.27 |
| 939 | condensed | 7 cans of the same brand | 82.2 | 1.4 | 4.6 | — | 0.41 |
| 940 | condensed, as served | Diluted with an equal volume of water | 91.1 | 0.7 | 2.3 | — | 0.20 |
| 941 | **Chicken noodle** dried | 10 packets, 5 brands | 4.8 | 10.2 | 50.7 | — | 2.20 |
| 942 | dried, as served | Calculated from 35 g soup powder to 570 ml water | 94.2 | 0.6 | 3.1 | — | 0.13 |
| 943 | **Lentil** | Recipe p 346 | 77.8 | 2.0 | 9.9 | 2.2 | 0.71 |
| 944 | **Minestrone** dried | 10 packets, 3 brands | 3.9 | 15.0 | 32.6 | 6.6 | 1.62 |
| 945 | dried, as served | Calculated from 45 g soup powder to 570 ml water | 92.6 | 1.2 | 2.5 | 0.5 | 0.12 |
| 946 | **Mushroom, cream of** canned, ready to serve | 10 cans, 3 brands | 89.2 | 0.8 | 3.1 | — | 0.17 |
| 947 | **Oxtail** canned, ready to serve | 10 cans, 3 brands | 88.5 | 0.9 | 4.2 | — | 0.38 |
| 948 | dried | 10 packets, 5 brands | 3.0 | 9.2 | 41.8 | 3.8 | 2.81 |
| 949 | dried, as served | Calculated from 45 g soup powder to 570 ml water | 92.5 | 0.7 | 3.2 | 0.3 | 0.22 |
| 950 | **Tomato, cream of** canned, ready to serve | 10 cans, 3 brands | 84.2 | 2.6 | 3.3 | — | 0.13 |
| 951 | condensed | 7 cans, 2 brands | 70.6 | 11.2 | 3.4 | — | 0.27 |
| 952 | condensed, as served | Diluted with an equal volume of water | 85.3 | 5.6 | 1.7 | — | 0.14 |
| 953 | **dried** | 10 packets, 4 brands | 2.8 | 36.1 | 28.9 | 3.3 | 1.05 |
| 954 | dried, as served | Calculated from 58 g soup powder to 570 ml water | 90.6 | 3.5 | 2.8 | 0.3 | 0.10 |
| 955 | **Vegetable** canned, ready to serve | 10 cans, 4 brands | 86.4 | 2.5 | 4.2 | — | 0.24 |

[a] See McCance, Sheldon and Widdowson (1934)

| No | Food | Energy value kcal | Energy value kJ | Protein (N × 6.25) g | Fat g | Carbo-hydrate g | Na mg | K mg | Ca mg | Mg mg | P mg | Fe mg | Cu mg | Zn mg | S mg | Cl mg |
|---|---|---|---|---|---|---|---|---|---|---|---|---|---|---|---|---|
| 937 | **Bone and vegetable broth** | 60 | 251 | 3.7 | 4.6 | 1.1 | 74 | 64 | 17 | 3 | 10 | 0.3 | 0.04 | — | — | 75 |
| | ***Soup*** | | | | | | | | | | | | | | | |
| 938 | **Chicken, cream of** canned, ready to serve | 58 | 242 | 1.7 | 3.8 | 4.5 | 460 | 41 | 27 | 5 | 27 | 0.4 | 0.02 | 0.3 | — | 700 |
| 939 | condensed | 98 | 407 | 2.6 | 7.2 | 6.0 | 710 | (62) | (41) | (7) | (41) | (0.5) | (0.03) | (0.5) | — | 1070 |
| 940 | condensed, as served | 49 | 203 | 1.3 | 3.6 | 3.0 | 350 | (31) | (20) | (4) | (20) | (0.3) | (0.02) | (0.3) | — | 530 |
| 941 | **Chicken noodle** dried | 329 | 1394 | 13.8 | 5.0 | 60.9 | 6120 | 270 | 45 | 44 | 160 | 2.7 | 0.26 | 1.2 | — | 9030 |
| 942 | dried, as served | 20 | 84 | 0.8 | 0.3 | 3.7 | 370 | 16 | 3 | 3 | 10 | 0.2 | 0.02 | 0.1 | — | 550 |
| 943 | **Lentil** | 99 | 402 | 4.4 | 3.7 | 11.9 | 190 | 160 | 40 | 16 | 59 | 1.2 | 0.11 | 0.5 | — | 290 |
| 944 | **Minestrone** dried | 298 | 1259 | 10.1 | 8.8 | 47.6 | 5600 | 800 | 120 | 48 | 160 | 2.8 | 0.29 | 1.0 | — | 7670 |
| 945 | dried, as served | 23 | 99 | 0.8 | 0.7 | 3.7 | 430 | 62 | 9 | 7 | 12 | 0.2 | 0.02 | 0.1 | — | 590 |
| 946 | **Mushroom, cream of** canned, ready to serve | 53 | 222 | 1.1 | 3.8 | 3.9 | 470 | 55 | 30 | 4 | 30 | 0.3 | 0.04 | 0.3 | — | 750 |
| 947 | **Oxtail** canned, ready to serve | 44 | 185 | 2.4 | 1.7 | 5.1 | 440 | 93 | 40 | 6 | 37 | 1.0 | 0.04 | 0.4 | — | 660 |
| 948 | dried | 356 | 1504 | 17.6 | 10.5 | 51.0 | 5250 | 700 | 140 | 44 | 260 | 4.3 | 0.25 | 2.4 | — | 7670 |
| 949 | dried, as served | 27 | 116 | 1.4 | 0.8 | 3.9 | 400 | 54 | 11 | 3 | 20 | 0.3 | 0.02 | 0.2 | — | 590 |
| 950 | **Tomato, cream of** canned, ready to serve | 55 | 230 | 0.8 | 3.3 | 5.9 | 460 | 190 | 17 | 8 | 20 | 0.4 | 0.06 | 0.2 | — | 740 |
| 951 | condensed | 123 | 514 | 1.7 | 6.8 | 14.6 | 830 | (360) | (32) | (15) | (38) | (0.7) | (0.11) | 0.3 | — | 1320 |
| 952 | condensed, as served | 62 | 258 | 0.9 | 3.4 | 7.3 | 410 | (180) | (16) | (8) | (19) | (0.3) | (0.06) | 0.2 | — | 660 |
| 953 | **dried** | 321 | 1359 | 6.6 | 5.6 | 65.0 | 4040 | 920 | 140 | 39 | 130 | 1.8 | 0.33 | 0.8 | — | 6620 |
| 954 | dried, as served | 31 | 130 | 0.6 | 0.5 | 6.3 | 390 | 89 | 14 | 4 | 13 | 0.2 | 0.03 | 0.1 | — | 640 |
| 955 | **Vegetable** canned, ready to serve | 37 | 159 | 1.5 | 0.7 | 6.7 | 500 | 140 | 17 | 10 | 27 | 0.6 | 0.06 | 0.3 | — | 750 |

| No | Food | Retinol µg | Carotene µg | Vitamin D µg | Thiamin mg | Riboflavin mg | Nicotinic acid mg | Potential nicotinic acid from tryptophan mgTrp ÷60 | Vitamin C mg | Vitamin E mg |
|---|---|---|---|---|---|---|---|---|---|---|
| 937 | **Bone and vegetable broth** | 0 | — | 0 | — | — | — | 0.8 | 0 | — |
| | ***Soup*** | | | | | | | | | |
| 938 | **Chicken, cream of** canned, ready to serve | 0 | 0 | 0 | 0.01 | 0.03 | 0.2 | 0.3 | 0 | — |
| 939 | condensed | 0 | 0 | 0 | (0.02) | 0.04 | 0.6 | 0.5 | 0 | — |
| 940 | condensed, as served | 0 | 0 | 0 | (0.01) | 0.02 | 0.3 | 0.2 | 0 | — |
| 941 | **Chicken noodle** dried | 0 | 0 | 0 | 0.23 | 0.08 | 2.2 | 2.6 | 0 | — |
| 942 | dried, as served | 0 | 0 | 0 | 0.01 | Tr | 0.1 | 0.2 | 0 | — |
| 943 | **Lentil** | 40 | 430 | 0.28 | (0.07) | (0.05) | (0.3) | 0.8 | Tr | — |
| 944 | **Minestrone** dried | 0 | — | 0 | 0.21 | 0.15 | 3.1 | 1.9 | 0 | — |
| 945 | dried, as served | 0 | — | 0 | 0.02 | 0.01 | 0.2 | 0.1 | 0 | — |
| 946 | **Mushroom, cream of** canned ready to serve | 0 | 0 | 0 | Tr | 0.05 | 0.3 | 0.2 | 0 | — |
| 947 | **Oxtail** canned, ready to serve | 0 | 0 | 0 | 0.02 | 0.03 | 0.7 | 0.5 | 0 | — |
| 948 | **dried** | 0 | 0 | 0 | 10.4[a] | 0.30 | 3.5 | 3.8 | 0 | — |
| 949 | dried, as served | 0 | 0 | 0 | 0.8[a] | 0.02 | 0.3 | 0.3 | 0 | — |
| 950 | **Tomato, cream of** canned, ready to serve | 0 | 210 | 0 | 0.03 | 0.02 | 0.5 | 0.1 | (Tr) | — |
| 951 | condensed | 0 | (400) | 0 | (0.06) | 0.05 | 1.0 | 0.2 | (Tr) | — |
| 952 | condensed, as served | 0 | (200) | 0 | (0.03) | 0.03 | 0.5 | 0.1 | (Tr) | — |
| 953 | **dried** | 0 | — | 0 | 0.23 | 0.18 | 1.9 | 0.9 | (Tr) | — |
| 954 | dried, as served | 0 | — | 0 | 0.02 | 0.02 | 0.2 | 0.1 | (Tr) | — |
| 955 | **Vegetable** canned, ready to serve | 0 | Tr[b] | 0 | 0.03 | 0.02 | 0.4 | 0.2 | (Tr) | — |

| No | Food | Vitamin $B_6$ mg | Vitamin $B_{12}$ µg | Folic acid Free µg | Folic acid Total µg | Pantothenic acid mg | Biotin µg |
|---|---|---|---|---|---|---|---|
| 937 | **Bone and vegetable broth** | — | 0 | — | — | — | — |
| | ***Soup*** | | | | | | |
| 938 | **Chicken, cream of** canned, ready to serve | 0.01 | 0 | — | — | — | — |
| 939 | condensed | — | 0 | — | — | — | — |
| 940 | condensed, as served | — | 0 | — | — | — | — |
| 941 | **Chicken noodle** dried | — | 0 | — | — | — | — |
| 942 | dried, as served | — | 0 | — | — | — | — |
| 943 | **Lentil** | (0.07) | 0 | — | — | — | — |
| 944 | **Minestrone** dried | — | 0 | — | — | — | — |
| 945 | dried, as served | — | 0 | — | — | — | — |
| 946 | **Mushroom, cream of** canned, ready to serve | 0.01 | 0 | (2) | — | — | — |
| 947 | **Oxtail** canned, ready to serve | 0.03 | 0 | (2) | — | — | — |
| 948 | dried | — | 0 | — | — | — | — |
| 949 | dried, as served | — | 0 | — | — | — | — |
| 950 | **Tomato, cream of** canned, ready to serve | 0.06 | 0 | 6 | 12 | — | — |
| 951 | condensed | — | 0 | — | — | — | — |
| 952 | condensed, as served | — | 0 | — | — | — | — |
| 953 | **dried** | — | 0 | 21 | 52 | — | — |
| 954 | dried, as served | — | 0 | — | — | — | — |
| 955 | **Vegetable** canned, ready to serve | 0.05 | 0 | 2 | 10 | — | — |

Notes

[a] This remarkably high content is derived from the flavouring agent.

[b] 36µg α-carotene per 100g was found, but no β-carotene.

| No | Food | Description and number of samples | Water g | Sugars g | Starch and dextrins g | Dietary fibre g | Total nitrogen g |
|---|---|---|---|---|---|---|---|
| 956 | **Baking powder** | 6 samples of the same brand | 6.3 | Tr | 37.8 | — | 0.91 |
| 957 | **Bovril** | 9 jars | 38.7 | 0 | 2.9 | 0 | 6.25[a] |
| 958 | **Curry powder** | 2 samples | —[b] | — | — | — | 1.52 |
| 959 | **Gelatin** | Literature sources | 13.0 | 0 | 0 | 0 | 15.20 |
| 960 | **Ginger** ground | 3 samples | —[b] | — | — | — | 1.19 |
| 961 | **Marmite** | 7 jars | 25.4 | 0 | 1.8 | — | 6.62[c] |
| 962 | **Oxo cubes** | 10 samples | 9.1 | — | 12.0 | 0 | 6.29 |
| 963 | **Mustard** powder | 2 brands | —[b] | — | — | — | 4.62 |
| 964 | **Pepper** | 3 samples | —[b] | — | — | — | 1.40 |
| 965 | **Salt** block | 2 samples | 0.2 | 0 | 0 | 0 | 0 |
| 966 | table | 2 samples | Tr | 0 | 0 | 0 | 0 |
| 967 | **Vinegar**[d] | 4 samples | — | 0.6 | 0 | 0 | 0.07 |
| 968 | **Yeast** bakers', compressed | Literature sources | 70.0 | Tr | 1.1 | 6.9 | 2.02[e] |
| 969 | dried | Literature sources | 5.0 | Tr | (3.5) | (21.9) | 6.32[e] |

[a] Includes 0.17 g purine nitrogen
[b] The loss of weight at 100°C cannot be used to determine the amount of water present, since these substances contain volatile essential oils
[c] Includes 0.27 g purine nitrogen
[d] Contains 4.8 ml acetic acid per cent
[e] Purine nitrogen forms about 10 per cent of the total nitrogen

| No | Food | Energy value | | Protein | Fat | Carbo-hydrate | mg | | | | | | | | | |
|---|---|---|---|---|---|---|---|---|---|---|---|---|---|---|---|---|
| | | kcal | kJ | g | g | g | Na | K | Ca | Mg | P | Fe | Cu | Zn | S | Cl |
| 956 | **Baking powder** | 163 | 693 | 5.2 | Tr | 37.8 | 11 800 [a] | 49 | 11300 [a] | 9 | 8430 [a] | Tr | Tr | — | — | 29 |
| 957 | **Bovril** | 174 | 737 | 39.1 [b] | 0.7 | 2.9 | 4800 | 1200 | 40 | 61 | 590 | 14.0 | 0.45 | 1.8 | — | 6800 |
| 958 | **Curry powder** | 233 | 979 | 9.5 | 10.8 | 26.1 | 450 | 1830 | 640 | 280 | 270 | 75.0 [c] | 1.04 | — | 86 | 470 |
| 959 | **Gelatin** | 338 | 1435 | 84.4 | Tr | 0 | — | — | — | — | — | — | — | — | — | — |
| 960 | **Ginger** ground | 258 | 1101 | 7.4 | 3.3 [d] | 60.0 | 34 | 910 | 97 | 130 | 140 | 17.2 | 0.45 | (6.8) | 150 | 40 |
| 961 | **Marmite** | 179 | 759 | 41.4 [b] | 0.7 | 1.8 | 4500 | 2600 | 95 | 180 | 1700 | 3.7 | 0.30 | 2.1 | — | 6600 |
| 962 | **Oxo cubes** | 229 | 969 | 38.3 [b] | 3.4 | 12.0 | 10 300 | 730 | 180 | 59 | 360 | 24.5 | 0.71 | — | — | 16 000 |
| 963 | **Mustard** powder | 452 | 1884 | 28.9 | 28.7 | 20.7 | 5 | 940 | 330 | 260 | 180 | 10.9 | 0.20 | (6.5) | 1280 | 62 |
| 964 | **Pepper** | 308 | 1312 | 8.8 | 6.5 [d] | 68.0 | 7 | 42 | 130 | 45 | 130 | 10.2 | 1.13 | (1.8) | 99 | 60 |
| 965 | **Salt** block | 0 | 0 | 0 | 0 | 0 | 38 700 | Tr | 230 | 140 | Tr | 0.3 | 0.39 | — | 400 | 59 600 |
| 966 | table | 0 | 0 | 0 | 0 | 0 | 38 850 | Tr | 29 | 290 | 8 | 0.2 | 0.10 | — | 23 | 59 900 |
| 967 | **Vinegar** | 4 | 16 | 0.4 | 0 | 0.6 | 20 | 89 | 15 | 22 | 32 | 0.5 | 0.04 | — | 19 | 47 |
| 968 | **Yeast** bakers', compressed | 53 | 226 | 11.4 [b] | 0.4 | 1.1 | 16 | 610 | 25 | 59 | 390 | 5.0 | (1.6) | (2.6) | — | — |
| 969 | dried | 169 | 717 | 35.6 [b] | 1.5 | 3.5 | (50) | (2000) | 80 | 230 | (1290) | 20.0 | 5.0 | 8.0 | — | — |

[a] The sodium, calcium and phosphorus content will depend on the brand

[b] (Total N − purine N) × 6.25

[c] This high value has been confirmed by a recent analysis giving 95 mg per 100 g

[d] By Soxhlet extraction. The figure for fat obtained by von Lieberman's method is 0.4 g per 100 g in ginger and 2.0 g per 100 g in pepper, and these have been used for calculating energy values

| No | Food | Retinol µg | Carotene µg | Vitamin D µg | Thiamin mg | Riboflavin mg | Nicotinic acid mg | Potential nicotinic acid from tryptophan mg Trp ÷ 60 | Vitamin C mg | Vitamin E mg |
|---|---|---|---|---|---|---|---|---|---|---|
| 956 | **Baking powder** | 0 | 0 | 0 | Tr | Tr | Tr | 1 | 0 | Tr |
| 957 | **Bovril** | 0 | 0 | 0 | 9.1 | 7.4 | 82 | 3 | 0 | — |
| 958 | **Curry powder** | 0 | — | 0 | — | — | — | — | 0 | — |
| 959 | **Gelatin** | 0 | 0 | 0 | Tr | Tr | Tr | 0 | 0 | 0 |
| 960 | **Ginger** ground | 0 | — | 0 | — | — | — | — | 0 | — |
| 961 | **Marmite** | 0 | 0 | 0 | 3.1 | 11 | 58 | 9 | 0 | — |
| 962 | **Oxo cubes** | 0 | 0 | 0 | — | — | — | — | 0 | — |
| 963 | **Mustard** powder | 0 | — | 0 | — | — | — | — | 0 | — |
| 964 | **Pepper** | 0 | — | 0 | — | — | — | — | 0 | — |
| 965 | **Salt**, block | 0 | 0 | 0 | 0 | 0 | 0 | 0 | 0 | 0 |
| 966 | table | 0 | 0 | 0 | 0 | 0 | 0 | 0 | 0 | 0 |
| 967 | **Vinegar** | 0 | 0 | 0 | 0 | 0 | 0 | 0 | 0 | 0 |
| 968 | **Yeast** bakers', compressed | 0 | Tr | 0 | 0.71 | 1.7 | 11 | 2 | Tr | Tr |
| 969 | dried | 0 | Tr | 0 | 2.33[a] | 4.0 | 36 | 7 | Tr | Tr |

| No | Food | Vitamin $B_6$ mg | Vitamin $B_{12}$ µg | Folic acid Free µg | Folic acid Total µg | Pantothenic acid mg | Biotin µg | Notes |
|---|---|---|---|---|---|---|---|---|
| 956 | **Baking powder** | Tr | 0 | Tr | Tr | Tr | Tr | [a] Value for bakers' yeast. Brewers' yeast contains 15.6 mg per 100 g. |
| 957 | **Bovril** | 0.53 | 8.3 | 750 | 1040 | — | — | |
| 958 | **Curry powder** | — | 0 | — | — | — | — | |
| 959 | **Gelatin** | Tr | 0 | Tr | Tr | Tr | Tr | |
| 960 | **Ginger** ground | — | 0 | — | — | — | — | |
| 961 | **Marmite** | 1.3 | 0.5 | 83 | 1010 | — | — | |
| 962 | **Oxo cubes** | — | — | — | — | — | — | |
| 963 | **Mustard** powder | — | 0 | — | — | — | — | |
| 964 | **Pepper** | — | 0 | — | — | — | — | |
| 965 | **Salt** block | 0 | 0 | 0 | 0 | 0 | 0 | |
| 966 | table | 0 | 0 | 0 | 0 | 0 | 0 | |
| 967 | **Vinegar** | 0 | 0 | 0 | 0 | 0 | 0 | |
| 968 | **Yeast** bakers', compressed | 0.6 | Tr | (42) | (1250) | 3.5 | (60) | |
| 969 | dried | 2.0 | Tr | 130 | 4000 | 11.0 | 200 | |

| No | Food | Description and number of samples | Water g | Sugars g | Starch and dextrins g | Dietary fibre g | Total nitrogen g |
|---|---|---|---|---|---|---|---|

| No | Food | Energy value kcal | Energy value kJ | Protein g | Fat g | Carbo-hydrate g | mg Na | mg K | mg Ca | mg Mg | mg P | mg Fe | mg Cu | mg Zn | mg S | mg Cl |
|---|---|---|---|---|---|---|---|---|---|---|---|---|---|---|---|---|

| No | Food | Retinol µg | Carotene µg | Vitamin D µg | Thiamin mg | Riboflavin mg | Nicotinic acid mg | Potential nicotinic acid from tryptophan mg Trp ÷ 60 | Vitamin C mg | Vitamin E mg |
|---|---|---|---|---|---|---|---|---|---|---|

| No | Food | Vitamin $B_6$ mg | Vitamin $B_{12}$ µg | Folic acid Free µg | Folic acid Total µg | Pantothenic acid mg | Biotin µg | Notes |
|---|---|---|---|---|---|---|---|---|

# Section 2
# Amino acid composition

mg per g nitrogen

| | | | |
|---|---|---|---|
| Isoleucine | Ile | Arginine | Arg |
| Leucine | Leu | Histidine | His |
| Lysine | Lys | Alanine | Ala |
| Methionine | Met | Aspartic acid | Asp |
| Cystine | Cys | Glutamic acid | Glu |
| Phenylalanine | Phe | Glycine | Gly |
| Tyrosine | Tyr | Proline | Pro |
| Threonine | Thr | Serine | Ser |
| Tryptophan | Trp | | |
| Valine | Val | | |

**Asterisk indicates new analytical data**

## **Amino acids** (mg per g nitrogen)

| No | Food | | Ile | Leu | Lys | Met | Cys | Phe | Tyr | Thr | Trp | Val | Arg | His | Ala | Asp | Glu | Gly | Pro | Ser |
|---|---|---|---|---|---|---|---|---|---|---|---|---|---|---|---|---|---|---|---|---|
| | ***Cereals*** | | | | | | | | | | | | | | | | | | | |
| 2002 | **Barley** pearl | | 220 | 420 | 160 | 100 | 140 | 320 | 190 | 210 | 100 | 310 | 300 | 130 | 260 | 350 | 1470 | 240 | 680 | 250 |
| 2005 | **Bran** wheat | | 210 | 410 | 270 | 100 | 170 | 260 | 200 | 220 | 80 | 310 | 490 | 190 | 350 | 510 | 1280 | 400 | 390 | 300 |
| 2006 | **Cornflour** maize | | 230 | 780 | 170 | 120 | 100 | 310 | 240 | 230 | 40 | 300 | 260 | 170 | 470 | 390 | 1180 | 230 | 560 | 310 |
| | **Flour** | | | | | | | | | | | | | | | | | | | |
| 2009 | wholemeal | | 210 | 420 | 150 | 100 | 160 | 280 | 190 | 170 | 70 | 280 | 290 | 130 | 230 | 310 | 1710 | 250 | 660 | 330 |
| 2010 | brown | | 210 | 420 | 140 | 100 | 160 | 280 | 190 | 170 | 70 | 270 | 260 | 130 | 190 | 270 | 2020 | 200 | 770 | 350 |
| 2011 | white | | 240 | 440 | 120 | 100 | 160 | 300 | 160 | 170 | 70 | 270 | 220 | 130 | 190 | 270 | 2060 | 200 | 790 | 350 |
| 2017 | **Oatmeal** | | 240 | 450 | 230 | 110 | 170 | 310 | 210 | 210 | 80 | 320 | 390 | 130 | 280 | 480 | 1310 | 290 | 320 | 290 |
| 2019 | **Rice** milled | | 240 | 510 | 230 | 130 | 100 | 300 | 250 | 210 | 80 | 360 | 470 | 150 | 360 | 600 | 1200 | 270 | 290 | 290 |
| 2021 | **Rye** whole | | 220 | 390 | 210 | 90 | 120 | 280 | 120 | 210 | 70 | 300 | 290 | 140 | 270 | 450 | 1510 | 270 | 590 | 240 |
| 2024 | **Soya** flour | | 280 | 490 | 400 | 80 | 100 | 310 | 200 | 240 | 80 | 300 | 450 | 160 | 270 | 730 | 1170 | 260 | 340 | 320 |
| | ***Milk and eggs*** | | | | | | | | | | | | | | | | | | | |
| 2123 | **Milk** cows' | | 350 | 640 | 510 | 180 | 60 | 340 | 280 | 310 | 90 | 460 | 250 | 190 | 240 | 530 | 1440 | 140 | 590 | 370 |
| 2138 | **Milk** human | * | 320 | 580 | 430 | 90 | 120 | 230 | 180 | 270 | 140 | 410 | 230 | 150 | 250 | 540 | 1070 | 150 | 580 | 260 |
| 2161 | **Yogurt** | * | 390 | 720 | 430 | 130 | 50 | 370 | 310 | 280 | 80 | 430 | 180 | 210 | 240 | 430 | 1150 | 160 | 480 | 360 |
| | **Eggs** | | | | | | | | | | | | | | | | | | | |
| 2165 | whole | * | 350 | 520 | 390 | 200 | 110 | 320 | 250 | 320 | 110 | 470 | 380 | 150 | 340 | 670 | 750 | 190 | 240 | 490 |
| 2166 | white | | 350 | 510 | 360 | 220 | 110 | 360 | 250 | 300 | 110 | 490 | 340 | 140 | 360 | 680 | 760 | 200 | 250 | 460 |
| 2167 | yolk | | 360 | 530 | 450 | 160 | 100 | 250 | 250 | 350 | 110 | 430 | 450 | 160 | 310 | 660 | 680 | 170 | 220 | 540 |

## **Amino acids** (mg per g nitrogen)

| No | Food | | Ile | Leu | Lys | Met | Cys | Phe | Tyr | Thr | Trp | Val | Arg | His | Ala | Asp | Glu | Gly | Pro | Ser |
|---|---|---|---|---|---|---|---|---|---|---|---|---|---|---|---|---|---|---|---|---|
| | ***Meat*** | | | | | | | | | | | | | | | | | | | |
| 2210 | **Bacon** lean | * | 300 | 460 | 530 | 160 | 80 | 270 | 220 | 270 | 70 | 320 | 400 | 200 | 380 | 560 | 1020 | 330 | 320 | 260 |
| 2237 | **Beef** lean | * | 320 | 500 | 570 | 170 | 80 | 280 | 240 | 290 | 80 | 330 | 420 | 230 | 400 | 600 | 1080 | 350 | 320 | 280 |
| 2266 | **Lamb** lean | * | 290 | 450 | 610 | 160 | 80 | 240 | 220 | 290 | 80 | 300 | 380 | 200 | 360 | 570 | 1050 | 310 | 290 | 270 |
| 2296 | **Pork** lean | * | 280 | 440 | 600 | 170 | 80 | 240 | 230 | 270 | 70 | 300 | 370 | 270 | 340 | 560 | 1000 | 330 | 300 | 260 |
| | ***Poultry and game*** | | | | | | | | | | | | | | | | | | | |
| 2314 | **Chicken** | * | 290 | 470 | 560 | 150 | 80 | 280 | 220 | 260 | 70 | 300 | 390 | 190 | 360 | 570 | 1030 | 310 | 260 | 250 |
| 2327 | **Duck** | * | 310 | 490 | 550 | 170 | 80 | 280 | 230 | 280 | 80 | 320 | 420 | 160 | 380 | 580 | 1040 | 320 | 310 | 260 |
| 2340 | **Turkey** | * | 310 | 480 | 560 | 180 | 70 | 280 | 210 | 260 | 70 | 320 | 390 | 180 | 360 | 580 | 990 | 310 | 310 | 260 |
| 2350 | **Rabbit** | * | 310 | 480 | 550 | 170 | 80 | 290 | 230 | 270 | 70 | 320 | 400 | 160 | 380 | 600 | 1030 | 320 | 320 | 260 |
| | ***Offal*** | | | | | | | | | | | | | | | | | | | |
| 2354 | **Brain,** calf and lamb | * | 270 | 510 | 560 | 130 | 110 | 320 | 240 | 320 | 80 | 360 | 390 | 250 | 340 | 570 | 870 | 290 | 340 | 330 |
| 2357 | **Heart,** lamb and ox | * | 330 | 570 | 540 | 140 | 100 | 290 | 210 | 290 | 80 | 350 | 400 | 160 | 390 | 530 | 950 | 380 | 220 | 330 |
| 2363 | **Kidney,** lamb, ox and pig | * | 260 | 490 | 510 | 130 | 90 | 310 | 200 | 270 | 80 | 350 | 350 | 220 | 330 | 550 | 770 | 370 | 350 | 300 |
| 2370 | **Liver,** calf, chicken, lamb ox and pig | * | 270 | 490 | 530 | 150 | 90 | 310 | 190 | 270 | 80 | 360 | 330 | 230 | 330 | 540 | 760 | 310 | 330 | 290 |
| 2381 | **Oxtail** | * | 300 | 430 | 560 | 120 | 80 | 250 | 210 | 260 | 80 | 300 | 380 | 250 | 360 | 520 | 980 | 390 | 400 | 250 |
| 2384 | **Sweetbread** | * | 220 | 400 | 540 | 90 | 80 | 210 | 150 | 230 | 80 | 270 | 370 | 180 | 320 | 430 | 870 | 390 | 320 | 250 |
| 2386 | **Tongue,** lamb and ox | * | 290 | 440 | 660 | 110 | 90 | 220 | 190 | 260 | 80 | 300 | 370 | 250 | 330 | 540 | 980 | 350 | 330 | 260 |
| 2391 | **Tripe** | * | 250 | 420 | 500 | 150 | 80 | 240 | 180 | 270 | 80 | 310 | 440 | 180 | 420 | 530 | 940 | 650 | 530 | 310 |

# **Amino acids** (mg per g nitrogen)

| No | Food | | Ile | Leu | Lys | Met | Cys | Phe | Tyr | Thr | Trp | Val | Arg | His | Ala | Asp | Glu | Gly | Pro | Ser |
|---|---|---|---|---|---|---|---|---|---|---|---|---|---|---|---|---|---|---|---|---|
| | ***Canned meats*** | | | | | | | | | | | | | | | | | | | |
| 2393 | **Beef,** corned | * | 290 | 460 | 580 | 150 | 90 | 260 | 240 | 280 | 90 | 330 | 410 | 180 | 390 | 580 | 1020 | 420 | 390 | 250 |
| 2394 | **Ham** | * | 290 | 480 | 560 | 170 | 80 | 250 | 200 | 270 | 60 | 310 | 410 | 230 | 380 | 570 | 1030 | 390 | 320 | 230 |
| 2395 | **Ham and pork** chopped | * | 270 | 430 | 530 | 140 | 80 | 230 | 210 | 270 | 70 | 300 | 410 | 200 | 370 | 570 | 1000 | 440 | 400 | 280 |
| 2396 | **Luncheon meat** | * | 230 | 390 | 410 | 120 | 90 | 240 | 170 | 220 | 80 | 290 | 380 | 150 | 390 | 480 | 960 | 540 | 550 | 270 |
| 2397 | **Stewed steak with gravy** | * | 270 | 440 | 540 | 140 | 70 | 250 | 180 | 280 | 70 | 290 | 400 | 210 | 370 | 530 | 1050 | 430 | 390 | 290 |
| 2398 | **Tongue** | * | 290 | 460 | 600 | 150 | 90 | 300 | 230 | 270 | 90 | 320 | 410 | 150 | 380 | 540 | 960 | 430 | 390 | 280 |
| 2400 | **Veal,** jellied | * | 300 | 450 | 540 | 150 | 80 | 270 | 210 | 270 | 70 | 310 | 430 | 180 | 360 | 550 | 990 | 390 | 340 | 270 |
| | ***Offal products*** | | | | | | | | | | | | | | | | | | | |
| 2401 | **Black pudding** | * | 140 | 610 | 460 | 90 | 80 | 360 | 150 | 250 | 80 | 450 | 300 | 310 | 460 | 590 | 930 | 400 | 440 | 300 |
| 2402 | **Faggots** | * | 250 | 440 | 420 | 100 | 90 | 300 | 140 | 220 | 70 | 320 | 400 | 140 | 450 | 480 | 1270 | 620 | 640 | 290 |
| 2403 | **Haggis** | * | 240 | 460 | 420 | 100 | 80 | 270 | 170 | 260 | 70 | 370 | 380 | 170 | 370 | 510 | 1010 | 440 | 420 | 300 |
| 2404 | **Liver sausage** | * | 250 | 470 | 490 | 120 | 80 | 270 | 170 | 340 | 70 | 370 | 370 | 210 | 370 | 520 | 980 | 490 | 380 | 310 |
| | ***Sausages*** | | | | | | | | | | | | | | | | | | | |
| 2405 | **Frankfurters** | * | 290 | 460 | 490 | 140 | 70 | 270 | 210 | 250 | 60 | 320 | 410 | 180 | 400 | 560 | 1070 | 480 | 490 | 280 |
| 2406 | **Polony** | * | 240 | 410 | 460 | 120 | 70 | 230 | 140 | 220 | 70 | 300 | 360 | 150 | 350 | 460 | 1340 | 490 | 550 | 250 |
| 2407 | **Salami** | * | 300 | 450 | 520 | 130 | 80 | 260 | 190 | 280 | 70 | 310 | 380 | 170 | 370 | 580 | 1060 | 430 | 370 | 250 |
| 2408 | **Sausages** beef | * | 260 | 430 | 380 | 120 | 100 | 260 | 160 | 240 | 80 | 310 | 380 | 160 | 400 | 500 | 1280 | 550 | 550 | 270 |
| 2411 | **Sausages** pork | * | 260 | 410 | 410 | 130 | 110 | 250 | 160 | 240 | 80 | 300 | 370 | 170 | 370 | 490 | 1150 | 460 | 510 | 270 |
| 2414 | **Saveloy** | * | 220 | 380 | 460 | 110 | 80 | 210 | 150 | 210 | 70 | 270 | 370 | 160 | 360 | 470 | 1000 | 530 | 510 | 240 |

## **Amino acids** (mg per g nitrogen)

| No | Food | | Ile | Leu | Lys | Met | Cys | Phe | Tyr | Thr | Trp | Val | Arg | His | Ala | Asp | Glu | Gly | Pro | Ser |
|---|---|---|---|---|---|---|---|---|---|---|---|---|---|---|---|---|---|---|---|---|
| | ***Meat products*** | | | | | | | | | | | | | | | | | | | |
| 2415 | **Beefburgers** | * | 280 | 450 | 490 | 160 | 70 | 270 | 200 | 250 | 70 | 310 | 400 | 200 | 400 | 540 | 1170 | 420 | 400 | 260 |
| 2417 | **Brawn** | * | 200 | 340 | 450 | 110 | 70 | 270 | 160 | 190 | 70 | 260 | 440 | 130 | 450 | 460 | 900 | 780 | 440 | 250 |
| 2418 | **Meat paste** | * | 300 | 450 | 490 | 150 | 80 | 240 | 140 | 400 | 70 | 330 | 390 | 170 | 410 | 580 | 1050 | 430 | 410 | 270 |
| 2419 | **White pudding** | * | 250 | 450 | 310 | 120 | 90 | 290 | 190 | 300 | 70 | 380 | 390 | 190 | 290 | 490 | 1330 | 370 | 400 | 340 |
| | ***Meat and pastry products*** | | | | | | | | | | | | | | | | | | | |
| 2420 | **Cornish pastie** | * | 230 | 400 | 250 | 110 | 100 | 290 | 170 | 200 | 80 | 280 | 260 | 140 | 250 | 400 | 1680 | 280 | 570 | 250 |
| 2421 | **Pork pie** | * | 260 | 400 | 330 | 120 | 100 | 310 | 170 | 210 | 80 | 280 | 330 | 160 | 320 | 430 | 1390 | 390 | 570 | 280 |
| 2425 | **Steak and kidney pie** individual | * | 290 | 510 | 340 | 120 | 110 | 380 | 130 | 250 | 70 | 360 | 380 | 190 | 360 | 450 | 1690 | 390 | 710 | 290 |
| | ***Fish*** | | | | | | | | | | | | | | | | | | | |
| 2435 | **White and fatty fish** all kinds | | 330 | 530 | 610 | 180 | 70 | 260 | 220 | 300 | 70 | 360 | 400 | 180 | 430 | 650 | 950 | 290 | 260 | 310 |
| 2516 | **Crustacea** all kinds | | 290 | 540 | 490 | 180 | 80 | 250 | 230 | 290 | 70 | 300 | 520 | 120 | 420 | 680 | 980 | 410 | 270 | 320 |
| 2530 | **Molluscs** all kinds | | 300 | 480 | 500 | 170 | 100 | 260 | 260 | 290 | 80 | 390 | 470 | 150 | 350 | 700 | 880 | 320 | 260 | 320 |

## **Amino acids** (mg per g nitrogen)

| No | Food | Ile | Leu | Lys | Met | Cys | Phe | Tyr | Thr | Trp | Val | Arg | His | Ala | Asp | Glu | Gly | Pro | Ser |
|---|---|---|---|---|---|---|---|---|---|---|---|---|---|---|---|---|---|---|---|
| | ***Vegetables*** | | | | | | | | | | | | | | | | | | |
| 2558 | **Asparagus** | 160 | 280 | 280 | 80 | 60 | 160 | 130 | 180 | 70 | 230 | 240 | 100 | 360 | 680 | 1300 | 210 | 360 | 200 |
| 2561 | **Beans, French** | 230 | 430 | 340 | 80 | 70 | 270 | 210 | 240 | 90 | 310 | 270 | 150 | 280 | 750 | 670 | 240 | 240 | 330 |
| 2564 | **broad** | 250 | 440 | 400 | 40 | 50 | 270 | 200 | 210 | 60 | 280 | 560 | 150 | 260 | 700 | 940 | 260 | 250 | 280 |
| 2565 | **butter** | 310 | 510 | 470 | 90 | 90 | 380 | 200 | 260 | 60 | 320 | 370 | 200 | 290 | 770 | 820 | 260 | 290 | 410 |
| 2567 | **haricot** | 260 | 480 | 450 | 70 | 50 | 330 | 160 | 250 | 60 | 290 | 360 | 180 | 260 | 750 | 920 | 240 | 220 | 350 |
| 2572 | **red kidney** | 260 | 480 | 450 | 70 | 50 | 330 | 160 | 250 | 60 | 290 | 360 | 180 | 260 | 750 | 920 | 240 | 220 | 350 |
| 2574 | **Beetroot** | 150 | 280 | 330 | 120 | 70 | 220 | 220 | 210 | 60 | 150 | 410 | 80 | 140 | 1130 | 950 | 130 | 160 | 220 |
| 2576 | **Broccoli tops** | 240 | 330 | 320 | 90 | 70 | 230 | — | 230 | 70 | 310 | 360 | 110 | — | — | — | — | — | — |
| 2578 | **Brussels sprouts** | 260 | 340 | 340 | 60 | 40 | 230 | — | 270 | 70 | 300 | 390 | 140 | — | — | — | — | — | — |
| 2585 | **Cabbage** | 190 | 330 | 190 | 60 | 70 | 190 | 120 | 230 | 60 | 260 | 520 | 160 | 320 | 410 | 540 | 300 | 230 | 260 |
| 2587 | **Carrots** | 190 | 280 | 240 | 70 | 70 | 170 | 140 | 180 | 50 | 280 | 280 | 90 | 300 | 730 | 1210 | 180 | 180 | 200 |
| 2591 | **Cauliflower** | 270 | 420 | 350 | 120 | — | 210 | 90 | 260 | 90 | 360 | 280 | 120 | 500 | 520 | 480 | 430 | — | — |
| 2594 | **Celery** | 240 | 430 | 130 | 110 | 30 | 280 | 80 | 210 | 70 | 300 | 250 | 90 | — | — | — | — | — | — |
| 2597 | **Cucumber** | 190 | 260 | 270 | 60 | — | 140 | — | 160 | 50 | 210 | 470 | 90 | — | — | — | — | — | — |
| 2603 | **Lentils** | 270 | 480 | 450 | 50 | 60 | 330 | 200 | 250 | 60 | 310 | 540 | 170 | 270 | 720 | 1040 | 260 | 270 | 330 |
| 2606 | **Lettuce** | 240 | 390 | 240 | 110 | — | 320 | 170 | 260 | 50 | 340 | 280 | 100 | 270 | 720 | 640 | 260 | 330 | 210 |
| 2609 | **Mushrooms** | 140 | 230 | 280 | 90 | 50 | 130 | 120 | 170 | 60 | 160 | 370 | 80 | 290 | 280 | 440 | 160 | 320 | 170 |
| 2613 | **Onions** | 90 | 170 | 280 | 70 | — | 170 | 210 | 90 | 90 | 140 | 800 | 60 | — | — | 930 | — | — | — |
| 2620 | **Peas** | 270 | 430 | 470 | 60 | 70 | 290 | 170 | 250 | 60 | 290 | 590 | 140 | 260 | 690 | 1010 | 250 | 240 | 270 |
| 2630 | **chick** | 280 | 470 | 430 | 80 | 90 | 360 | 180 | 240 | 50 | 280 | 590 | 170 | 270 | 730 | 990 | 250 | 260 | 320 |
| 2633 | **red pigeon** | 190 | 390 | 480 | 80 | 70 | 520 | 130 | 180 | 30 | 230 | 300 | 230 | 260 | 600 | 1170 | 200 | 250 | 260 |

**Amino acids** (mg per g nitrogen)

| No | Food | Ile | Leu | Lys | Met | Cys | Phe | Tyr | Thr | Trp | Val | Arg | His | Ala | Asp | Glu | Gly | Pro | Ser |
|---|---|---|---|---|---|---|---|---|---|---|---|---|---|---|---|---|---|---|---|
| | ***Vegetables** contd* | | | | | | | | | | | | | | | | | | |
| 2639 | **Potatoes** | 260 | 380 | 340 | 100 | 80 | 270 | 190 | 240 | 90 | 320 | 310 | 120 | 230 | 1150 | 800 | 210 | 240 | 260 |
| 2657 | **Spinach** | 300 | 590 | 450 | 110 | 100 | 380 | 310 | 330 | 100 | 380 | 400 | 160 | 400 | 620 | 730 | 320 | 300 | 300 |
| 2664 | **Sweet potatoes** | 230 | 340 | 210 | 100 | 70 | 240 | 150 | 240 | 110 | 280 | 310 | 80 | 300 | 830 | 540 | 230 | 220 | 260 |
| 2666 | **Tomatoes** | 120 | 170 | 180 | 40 | 40 | 110 | 80 | 140 | 50 | 130 | 130 | 90 | 150 | 720 | — | 110 | 100 | 160 |
| 2669 | **Turnips** | 160 | 260 | 120 | 70 | — | 130 | 90 | 180 | 80 | 160 | 100 | 50 | 290 | 360 | 580 | 160 | 220 | 210 |
| 2671 | **Turnip tops** | 210 | 420 | 310 | 90 | 80 | 280 | 170 | 250 | 80 | 270 | 240 | 110 | 330 | 490 | 680 | 270 | 250 | 230 |
| 2673 | **Yam** | 220 | 380 | 260 | 90 | 80 | 290 | 200 | 210 | 80 | 270 | 480 | 120 | 270 | 660 | 780 | 220 | 230 | 320 |
| | ***Fruit*** | | | | | | | | | | | | | | | | | | |
| 2675 | **Apples** | 220 | 390 | 370 | 50 | 80 | 160 | 90 | 230 | 60 | 250 | 170 | 120 | 280 | 1300 | 700 | 240 | 200 | 270 |
| 2682 | **Apricots** | 110 | 180 | 180 | 30 | — | 100 | 80 | 130 | 50 | 150 | 80 | 100 | 220 | 1470 | 370 | 110 | 170 | 180 |
| 2692 | **Avocado pears** | 210 | 340 | 310 | 100 | — | 220 | 140 | 180 | 70 | 290 | 210 | 110 | 380 | 1410 | 770 | 250 | 240 | 260 |
| 2693 | **Bananas** | 250 | 320 | 270 | 80 | 170 | 260 | 160 | 190 | 70 | 260 | 360 | 380 | 280 | 660 | 580 | 260 | 260 | 240 |
| 2724 | **Dates** | 140 | 270 | 170 | 80 | 130 | 180 | 90 | 170 | 170 | 200 | 210 | 90 | 290 | 370 | 650 | 280 | 360 | 210 |
| 2726 | **Figs** | 190 | 270 | 250 | 50 | 100 | 150 | 270 | 200 | 50 | 240 | 140 | 90 | 380 | 1500 | 600 | 210 | 410 | 310 |
| 2736 | **Grapes** | 50 | 130 | 140 | 210 | 100 | 130 | 110 | 170 | 30 | 170 | 460 | 230 | 260 | 760 | 1300 | 190 | 210 | 300 |
| 2762 | **Melons, Canteloupe** | — | — | 160 | 20 | — | 190 | — | — | 10 | — | — | — | — | — | — | — | — | — |
| 2766 | **watermelon** | — | — | — | — | — | 150 | 150 | — | — | — | — | — | — | — | — | — | — | — |
| 2773 | **Oranges** | 180 | 170 | 330 | 90 | 80 | 230 | 130 | 90 | 40 | 240 | 400 | 90 | 390 | 880 | 760 | 640 | 350 | 180 |
| 2779 | **Peaches** | 100 | 220 | 230 | 240 | 70 | 140 | 160 | 210 | 30 | 310 | 130 | 130 | 310 | 710 | 1100 | 120 | 210 | 260 |
| 2785 | **Pears** | — | — | — | — | — | 150 | 240 | — | — | — | — | — | — | — | — | — | — | — |
| 2791 | **Pineapple** | — | — | 140 | 20 | — | 160 | 160 | — | 80 | — | — | — | — | — | — | — | — | — |
| 2817 | **Strawberries** | 140 | 320 | 250 | 10 | 50 | 180 | 210 | 190 | 70 | 180 | 270 | 120 | 320 | 1400 | 920 | 250 | 200 | 240 |

## **Amino acids** (mg per g nitrogen)

| No | Food | | Ile | Leu | Lys | Met | Cys | Phe | Tyr | Thr | Trp | Val | Arg | His | Ala | Asp | Glu | Gly | Pro | Ser |
|---|---|---|---|---|---|---|---|---|---|---|---|---|---|---|---|---|---|---|---|---|
| | ***Nuts*** | | | | | | | | | | | | | | | | | | | |
| 2822 | **Almonds** | | 220 | 390 | 140 | 80 | 90 | 300 | 180 | 150 | 50 | 320 | 610 | 140 | 240 | 590 | 1370 | 330 | 300 | 220 |
| 2826 | **Brazil nuts** | | 180 | 430 | 170 | 360 | 130 | 240 | 170 | 160 | 70 | 270 | 830 | 140 | 220 | 460 | 1160 | 280 | 300 | 270 |
| 2830 | **Cob** or **hazel nuts** | | 360 | 390 | 180 | 60 | 70 | 230 | 230 | 180 | 90 | 390 | 910 | 120 | — | 440 | 1280 | 590 | 350 | 600 |
| 2832 | **Coconut** | | 240 | 420 | 220 | 110 | 100 | 280 | 170 | 210 | 70 | 340 | 820 | 130 | 280 | 550 | 1170 | 280 | 230 | 300 |
| 2835 | **Peanuts** | | 210 | 400 | 220 | 70 | 80 | 310 | 240 | 160 | 70 | 260 | 700 | 150 | 240 | 710 | 1140 | 350 | 270 | 300 |
| 2838 | **Peanut butter** | * | 230 | 420 | 210 | 80 | 80 | 310 | 210 | 160 | 90 | 280 | 750 | 150 | 280 | 760 | 1240 | 360 | 290 | 360 |
| 2839 | **Walnuts** | | 250 | 450 | 120 | 90 | 110 | 270 | 210 | 190 | 60 | 300 | 790 | 130 | — | — | — | — | — | — |
| | ***Confectionery*** | | | | | | | | | | | | | | | | | | | |
| 2857 | **Chocolate** milk | * | 400 | 680 | 480 | 160 | 80 | 410 | 200 | 300 | 120 | 440 | 270 | 220 | 280 | 550 | 1390 | 180 | 660 | 440 |
| 2858 | plain | * | 240 | 400 | 260 | 120 | 120 | 340 | 130 | 260 | 90 | 360 | 400 | 120 | 290 | 620 | 1160 | 260 | 350 | 330 |
| | ***Beverages*** | | | | | | | | | | | | | | | | | | | |
| 2868 | **Cocoa powder** | * | 180 | 290 | 190 | 80 | 100 | 210 | 140 | 190 | 80 | 280 | 340 | 80 | 220 | 480 | 820 | 210 | 280 | 280 |
| 2872 | **Coffee** instant | * | 110 | 250 | 20 | 90 | 30 | 160 | 100 | 80 | 80 | 170 | 0 | 70 | 180 | 290 | 910 | 230 | 170 | 70 |
| | ***Beers*** | | | | | | | | | | | | | | | | | | | |
| 2895 | **Keg** bitter | * | 90 | 180 | 140 | 60 | 140 | 140 | 160 | 170 | 190 | 180 | 190 | 120 | 250 | 350 | 1050 | 270 | 890 | 210 |
| 2896 | **Lager** | * | 100 | 180 | 230 | 80 | 130 | 140 | 150 | 180 | 410 | 180 | 180 | 120 | 270 | 350 | 1190 | 290 | 880 | 240 |

## **Amino acids** (mg per g nitrogen)

| No | Food | | Ile | Leu | Lys | Met | Cys | Phe | Tyr | Thr | Trp | Val | Arg | His | Ala | Asp | Glu | Gly | Pro | Ser |
|---|---|---|---|---|---|---|---|---|---|---|---|---|---|---|---|---|---|---|---|---|
| | ***Miscellaneous*** | | | | | | | | | | | | | | | | | | | |
| 2957 | **Bovril** | * | 160 | 290 | 330 | 80 | 20 | 190 | 110 | 220 | 30 | 250 | 350 | 140 | 480 | 440 | 750 | 710 | 530[a] | 240 |
| 2959 | **Gelatin** | | 90 | 180 | 250 | 50 | Tr | 130 | 20 | 120 | 0 | 140 | 490 | 40 | 610 | 370 | 630 | 1510 | 860[b] | 230 |
| 2961 | **Marmite** | * | 290 | 360 | 430 | 80 | 60 | 240 | 110 | 310 | 80 | 370 | 160 | 140 | 410 | 580 | 780 | 310 | 300 | 310 |
| 2968 | **Yeast** | | 310 | 450 | 510 | 110 | 60 | 270 | 230 | 300 | 70 | 400 | 320 | 180 | 400 | 620 | 670 | 290 | 260 | 340 |

[a] Also contains 340 mg hydroxyproline    [b] Also contains 730 mg hydroxyproline

# The tables

*continued*

## Section 3
## Fatty acid composition

g fatty acids per 100g total fatty acids

*Common names of the most frequently occurring fatty acids*

| Carbon : Double bonds | Common name |
|---|---|
| Saturated | |
| C4 : 0 | Butyric |
| C6 : 0 | Caproic |
| C8 : 0 | Caprylic |
| C10 : 0 | Capric |
| C12 : 0 | Lauric |
| C14 : 0 | Myristic |
| C16 : 0 | Palmitic |
| C18 : 0 | Stearic |
| C20 : 0 | Arachidic |
| C22 : 0 | Behenic |
| C24 : 0 | Lignoceric |
| Mono-unsaturated | |
| C16 : 1 | Palmitoleic |
| C18 : 1 | Oleic |
| C20 : 1 | Eicosenoic |
| C22 : 1 | Erucic |
| Polyunsaturated | |
| C18 : 2 | Linoleic |
| C18 : 3 | Linolenic |
| C20 : 4 | Arachidonic |

**Asterisk indicates new analytical data**

| No | Food | | Saturated | | | | | | Mono-unsaturated | | | | Polyunsaturated | | | |
|---|---|---|---|---|---|---|---|---|---|---|---|---|---|---|---|---|
| | | | 10:0 | 12:0 | 14:0 | 16:0 | 18:0 | 20:0 | 16:1 | 18:1 | 20:1 | 22:1 | 18:2 | 18:3 | 20:4 | Other |
| 3002 | **Barley** | | 0 | Tr | 0.4 | 23.6 | 0.7 | 0 | 0.1 | 11.8 | Tr | 0 | 57.4 | 6.1 | 0 | |
| 3005 | **Bran** wheat | | 0 | Tr | Tr | 18.4 | 1.0 | 0.8 | 0.5 | 15.3 | 0.4 | 0 | 59.4 | 4.1 | 0.2 | |
| 3008 | **Flour** wholemeal, brown and white | | 0 | Tr | Tr | 18.4 | 1.0 | 0.8 | 0.5 | 15.3 | 0.4 | 0 | 59.4 | 4.1 | 0.2 | |
| 3017 | **Oatmeal** | | 0 | Tr | Tr | 17.0 | 1.1 | 0.5 | 0.2 | 38.4 | Tr | 0 | 40.7 | 2.2 | Tr | |
| 3019 | **Rice** | | 0 | Tr | 0.9 | 24.0 | 2.5 | 0.4 | 0.1 | 29.6 | 0 | 0 | 41.2 | 1.1 | Tr | |
| 3021 | **Rye** | | 0 | Tr | Tr | 18.8 | 0.6 | Tr | 0.5 | 13.7 | 0.8 | 0 | 56.8 | 8.8 | 0 | |
| 3030 | **Bread** wholemeal | * | 0 | Tr | 1.7 | 19.2 | 4.2 | Tr | 1.9 | 16.9 | Tr | 0 | 50.2 | 3.6 | Tr | |
| 3033 | white | * | 0 | 0.7 | 1.6 | 23.0 | 5.0 | Tr | 1.1 | 17.7 | Tr | 0 | 45.4 | 3.3 | Tr | |
| | ***Biscuits*** | | | | | | | | | | | | | | | |
| 3058 | **chocolate** full coated [a] | * | 1.0 | 10.7 | 5.1 | 25.7 | 20.1 | 0.5 | 0.7 | 29.4 | 0.3 | 0 | 4.1 | 0.2 | 0 | |
| 3060 | **crispbread** rye | * | 0 | 0.2 | 0.2 | 18.2 | 0.7 | 0 | 0.5 | 14.8 | 1.6 | 0 | 56.2 | 7.2 | 0 | |
| 3061 | wheat, starch reduced [a] | * | 0 | 0.6 | 0.9 | 32.4 | 3.3 | 0.2 | 0.3 | 27.4 | 0.6 | 0 | 32.7 | 1.6 | 0 | |
| 3063 | **digestive** chocolate [a] | * | 0 | 0.6 | 2.2 | 31.1 | 17.7 | 0.9 | 1.0 | 35.2 | 1.6 | 1.6 | 6.6 | 0.2 | 0 | |
| 3064 | **ginger nuts** [a] | * | 0 | 1.1 | 2.8 | 35.8 | 9.2 | 0.6 | 1.6 | 36.6 | 1.0 | 0.8 | 9.1 | 0.5 | 0 | |
| 3066 | **Matzo** | * | 0 | 0.8 | 0.3 | 20.3 | 0.7 | 0 | 0.2 | 10.0 | 0.8 | 0 | 62.6 | 4.0 | 0 | |
| 3067 | **oatcakes** [a] | * | 0 | 0.3 | 1.9 | 15.4 | 4.3 | 0.6 | 1.4 | 38.1 | 4.2 | 3.1 | 27.2 | 2.4 | 0 | |
| 3068 | **sandwich** [a] | * | 1.5 | 14.0 | 5.9 | 26.9 | 8.5 | 0.4 | 0.7 | 31.0 | — | 0.5 | 6.0 | 0 | — | 8:0 1.4<br>20:1–20:5 1.4 |
| 3069 | **semi-sweet** [a] | * | 0 | 2.2 | 3.1 | 35.5 | 8.8 | 0.6 | 1.2 | 35.6 | — | 0.5 | 9.4 | 0 | — | 20:1–20:5 1.4 |
| 3070 | **short-sweet** [a] | * | 0 | 3.0 | 3.8 | 36.5 | 8.2 | 0.9 | 1.4 | 34.0 | — | 0 | 8.2 | 0.5 | — | 20:1–20:5 2.2 |
| 3072 | **wafers** filled [a] | * | 2.8 | 28.7 | 10.5 | 14.4 | 5.1 | 0 | 0.3 | 28.5 | 0 | 0 | 3.1 | 0 | 0 | 10:0 3.4 |

[a] The composition may vary according to type of fat used in the manufacture of the biscuits

| No | Food | | Saturated | | | | | | | Mono-unsaturated | | | | Polyunsaturated | | | Other |
|---|---|---|---|---|---|---|---|---|---|---|---|---|---|---|---|---|---|
| | | | 8:0 | 10:0 | 12:0 | 14:0 | 16:0 | 18:0 | 20:0 | 16:1 | 18:1 | 20:1 | 22:1 | 18:2 | 18:3 | 20:4 | |
| | ***Cakes*** | | | | | | | | | | | | | | | | |
| 3074 | **Fancy iced cakes** [a] | * | 2.5 | 2.1 | 21.6 | 9.4 | 18.1 | 11.9 | Tr | 2.6 | 20.5 | 1.6 | 3.1 | 5.1 | 0.7 | 0 | |
| 3077 | **Fruit cake** plain [a] | * | 0 | 0 | 0.5 | 5.2 | 30.6 | 10.0 | 0.8 | 6.4 | 29.4 | 4.0 | 2.4 | 8.5 | 0.7 | 0 | |
| 3079 | **Madeira cake** [a] | * | 1.7 | 1.6 | 10.1 | 8.3 | 22.7 | 9.1 | 0.7 | 4.9 | 22.8 | 2.8 | 4.6 | 9.1 | 0 | 0 | 22:0 0.6 |
| 3083 | **Spongecake** jam filled [a] | * | 0 | 0 | Tr | 3.4 | 25.7 | 10.1 | 0.8 | 4.6 | 26.0 | 3.3 | 7.3 | 14.0 | 2.9 | Tr | |
| | ***Puddings*** | | | | | | | | | | | | | | | | |
| 3108 | **Ice cream** non-dairy [a] | * | 0 | 0 | Tr | 2.5 | 43.2 | 7.6 | Tr | 0.8 | 35.0 | 1.7 | 1.1 | 7.1 | 0 | 0 | |

[a] The composition may vary according to type of fat used in the manufacture of these foods

| | | | Saturated | | | | | | | | Mono-unsaturated | | | Polyunsaturated | | |
|---|---|---|---|---|---|---|---|---|---|---|---|---|---|---|---|---|
| No | Food | | 4:0 | 6:0 | 8:0 | 10:0 | 12:0 | 14:0 | 16:0 | 18:0 | 14:1 | 16:1 | 18:1 | 18:2 | 18:3 | Other |
| 3107 | **Ice cream** dairy | * | 2.9 | 2.0 | 1.1 | 2.8 | 3.7 | 10.7 | 31.8 | 12.4 | 0.8 | 1.8 | 23.7 | 1.6 | 1.0 | 15:0 1.1<br>17:0 0.5<br>17:1 1.0 |
| 3123 | **Milk, cows'** | | 3.2<br>*(2.6–3.9)* | 2.0<br>*(1.5–2.3)* | 1.2<br>*(0.9–1.4)* | 2.8<br>*(2.5–3.2)* | 3.5<br>*(3.1–4.0)* | 11.2<br>*(10.4–12.4)* | 26.0<br>*(24.1–32.0)* | 11.2<br>*(9.2–13.2)* | 1.4<br>*(1.1–1.6)* | 2.7<br>*(2.1–3.1)* | 27.8<br>*(22.0–30.7)* | 1.4<br>*(0.8–1.9)* | 1.5<br>*(0.6–2.5)* | 15:0 1.1<br>15:1 0.7<br>17:0 1.0<br>17:1 1.1 |
| 3137 | **Milk, goats'** | | 2.1 | 2.4 | 3.2 | 9.1 | 4.5 | 11.3 | 27.0 | 9.6 | Tr | 2.4 | 26.0 | 2.3 | — | |
| 3138 | **Milk, human** | * | 0 | 0 | Tr | 1.4<br>*(0.5–2.0)* | 5.4<br>*(3.3–8.2)* | 7.3<br>*(5.6–8.5)* | 26.5<br>*(20.2–26.8)* | 9.5<br>*(4.7–10.3)* | Tr | 4.0<br>*(2.4–5.7)* | 35.4<br>*(35.4–46.4)* | 7.2<br>*(4.1–13.0)* | 0.8<br>*(0.4–3.4)* | 17:1 0.6<br>20:1 0.5 |
| 3165 | **Eggs** | | 0 | 0 | 0 | 0 | 0 | Tr | 28.6 | 9.3 | Tr | 4.2 | 42.9 | 11.1 | Tr | 20:4 0.8<br>22:6 1.2 |

| | | Saturated | | | | | | Mono-unsaturated | | | | Polyunsaturated | | | | |
|---|---|---|---|---|---|---|---|---|---|---|---|---|---|---|---|---|
| No | Food | 12:0 | 14:0 | 16:0 | 18:0 | 20:0 | 22:0 | 16:1 | 18:1 | 20:1 | 22:1 | 18:2 | 18:3 | 20:4 20:5 | 22:5 22:6 | Other |
| 3183 | **Compound cooking fat** [a] | 0.4 | 6.2 | 22.2 | 8.5 | 2.6 | 2.2 | 6.5 | 19.5 | 8.0 | 8.3 | 5.0 | 0.5 | 6.3 | 3.0 | |
| 3184 | **Dripping, beef** | Tr | 3.2 | 26.9 | 13.0 | Tr | 0 | 6.3 | 42.0 | 0 | 0 | 2.0 | 1.3 | 1.0[b] | 0 | 14:1 1.5<br>15:0 0.6<br>17:0 1.2<br>17:1 1.0 |
| 3185 | **Lard** | Tr | 1.6 | 26.8 | 15.6 | Tr | 0 | 2.5 | 40.7 | 0.8 | 0 | 8.7 | 0.8 | Tr | 0 | 17:0 0.2 |
| 6186 | **Low fat spread** [a] | 5.8 | 2.9 | 13.7 | 4.8 | 0.5 | 0.5 | 0.6 | 31.2 | 1.9 | 6.2 | 27.7 | 2.8 | 0.5 | Tr | |
| | ***Margarine*** [a] | | | | | | | | | | | | | | | |
| 3188 | **hard** animal and vegetable oils | 0.3 | 5.8 | 19.6 | 7.8 | 2.0 | 2.0 | 5.8 | 21.6 | 8.5 | 8.8 | 4.6 | 0.2 | 7.2 | 4.0 | 17:0 1.0 |
| 3189 | vegetable oils only | 0.1 | 1.2 | 28.0 | 7.4 | 1.0 | 0.5 | 1.2 | 42.6 | 1.6 | 3.5 | 9.9 | 0.5 | 1.2 | 1.0 | 17:0 0.3 |
| 3190 | **soft** animal and vegetable oils | 1.0 | 4.5 | 15.7 | 5.3 | 1.7 | 2.5 | 5.5 | 25.7 | 6.5 | 9.4 | 8.8 | 0.4 | 6.7 | 4.5 | 17:0 0.9 |
| 3191 | vegetable oils only | 1.5 | 1.4 | 23.7 | 5.2 | 0.8 | 0.5 | 1.4 | 36.9 | 1.4 | 3.8 | 21.1 | 2.0 | Tr | Tr | |
| 3192 | **polyunsaturated** vegetable oils only | 2.6 | 1.4 | 10.8 | 8.7 | 0.5 | 0.7 | 0.4 | 18.8 | 0.6 | 0.7 | 53.7 | 0.7 | 0.2 | Tr | |
| 3194 | **Suet** shredded * | Tr | 3.3 | 27.8 | 26.6 | Tr | 0 | 2.2 | 34.3 | Tr | 0 | 1.3 | 0 | Tr | Tr | 15:0 0.5<br>17:0 1.2<br>15:1 0.6<br>17:1 1.6 |

[a] As these products are made from a mixture of oils and fats, the composition may vary throughout the year depending on raw materials
[b] Only 20:4

| No | Food | Saturated | | | | | | | Mono-unsaturated | | | | Poly-unsaturated | |
|---|---|---|---|---|---|---|---|---|---|---|---|---|---|---|
| | | 12:0 | 14:0 | 16:0 | 18:0 | 20:0 | 22:0 | 24:0 | 16:1 | 18:1 | 20:1 | 22:1 | 18:2 | 18:3 |
| | ***Vegetable oils*** | | | | | | | | | | | | | |
| 3196 | **coconut**[a] | 47.7 *(44–51)* | 15.8 | 9.0 | 2.4 | 1.0 | 0 | 0 | 0.4 | 6.6 | 0 | 0 | 1.8 | 0 |
| 3197 | **cottonseed** | 0.4 | 0.8 | 23.0 *(15–28)* | 2.4 | 0.2 | Tr | Tr | 1.3 | 21.0 *(13–27)* | Tr | Tr | 49.0 *(33–64)* | 1.4 |
| 3198 | **maize, corn** | 0 | 0.6 | 14.0 *(6–22)* | 2.3 | 0.3 | Tr | Tr | 0.3 | 30.0 *(19–50)* | 0.2 | 0.2 | 50.0 *(34–62)* | 1.6 |
| 3199 | **olive** | 0 | Tr | 12.0 *(7–20)* | 2.3 | 0.4 | 0 | 0 | 1.0 | 72.0 *(65–85)* | 0 | 0 | 11.0 *(4–20)* | 0.7 |
| 3200 | **palm** | 0.2 | 1.1 | 41.5 *(32–51)* | 4.3 | 0.3 | 0 | 0 | 0.3 | 43.3 *(35–52)* | 0 | 0 | 8.4 *(5–12)* | 0.3 |
| 3201 | **peanut, groundnut, arachis** | 0.1 | 0.5 | 10.7 *(6–15)* | 2.7 | 1.2 | 3.4 | 1.1 | Tr | 49.0 *(35–72)* | 1.1 | Tr | 29.0 *(13–45)* | 0.8 |
| 3202 | **rapeseed** high erucic acid | 0 | Tr | 3.5 | 1.0 | 0.8 | 0.2 | 0.1 | 0.2 | 24.1 *(3–45)* | 10.0 *(3–15)* | 33.0 *(12–61)* | 15.5 *(11–29)* | 10.5 *(5–16)* |
| 3203 | low erucic acid | 0 | Tr | 4.5 | 1.2 | 0.8 | 0.3 | 0.1 | 2.4 | 54.0 *(43–70)* | 1.5 | 2.0 *(0–11)* | 23.0 *(15–31)* | 10.0 *(6–15)* |
| 3204 | **safflowerseed** | 0 | Tr | 8.0 | 2.5 | 0.2 | Tr | 0 | 0.1 | 13.0 *(7–42)* | 0.1 | 0 | 75.0 *(55–81)* | 0.5 |
| 3205 | **soyabean** | 0.1 | 0.2 | 10.0 *(6–19)* | 4.0 | 0.3 | 0.1 | Tr | 0.2 | 25.0 *(14–35)* | 0.2 | Tr | 52.0 *(40–62)* | 7.4 *(4–11)* |
| 3206 | **sunflowerseed** | 0 | 0.1 | 5.8 | 6.3 *(0.2–12)* | 0.6 | 0.7 | 0.2 | 0.1 | 33.0 *(5–60)* | 0.2 | Tr | 52.0 *(17–78)* | 0.3 |

[a] 8:0 7.5, 10:0 7.1

| No | Food | | Saturated | | | | | Mono-unsaturated | | | | Polyunsaturated | | | | | | Other | |
|---|---|---|---|---|---|---|---|---|---|---|---|---|---|---|---|---|---|---|---|
| | | | 14:0 | 15:0 | 16:0 | 17:0 | 18:0 | 16:1 | 17:1 | 18:1 | 20:1 | 18:2 | 18:3 | 20:3 | 20:4 | 20:5 | 22:5 | | |
| 3209 | **Bacon** | * | 1.6 | Tr | 27.4 | Tr | 14.3 | 3.5 | Tr | 43.8 | 0.6 | 7.2 | 0.6 | 0 | Tr | Tr | 0 | | |
| 3240 | **Beef** | | 3.2 | 0.6 | 26.9 | 1.2 | 13.0 | 6.3 | 1.0 | 42.0 | Tr | 2.0 | 1.3 | Tr | 1.0 | Tr | Tr | 14:1 | 1.5 |
| 3269 | **Lamb** | | 5.4 | 0.6 | 24.2 | 1.0 | 20.9 | 1.3 | 1.0 | 38.2 | Tr | 2.5 | 2.5 | 0 | 0 | Tr | Tr | | |
| 3299 | **Pork** [a] | | 1.6 | Tr | 27.1 | Tr | 13.8 | 3.4 | Tr | 43.8 | 0.7 | 7.4 | 0.9 | 0 | Tr | Tr | Tr | | |
| 3314 | **Chicken** [a] | * | 1.3 | Tr | 26.7 | Tr | 7.1 | 7.2 | Tr | 39.8 | 0.6 | 13.5 | 0.7 | Tr | 0.7 | | Tr | 22:6 | 1.0 |
| 3328 | **Duck** | * | 0.6 | Tr | 22.8 | Tr | 5.5 | 4.4 | Tr | 52.8 | Tr | 12.1 | 0.6 | Tr | Tr | Tr | Tr | | |
| 3332 | **Grouse** | | 0.6 | 0.1 | 16.7 | 1.5 | 5.7 | 1.9 | 0.3 | 10.7 | 0.1 | 31.9 | 30.3 | Tr | Tr | Tr | Tr | | |
| 3334 | **Partridge** | | 0.9 | 0.1 | 21.0 | 1.8 | 3.8 | 7.6 | 1.8 | 39.8 | 0.1 | 15.5 | 9.6 | Tr | Tr | Tr | Tr | | |
| 3336 | **Pheasant** | | 1.0 | 0.1 | 28.1 | 0.1 | 5.9 | 11.4 | 0.1 | 40.4 | 0.1 | 6.1 | 6.7 | Tr | Tr | Tr | Tr | | |
| 3340 | **Turkey** [a] | | 1.0 | Tr | 25.0 | 0.5 | 10.0 | 5.0 | Tr | 21.5 | 0.4 | 20.0 | 1.0 | Tr | 5.0 | 1.5 | 2.0 | 22:6 | 5.0 |
| 3350 | **Rabbit** | * | 2.6 | 0.7 | 30.0 | 0.8 | 9.2 | 2.1 | Tr | 18.7 | Tr | 20.9 | 9.9 | Tr | 1.9 | 0 | 1.3 | | |
| | ***Offal*** | | | | | | | | | | | | | | | | | | |
| 3356 | **Brain, lamb** | * | 0.8 | 0.5 | 21.5 | 0.5 | 18.1 | 1.4 | 1.9 [b] | 28.4 | 3.3 | 0.4 | 0 | 1.5 | 4.2 | 0.7 | 3.4 | 22:1 | 0.6 |
| | | | | | | | | | | | | | | | | | | 22:4 | 0.8 |
| | | | | | | | | | | | | | | | | | | 22:6 | 9.5 |
| 3358 | **Heart, lamb** | * | 3.3 | 0.5 | 19.7 | 1.1 | 24.2 | 2.1 | 2.4 | 33.1 | Tr | 7.3 | 2.7 | Tr | 2.1 | | Tr | | |
| 3360 | **ox** | * | 3.3 | 0.8 | 27.4 | 1.3 | 29.2 | 1.9 | 1.8 | 29.2 | Tr | 2.5 | 0.5 | Tr | 0.7 | | Tr | 15:1 | 0.6 |
| 3364 | **Kidney, lamb** | * | 2.3 | Tr | 19.9 | 1.0 | 22.2 | 2.1 | 1.3 [b] | 28.2 | Tr | 8.1 | 4.0 | 0.5 | 7.1 | Tr | Tr | | |
| 3366 | **ox** | * | 2.7 | 0.7 | 25.0 | 1.0 | 26.9 | 2.0 | 1.4 [b] | 31.0 | Tr | 4.8 | 0.5 | Tr | 2.6 | Tr | Tr | 15:1 | 0.6 |
| 3368 | **pig** | * | 1.0 | Tr | 24.8 | Tr | 17.7 | 2.0 | Tr | 32.3 | 0.5 | 11.7 | 0.5 | 0.6 | 6.7 | Tr | Tr | | |
| 3371 | **Liver, calf** | * | 0.8 | Tr | 16.5 | 0.6 | 23.3 | 1.9 | 0.7 | 20.8 | Tr | 15.0 | 1.4 | 2.1 | 9.0 | 0.3 | 4.0 | 22:6 | 2.5 |
| 3373 | **chicken** | * | 0.5 | 0 | 24.6 | Tr | 17.0 | 3.2 | Tr | 26.3 | Tr | 14.8 | 0.6 | 0.7 | 5.5 | 0 | 0.9 | 22:6 | 4.8 |
| 3375 | **lamb** | * | 1.3 | 0.5 | 20.4 | 1.0 | 18.3 | 3.5 | 1.6 | 29.7 | 0 | 5.0 | 3.8 | 0.6 | 5.1 | 0 | 3.0 | 15:1 [c] | 0.5 |
| | | | | | | | | | | | | | | | | | | 22:6 | 2.4 |
| 3377 | **ox** | * | 0.9 | 0.8 | 17.2 | 0.6 | 30.1 | 1.4 | 1.2 | 18.2 | 0 | 7.4 | 2.5 | 4.6 | 6.4 | 0.7 | 5.6 | 15:1 | 0.8 |
| | | | | | | | | | | | | | | | | | | 22:6 | 1.2 |
| 3379 | **pig** | * | Tr | Tr | 17.7 | 0.5 | 23.4 | 1.7 | Tr | 19.2 | Tr | 14.7 | 0.5 | 1.3 | 14.3 | 0 | 2.3 | 22:6 | 3.8 |

[a] The fatty acid composition varies according to the diet fed to the animal

[b] Includes branch chain C17

[c] Also contains 3.2 g C18: unidentified polyunsaturated fatty acids

| No | Food | | Saturated | | | | | Mono-unsaturated | | | | Polyunsaturated | | | | |
|---|---|---|---|---|---|---|---|---|---|---|---|---|---|---|---|---|
| | | | 14:0 | 15:0 | 16:0 | 17:0 | 18:0 | 16:1 | 17:1 | 18:1 | 20:1 | 18:2 | 18:3 | 20:4 | 20:5 | Other |
| | ***Offal** contd* | | | | | | | | | | | | | | | |
| 3384 | **Sweetbread, lamb** | * | 4.9 | 0.6 | 21.7 | 1.1 | 22.4 | 2.6 | 1.3 | 37.1 | Tr | 2.1 | 2.2 | 1.3 | Tr | 12:0 0.7 |
| 3391 | **Tripe, ox** | * | 2.8 | 0.9 | 23.4 | 1.3 | 30.5 | 2.2 | 1.5 | 33.3 | 0 | 1.5 | 0.6 | Tr | Tr | 15:1 1.0 |
| | ***Canned meats*** | | | | | | | | | | | | | | | |
| 3394 | **Ham** | * | 1.5 | Tr | 26.1 | Tr | 11.6 | 3.8 | Tr | 44.4 | 0.6 | 9.5 | Tr | 0.9 | | |
| 3395 | **Ham and pork** chopped | * | 1.6 | Tr | 25.0 | Tr | 12.5 | 3.4 | Tr | 45.6 | 0.8 | 9.6 | 0.5 | 0.3 | | |
| 3396 | **Luncheon meat** | * | 1.9 | Tr | 26.7 | 0.3 | 11.5 | 3.8 | 0.4 | 45.0 | 1.1 | 7.8 | 0.7 | 0.2 | | 20:3 0.1 |
| | | | | | | | | | | | | | | | | 22:5 0.3 |
| 3399 | **Tongue, lamb** | * | 2.7 | 0.5 | 19.7 | 1.0 | 16.9 | 2.9 | 1.4 | 46.2 | 0 | 4.0 | 3.4 | Tr | | |
| | ***Sausages*** | | | | | | | | | | | | | | | |
| 3404 | **Liver sausage** | * | 1.6 | Tr | 25.4 | Tr | 12.3 | 3.9 | Tr | 44.7 | 0.8 | 9.1 | 0.5 | Tr | | |
| 3408 | **Sausages**, beef | * | 3.6 | Tr | 25.5 | 0.5 | 14.8 | 4.2 | 0.9 | 44.0 | Tr | 3.9 | 1.1 | 0 | | |
| 3411 | pork | * | 1.9 | Tr | 25.8 | Tr | 13.6 | 3.6 | Tr | 45.4 | 0.5 | 7.7 | 0.6 | 0 | | |
| | ***Other products*** | | | | | | | | | | | | | | | |
| 3425 | **Steak and kidney pie** individual | * | 3.1 | Tr | 25.7 | Tr | 14.0 | 3.3 | Tr | 37.3 | 1.3 | 10.0 | 0.9 | Tr | | 20:0 0.6 |
| | | | | | | | | | | | | | | | | 22:0 0.5 |
| | | | | | | | | | | | | | | | | 22:1 1.1 |

| No | Food | Saturated 14:0 | 15:0 | 16:0 | 17:0 | 18:0 | Mono-unsaturated 16:1 | 18:1 | 20:1 | 22:1 | Polyunsaturated 18:2 | 18:3 | 18:4 | 20:4 | 20:5 | 22:5 | 22:6 | Other |
|---|---|---|---|---|---|---|---|---|---|---|---|---|---|---|---|---|---|---|
| | ***White fish*** | | | | | | | | | | | | | | | | | |
| 3438 | **Cod** raw | 0.9 | 0.2 | 21.5 | Tr | 3.5 | 2.3 | 11.0 | 1.8 | 0.8 | 0.5 | 0.1 | 0.2 | 3.9 | 17.2 | 1.5 | 33.4 | |
| 3451 | **Haddock** raw | 1.5 | 0.5 | 20.0 | 1.5 | 6.1 | 4.0 | 14.2 | 2.6 | 0.1 | 2.2 | 0.4 | 0.5 | 3.3 | 12.0 | 2.4 | 24.5 | 22:4 1.8 |
| 3458 | **Halibut** raw | 2.8 | 0.3 | 10.3 | 0.8 | 2.4 | 8.1 | 17.5 | 6.1 | Tr | 1.6 | 3.5 | 1.9 | 8.5[a] | 10.3 | 4.9 | 15.0 | 17:1 0.5<br>20:2 0.5<br>22:4 2.3 |
| 3461 | **Lemon sole** raw | 2.7 | 0.8 | 12.5 | 0.8 | 3.3 | 8.1 | 13.2 | 4.8 | 1.3 | 0.5 | 0.5 | 1.7 | 30.3 (20:4 and 20:5 bracketed together) | | 3.4 | 11.2 | 17:1 1.8 |
| 3466 | **Plaice** raw | 3.5 | 0.5 | 16.4 | 0.4 | 2.6 | 14.7 | 17.9 | 3.7 | 2.2 | 0.7 | 0.7 | 2.1 | 16.3 | | 3.6 | 10.3 | 16:2 1.1<br>17:1 1.0<br>20:3 0.7 |
| 3471 | **Saithe** raw | 1.4 | 0.2 | 9.9 | 0.2 | 5.3 | 3.7 | 20.5 | 5.1 | 6.2 | 1.1 | 0.6 | 0.7 | 13.9 | | 1.8 | 27.1 | 17:1 1.6 |
| 3474 | **Whiting** raw | 2.7 | 0.3 | 13.3 | 0.2 | 3.9 | 5.2 | 20.8 | 7.9 | 6.3 | 1.5 | 0.5 | 1.8 | 12.3 | | 2.1 | 18.0 | 17:1 0.8 |
| | ***Fatty fish*** | | | | | | | | | | | | | | | | | |
| 3482 | **Herring** raw | 6.7 | 0.5 | 13.7 | 0.2 | 1.2 | 10.0 | 15.2 | 13.2 | 17.4 | 1.4 | 1.2 | 1.8 | 0.6 | 7.0 | 1.1 | 6.5 | |
| 3491 | **Mackerel** raw | 5.0 | 0.5 | 17.6 | 0.4 | 3.5 | 5.9 | 18.4 | 7.1 | 9.9 | 1.6 | 1.1 | 1.9 | 1.0 | 7.3 | 1.6 | 12.6 | 16:2 0.7<br>24:1 1.5 |
| 3494 | **Pilchards** canned in tomato sauce * | 8.6 | Tr | 20.1 | Tr | 6.4 | 11.3 | 12.4 | 1.1 | 0.5 | 1.2 | 0.6 | 1.5 | 0.6 | 21.5 | 2.5 | 4.1 | 16:2 5.2<br>20:3 0.8 |
| 3498 | **Salmon** canned * | 4.8 | Tr | 18.8 | Tr | 3.9 | 6.0 | 22.8 | 8.4 | 5.4 | 1.4 | 0.8 | 1.7 | 0.5 | 8.2 | 2.7 | 11.0 | 16:2 0.6<br>20:3 1.4 |
| 3501 | **Sardines** canned in oil (fish plus oil) * | 3.1 | Tr | 14.0 | Tr | 3.5 | 4.3 | 49.7 | 1.4 | 2.0 | 7.4 | 1.0 | 1.1 | 0 | 5.5 | 0.7 | 4.3 | 16:2 0.8 |
| 3502 | canned in tomato sauce * | 5.2 | Tr | 21.1 | Tr | 5.0 | 6.2 | 22.8 | 1.4 | 0.5 | 6.6 | 1.7 | 2.5 | 0 | 9.5 | 1.3 | 12.3 | 16:2 1.1<br>20:3 0.8 |
| 3503 | **Sprats** raw | 7.9 | 0.6 | 20.8 | 0.3 | 2.0 | 5.8 | 18.2 | 8.9 | 13.9 | 1.4 | 1.1 | 1.9 | 0.7 | 6.0 | 0.7 | 7.7 | 24:1 2.1 |
| 3508 | **Tuna** canned in oil * | Tr | 0 | 17.1 | Tr | 1.7 | Tr | 41.0 | Tr | 0 | 36.6 | 0.9 | 0 | Tr | Tr | 0 | 0.8 | |

[a] Includes 20:3

| No | Food | Saturated | | | | | Mono-unsaturated | | | | Polyunsaturated | | | | | | | Other |
|---|---|---|---|---|---|---|---|---|---|---|---|---|---|---|---|---|---|---|
| | | 14:0 | 15:0 | 16:0 | 17:0 | 18:0 | 16:1 | 18:1 | 20:1 | 22:1 | 18:2 | 18:3 | 18:4 | 20:4 | 20:5 | 22:5 | 22:6 | |
| | ***Cartilaginous fish*** | | | | | | | | | | | | | | | | | |
| 3510 | **Dogfish** raw | 1.7 | 0.5 | 15.4 | 0.3 | 2.2 | 6.3 | 20.1 | 6.7 | 4.9 | 1.7 | 1.1 | 1.4 | 11.8 (20:4 + 20:5) | | 2.9 | 20.3 | 17:1 1.1<br>20:3 1.2 |
| 3513 | **Skate** raw | 1.9 | 0.3 | 11.1 | 0.3 | 2.7 | 6.0 | 13.2 | 3.6 | 2.8 | 1.2 | 0.5 | 1.6 | 13.6 (20:4 + 20:5) | | 4.2 | 34.2 | 17:1 0.8<br>20:3 0.8 |
| | ***Crustacea*** | | | | | | | | | | | | | | | | | |
| 3517 | **Crab** raw | 1.4 | 0.7 | 9.2 | 1.2 | 4.3 | 5.0 | 15.0 | 3.5 | 3.9 | 3.2 | 4.6 | 2.3 | 0.6 | 21.5 | 1.4 | 10.2 | 16:2 2.9<br>20:2 2.4<br>22:3 1.6<br>22:4 1.1<br>24:6 1.0 |
| 3526 | **Shrimps** raw | 2.5 | 0.6 | 15.8 | 0.5 | 2.4 | 5.9 | 18.8 | 2.6 | 1.7 | 1.4 | 1.3 | 1.1 | 1.3 | 21.6 | 1.2 | 15.4 | 17:1 1.1<br>22:3 1.6<br>22:4 1.1 |
| | ***Molluscs***[a] | | | | | | | | | | | | | | | | | |
| 3532 | **Mussels** raw | 2.5 | 0.8 | 12.2 | 1.3 | 7.4 | 6.6 | 7.1 | 7.5 | 5.2 | 2.0 | 1.6 | 5.5 | 4.5 | 11.3 | 2.0 | 4.6 | 16:2 1.8<br>16:4 1.0<br>19:3 1.3<br>20:2 1.2<br>22:2 1.5<br>22:3 1.0<br>24:0 1.1 |

[a] These fish also contain small quantities (less than 1 per cent) of other branch chain and polyunsaturated fatty acids which are not listed here

| | | | | | | | | | | | | | | | | | | |
|---|---|---|---|---|---|---|---|---|---|---|---|---|---|---|---|---|---|---|
| | ***Molluscs** contd* | | | | | | | | | | | | | | | | | |
| 3535 | **Oysters** raw | 4.6 | 1.1 | 20.2 | 1.6 | 4.0 | 3.8 | 5.8 | 2.8 | 3.0 | 1.9 | 1.5 | 4.5 | 1.6 | 15.2 | 1.8 | 17.2 | 22:4 1.8 |
| 3537 | **Scallops** raw | 4.3 | 1.2 | 17.6 | 0.8 | 4.1 | 3.9 | 5.1 | 3.1 | 2.0 | 0.8 | 1.5 | 3.5 | 3.8 | 11.6 | 0.5 | 8.2 | 12:0 5.4<br>13:0 3.0<br>16:2 1.9<br>22:2 1.4<br>22:3 2.7 |
| | ***Fish products*** | | | | | | | | | | | | | | | | | |
| 3550 | **Roe, cod** hard, raw | 1.3 | 0.2 | 21.8 | — | 1.8 | 6.4 | 19.4 | 1.9 | 0.7 | 0.5 | 0.1 | 0.2 | 3.1 | 16.8 | 1.4 | 23.3 | |

## Vegetables and fruit

Fatty acids g per 100 g total fatty acids

| | | Saturated | | | | | | Mono-unsaturated | | | Polyunsaturated | | | |
|---|---|---|---|---|---|---|---|---|---|---|---|---|---|---|
| No | Food | 12:0 | 14:0 | 16:0 | 17:0 | 18:0 | 20:0 | 16:1 | 18:1 | 20:1 | 18:2 | 18:3 | 20:4 | Other |
| | ***Vegetables*** | | | | | | | | | | | | | |
| 3562 | **Beans, runner** | 0 | 0 | 21.8 | Tr | 4.0 | 0 | 0.5 | 3.6 | 0 | 28.2 | 40.0 | 0 | |
| 3569 | **baked** canned in tomato sauce | 0 | 0 | 19.3 | Tr | 2.0 | 0 | 0 | 12.1 | 0 | 24.9 | 38.1 | 0 | |
| 3597 | **Cucumber** | 0.2 | 0.8 | 36.8 | Tr | 3.7 | 0 | 0.2 | 3.2 | 0 | 29.0 | 26.3 | 0 | |
| 3609 | **Mushrooms** | 0 | 0.4 | 27.4 | Tr | 1.9 | 0 | 0.3 | 1.3 | 0 | 13.2 | 55.4 | 0 | |
| 3620 | **Peas** fresh | 0 | 2.4 | 29.7 | Tr | 14.6 | 0 | 2.6 | 36.3 | 0.5 | 10.9 | 3.1 | 0 | |
| 3634 | **Peppers, green** | 0.1 | 2.9 | 15.4 | Tr | 4.2 | 0.1 | 0.5 | 7.3 | 0 | 56.3 | 12.0 | 0 | |
| 3639 | **Potatoes** | 0 | 0 | 17.8 | Tr | 5.4 | 0 | 1.3 | 1.9 | 0 | 56.5 | 17.2 | 0 | |
| 3657 | **Spinach** | 0 | 1.0 | 12.1 | Tr | — | 0 | 1.9 | 7.3 | 0 | 12.5 | 62.1 | 0 | |
| 3664 | **Sweet potatoes** | 5.5 | 0.7 | 35.0 | 1.5 | 3.4 | 1.2 | 1.5 | 6.7 | 0 | 34.3 | 6.9 | 0 | 10:0 1.5 |
| 3669 | **Turnips** | 0 | 0 | 14.1 | Tr | 1.4 | 0 | 0.8 | 8.0 | 0 | 16.4 | 57.8 | 0 | 17:1 1.7 |
| | ***Fruit*** | | | | | | | | | | | | | |
| 3675 | **Apples** | 0 | 0 | 24.5 | Tr | 3.8 | 0 | 0 | 6.9 | 0 | 54.0 | 10.8 | 0 | |
| 3692 | **Avocado pears** | 0 | Tr | 12.3 *(7–22)* | Tr | Tr | Tr | 3.5 *(3–11)* | 75.1 *(59–81)* | 0 | 8.6 *(7–14)* | 0.4 | 0.1 | |
| 3693 | **Bananas** | 0 | Tr | 41.9 | Tr | 3.8 | Tr | 2.1 | 14.4 | 0 | 16.1 | 21.7 | 0 | |

| | | | Saturated | | | | | | Mono-unsaturated | | | Polyunsaturated | | |
|---|---|---|---|---|---|---|---|---|---|---|---|---|---|---|
| No | Food | | 10:0 | 12:0 | 14:0 | 16:0 | 18:0 | 20:0 | 16:1 | 18:1 | 20:1 | 18:2 | 18:3 | Other |
| | ***Nuts*** | | | | | | | | | | | | | |
| 3822 | **Almonds** | | 0 | 0 | 0.1 | 6.3 | 1.7 | 0.2 | 0.7 | 70.9 | Tr | 19.1 | 0.5 | |
| 3826 | **Brazil nuts** | | 0 | 0 | 0.2 | 15.6 | 10.9 | 0 | 0.4 | 33.9 | Tr | 39.0 | 0 | |
| 3828 | **Chestnuts** | | 0 | 0 | 0 | 16.7 | 1.0 | 0.5 | 0.7 | 38.5 | Tr | 37.7 | 4.2 | |
| 3830 | **Cob** or **hazel nuts** | | 0 | 0 | 0.3 | 5.2 | 1.8 | 0.2 | 0.3 | 80.7 | 0.1 | 10.7 | 0.2 | |
| 3832 | **Coconut** | | 7.1 | 47.7 | 15.8 | 9.0 | 2.4 | 1.0 | 0.4 | 6.6 | 0 | 1.8 | 0 | 6:0 0.7<br>8:0 7.5 |
| 3835 | **Peanuts** | | Tr | 0.1 | 0.5 | 10.7 | 2.7 | 1.2 | Tr | 49.0 | 1.1 | 29.0 | 0.8 | 22:0 3.4<br>24:0 1.1 |
| 3838 | **Peanut butter** | * | 0 | 0 | 0 | 11.3 | 5.5 | 1.4 | Tr | 51.6 | 1.4 | 26.2 | 0 | 22:0 2.5 |
| 3839 | **Walnuts** | | 0 | 0 | 1.1 | 7.5 | 2.1 | 0.7 | 0.2 | 16.1 | Tr | 60.0 | 11.4 | |
| | ***Chocolate products*** | | | | | | | | | | | | | |
| 3857 | **Chocolate**, milk | * | 0.6 | 0.9 | 3.4 | 28.2 | 26.8 | 0.6 | 0.6 | 33.1 | Tr | 2.9 | 0.8 | 4:0 0.5<br>6:0 0.4 |
| 3858 | plain | * | Tr | 0.5 | 1.6 | 26.8 | 32.9 | 0.5 | Tr | 33.6 | 0 | 3.3 | 0 | |
| 3868 | **Cocoa powder** | * | 0 | Tr | Tr | 26.2 | 34.5 | 0.9 | Tr | 34.8 | 0 | 3.0 | 0 | |
| 3873 | **Drinking chocolate** | * | 0 | Tr | 0.5 | 26.6 | 33.5 | 0.8 | Tr | 34.7 | 0 | 3.2 | 0 | |

# The tables

*continued*

## Section 4
## Subsidiary data:
## cholesterol,
## phytic acid phosphorus,
## iodine,
## organic acids

# Cholesterol

A number of sterols (Kritchevsky, 1963; Lange, 1950) are found in foods either in the free form or esterified with fatty acids.

Although a range of sterols (the phytosterols) can be isolated from individual plants, most animal tissues and products contain virtually only one—cholesterol. Cholesterol is therefore the characteristic sterol of the animal kingdom and does not appear to occur in plants. Molluscs appear to be an exception in this matter and a number of different sterols have been found in the species examined.

A number of phytosterols are known and of these the most common is β-sitosterol; α-spinasterol occurs in spinach and stigmasterol is also widely distributed. Traces of other sterols are found in many plant oils. The phytosterols do not appear to be absorbed by the mammalian digestive tract and can often be recovered unchanged in faeces. The values in this section are therefore restricted to animal products. Lange (1950) gives some values for the phytosterol content of a range of plant foods.

*Sources of values*

The figures given are derived from two sources, direct analyses of samples collected for this edition and selected values derived from the literature (see Appendix 6). The values are given as mg cholesterol per 100g and can be converted to mmol cholesterol by dividing by 386.6.

**Asterisk indicates new analytical data**

**Table 4.1**
*Cholesterol per 100g*

| No | Food | Cholesterol mg per 100g | No | Food | Cholesterol mg per 100g |
|---|---|---|---|---|---|
| | **Cereal products** | | | | |
| | ***Cakes*** | | 4089 | **Pastry, choux** raw | 110 |
| 4074 | **Fancy iced cakes** | — | 4090 | cooked | 170 |
| 4075 | **Fruit cake** rich | 50 | 4091 | **flaky** raw | —[a] |
| 4076 | rich, iced | 40 | 4092 | cooked | —[a] |
| 4077 | plain | — | 4093 | **shortcrust** raw | —[a] |
| 4078 | **Gingerbread** | 60 | 4094 | cooked | —[a] |
| 4079 | **Madeira cake** | — | 4095 | **Scones** | (5) |
| 4080 | **Rock cakes** | 40 | 4096 | **Scotch pancakes** | 50 |
| 4081 | **Sponge cake** with fat | 130 | | ***Puddings*** | |
| 4082 | without fat | 260 | | | |
| 4083 | jam filled | — | 4097 | **Apple crumble** | —[a] |
| | ***Buns and Pastries*** | | 4098 | **Bread and butter pudding** | 100 |
| 4084 | **Currant buns** | — | 4099 | **Cheesecake** | 95 |
| 4085 | **Doughnuts** | — | 4100 | **Christmas pudding** | 60 |
| 4086 | **Eclairs** | 90 | 4101 | **Custard** egg | 100 |
| 4087 | **Jam tarts** | —[a] | 4102 | made with powder | 16 |
| 4088 | **Mince pies** | —[a] | 4103 | **Custard tart** | 60 |

| No | Food | Cholesterol mg per 100g | No | Food | Cholesterol mg per 100g |
|---|---|---|---|---|---|
| 4104 | **Dumpling** | 8 | 4113 | **Meringues** | 0 |
| 4105 | **Fruit pie** individual, with pastry top and bottom | — | 4114 | **Milk pudding** | 15 |
| | | | 4115 | canned, rice | — |
| 4106 | **Fruit pie** with pastry top | —[a] | 4116 | **Pancakes** | 65 |
| 4107 | **Ice cream** dairy | * 21 | 4117 | **Queen of puddings** | 100 |
| 4108 | non-dairy | * 11 | 4118 | **Sponge pudding** steamed | 80 |
| 4109 | **Jelly** packet, cubes | 0 | 4119 | **Suet pudding** steamed | 4 |
| 4110 | made with water | 0 | 4120 | **Treacle tart** | —[a] |
| 4111 | made with milk | 6 | 4121 | **Trifle** | 50 |
| 4112 | **Lemon meringue pie** | 90 | 4122 | **Yorkshire pudding** | 70 |

[a] Contains only a trace if made with vegetable fats

## Milk, milk products and eggs

| No | Food | Cholesterol mg per 100g |
|---|---|---|
| | ***Milk*** | |
| 4123 | **cows'** fresh, whole | 14 |
| 4126 | fresh, whole, Channel Islands | 18 |
| 4129 | sterilized | 14 |
| 4130 | longlife | 14 |
| 4131 | fresh, skimmed | 2 |
| 4132 | condensed, whole, sweetened | 34 |
| 4133 | condensed, skimmed, sweetened | 3 |
| 4134 | evaporated, whole, unsweetened | 34 |
| 4135 | dried, whole | * 120 |
| 4136 | dried, skimmed | 18 |
| 4137 | **Milk, goats'** | — |
| 4138 | **Milk, human** mature | * 16 |
| 4139 | transitional | — |
| 4140 | **Butter** salted | 230 |
| 4141 | **Cream** single | 66 |
| 4144 | double | 140 |
| 4147 | whipping | 100 |
| 4150 | sterilized, canned | 73 |
| | ***Cheese*** | |
| 4151 | Camembert type | 72 |
| 4152 | Cheddar type | * 70 |
| 4153 | Danish Blue type | 88 |
| 4154 | Edam type | 72 |
| 4155 | Parmesan | 90 |
| 4156 | Stilton | 120 |
| 4157 | cottage cheese | * 13 |
| 4158 | cream cheese | * 94 |
| 4159 | processed cheese | 88 |
| 4160 | cheese spread | 71 |
| | ***Yogurt*** low fat | |
| 4161 | natural | * 7 |
| 4162 | flavoured | * 7 |
| 4163 | fruit | * 6 |
| 4164 | hazelnut | * 7 |
| | ***Eggs*** | |
| 4165 | whole, raw | * 450 |
| 4166 | white, raw | 0 |
| 4167 | yolk, raw | 1260 |
| 4168 | dried | 1780 |
| 4169 | boiled | 450 |
| 4170 | fried | —[a] |
| 4171 | poached | 480 |
| 4172 | omelette | 410 |
| 4173 | scrambled | 410 |
| | ***Egg and cheese dishes*** | |
| 4174 | **Cauliflower cheese** | 17 |
| 4175 | **Cheese pudding** | 130 |
| 4176 | **Cheese soufflé** | 180 |
| 4177 | **Macaroni cheese** | 20 |
| 4178 | **Pizza, cheese and tomato** | 20 |
| 4179 | **Quiche Lorraine** | 130 |
| 4180 | **Scotch egg** | 220 |
| 4181 | **Welsh rarebit** | 67 |

[a] The cholesterol content will depend on the fat used for frying

## Fats and oils

| No | Food | Cholesterol mg per 100g | No | Food | Cholesterol mg per 100g |
|---|---|---|---|---|---|
| 4183 | **Compound cooking fat** | —[a] | 4187 | **Margarine** | —[a] |
| 4184 | **Dripping, beef** | (60) | 4193 | **Suet** block | (60) |
| 4185 | **Lard** | (70) | 4194 | shredded | * 74 |
| 4186 | **Low fat spread** | Tr | 4195 | **Vegetable oils** | Tr |

[a] The cholesterol content will depend on the blend of oils used. If made with vegetable oils only, these foods will contain only a trace of cholesterol

## Meat

| No | Food | | Cholesterol mg per 100g | No | Food | | Cholesterol mg per 100g |
|---|---|---|---|---|---|---|---|
| 4209 | **Bacon** raw, lean and fat | * | 57 | | *Offal* | | |
| 4210 | lean only | * | 51 | 4354 | **Brain, calf** and **lamb** | | |
| 4224 | fried, lean and fat | * | 80 | | raw | * | 2200 |
| 4225 | lean only | * | 87 | 4355 | **calf** boiled | * | 3100 |
| 4229 | grilled, lean and fat | * | 74 | 4356 | **lamb** boiled | * | 2200 |
| 4230 | lean only | * | 77 | 4358 | **Heart, lamb** raw | * | 140 |
| 4236 | **Beef** raw, lean and fat | * | 65 | 4359 | **sheep** roast | | 260 |
| 4237 | lean only | * | 59 | 4360 | **ox** raw | * | 140 |
| 4238 | cooked, lean and fat | * | 82 | 4361 | stewed | * | 230 |
| 4239 | lean only | * | 82 | 4364 | **Kidney, lamb** raw | * | 400 |
| 4265 | **Lamb** raw, lean and fat | * | 78 | 4365 | fried | * | 610 |
| 4266 | lean only | * | 79 | 4366 | **ox** raw | * | 400 |
| 4267 | cooked, lean and fat | * | 110 | 4367 | stewed | * | 690 |
| 4268 | lean only | * | 110 | 4368 | **pig** raw | * | 410 |
| 4295 | **Pork** raw, lean and fat | * | 72 | 4369 | stewed | * | 700 |
| 4296 | lean only | * | 69 | 4371 | **Liver, calf** raw | * | 370 |
| 4297 | cooked, lean and fat | * | 110 | 4372 | fried | * | 330 |
| 4298 | lean only | * | 110 | 4373 | **chicken** raw | * | 380 |
| 4316 | **Chicken** raw, light meat | * | 69 | 4374 | fried | * | 350 |
| 4317 | dark meat | * | 110 | 4375 | **lamb** raw | * | 430 |
| 4319 | boiled, light meat | * | 80 | 4376 | fried | * | 400 |
| 4320 | dark meat | * | 110 | 4377 | **ox** raw | * | 270 |
| 4323 | roast, light meat | * | 74 | 4378 | stewed | * | 240 |
| 4324 | dark meat | * | 120 | 4379 | **pig** raw | * | 260 |
| 4327 | **Duck** raw, meat only | * | 110 | 4380 | stewed | * | 290 |
| 4329 | roast, meat only | * | 160 | 4381 | **Oxtail** raw | * | 75 |
| 4342 | **Turkey** raw, light meat | * | 49 | 4382 | stewed | * | 110 |
| 4343 | dark meat | * | 81 | 4384 | **Sweetbread, lamb** | | |
| 4346 | roast, light meat | * | 62 | | raw | * | 260 |
| 4347 | dark meat | * | 100 | 4385 | fried | * | 380 |
| 4350 | **Rabbit** raw | * | 71 | | | | |

| No | Food | | Cholesterol mg per 100 g |
|---|---|---|---|
| | ***Offal** contd* | | |
| 4387 | **Tongue, lamb** raw | * | 180 |
| 4388 | **sheep** stewed | | (270) |
| 4389 | **ox** pickled, raw | * | 78 |
| 4390 | boiled | | (100) |
| 4391 | **Tripe**, dressed | * | 95 |
| 4392 | stewed | * | 160 |
| | ***Meat products and dishes*** | | |
| | ***Canned meats*** | | |
| 4393 | **Beef, corned** | * | 85 |
| 4394 | **Ham** | * | 33 |
| 4395 | **Ham and pork** chopped | * | 60 |
| 4396 | **Luncheon meat** | * | 53 |
| 4397 | **Stewed steak with gravy** | * | 44 |
| 4398 | **Tongue** | * | 110 |
| 4400 | **Veal,** jellied | * | 97 |
| | ***Offal products*** | | |
| 4401 | **Black pudding** fried | * | 68 |
| 4402 | **Faggots** | * | 79 |
| 4403 | **Haggis** boiled | * | 91 |
| 4404 | **Liver sausage** | * | 120 |
| | ***Sausages*** | | |
| 4405 | **Frankfurters** | * | 46 |
| 4406 | **Polony** | * | 40 |
| 4407 | **Salami** | * | 79 |
| 4408 | **Sausages, beef** raw | * | 40 |
| 4409 | fried | * | 42 |
| 4410 | grilled | * | 42 |
| 4411 | **pork** raw | * | 47 |
| 4412 | fried | * | 53 |
| 4413 | grilled | * | 53 |
| 4414 | **Saveloy** | * | 45 |
| | ***Other products*** | | |
| 4415 | **Beefburgers** frozen, raw | * | 59 |
| 4416 | fried | * | 68 |
| 4417 | **Brawn** | * | 52 |
| 4418 | **Meat paste** | * | 68 |
| 4419 | **White pudding** | * | 22 |
| | ***Meat and pastry products*** | | |
| 4420 | **Cornish pastie** | * | 49 |
| 4421 | **Pork pie** individual | * | 52 |
| 4422 | **Sausage roll** flaky pastry | | 20 |
| 4423 | short pastry | | 30 |
| 4424 | **Steak and kidney pie** pastry top only | | 125 |
| | ***Cooked dishes*** | | |
| 4426 | **Beef steak pudding** | | 30 |
| 4427 | **Beef stew** | | 30 |
| 4428 | **Bolognese sauce** | | 25 |
| 4429 | **Curried meat** | | 25 |
| 4430 | **Hot pot** | | 25 |
| 4431 | **Irish stew** | | 35 |
| 4433 | **Moussaka** | | 40 |
| 4434 | **Shepherd's pie** | | 25 |

## Fish

| No | Food | Cholesterol mg per 100 g |
|---|---|---|
| | ***White fish*** | |
| 4438 | **Cod** fresh, raw | 50 |
| 4440 | baked | 60 |
| 4442 | fried | — |
| 4443 | grilled | 60 |
| 4444 | poached | 60 |
| 4446 | steamed | 60 |
| 4448 | **Cod, smoked** raw | (50) |
| 4449 | poached | (60) |
| 4451 | **Haddock, fresh** raw | 60 |
| 4452 | fried | — |
| 4454 | steamed | 75 |
| 4456 | **smoked** steamed | (75) |
| 4458 | **Halibut** raw | 50 |
| 4459 | steamed | 60 |
| 4461 | **Lemon sole** raw | 60 |
| 4462 | fried | — |
| 4464 | steamed | 60 |
| 4466 | **Plaice** raw | 70 |
| 4467 | fried in batter | — |
| 4468 | fried in crumbs | — |
| 4469 | steamed | 90 |
| 4471 | **Saithe** raw | 60 |
| 4472 | steamed | 75 |
| 4477 | **Whiting** steamed | 110 |

| No | Food | Cholesterol mg per 100g |
|---|---|---|
| | ***Fatty fish*** | |
| 4480 | **Eel** raw | — |
| 4481 | stewed | — |
| 4482 | **Herring** raw | 70 |
| 4483 | fried | (80) |
| 4485 | grilled | 80 |
| 4487 | **Bloater** grilled | 80 |
| 4489 | **Kipper** baked | 80 |
| 4491 | **Mackerel** raw | 80 |
| 4492 | fried | (90) |
| 4494 | **Pilchards** canned in tomato sauce | (70) |
| 4495 | **Salmon** raw | (70) |
| 4496 | steamed | (80) |
| 4498 | canned | 90 |
| 4499 | smoked | (70) |
| 4500 | **Sardines** canned in oil, fish only | 100 |
| 4501 | fish plus oil | 80 |
| 4502 | canned in tomato sauce | (100) |
| 4504 | **Sprats** fried | — |
| 4506 | **Trout** steamed | (80) |
| 4508 | **Tuna** canned in oil | 65 |
| | ***Cartilaginous fish*** | |
| 4510 | **Dogfish** | — |
| 4513 | **Skate** | — |
| | ***Crustacea*** | |
| 4517 | **Crab** fresh | 100 |
| 4520 | canned | 100 |
| 4521 | **Lobster** | 150 |
| 4523 | **Prawns** | 200 |
| 4525 | **Scampi** | 110 |
| 4526 | **Shrimps** | 200 |
| | ***Molluscs*** [a] | |
| 4531 | **Cockles** | 40 |
| 4532 | **Mussels** raw | 100 |
| 4535 | **Oysters** raw | 50 |
| 4537 | **Scallops** raw | 40 |
| 4539 | **Whelks** | 100 |
| 4541 | **Winkles** | 100 |
| | ***Fish products and dishes*** | |
| 4543 | **Fish cakes** frozen | — |
| 4544 | fried | — |
| 4545 | **Fish fingers** frozen | (50) |
| 4546 | fried | (50) |
| 4547 | **Fish paste** | — |
| 4548 | **Fish pie** | 20 |
| 4549 | **Kedgeree** | 120 |
| 4550 | **Roe, cod** hard, raw | (500) |
| 4551 | fried | (500) |
| 4552 | **herring** soft, raw | 700 |
| 4553 | fried | (700) |

## Products containing eggs

| | | |
|---|---|---|
| 4852 | **Lemon curd** home made | 150 |
| 4854 | **Marzipan** home made | 35 |
| 4926 | **Mayonnaise** home made | 260 |

[a] Other sterols are present in these fish, cholesterol forms about 40 per cent of the total sterol in cockles, mussels, oysters and scallops. It forms about 90 per cent of the total sterol in whelks and about 70 per cent in winkles.

# Phytic acid phosphorus

**Table 4.2*** *Phytic acid phosphorus*

| | Phytic acid phosphorus as per cent of total phosphorus | | Phytic acid phosphorus as per cent of total phosphorus |
|---|---|---|---|
| ***Cereals and cereal foods*** | | ***Nuts*** | |
| **All-Bran** Kellogg's | 76 | **Almonds** | 82 |
| **Barley, pearl** | 66 | **Barcelona nuts** | 83 |
| **Biscuits, digestive** | 61 | **Brazil nuts** | 86 |
| **Bread** brown (92%) | 55 | **Chestnuts** | 18 |
| national wheatmeal (85%) | 30 | **Cob nuts** | 74 |
| white | 15 | **Coconuts** | 81 |
| Hovis | 38 | **Peanuts** | 57 |
| **Cornflakes** | 25 | **Walnuts** | 42 |
| **Flour** English or Manitoba, | | | |
| 100% extraction | 70 | ***Vegetables*** | |
| 85% extraction | 55 | **Artichokes, Jerusalem** | |
| 80% extraction | 47 | boiled | 25 |
| white | 30 | **Beans, broad** boiled | 5 |
| **Oatmeal** raw | 70 | **butter,** raw | 84 |
| **Rice** polished | 61 | **haricot,** raw | 73 |
| **Rye** 100% extraction | 72 | **Carrots** raw | 16 |
| 85% extraction | 54 | **Cauliflower** boiled | 0 |
| 75% extraction | 44 | **Celery** raw | 0 |
| 60% extraction | 31 | **Lentils** raw | 51 |
| **Ryvita** | 54 | **Mushrooms** raw | 0 |
| **Sago** | Tr | **Onions** raw | 0 |
| **Shredded Wheat** | 80 | **Parsnips** raw | 31 |
| **Soya** full fat or low fat | | **Peas** fresh, raw | 11 |
| flour or grits | 31 | dried, raw | 80 |
| **Tapioca** | 0 | split, raw | 57 |
| **Vita-Wheat** | 59 | canned | 17 |
| | | **Potatoes** old, boiled | 19 |
| | | new, boiled | 23 |
| ***Fruit*** | | **Spinach** boiled | 0 |
| | | **Swedes** raw | 0 |
| **Apples** | 0 | **Turnips** raw | 0 |
| **Bananas** | 0 | | |
| **Blackberries** | 16 | ***Cocoa and chocolate*** | |
| **Figs** dried | 13 | **Chocolate, milk** | 18 |
| **Prunes** dried | 0 | **Cocoa** | 15 |

*Reprinted from the third edition of these tables. For further discussion of phytic acid in foods see McCance and Widdowson 1935 and 1942.

# Iodine

## Occurrence

Iodine occurs in foods almost entirely as the inorganic iodide. Seafoods are by far the richest sources. Some green vegetables, notably spinach, lettuce and watercress, contain moderate amounts; most other foods contain only small amounts. The occurrence of iodine in foods is extremely variable, depending on the locality where it is produced. The small quantities that are present led to difficulties in earlier methods of analysis, and methods used after about 1932 are held to be more reliable. A commonly used method is that employing the colour reaction of ceric sulphate and arsenious acid (Broadhead, Pearson and Wilson, 1965; Rodgers and Poole 1958); alternative methods using neutron activation analysis have also been described (Bowen 1959; Johansen and Steinnes, 1976).

## Amounts in foods

The most comprehensive study of the iodine content of foods is the annotated bibliography of the Chilean Iodine Educational Bureau (1952). Since the 1950's there have been relatively few reports on the iodine content of foods (Vought and London 1964). The Chilean Iodine Educational Bureau closed down in 1971, and there has been no study on foods by the Bureau since the 1952 publication. Some of the more important studies on British and Irish foods are discussed below.

*Milk*

Iodine crosses the mammary barrier very readily; consequently the iodine in milk closely reflects the iodine in the cow's diet. Iodine is commonly added to the winter feed of cows, and winter milk has a higher iodine content than does summer milk (Alderman and Stranks, 1967; Broadhead *et al.*, 1965).

*Fish*

The iodine content of fish has been reported by Broadhead *et al.* (1965) and Wayne, Koutras and Alexander (1964). The losses of iodine during the cooking of fish were found to be about 20 per cent in grilling and frying and 60 per cent in boiling (Harrison, McFarlane, Harden and Wayne, 1965).

*Other foods*

There is one recent report in Great Britain on the iodine content of *eggs* (Wayne *et al.*, 1964). There are very few studies on *meat*, the most useful one being for a number of cooked meats and meat products in Ireland (Mason, O'Donovan and Kilbride, 1945). *Cereals* also have not been studied in this country to any great extent. The iodine content of *vegetables* has been reported in more detail because of their content of goitrogens, particularly in the *Brassica* genus. There are no recent British studies, but values for cabbages, carrots, lettuce, onions, potato and watercress were reported in detail by Orr (1931), and some cooked vegetables by Mason *et al.* (1945).

## Goitrogens

There are a number of substances present in plants of the *Brassica* and other Cruciferae and some Leguminosae genera which interfere with the uptake and utilisation of iodine. The goitrogens also pass into milk. The occurrence and mode of action of a number of goitrogenic substances have been described by Gontzea and Sutzescu (1968).

# Organic acids

Organic acids are found in many foods and, while for the most part they are minor constituents, in some foods the concentrations of individual acids may be nutritionally significant. The major organic acids most frequently found in foods are given in table 4.3. This list is not exclusive and many hydroxy and other organic acids are found in some foods, usually in low concentrations.

## Occurrence

The organic acids are quantitatively more important in fruits and fruit products and in the majority of vegetables the concentrations are quite low. Many manufactured products contain added citric acid and acetic acid is widely used as a preservative in pickling. Lactic acid is found in fermented products such as yogurt and sauerkraut and at low concentrations in cheese.

*Citric* and *malic* acids are the major organic acids in most fruits and vegetables and the many other organic acids are residual components of the various oxidative and other metabolic pathways in the plant. The concentrations of all these organic acids depend very greatly on the state of maturity of the food and the conditions under which it has been grown. One factor which may be of special importance is the level of illumination the plant has received. The concentrations of organic acids are furthermore dependent on the post-harvest metabolism of the plant and in fruits the changes during the interval between harvest and consumption are often very large (Hulme, 1971).

*Tartaric* acid is the major organic acid in wines and in the fruit of the tamarind and the beobab tree.

*Oxalic acid*, often as the calcium salt, is found in many vegetables and some fruits and inclusions of oxalate crystals can frequently be seen in sections of plant tissue.

## Absorption and metabolism

The organic acids are usually well absorbed, although oxalic acid may be an exception as it forms insoluble salts with calcium at the pH of the intestinal contents and some oxalate is excreted in this way. The toxicity of oxalate shows, however, that some absorption does occur.

Many of the organic acids in foods are intermediates in metabolic processes common to most living cells and it is reasonable to assume that they are completely metabolised within the body. The extent to which tartaric acid is metabolised is uncertain but it is believed that digestion mainly occurs as a result of fermentation in the large intestine by the microflora and that any absorbed tartrate is excreted unchanged.

## Energy value

The organic acids that are normal constituents of metabolic pathways will provide energy to the body and should therefore not be ignored in the calculation of the energy value of foods. The energy conversion factors suggested in table 4.3 are the heats of combustion of the acids as it is reasonable to expect these acids to be completely absorbed and metabolised to carbon dioxide and water.

## Amounts in foods

Few detailed studies of the concentrations of organic acids in foods in themselves have been reported, although there is a large body of work on the concentration and metabolism of organic acids in fruits.

*Vegetables*

Before the development of chromatographic methods, separation of the individual acids was difficult and most estimates were based on total titratable acidity. This procedure may underestimate total organic anions but the errors involved are thought to be small for most foods. Using this technique, Hartmann and Hillig (1934) showed that the total organic acids in vegetables ranged between 0.1 and 0.8 g/100 g, and in most of those examined the concentration did not exceed 0.5 g/100 g. For practical nutritional purposes the organic acids in vegetables can therefore be discounted in energy calculations.

*Fruits*

In fruits the situation is more complex; Merrill and Watt (1955) grouped the fruits into five classes depending on the range of reported values for total organic acids present. A large number of fruits contained less than 1 g/100 g and only in lemons and limes did the concentrations exceed 3 g/100 g. Actual values reported in the literature are very variable and depend on variety, state of maturity and especially on the extent of post-harvest metabolism. It is therefore very difficult to give meaningful typical values and the method adopted by Merrill and Watt is probably the best practical guide.

This shows that lemons and limes have more than 3 g/100 g; cranberries, currants (black, red or white) and gooseberries between 2 and 3 g/100 g; and apricots, grapefruit, loganberries, nectarines, oranges, plums, pomegranates, raspberries, strawberries and tangerines between 1 and 2 g/100 g.

*Beverages*

Citric acid is added to many types of beverage, especially those with a fruit character. In most fruit drinks the concentrations are less than 1 g/100 ml in the ready-to-consume drink, but lemon juices may contain up to 6 g/100 ml of mainly citric acid (≡14.8 kcal). Beverages designated as 'low calorie' may have only minor amounts of energy from organic acids (usually less than 1 kcal/100 ml) but some have citric acid concentrations which would provide up to 7 kcal/100 ml.

*Vinegar*

Vinegar contains about 5 g acetic acid/100 ml and this will provide 17 kcal/100 ml.

**Conclusions**

For most nutritional purposes the concentrations of organic acids in foods are of academic interest. Oxalate concentrations are of course of great significance in the toxicological properties of foods. Organic acids can, in certain fruits and beverages, make a significant contribution to the energy value and it is hoped that as more values become available it will be possible to include this contribution in the total calculated energy contents given in section 1. For this edition it was considered that the data were too fragmentary to adopt this approach and the contributions from organic acids have not been included.

**Table 4.3**
*Major organic acids in foods*[a]

| Acid | Energy value[b] (per g) kcal | kJ | Occurrence |
|---|---|---|---|
| Acetic acid | 3.49 | 14.6 | Fermented products, vinegar, pickles etc |
| Citric acid | 2.47 | 10.3 | Most fruits and fruit products; low concentrations in vegetables, many processed foods and drinks |
| Lactic acid | 3.62 | 15.1 | Fermented products, yogurts, sauerkraut |
| Malic acid | 2.39 | 10.0 | Many fruits and fruit products—major acid in many fruits, low concentrations in vegetables |
| Oxalic acid | [c] | [c] | Many vegetables and some fruits |
| Tartaric acid | [c] | [c] | Some fruits, major acid in wines and a few fruits |

[a] Many other hydroxy and other organic acids occur in foods usually at low concentrations (less than 0.1 g/100 g)

[b] Based on heats of combustion

[c] These acids are probably not metabolised to any significant extent to provide energy

# Appendix I: Details of analytical procedures

The analytical methods used to obtain the values presented in the tables are described in this appendix. The aim of this is to enable the user to see the principles behind the methods and, by having procedural details or references to the literature, to set up and use similar methods.

Analytical methods for foods, despite many contrary impressions, are in a continuous state of development, modification and appraisal. In most the principle of the method used is more important than the precise technical procedure. Instrumental methods have transformed many determinations that were difficult or time-consuming into simple rapid procedures, and in a few cases have made determinations that were impracticable or virtually impossible to perform on more than the occasional sample routine procedures. Although instrumental analysis is rapidly becoming the rule it is incorrect to assume that these modern procedures are, in themselves, more accurate or precise than the methods they have replaced. In most cases they enable more samples to be analysed in a given time or make fewer demands on the manipulative skills of the analyst. In the course of this revision many comparisons between results obtained by new and older methods have been made. These have shown that in the majority of cases the skill and care of the analysts in the past has compensated for the technical difficulties associated with the methods they had to use.

## Water

The values for water content in the earlier editions were obtained by drying; foods rich in sugars, such as fruits and vegetables, were dried at 50°C and other foods at around 100°C. This method measures the loss of all volatile constituents and could not be used where alcohol, acetic acid or volatile oils were present. Accordingly values for total solids were given for the alcoholic beverages and omitted for condiments with volatile oils. In the analyses for the third edition samples rich in sugar either were dried in a vacuum oven at 60°C or else had water measured by distillation with benzene in a Dean and Stark type apparatus (AOAC 1955). The two procedures gave similar results.

### Methods used for this edition

The water content was calculated in most foods from the loss in mass on freeze-drying, and the moisture content of the freeze-dried solids determined by drying in an oven at 100°C until constant in mass. Samples rich in sugar and some beverages were dried in a vacuum oven at 70°C. Other samples that were not freeze-dried, such as Marmite and Bovril, were mixed with sand and ethanol, pre-dried on a water bath and heated to constant mass in an oven at 100°C.

## Total nitrogen

In all the previous editions total nitrogen was measured by a micro-Kjeldahl method. There were some differences in the 'catalyst' mixtures used, which tended to follow the fashion of the day. Copper sulphate was used by McCance and Shipp (1933) for the meats and fish, and by McCance, Widdowson and Shackleton (1936) for the fruits, vegetables and nuts. In the analyses for the third edition the Chibnall, Rees and Williams (1943) catalyst was used (potassium sulphate/copper sulphate/sodium selenite).

The preparation of the sample for digestion differed according to the food. The measurements on the fruits, vegetables and nuts were made on small subsamples weighed out directly; for the other foods a large sample (10–20 g) was refluxed in dilute sulphuric acid to produce a homogeneous suspension from which aliquots were taken for digestion.

### Methods used for this edition

Nitrogen was determined by a Kjeldahl procedure similar to the methods given in British Standards for meat and meat products (BS 4401 : 1969), milk (BS 1741 : 1963) and cheese (BS 770 : 1963).

## Fat

Two types of procedure were used for the first and second editions. One was the conventional Soxhlet extraction of a dried sample of the food with petroleum spirit, and the other was a procedure devised by von Lieberman and Szekely (1898). In this the food was saponified in strong alkali and the fatty acids subsequently released by acidification. The fatty acids were extracted into petroleum spirit and the total fatty acids measured by titration. McCance and Widdowson (1940) found that the Soxhlet method underestimated fat in many foods and preferred the alkaline extraction method because they felt that it measured triglycerides more nearly, in addition to giving a more complete extraction.

In the analyses for the third edition an alkaline extraction method was found to be suitable for many animal products, but with other foods an acid hydrolysis before extraction gave the most complete extraction of fat. The method used was a modification of the AOAC (1955) procedure for cereals followed by saponification of the total lipid and measurement of the fatty acids. In both these approaches it was found technically easier to measure the total fatty acids gravimetrically.

### Methods used for this edition

Several types of procedure were used for the determination of fat. For meat and meat products the Werner Schmid method, which involved acid hydrolysis followed by extraction of the fat with diethyl ether, was found to be suitable (BS 4401, Pt 4, 1970 Method B). Another acid hydrolysis procedure, that of Weibull Stoldt, was found to be preferable to the Werner Schmid for certain products, such as some cakes, canned and dried soups and beverages (BS 4401, Pt 4, 1970 Method A). Free fat in the fat separated from meat and bacon was determined by Soxhlet extraction with light petroleum (BS 4401, Pt 5 1970). For milk and some milk products a Rose–Gottlieb procedure, now adopted as an international standard method, was used (BS 1743 : 1968), and for cheese Method 16.230 of the Official Methods of Analysis of the Association of Official Analytical Chemists (12th edition, 1975) was employed.

AOAC methods were also found to be applicable to fish (Method 18.040) and biscuits and breakfast cereals (14.019). The rapid method of Southgate (1971), modified by the use of chloroform instead of petroleum spirit for the final fat extraction, was used for liver and gave values higher than those obtained with the Werner Schmid method, similarly modified. However, for other offal the two methods gave similar values.

**Carbohydrate**

*Available carbohydrate*

The values in the first and second editions were obtained using methods based on those described by Widdowson and McCance (1935). These involved extraction of free sugars with aqueous ethanol in a Soxhlet extractor and measurement of the free sugars. Two types of reducing sugar method were used and the results obtained were used, by solving simultaneous equations, to give the glucose and fructose concentrations in the extract. Sucrose was measured by inversion, with either dilute citric acid or an invertase preparation. It is interesting to note that this procedure gave results very similar to those obtained with quantitative paper chromatography or specific enzymatic methods in the hand of modern authors (Southgate, 1976). Starch was measured in most foods after hydrolysis with takadiastase, again using two reducing sugar methods, in order to estimate the glucose : maltose ratio in the hydrolysate. The starch in some refined cereal foods was measured as reducing sugars after dilute acid hydrolysis.

In the third edition a similar approach was adopted, a combination of reducing sugar methods, inversion and paper chromatography being used for the analysis of the sugars in an aqueous alcoholic extract. Starch was measured by the use of a takadiastase preparation which gave very nearly complete conversion of starch to glucose (Southgate, 1969a), with dilute acid hydrolysis for some cereal foods as in earlier editions.

## Methods used for this edition

The principles used for the new analyses were the same as those in earlier editions. They are described in some detail here as they are awaiting publication (Dean, in preparation). A preliminary examination of the foodstuff by paper chromatography was made to obtain an indication of the sugars that were present and their approximate concentration. This information also enabled a suitable standard for quantitative measurements to be selected—this needed to be a sugar not present in the sample and well separated on the chromatogram from other sugars that were present.

*Sugars*

For quantitative work the sugars were extracted from the foodstuffs either by treatment with 80 per cent v/v ethanol in a Soxhlet extraction apparatus for 3 hours or by boiling with 80 per cent v/v ethanol for 20 minutes. A known amount of a suitable internal standard was then added to the extract and the residue was set aside for starch determination. The ethanol was removed from the extract by rotary evaporation under reduced pressure and the residue obtained was dissolved in distilled water. This solution was then deproteinised by adding equivalent amounts of cadmium sulphate and barium hydroxide solutions and after filtration was concentrated by rotary evaporation. The solution was then deionised by passage through a mixed bed ion-exchange column; the eluant was reduced in volume to 50 ml and 1 ml of boric acid (0.2 M) was added to 1 ml of this solution. An aliquot of this mixture, usually 100 μl, containing about 50 μg of each sugar was then injected on to the column of an autoanalyser. The sugars were eluted from the anion-exchange column with boric acid solutions of increasing molarity, pH and chloride ion concentration from an autograd. The eluate from the column was mixed with orcinol in 70% v/v sulphuric acid (1 g per litre) in a bubble-segmented stream, and the colour developed at 95°C and measured continuously at

420 nm. The areas of the peaks on the chromatogram representing the various sugars were then converted to microgram amounts of sugar from previously prepared calibration lines and finally expressed as percentages of the sugar in the sample.

*Starch*

The residue remaining after extraction of the free sugars was further examined for starch and dextrin content. Both were hydrolysed with the selective enzyme glucamylase to glucose. After filtration of the digest the liberated glucose was treated with glucose oxidase and estimated colorimetrically at 37°C in an autoanalyser. For some products, such as some biscuits and breakfast cereals, the procedure was modified by heating the residue (50–200 mg) for 3 minutes with 20 ml distilled water in a boiling water bath and then autoclaving it for 1 hour at 121°C before proceeding with the enzymatic hydrolysis and colour reaction. Acid hydrolysis, in which 100 mg of the residue was heated with 10 ml 0.75 M sulphuric acid for 3 hours, was used before glucose determination for certain products, such as some cakes, breakfast cereals and dried soups.

*Unavailable carbohydrates/dietary fibre*

The method used for the unavailable carbohydrates or dietary fibre in fruit, vegetables and nuts in the earlier editions was to measure the weight of the residue insoluble in the 80 per cent v/v ethanol used to extract the free sugars. The values for starch and protein were then deducted from this residue to give a value for *unavailable carbohydrates*.

**Method used for this edition**

Unavailable carbohydrates were measured by the method of Southgate (1969b) as later modified (Southgate 1976). This method includes a starch hydrolysis and accounts for substantially all the residue insoluble in 80 per cent v/v ethanol except protein and ash, and it therefore gives total values that are virtually identical with those obtained by the previous method.

**Alcohol**

In the previous editions alcohol was measured by the standard Inland Revenue distillation method.

**Method used for this edition**

A similar method was used for the new analyses.

**Inorganic constituents**

In the first and second editions the values for inorganic constituents were obtained by microchemical methods (either colorimetric or titrimetric) on either a solution of the ash in dilute acid or an acid digestion (wet oxidation) of the sample.

Samples of the food were dried in silica crucibles and heated to drive off fumes; they were then heated in a special incinerative apparatus (McCance and Shipp, 1933) or a muffle furnace. Sodium, potassium, calcium, magnesium, iron and copper were measured on the acid extract of the ash.

*Sodium* was precipitated as the zinc uranyl acetate and the uranium measured colorimetrically by reaction with potassium ferrocyanide; *potassium* was precipitated as the cobalti-nitrite and the precipitate titrated with permanganate; *calcium* was precipitated as the oxalate and titrated with permanganate; *magnesium* was precipitated as the ammonium phosphate; *iron* was measured colorimetrically by reaction with thioglycollic acid or with thiocyanate, and *copper* colorimetrically after reaction with sodium diethyl dithiocarbamate.

*Phosphorus* was measured after oxidation of the sample in a perchloric/ sulphuric acid mixture by a colorimetric method involving reduction of the phosphomolybdic acid complex.

*Chloride* was measured by titration using Volhard's method after oxidation of the sample with nitric acid in the presence of excess silver nitrate.

*Sulphur* was measured by the method of Masters and McCance (1939).

For the third edition some modifications were introduced but the same overall principles were retained.

The samples were ashed in silica crucibles in an electric muffle furnace at 450°C after a preliminary heating to drive off fumes. This usually produced a light grey or white ash, but if the ash was still dark it was treated with nitric acid and reheated. The ash was extracted with acid as described by McCance, Widdowson and Shackleton (1936).

*Sodium* was then measured gravimetrically as the zinc uranyl acetate (Widdowson and Southgate, 1959); *potassium* was precipitated as the cobalti-nitrite and the precipitate titrated with permanganate or ceric sulphate (some measurements were also made with a flame photometer); *calcium* was precipitated as the oxalate and titrated with either permanganate or ceric sulphate; *magnesium* was precipitated as the ammonium phosphate and the phosphate measured by the Fiske and Subbarow (1925) method. *Iron* was measured by two colorimetric procedures, with thioglycollic acid or *ortho*-phenanthroline; these methods gave virtually identical results. *Copper* was measured colorimetrically after reaction with sodium diethyl dithiocarbamate. *Phosphorus* was measured by the Fiske and Subbarow (1925) method. The last three constituents were measured both in the ash extract and on perchloric/sulphuric acid oxidations of the food. No differences between the two results were seen provided that all the pyrophosphate formed in dry ashing had been hydrolysed before measurement of phosphorus was attempted. *Chloride* was measured by a procedure virtually identical with that used for the first and second editions. *Sulphur* values were obtained by the method of Masters and McCance (1939).

### Methods used for this edition

A suitable portion of dried material was weighed into a silica dish and most of the organic matter was destroyed at low temperature either on a hot plate or under an infrared lamp. The dish was then brought slowly to 550°C in a muffle furnace and the sample allowed to ash overnight. The residue was extracted by heating it with dilute hydrochloric acid and the solution was filtered into a graduated flask. The filter paper and residue were ashed overnight as before at 550°C, the extract of the residue was combined with the first extract and the solution was diluted to 100 ml. After the solution had been thoroughly mixed it was used either directly or after dilution for the determination of *calcium, copper, iron, magnesium* and *zinc* by atomic absorption spectrometry, and for *sodium* and *potassium* determination by emission spectrometry, with a Perkin Elmer instrument Model 403. A portion of the extract was also used for the colorimetric determination of *phosphorus* by reduction of the complex formed wtih ammonium molybdate with hydroquinone and sodium sulphite.

*Chloride* A known weight of dried material was moistened with a solution of sodium carbonate and heated first under an infrared lamp and then in a muffle furnace at a temperature not exceeding 500°C. The residue was extracted with water and diluted to about 100 ml. Chloride was then determined according to the Volhard procedure by treating this solution with an excess of 0.1 N silver nitrate solution, adding 2 ml of nitrobenzene and determining the residual silver nitrate by titration with 0.1 N potassium thiocyanate solution, ferric alum being used as indicator.

*Sulphur* The dried sample was heated with sodium carbonate and sodium peroxide in a nickel crucible to destroy organic matter and convert sulphur to sulphate. After it had cooled, the fused mass was extracted with water and dilute hydrochloric acid, barium chloride solution was added and sulphur was determined gravimetrically as barium sulphate. Confirmation of the results was obtained by X-ray fluorescence (Isherwood and King, 1976).

## Vitamins

The values for vitamins in the previous editions were taken from the literature with very few exceptions. The B vitamins in the bread samples were measured by methods similar to those used in this edition.

### Methods used for this edition

*Vitamin A: retinol and β-carotene*

A suitable weight of sample was saponified with ethanolic potassium hydroxide solution and the unsaponifiable matter containing retinol and β-carotene was extracted with diethyl ether. Retinol was then separated from β-carotene, sterols and vitamins D and E by partition chromatography between a mobile phase of 2,2,4-trimethylpentane and a stationary phase of methanol containing 10 per cent water, Sephadex LH20 being used as the inert support for the stationary phase (Bell, 1971). Measurement of the absorbance of the retinol fraction in isopropyl alcohol (propan-2-ol) at 325 nm and of the β-carotene fraction in cyclohexane at 455 nm now enabled the vitamin content to be calculated, allowance for any irrelevant absorption in the ultraviolet being made by the correction of Wilkie (1964). In some cases such as canned fish, where purification of the extract by column chromatography on Sephadex LH20 was inadequate, an additional column of calcium phosphate was also employed.

*Vitamins of the B group other than thiamin*

Nicotinic acid, riboflavin, vitamin $B_6$, vitamin $B_{12}$, folic acid, pantothenic acid and biotin were determined by microbiological assay. The general scheme involved liberation of the vitamin from the sample by acid or enzymatic hydrolysis, dilution with nutrient medium, sterilisation of the solutions, inoculation with a suitable culture of microorganisms as shown in the table, and incubation and estimation of the growth of the microorganisms by turbidimetry. In some instances a microbiological assay technique was used to confirm values for thiamin obtained by the standard fluorimetric procedure. A detailed description of all the techniques employed has been given by Bell (1974).

| Vitamin | Microorganism | Culture number | | |
|---|---|---|---|---|
| | | ATCC | NCIB | NCYC |
| Nicotinic acid | *Lactobacillus plantarum* | 8014 | 6376 | — |
| Riboflavin | *Streptococcus zymogenes* | 10100 | 7432 | — |
| Vitamin $B_6$ | *Saccharomyces carlsbergensis* | 9080 | — | 74 |
| Vitamin $B_{12}$ | *Lactobacillus leichmannii* | 7830 | 8118 | — |
| Folic acid | *Lactobacillus casei* | 7469 | 6375 | — |
| Pantothenic acid | *Lactobacillus plantarum* | 8014 | 6376 | — |
| Biotin | *Lactobacillus plantarum* | 8014 | 6376 | — |
| Thiamin | *Lactobacillus viridescens* | 12706 | 8965 | — |

*Thiamin*

Thiamin was determined by the fluorimetric method recommended by the Society of Public Analysts and Other Analytical Chemists: Analytical Methods Committee (1951).

*Vitamin C*

*Preparation of extract* The vitamin was extracted from the food by mixing an extracting solution consisting of 3 per cent acetic acid and 8 per cent metaphosphoric acids with a suitable amount of the sample in a Sunbeam blender for 2 minutes, centrifuging the mixture at 3000 revolutions per minute for 10 minutes and filtering the supernatant liquid through a filter paper.

*Ascorbic acid* A suitable aliquot of the prepared extract was titrated with a solution of 2,6-dichlorophenolindophenol that had been standardised against pure ascorbic acid. The procedure was similar to that described in the Official Methods of Analysis of the AOAC (1975).

*Ascorbic plus dehydroascorbic acids* Ascorbic acid was converted to dehydroascorbic acid by shaking an aliquot of the prepared extract with Norit charcoal. The solution was then filtered and an aliquot was reacted with *o*-phenylenediamine reagent to form a fluorescent compound which was measured on a fluorimeter at 455 nm using an exciting wavelength of 365 nm. Any fluorescence due to interfering substances was determined after complexing the dehydroascorbic acid with boric acid and an allowance was made for this interference. The procedure was similar to that described in the Official Methods of Analysis of the AOAC (1975).

*Vitamin E*

A suitable quantity of the sample was saponified with ethanolic potassium hydroxide solution in the presence of ascorbic acid and nitrogen. The unsaponifiable matter was extracted with diethyl ether and the extract was purified on a column of neutral alumina deactivated with 10 per cent water. Tocopherols were then determined colorimetrically by reaction with ferric chloride and 4,7-diphenyl-1,10-phenanthroline reagents. Gas–liquid chromatography on 2-metre glass columns of 3 per cent OV17 on Gas Chrom Q at 235° was used to confirm some of the results obtained by colorimetry and to provide information on the nature of the individual tocopherols present (Christie, Dean and Millburn, 1973).

**Amino acids**

The values in the previous editions were in the main derived from the literature. The values for potato that were included were obtained by a manual version of the procedure used for the new analyses.

**Method used for this edition**

A sample of the freeze-dried food was defatted in a Soxhlet apparatus with light petroleum (BP40–60°) for 2 hours and then thoroughly mixed. 200 mg of the defatted material was hydrolysed with 5 ml 6N hydrochloric acid in an evacuated sealed tube for 16 hours at 125°C. The liberated amino acids were separated by ion-exchange chromatography on a Technicon autoanalyser and determined by colorimetric reaction with ninhydrin. Cystine and methionine were determined on pre-oxidised samples by the method of Moore (1963); tryptophan was determined after alkaline hydrolysis by the method of Miller (1967). Results were corrected for hydrolytic losses, and after the nitrogen content of the defatted material had been determined values were calculated as mg of amino acid per g of nitrogen.

**Fatty acids**

No values for fatty acid composition were given in the previous editions. For this edition the fat was isolated by a chloroform–methanol–water extraction process (Bligh and Dyer, 1959). Solutions of the methyl esters of the fatty acids were prepared from the fat by conventional methods (IUPAC, 1976). The methyl esters of the fatty acids were separated and determined by gas–liquid chromatography (IUPAC, 1976).

**Cholesterol**

No values were given previously. For this edition a known weight of dried material was saponified with ethanolic potassium hydroxide solution for 1 hour and the unsaponifiable material was extracted with diethyl ether. The ether extract was washed with water and the traces of water were removed from the ether by rotary evaporation in the presence of ethanol. After removal of traces of ethanol by a further evaporation with light petroleum, the residue was dissolved in 10 ml of iso-octane (2,2,4,-trimethylpentane). An appropriate amount of an internal standard (5α-cholestan-3-one) was added to the extract and cholesterol was determined by gas–liquid chromatography on a 2-metre glass column, internal diameter 2 mm, containing 3 per cent OV17 on Gas Chrom Q at a temperature of 220°C.

## References to appendix 1


AOAC (1955) *Official methods of analysis*, 8th edition. Association of Official Agricultural Chemists. Washington DC

AOAC (1975) *Official methods of analysis*, 12th edition. Association of Official Analytical Chemists. Washington, DC

Bell, J. G. (1971) Separation of oil-soluble vitamins by partition chromatography on Sephadex LH20. *Chem. and Ind.* 201–202

Bell, J. G. (1974) Microbiological assay of vitamins of the B group in foodstuffs *Lab. Pract.* **23**, 235–242, 252

Bligh, E. G., and Dyer, W. J. (1959) A rapid method of total lipid extraction and purification, *Canad. J. Biochem. Physiol.* **37**. 911–917

Chibnall, A. C., Rees, M. W., and Williams, E. F. (1943) The total nitrogen content of egg albumin and other proteins. *Biochem. J.* **37**, 354–359

Christie, A. A., Dean, A. C., and Millburn, B. A. (1973) The determination of vitamin E in food by colorimetry and gas–liquid chromatography *Analyst* **98**, 161–167

Dean, A. C. (in preparation)

Fiske, C. H., and Subbarow, Y. (1925) The colorimetric determination of phosphorus *J. biol. Chem.* **66**, 375–400

Isherwood, S. A., and King, R. T. (1976) Determination of calcium, potassium, chlorine, sulphur and phosphorus in meat and meat products by X-ray fluorescence spectroscopy *J. Sci. Food Agric.* **27**, 831–837

IUPAC (1977) Standard methods for the analysis of oils, fats and soaps 4th supplement to 5th edition. Method II D.19 Preparation of fatty acid methyl eters. Method II D.25 Gas liquid chromatography of fatty acid methyl esters

Masters, M., and McCance, R. A. (1939) The sulphur content of foods. *Biochem. J.* **33**, 1304–1312

McCance, R. A., and Shipp, H. L. (1933) *The chemistry and flesh foods and their losses on cooking.* Medical Research Council Special Report Series No. 187. HMSO, London

McCance, R. A., and Widdowson, E. M. (1940) *The chemical composition of foods.* Medical Research Council Special Report Series No. 235. HMSO, London

McCance, R. A., and Widdowson, E. M., and Shackleton, L. R. B. (1936) *The nutritive value of fruits, vegetables and nuts.* Medical Research Council Special Report Series No. 213. HMSO, London

Miller, E. L. (1967) Determination of the tryptophan content of feedingstuffs with particular reference to cereals. *J. Sci. Food Agric.* **18**, 381–386

Moore, S. M. (1963) On the determination of cystine as cysteic acid. *J. biol. Chem.* **238**, 235–237

Society of Public Analysts and Other Analytical Chemists: Analytical Methods Committee (1951) The chemical assay of aneurine in foodstuffs. *Analyst* **76**, 127–133

Southgate, D. A. T. (1969a) Determination of carbohydrates in foods. I Available carbohydrates. *J. Sci. Food Agric.* **20**, 326–330

Southgate, D. A. T. (1969b) Determination of carbohydrates in foods. II Unavailable carbohydrates. *J. Sci. Food Agric.* **20**, 331–335

Southgate, D. A. T. (1971) A procedure for the measurement of fats in foods. *J. Sci. Food Agric.* **22**, 590–591

Southgate, D. A. T. (1976) *Determination of food carbohydrates.* Applied Science Publishers, London

Von Lieberman, L., and Szekely, S. (1898) Eine neue Methode der Fettbestimmung in Futtermitteln, Fleisch, Koth, u.s.w. *Pflüg. Arch. ges. Physiol.* **72**, 360

Widdowson, E. M., and McCance, R. A. (1935) The available carbohydrates of fruits. Determination of glucose, fructose, sucrose, and starch. *Biochem. J.* **29**, 151–156

Widdowson, E. M., and Southgate, D. A. T. (1959) Haemorrhage and tissue electrolytes. *Biochem. J.* **72**, 200–204

Wilkie, J. B. (1964) Corrections for background in spectrophotometry using difference-in-absorbance values. Application to vitamin A. *Anal. Chem.* **36**, 896–900

# Appendix 2: Note on the calculation of the energy value of foods and of diets*

**by E. M. Widdowson**

The energy value of a food is measured in Calories, which are physical units of heat. The number of Calories the body can derive from a food is, however, less than the number of Calories produced when the food is burned in a calorimeter because the calorie-producing nutrients, which are mainly protein, fat and carbohydrate, are not completely digested; the products of digestion, moreover, are not completely absorbed in the human gut, and the portion of the protein which is digested and absorbed is not completely oxidised to yield energy in the body.

The calorific value of a food is usually calculated from the amounts of protein, fat and carbohydrate it contains: these amounts are determined by chemical methods and the values are then multiplied by factors representing the number of Calories thought to be produced in the body by 1 gram of protein, fat or carbohydrate. The sum of these products gives the calorific value of the food. These calorie conversion factors do not represent the number of Calories which 1 gram of protein, fat, or carbohydrate would produce in a calorimeter. They are arrived at by applying to the values found by physical calorimetry various corrections allowing for losses occurring in digestion and absorption, and through incomplete oxidation. Since no two foods and no two people are ever exactly alike, and since these physiological corrections are based on averages the calorie conversion factors do not have the same accuracy as the values for Calories arrived at by physical calorimetry, or the values for protein, fat and carbohydrate found by chemical determination. Furthermore, different corrections are applied in different countries; and even within one country the method used may vary from one set of tables to another, and individual workers may use different methods from time to time. The problem is a complicated one, and there is no clear-cut answer to it.

The difference between the number of Calories which a diet would provide were the protein, fat and carbohydrate in it completely digested, and the number of Calories which it does in fact provide, is mainly due to the so-called 'unavailable carbohydrates' which are contained in plant foods. These are made up of hemicelluloses and fibre, and the digestive tract of man secretes no enzymes capable of digesting them, though micro-organisms in the gut may break down some of them and convert them to lower fatty acids, part of which may be absorbed and become a minor source of energy (McCance and Lawrence, 1929). In sheep and cattle, however, the large rumen provides space in which bacteria and protozoa can break down the hemicelluloses

* Reprinted from third edition

present in grasses and these contribute considerably to the nutrition of the animal. Although complex carbohydrates may, therefore, contribute a few Calories to man, their chief importance to the calorific value of a diet is a negative one. Fibre reduces the calorific value of a food or diet by hastening transport through the gut, and increasing the weight of the stools and the amount of nitrogen and fat in them. The more fibre a food or diet contains, the more nitrogen and fat will be excreted in the faeces and the less energy will therefore be derived from the protein and fat of the food or diet (McCance and Widdowson, 1947; McCance and Walsham 1948; McCance and Glaser, 1948).

## History of calorie conversion factors

Most of the fundamental work on the calorific value of foods was carried out by Rubner and by Atwater and his colleagues more than 50 years ago. Rubner worked in Germany and Atwater in America during the last 20–25 years of the 19th century and the first part of the present one. In his early days, Atwater spent some time in Germany as Rubner's pupil, and it was undoubtedly this experience that inspired his later work. Rubner's most important papers for the present purpose were published in 1885 and 1901. He measured the heats of combustion of a number of different proteins, fats and carbohydrates in a bomb calorimeter, and also studied the heat of combustion of urine passed by a dog, a man, a boy and a baby. He realised that the heat of combustion of protein in the bomb calorimeter was greater than its calorific value to the body because the body oxidises protein only to urea, creatinine, uric acid and other nitrogenous end-products which are themselves capable of further oxidation. Rubner also analysed the faeces of the man who acted as his experimental subject and he found that the loss of energy in the nitrogenous substances in the urine and faeces were 16.3 and 6.9 per cent of the intake respectively, making a total loss of about 23 per cent. He deducted 23 per cent from the heats of combustion of animal and vegetable protein and arrived at a figure of 4.1 Calories per gram of mixed protein. Rubner made no allowances for losses in digestion and absorption of fat and carbohydrate, and his factors (9.3 Calories per gram of fat and 4.1 Calories per gram of carbohydrate) represent the average heats of combustion of a variety of fats and carbohydrates.

Atwater, working over 50 years ago, contributed more to our knowledge about the energy value of foods than any one else before or since his time. The heats of combustion of different proteins, fats and carbohydrates were measured in a bomb calorimeter (Atwater and Bryant, 1900). These authors also analysed the urine from forty-six persons and measured its heat of combustion. They found that for every gram of nitrogen in the urine there was unoxidized material sufficient to yield an average of 7.9 Calories. This is equivalent to 1.25 Calories per gram of protein in the food, if the person is in nitrogen equilibrium.

Atwater (1902) also made extensive studies of the 'availability' of nutrients, and he was careful to distinguish between what he called 'available' and 'digestible'. He regarded the faeces as being made up of two parts, the undigested and therefore unabsorbed food residues, and the 'metabolic products' of digestion, consisting of desquamated cells, bacteria and nitrogenous substances in the digestive juices. By 'digestible' nitrogen he meant the nitrogen in the food minus the nitrogen in the undigested, unabsorbed food residues, and this he could not measure. By 'available' nitrogen he meant the nitrogen in the food minus the nitrogen in the food residues together with the metabolic products of digestion, that is, the nitrogen in the food minus the nitrogen in the faeces.

Three men, aged 32, 29 and 22 years, served as subjects for Atwater's studies on 'availability'. Atwater made a total of fifty experiments on these men, each lasting for 3–8 days. The subjects ate what were described as mixed diets, which varied in the amount of fat and carbohydrate they contained, but none of the diets contained much roughage, i.e., unavailable carbohydrate. The foods were analysed for nitrogen and fat, and the faeces were analysed also.

Atwater and Bryant (1900) collected what they could find in the literature, including the results of their own work (Atwater and Benedict, 1897) on the 'availability' to man of single foods. From these data they prepared tentative coefficients for the 'availability' of the protein, fat and carbohydrate in the common classes of food, and they applied these coefficients to the mixed diets that their own subjects had eaten. They then compared the calculated 'availability' of the protein, fat and carbohydrate of the mixed diets with the 'availability' of these nutrients in the diets as found by experiment. They did the same with the results of sixty-one other experiments in which, apparently, ten men served as subjects, though no detailed description of these experiments was published. They found the 'coefficients of availability' of the protein, fat and carbohydrate in the mixed diets as determined by experiment to agree very well with the values as calculated by the proposed factors for availability of the protein, fat and carbohydrate in separate classes of foods.

For the calculation of the 'available energy' from mixed diets Atwater and Bryant (1900) suggested the use of the average factors 4.0, 8.9 and 4.0 for protein, fat and carbohydrate respectively. The figure 8.9 was later rounded off to 9.0 (Atwater, 1910). These factors, which Atwater had intended should be used only for calculating the Calories to be obtained from the protein, fat and carbohydrate in mixed diets, came to be widely used for calculating the available energy value of individual foods (Sherman, 1911, 1952; Chatfield and Adams, 1940; Platt, 1945).

In 1936, Morey published a paper in which she reviewed the work done by Rubner and Atwater at the turn of the century, and showed how the calorie conversion factors suggested by these two pioneers had been derived. It was Maynard (1944), however, who really opened up the whole subject again, and he was the first to draw attention to Atwater's original intention that the calorie conversion factors for protein, fat and carbohydrate should not be the same for all foods. Osmond (1948) was the first to adopt Maynard's suggestions as to the correct use of Atwater's factors in his tables of composition of Australian foods. Shortly after Maynard's paper was published, the Nutrition Division of the Food and Agriculture Organization of the United Nations appointed a Committee to discuss the question of calorie conversion factors, and the conclusions of the Committee were set out in a Report (1947), in which a table was given showing Atwater's suggested factors for calculating the physiological energy values of different classes of foods.

In 1955, the United States Department of Agriculture issued a handbook entitled *Energy Value of Foods* (Merrill and Watt, 1955) in which the fundamental work of Atwater was described in some detail, and the steps followed in his procedure for determining the energy value of foods were set out. The authors examined the results of work done since Atwater's time on the availability of the protein, fat and carbohydrate in individual foods, and prepared a more detailed table of factors for different classes of food. This table had formed the basis of the calculation of calorific values of foods in the current US Department of Agriculture's publication *Composition of Foods* (Watt and Merrill, 1950). At about the time that Merrill and Watt's (1955) handbook was published the British Nutrition Society held a symposium on the 'Assessment of the energy value of human and animal foods', when the differences and difficulties of the problem were discussed from a more general point of view (Blaxter and Graham, 1955; Widdowson, 1955; Hollingsworth, 1955).

**Choice of calorie conversion factors for the 1st and 2nd editions of the present report**

In the first edition of these tables an important departure from traditional practice was the method used for the determination of carbohydrate. In Atwater's own work, and in the work of those who followed him, the percentage of carbohydrate in foods was generally not determined directly but was calculated 'by difference', ie as the difference between 100 and the sum of the percentage of water, protein, fat and ash in the food. Thus it included not only sugars, dextrins and starch, which are known to be available to man, but also all the complex carbohydrates, most of which are not available as carbohydrate at all. When the first edition of this report was being prepared it was decided that the values found by direct determination of the available carbohydrates were likely to approximate more closely to the physiological values, and the method of calculating carbohydrate 'by difference' was abandoned. The glucose, fructose, sucrose, dextrins and starch were separately determined and their sum, expressed in terms of 'monosaccharides', was given as 'available carbohydrate'. Glucose and other monosaccharides have a heat of combustion of 3.75 Calories per gram, and this was the value assigned to the available carbohydrate fraction in the second edition of the present publication. The unavailable carbohydrate was considered to contribute no Calories to the diet.

The figure chosen for protein in the first and second editions was 4.1 Calories per gram, which was Rubner's factor for mixed meat and vegetable protein; this makes an allowance of about 7 per cent for nitrogen lost in the faeces, and the correction for unoxidized nitrogenous material in the urine is the same as Atwater's. Rubner's factor of 9.3 was chosen for fat; this is the average heat of combustion of animal and vegetable fats, and it makes little or no allowance for losses of fat in the faeces. The heat of combustion of ethyl alcohol is 7.07 Calories per gram, and a factor of 7.0 was used in the first and second edition of these tables.

**Factors used in *Nutritive Values of Wartime Foods***

The second World War brought a need for tables giving the composition of the foods which were being produced and imported at that time, and the Council's Accessory Food Factors Committee undertook to compile such tables. These were published under the title *Nutritive Values of Wartime Foods* (Medical Research Council: Accessory Food Factors Committee, 1945). The figures for the protein, fat and carbohydrate in many of the foods were taken from the first edition of the present tables, the values for carbohydrate being based on direct chemical estimations of 'available carbohydrate', but expressed in terms of starch. To calculate the calorific value of the protein, fat and carbohydrate the factors 4, 9 and 4 Calories per gram respectively were used. In that publication the calorific value of the carbohydrate fraction of foods was definitely under-estimated since only the available fraction was considered, and a figure even lower than the physical, and probably also physiological, calorific value of starch (4.2 Calories per gram) was applied to it.

**Choice of calorie conversion factors for the 3rd edition**

Much thought has been given to the calorie conversion factors that should be used in the present edition of these tables. All the methods in current use are open to criticism. The use of different factors for protein and fat from various sources as worked out by Atwater and recommended by Maynard (1944), the FAO Committee (1947) and Merrill and Watt (1955) is undoubtedly a more correct approach than the use of the same factors for all foods, whether

4 and 9 or 4.1 and 9.3. On the other hand, the determination of the available carbohydrate fractions directly is acknowledged to be the better method, though there are few published tables in which this method has been used. The FAO Committee (1947) concluded that 'the correct chemical approach is by the extension of analytical work to include all substances covered by carbohydrates by difference'. Further studies of the digestibility of these substances are also required. Only when all the constituents of food have been determined and their physiological effects defined can their role in metabolism and their fuel value be accurately described'.

Work is in progress* along both lines suggested by the FAO Committee at the present time and, after much consideration, and with the advice of the Council's Diet and Energy Committee, the authors have decided that in order to avoid confusion the method of calculating the calorific values of foods shall remain unchanged in the present edition of these tables. The factors used, therefore, are 4.1 Calories per gram of protein, 9.3 Calories per gram of fat, 3.75 Calories per gram of available carbohydrate expressed as monosaccharides and 7.0 Calories per gram of alcohol. It is hoped that, when further evidence is available, a uniform method will be agreed upon, and used internationally.

Table 1 gives the calorific values of various foods as calculated by three different methods. It shows that in fact the agreement between the values arrived at by the different methods is in most instances quite close. The use of the factor 9.3 instead of 9 gives a slightly higher value for butter and other fats, but only in the case of fruit and vegetables where much of the carbohydrate is present in an 'unavailable' form do the figures really differ. Since these foods contribute a relatively small proportion of the calorific value of a whole diet it will not make much difference which factors are used to calculate the calorific value of mixed diets. In this respect it is of interest to note that calculations of the calorific value of National Food Supplies for the years 1947, 1955, 1956 and 1957 have been made by the various methods, and the results compared. The difference between the highest and lowest value was of the order of 2 per cent.

* Now published (Southgate and Durnin, 1970)

**Table 1**
*Comparison of the calorific values of foods calculated by three methods*
(Calories per 100 g)

| | Third edition of the present tables: protein × 4.1 fat × 9.3 available carbohydrate (as monosaccharides) × 3.75 | MRC War Memorandum No. 14 (1945): protein × 4.0 fat × 9.0 available carbohydrate (as starch) × 4.2 | FAO (1947) Merrill and Watt (1955): specific factors for different foods |
|---|---|---|---|
| *Cereals* | | | |
| Bread, brown | 242 | 245 | 251 |
| Bread, white | 243 | 242 | 242 |
| Flour, Manitoba, wholemeal | 339 | 336 | 327 |
| Flour, Manitoba, white | 352 | 350 | 353 |
| Oatmeal | 404 | 400 | 399 |
| Rice, polished | 361 | 359 | 368 |
| *Dairy-products* | | | |
| Butter | 793 | 768 | 748 |
| Cheese, Cheddar | 425 | 412 | 414 |
| Cheese, Gorgonzola | 393 | 380 | 382 |
| Eggs | 163 | 158 | 169 |
| Milk, fresh, whole | 66 | 65 | 68 |
| *Meat* | | | |
| Beef, corned | 231 | 224 | 231 |
| Beef, frozen, raw | 151 | 147 | 153 |
| Beef, steak, raw | 177 | 172 | 177 |
| Liver, raw | 143 | 139 | 144 |
| *Fruit* | | | |
| Apples, English, eating | 45 | 45 | 55 |
| Apricots, dried | 183 | 182 | 297 |
| Bananas | 77 | 76 | 103 |
| Currants, black, raw | 29 | 28 | 79 |
| Currants, red, raw | 21 | 21 | 60 |
| Gooseberries, green, raw | 17 | 17 | 35 |
| Grapefruit | 22 | 22 | 32 |
| Oranges | 35 | 35 | 49 |
| *Vegetables* | | | |
| Beans, butter, raw | 266 | 264 | 350 |
| Beans, runner, raw | 15 | 15 | 31 |
| Cabbage, Savoy, raw | 26 | 26 | 30 |
| Carrots, old, raw | 23 | 23 | 32 |
| Peas, fresh, raw | 64 | 63 | 81 |
| Potatoes, old, raw | 87 | 86 | 92 |
| *Nuts* | | | |
| Peanuts | 603 | 586 | 576 |
| Walnuts | 549 | 535 | 519 |

## References to appendix 2


Atwater, W. O. (1902) On the digestibility and availability of food materials. *Conn.* (*Storrs*) *Agric. Exp. Sta. 14th Annu. Rep.*, 1901

Atwater, W. O. (1910) Principles of nutrition and nutritive value of food. *Fmrs' Bull. US Dep. Agric.* No. 142 (2nd review)

Atwater, W. O., and Benedict, F. G. (1897) Experiments on the digestion of food by man. *Conn.* (*Storrs*) *Agric. Exp. Sta. Bull.* No. 18

Atwater, W. O., and Bryant, A. P. (1900) The availability and fuel value of food materials. *Conn.* (*Storrs*) *Agric. Exp. Sta., 12th Annu. Rep.*, 1899

Blaxter, K. L., and Graham, N. McC. (1955) Methods of assessing the energy values of foods for ruminant animals. *Proc. Nutr. Soc.* **14**, 131–139

Chatfield, C., and Adams, G. (1940) Proximate composition of American food materials. *Circ. US Dep. Agric.* No. 549.

Food and Agriculture Organization of the United Nations. Committee on Calorie Conversion Factors and Food Composition Tables (1947) *Energy-yielding components of food and computation of calorie values*. United Nations, Food and Agriculture Organization, Washington DC

Hollingsworth, D. F. (1955) Some difficulties in estimating the energy values of human diets. *Proc. Nutr. Soc.* **14**, 154–160

McCance, R. A., and Glaser, E. M. (1948) The energy value of oatmeal and the digestibility and absorption of its proteins, fats and calcium. *Brit. J. Nutr.* **2**, 221–228

McCance, R. A., and Lawrence, R. D. (1929) *The carbohydrate content of foods*. Medical Research Council Special Report Series No. 135. HMSO, London

McCance, R. A., and Walsham, C. M. (1948) The digestibility and absorption of the calories, proteins, purines, fat and calcium in wholemeal wheaten bread. *Brit. J. Nutr.* **2**, 26–41

McCance, R. A., and Widdowson, E. M. (1947) The digestibility of English and Canadian wheats, with special reference to the digestibility of wheat protein by man. *J. Hyg. Camb.* **45**, 59–64

Maynard, L. A. (1944) The Atwater system of calculating the caloric value of diets. *J. Nutr.* **28**, 443–452

Medical Research Council: Accessory Food Factors Committee (1945) *Nutritive values of wartime foods*. Medical Research Council War Memorandum No. 14. HMSO, London

Merrill, A. L., and Watt, B. K. (1955) *Energy value of foods—basis and derivation*. US Department of Agriculture, Agriculture Handbook No. 74, Washington DC

Morey, N. B. (1936) An analysis and comparison of different methods of calculating the energy value of diets. *Nutr. Abstr. Rev.* **6**, 1–12

Osmond, A. (1946) *Tables of composition of Australian foods*. Special Report Series No. 2 of the National Health and Medical Research Council Nutrition Committee, Canberra

Platt, B. S. (1945) *Tables of representative values of foods commonly used in tropical countries*. Medical Research Council Special Report Series No. 253. HMSO, London

Rubner, M. (1885) Calorimetrische Untersuchungen. *Z. Biol.* **21**, 250

Rubner, M. (1901) Der Energiewert der Kost des Menschen. *Z. Biol.* **42**, 261

Sherman, H. C. (1911) *The chemistry of food and nutrition*. Macmillan Co., New York

Sherman, H. C. (1952) *The chemistry of food and nutrition*, 8th edition. Macmillan Co., New York

Southgate, D. A. T., and Durnin, J. V. G. A. (1970) Calorie conversion factors: an experimental reassessment of the factors used in calculation of the energy value of human diets. *Br. J. Nutr.* **24**, 517–535

Watt, B. J., and Merrill, A. L. (1950) *Composition of foods—raw, processed, prepared.* US Department of Agriculture, Agriculture Handbook No. 8, Washington DC

Widdowson, E. M. (1955) Assessment of the energy value of human foods. *Proc. Nutr. Soc.* **14**, 142–154

# Appendix 3: Systematic names for fish and plant foods

## Fish

| Common name | Systematic name |
|---|---|
| **White fish** | |
| Cod | *Gadus morhua* |
| Haddock | *Melanogrammus aeglefinus* |
| Halibut | *Hippoglossus hippoglossus* |
| Lemon sole | *Microstomus kitt* |
| Plaice | *Pleuronectes platessa* |
| Saithe | *Pollachius virens* |
| Whiting | *Merlangius merlangus* |
| **Fatty fish** | |
| Eel | *Anguilla anguilla* |
| Herring, Bloater, Kipper | *Clupea harengus* |
| Mackerel | *Scomber scombrus* |
| Pilchards | *Sardinops sagax ocellata* |
| Salmon, Atlantic | *Salmo salar* |
| Salmon, red | *Oncorhynchus nerka* |
| Sardines | *Sardina pilchardus* |
| Sprats | *Sprattus sprattus* |
| Trout | *Salmo trutta* |
| Tuna, skipjack | *Euthynnus* sp<br>*Katsuwonus pelamis* |
| Whitebait | Young of *Clupea harengus* and *Sprattus sprattus* |
| **Cartilaginous fish** | |
| Dogfish | Probably *Squalus acanthias* |
| Skate | *Raja* sp |
| **Crustacea** | |
| Crab | *Cancer pagurus* |
| Lobster | *Homarus vulgaris* |
| Prawns | *Paleamon serratus* |
| Scampi | *Nephrops norvegicus* |
| Shrimps, brown | *Crangon crangon* |
| pink | *Pandalus montagui* |
| deep water | *Pandalus borealis* |

| | Common name | Systematic name |
|---|---|---|
| Fish *continued* | **Molluscs** | |
| | Cockles | *Cardium edule* |
| | Mussels | *Mytilus edulis* |
| | Oysters | *Ostrea edulis* |
| | Scallops | *Pecten maximus* |
| | Whelks | *Buccinum undatum* |
| | Winkles | *Littorina littorea* |
| Vegetables | Ackee | *Blighia sapida* |
| | Artichokes, globe | *Cynara scolymus* |
| | Artichokes, Jerusalem | *Helianthus tuberosus* |
| | Asparagus | *Asparagus officinalis* var *altilis* |
| | Aubergine | *Solanum melongena* var *ovigerum* |
| | Beans, French | *Phaseolus vulgaris* |
| | Beans, runner | *Phaseolus coccineus* |
| | Beans, broad | *Vicia faba* |
| | Beans, butter | *Phaseolus lunatus* |
| | Beans, haricot | *Phaseolus vulgaris* |
| | Beans, mung (green) | *Phaseolus aureus* |
| | Beans, red kidney | *Phaseolus vulgaris* |
| | Beansprouts | *Phaseolus aureus* |
| | Beetroot | *Beta vulgaris* |
| | Broccoli tops | *Brassica oleracea* var *botrytis* |
| | Brussels sprouts | *Brassica oleracea* |
| | Cabbage, red | *Brassica oleracea* |
| | Cabbage, Savoy | var of *Brassica oleracea* |
| | Cabbage, spring | *Brassica oleracea* var *capitata* |
| | Cabbage, white | var of *Brassica oleracea* |
| | Cabbage, winter | *Brassica oleracea* var *capitata* |
| | Carrots | *Daucus carota* |
| | Cauliflower | *Brassica oleracea* var *botrytis* |
| | Celeriac | *Apium graveolens* var *rapaceum* |
| | Celery | *Apium graveolens* |
| | Chicory | *Cichorium intybus* |
| | Cucumber | *Cucumis sativus* |
| | Endive | *Cichorium endivia* |
| | Horseradish | *Armoracia rusticana* |
| | Laverbread | *Porphyra umbilicalis* |
| | Leeks | *Allium ampelosprasum* var *porrum* |
| | Lentils | *Lens culinaris* |
| | Lettuce | *Lactuca sativa* |
| | Marrow | *Cucurbita pepo* |
| | Mushrooms | *Agaricus campestris* |
| | Mustard and cress | *Brassica* and *Lepidium* spp |
| | Okra | *Hibiscus esculentus* |
| | Onions | *Allium sepa* |
| | Parsley | *Petroselinum crispum* |
| | Parsnips | *Pastinaca sativa* |
| | Peas | *Pisum sativum* |
| | Peas, chick | *Cicer arietinum* |
| | Peas, red, pigeon | *Cajanus cajan* |
| | Peppers, green | *Capsicum annum* |

| | Common name | Systematic name |
|---|---|---|
| **Vegetables** *continued* | | |
| | Plantain | *Musa paradisiaca* |
| | Potatoes | *Solanum tuberosum* |
| | Pumpkin | *Cucurbito pepo* |
| | Radishes | *Raphanus sativus* |
| | Salsify | *Tragopogon porrifolius* |
| | Seakale | *Crambe maritima* |
| | Spinach | *Spinacia oleracea* |
| | Spring greens | var *Brassica oleracea* |
| | Swedes | *Brassica napus* var *napobrassica* |
| | Sweet potatoes | *Ipomaea batatas* |
| | Sweetcorn | *Zea mays* |
| | Tomatoes | *Lycopersicon esculentum* |
| | Turnips | *Brassica rapa* |
| | Watercress | *Nasturtium officinale* |
| | Yam | *Dioscorea* sp |
| **Fruit** | Apple | *Malus pumila* |
| | Apricot | *Prunus armeniaca* |
| | Avocado pear | *Persea americana* |
| | Banana | *Musa* sp |
| | Bilberry | *Vaccinium myrtillus* |
| | Blackberry | *Rubus ulmifolius* |
| | Cherry | *Prunus avium* |
| | Cranberry | *Vaccinium oxycoccus* |
| | Currants, black | *Ribes nigrum* |
| | Currants, red | *Ribes rubrum* |
| | Currants, white | *Ribes sativum* |
| | Currants, dried | *Vitis vinifera* |
| | Damson | *Prunus domestica* subsp *insititia* |
| | Date | *Phoenix dactylifera* |
| | Fig | *Ficus carica* |
| | Gooseberry | *Ribes grossularia* |
| | Grape | *Vitis vinifera* |
| | Grapefruit | *Citrus paradisi* |
| | Greengage | *Prunus domestica* subsp *italica* |
| | Guava | *Psidiom guajava* |
| | Lemon | *Citrus limon* |
| | Loganberry | *Rubus loganobaccus* |
| | Lychee | *Litchi chinensis* |
| | Mango | *Mangifera indica* |
| | Medlar | *Mespilus germanica* |
| | Melon, Cantaloupe | *Cucumis melo* |
| | Melon, yellow | *Cucumis citrallus* and *C. melo* |
| | Melon, watermelon | *Citrullus lanatus* |
| | Mulberry | *Morus nigra* |
| | Nectarine | *Prunus persica* var *nectarina* |
| | Olive | *Olea europaea* |
| | Orange | *Citrus sinensis* |
| | Passion fruit | *Passiflora edulis* |
| | Paw paw | *Carica papaya* |
| | Peach | *Prunus persica* |
| | Pear | *Pyrus communis* |
| | Pineapple | *Ananas comosus* |

| | Common name | Systematic name |
|---|---|---|
| **Fruit** *continued* | Plum | *Prunus domestica* subsp *domestica* |
| | Pomegranate | *Punica granatum* |
| | Quince | *Cydonia vulgaris* |
| | Raisin | *Vitis vinifera* |
| | Raspberry | *Rubus idaeus* |
| | Rhubarb | *Rheum rhaponticum* |
| | Strawberry | *Fragaria* sp |
| | Sultana | *Vitis vinifera* |
| | Tangerine | *Citrus reticulata* |
| **Nuts** | Almonds | *Prunus amygdalus* |
| | Barcelona nuts | *Corylus maxima barcelonensis* |
| | Brazil nuts | *Bertholletia excelsa* |
| | Chestnuts | *Castanea vulgaris* |
| | Cob/hazel | *Corylus avellana* and *C. maxima* |
| | Coconut | *Cocos nucifera* |
| | Peanuts | *Arachis hypogoea* |
| | Walnuts | *Juglans regia* |

## References to appendix 3

*Fish*

Labelling of Food (Amendment) Regulations 1972. Statutory Instruments 1972 No. 1510 HMSO, London

McCance, R. A., and Shipp, H. L. (1933). *The chemistry of flesh foods and their losses on cooking.* Medical Research Council Special Report Series No. 187. HMSO, London

*Vegetables, fruit and nuts*

Bailey, L. H. (1949) *Manual of cultivated plants most commonly found in the continental United States and Canada*, Macmillan & Co. New York

Tutin, T. G., Heywood, V. H., Burgess, N. A., Valentine, D. H., Walters, S. M., and Webb, D. A., and Moore, D. M. (editors) *Flora Europaea* Vol. I: Lycopodiaceae to Plantaceae (1964); Vol. II: Rosaceae to Umbelliferae (1968). Cambridge University Press, Cambridge

# Appendix 4: Recipes for cooked dishes

## Revised by J. Thorn and A. A. Paul

Bread

### 39 Soda bread

500g flour
1 level teaspoon salt
1 level teaspoon bicarbonate of soda
1 level teaspoon cream of tartar
290ml milk

Sift the dry ingredients and quickly knead to a soft dough with the milk. Bake for 35 minutes at Mark 7, 220°C.

Biscuits

### 65 Biscuits, home made basic mixture

100g margarine
100g caster sugar
200g flour
1 egg

Cream the fat and sugar. Mix in the egg, then the flour and knead the dough lightly until smooth. Roll out thinly, prick and shape. Bake 10-15 minutes at Mark 4, 180°C.

### 71 Shortbread

200g flour
100g butter
50g caster sugar

Beat the butter and sugar to a cream. Mix in the flour and knead till smooth. Press into a flat tin to about 2cm in thickness. Bake for about 45 minutes at Mark 3, 170°C.

Cakes

### 75 Fruit cake rich

200g margarine
200g brown sugar
4 eggs
20g black treacle
20ml brandy
250g flour
$\frac{1}{4}$ level teaspoon salt
750g mixed dried fruit
150g mixed glacé fruit, chopped
1 level teaspoon mixed spice

Cream the fat and sugar. Beat in the eggs, treacle and brandy. Fold in the sifted flour and spices, and mix in the fruit. Turn into a 20cm cake tin. Bake for 4 hours at Mark 2, 150°C.

### 76 Fruit cake rich, iced

1680g fruit cake, rich
70g apricot jam
410g marzipan

*Royal icing*
300g icing sugar
1 egg white
1 teaspoon lemon juice

Make the cake as in Recipe no 75. When cold spread with a thin layer of apricot jam and cover with marzipan. Make the royal icing by beating the egg whites and icing sugar; finally add the lemon juice.

Cakes *continued*

### 78 Gingerbread

300g flour
100g margarine
100g sugar
200g treacle
2 eggs
2 level teaspoons ground ginger
$\frac{1}{2}$ level teaspoon bicarbonate of soda
75ml milk

Melt the margarine, sugar and treacle in a pan, heating gently. Beat the egg well. Mix all the ingredients together and bake for about $1\frac{1}{4}$ hours at Mark 4, 180°C.

### 80 **Rock cakes** (basic recipe, rubbing-in method)

200g flour
3 level teaspoons baking powder
100g margarine
100g sugar
1 egg
50ml milk
100g currants

Sift together the flour and baking powder, and rub in the fat, add the currants. Mix to a soft dropping consistency with the egg and milk. Drop the mixture in small portions on to a baking sheet. Bake for about 15 minutes at Mark 8, 230°C.

### 81 **Sponge cake** with fat (basic recipe, creaming method)

150g flour
1 level teaspoon baking powder
150g margarine
150g caster sugar
3 eggs

Cream the fat and sugar until light and fluffy. Add the beaten egg a little at a time and beat well. Fold in the sifted flour and baking powder. Bake for about 20 minutes at Mark 5, 190°C.

### 82 **Sponge cake** without fat (basic recipe, whisking method)

4 eggs
100g caster sugar
100g flour

Whisk the eggs and sugar in a basin over hot water until stiff. Fold in the flour. Bake for about 25 minutes at Mark 5, 190°C, or, for Swiss rolls, 7 minutes at Mark 8, 230°C.

Buns and pastries

### 86 Eclairs

200g choux pastry, cooked
150g double cream

*Icing*
100g icing sugar
50g plain chocolate
30ml water

Make the choux pastry (see below) into eclairs. Slit, fill with whipped cream and top with chocolate icing.

### 87 Jam tarts

200g raw shortcrust pastry
200g jam

Line about ten tart tins with thinly rolled pastry. Fill each tart with jam and bake in a hot oven, Mark 6, 200°C, for 10–15 minutes.

### 88 Mince pies

300g raw shortcrust pastry
200g mincemeat

Roll out the pastry and cut into rounds. Place half the rounds in tart tins. Fill with mincemeat and cover with remaining pastry. Bake for about 20 minutes at Mark 5, 190°C.

Buns and pastries *continued*

### 89 and 90 **Pastry, choux**

100 g flour
50 g margarine
150 ml water
2 eggs
¼ level teaspoon salt

Boil the water, salt and margarine, add the flour and beat over heat to form a ball of smooth mixture. Cool and beat in the eggs. Pipe out as desired and bake for about 30 minutes at Mark 6, 200°C.

### 91 and 92 **Pastry, flaky**

200 g flour
75 g margarine
75 g lard
½ level teaspoon salt
10 ml lemon juice
80 ml water to bind

Make the pastry in the normal way, baking it at Mark 7, 220°C, or as directed.

### 93 and 94 **Pastry, shortcrust**

200 g flour
50 g margarine
50 g lard
½ level teaspoon salt
30 ml water to bind

Make the pastry in the normal way, baking it at Mark 6, 200°C, or as directed.

### 95 **Scones**

200 g flour
4 level teaspoons baking powder
¼ level teaspoon salt
50 g margarine
10 g sugar
125 ml milk

Sift the flour, sugar and baking powder and rub in the fat. Mix in the milk. Roll out and cut into rounds. Bake in a hot oven, Mark 7, 220°C, for about ten minutes.

### 96 **Scotch pancakes** (**Drop scones**)

200 g flour
½ level teaspoon salt
½ level teaspoon bicarbonate of soda
1 level teaspoon cream of tartar
50 g margarine
25 g caster sugar
1 egg
200 ml milk
15 g margarine for griddle

Sift flour with salt and raising agent, rub in fat and mix in sugar. Add egg and milk to give a stiff batter. Cook by spoonfuls on hot greased griddle.

Puddings

### 97 **Apple crumble**

400 g cooking apples, weighed after preparation
100 g flour
½ level teaspoon cinnamon
50 g margarine
100 g sugar

Peel, core and slice the apples. Arrange in a dish and sprinkle with half the sugar. Rub the other ingredients together and pile on top. Bake for 40 minutes at Mark 5, 190°C.

### 98 **Bread and butter pudding**

75 g bread
20 g butter
500 ml milk
30 g sugar
2 eggs
30 g currants

Cut the bread very thinly and spread with butter. Beat the eggs with the sugar and add the milk. Place layers of bread and currants in a pie dish and pour the eggs and milk over the bread. Leave to soak for 30 minutes and then bake at Mark 4, 180°C, for 30–40 minutes.

## 99 Cheesecake

*Base, for 18 cm tin*
150 g digestive biscuit crumbs
75 g margarine

*Top*
350 g cream or curd cheese
2 eggs
100 g caster sugar
25 g cornflour
1 lemon (juice = 40 g) and finely grated rind
150 g double cream
½ teaspoon vanilla essence

Melt the margarine in a pan and combine with the biscuit crumbs. Press into the base of the tin. Combine the topping ingredients, beat well and pour into base. Bake for 45 minutes at Mark 4, 180°C, until only just firm in the centre.

## 100 Christmas pudding

100 g flour
300 g breadcrumbs, fresh
1 level teaspoon mixed spices
½ level teaspoon salt
125 g suet
150 g raisins
150 g sultanas
150 g currants
50 g chopped mixed peel
30 g ground almonds
150 g brown sugar
3 eggs
15 g treacle
150 ml stout

Sift the flour, spices and salt into a basin and mix in all dry ingredients. Whisk the eggs, treacle and stout and stir thoroughly into dry ingredients. Put into well greased basins, cover with greased paper and foil. Boil for 6 hours. Renew foil and store. Re-boil for about 2 hours when required.

## 101 **Custard, egg** baked or sauce

500 ml milk
2 eggs
30 g sugar
vanilla essence

Beat the eggs and sugar together. Add the milk and vanilla essence. Either stir over gentle heat until mixture thickens or bake in a dish standing in a pan of water at Mark 3, 170°C, for 40 minutes.

## 102 **Custard** made with powder

500 ml milk
25 g custard powder
25 g sugar

Blend the custard powder with a little of the milk. Add the sugar to the remainder of the milk and bring to the boil. Pour immediately over the paste, stirring all the time. Return to the pan, bring back to boiling point, stirring, then serve.

## 103 Custard tart

300 g raw shortcrust pastry
250 ml milk
1 egg
15 g sugar

Make the pastry and line a shallow tin. Make the custard and use as filling. Bake at Mark 6, 200°C, lowering to Mark 5, 190°C until the custard is set (about 40 minutes).

## 104 Dumpling

100 g flour
45 g suet
75 g water
1 level teaspoon baking powder
½ level teaspoon salt

Mix the dry ingredients together with the cold water to form a soft dough. Divide into balls, flour them and place in boiling water. Boil for 30 minutes.

### 106 **Fruit pie** with pastry top

200g raw shortcrust pastry
450g fruit (prepared)
80g sugar
a little water if required

Place the prepared fruit, sugar and water in a pie dish. Cover with the pastry. Bake for 10 to 15 minutes at Mark 6, 200°C, to set the pastry, then about 20 minutes at Mark 4, 180°C, to cook the fruit.

### 110 **Jelly** made with water

130g jelly cubes
440ml water

Dissolve the jelly cubes in hot water. Add the rest of the cold water. Pour into a mould and allow to set.

### 111 **Jelly** made with milk

130g jelly cubes
250ml milk
200ml water

Dissolve the jelly cubes in hot water. Cool, add milk slowly, stirring constantly. Leave to set in a mould.

### 112 **Lemon meringue pie**

200g raw shortcrust pastry
2 lemons (juice = 80g)
2 eggs
125g caster sugar
25g cornflour
15g margarine
125ml water

Boil the cornflour, water, grated rind and juice of lemons and 25g of the sugar. Cool, stir in the egg yolks, and pour the mixture into the flan case. Make a meringue with the egg whites and the rest of the sugar; pile on top of the lemon mixture. Bake for 30 minutes at Mark 4, 180°C, until crisp and brown on top.

### 113 **Meringues**

4 egg whites
200g caster sugar

Whisk the egg whites until stiff. Fold in the sugar. Pipe onto the baking sheet. Bake for 3 hours at Mark $\frac{1}{2}$, 130°C.

### 114 **Milk puddings**

500ml milk
50g cereal (eg rice, sago, semolina, tapioca)
25g sugar

Simmer until cooked or bake in a moderate oven Mark 4, 180°C, according to type of cereal.

### 116 **Pancakes**

100g flour
250ml milk
1 egg
50g lard
50g sugar

Sieve the flour into a basin. Break in the egg and add about 100ml of the milk, stirring until smooth. Add the rest of the milk and beat to a smooth batter. Heat a little lard in a frying pan and pour in enough batter to cover the bottom. Cook both sides and turn onto sugared paper. Dredge lightly with sugar. Repeat until all the batter is used, to give about 10 pancakes.

### 117 Queen of puddings

250 ml milk
25 g butter
50 g breadcrumbs, fresh
100 g sugar
2 eggs, separated
rind of 1 lemon
50 g jam

Heat the milk and butter and pour over the breadcrumbs and 30 g of the sugar. Leave to soak for 30 minutes. Add the beaten egg yolks and grated lemon rind, and pour into a greased pie dish. Bake for about 20 minutes at Mark 4, 180°C. Spread the top with jam. Whisk the egg whites stiffly, then whisk in the rest of the sugar one teaspoonful at a time. Pile on top and bake at Mark 1, 140°C, until crisp and golden brown.

### 118 Sponge pudding steamed, basic mixture

100 g flour
1 level teaspoon baking powder
50 g margarine
50 g caster sugar
1 egg
30 ml milk

Cream the fat and sugar. Beat in the eggs a little at a time. Fold in the sifted flour and baking powder, adding milk to give a soft dropping consistency. Turn the mixture into a greased basin and steam for 1½ to 2 hours.

### 119 Suet pudding steamed, basic mixture

50 g flour
50 g breadcrumbs, fresh
50 g suet, shredded
30 g sugar
1 level teaspoon baking powder
¼ level teaspoon salt
80 ml milk

Mix the dry ingredients to a soft paste with the milk. Pour into a greased basin, cover with greased paper and steam for about 2½ hours.

### 120 Treacle tart

300 g raw shortcrust pastry
250 g golden syrup
50 g breadcrumbs, fresh

Line shallow tins with pastry, pour in the syrup and sprinkle with the breadcrumbs. Bake for 20–30 minutes at Mark 6, 200°C.

### 121 Trifle

75 g sponge cake
25 g jam
50 g fruit juice
75 g tinned fruit
25 ml sherry
250 g custard (made with powder)
25 g double cream
10 g nuts
10 g cherries
angelica

Slit the sponge cake, spread with jam and sandwich together. Cut into 4 cm cubes. Soak in the fruit juice and sherry. Mix with the fruit, cover with cold custard and decorate with the whipped cream, nuts and angelica.

### 122 Yorkshire pudding

100 g flour
1 level teaspoon salt
1 egg
250 ml milk
20 g dripping

Sieve flour and salt into a basin. Break in the egg and add about 100 ml of the milk, stirring until smooth. Add the rest of the milk and beat to a smooth batter. Pour into a tin containing very hot dripping. Bake for about 40 minutes at Mark 7, 220°C.

## 172 Omelette

2 eggs
10 ml water
10 g butter
$\frac{1}{2}$ level teaspoon salt
pepper

Beat the eggs with the salt and water. Heat the butter in an omelette pan. Pour in the mixture and stir until it begins to thicken evenly. While still creamy, fold the omelette and serve.

## 173 Scrambled eggs

2 eggs
15 g butter
20 ml milk
1 level teaspoon salt

Melt the butter in a small pan, stir in the beaten egg, milk and seasoning. Cook over gentle heat until the mixture thickens.

## 174 Cauliflower cheese

1 small cauliflower (700 g)
250 ml milk
100 ml cauliflower water
25 g margarine
25 g flour
100 g cheddar cheese, grated
$\frac{1}{2}$ level teaspoon salt
pepper

Prepare cauliflower and boil in water until just tender. Drain, saving 100 ml of the water, place cauliflower in a dish and keep warm. Make a white sauce from the margarine, flour, milk and cauliflower water. Add 75 g of the cheese and season. Pour over the cauliflower and sprinkle with the remaining cheese. Brown under the grill or in a hot oven, Mark 7, 220°C.

## 175 Cheese pudding

50 g breadcrumbs, fresh
250 ml milk
$\frac{1}{2}$ level teaspoon salt
cayenne pepper
75 g grated cheese
2 eggs

Heat the milk, pour over the breadcrumbs and allow to soak for about 30 minutes. Add the grated cheese, seasoning and egg yolks. Fold in the stiffly whipped whites and pour into a greased pie dish. Bake in a moderate oven, Mark 4, 180°C, for half an hour until well risen and golden brown.

## 176 Cheese soufflé

50 g margarine
50 g flour
250 ml milk
$\frac{1}{2}$ level teaspoon cayenne pepper
$\frac{1}{2}$ level teaspoon dry mustard
4 eggs
100 g cheese, grated

Melt the butter over gentle heat; stir in the flour and add the milk slowly. Cook for a minute or two. Cool slightly, beat in egg yolks, seasoning and cheese. Whisk egg whites stiffly and fold into mixture. Bake in a greased 17 cm soufflé dish at Mark 6, 200°C, for about 35 minutes.

## 177 Macaroni cheese

100 g macaroni
350 ml milk
25 g margarine
25 g flour
100 g cheese, grated
1 level teaspoon salt

Boil the macaroni and drain well. Make a white sauce from the margarine, flour and milk. Add 75 g of the cheese and season. Add the macaroni and put into a pie dish. Sprinkle with the remaining cheese and brown under the grill or in a hot oven Mark 7, 220°C.

Egg and cheese dishes *continued*

## 178 **Pizza** cheese and tomato

*Dough*

200 g flour
1 level teaspoon salt
1 level teaspoon sugar
15 g fresh yeast or 2 level teaspoons dried yeast
150 ml warm water

200 g tomatoes
150 g cheese
8 black olives (40 g)
20 g oil

Make the dough in the usual way, proving once. Knead and roll out to shape. Leave for 10 minutes. Arrange sliced or pulped tomatoes on top, then cheese and olives. Brush with oil. Bake for 30 minutes at Mark 8, 230°C.

## 179 **Quiche Lorraine**

200 g raw, shortcrust pastry
100 g bacon, streaky
100 g cheese

2 eggs
200 ml milk

Line a 20 cm flan ring with shortcrust pastry. Fill with the chopped bacon, fried and grated cheese. Beat the eggs in warmed milk and pour into the pastry case. Bake for 10 minutes at Mark 6, 200°C, then for 30 minutes at Mark 4, 180°C.

## 180 **Scotch eggs**

4 eggs
250 g raw pork sausage meat
25 g breadcrumbs, dried

20 g flour
15 g beaten egg

Hard boil the eggs, cool and shell. Dip in seasoned flour and cover with sausage meat. Brush with beaten egg and coat with crumbs. Deep fry for 8–10 minutes.

## 181 **Welsh rarebit**

2 slices buttered toast (50 g)
50 g grated cheese
$\frac{1}{4}$ level teaspoon dry mustard

20 ml milk
$\frac{1}{4}$ level teaspoon salt
cayenne pepper and pepper

Mix the cheese and seasoning with the milk. Spread on the toast and brown under the grill.

Meat dishes

## 422 and 423 **Sausage rolls** flaky and short

100 g raw flaky pastry
40 g pork sausage meat

*or*

100 g raw shortcrust pastry
50 g pork sausage meat

Make the pastry, roll out and cut into 10 cm squares. Place some sausage meat into the middle of each. Fold over and seal. Bake for 20–30 minutes at Mark 7, 220° C.

## 424 **Steak and kidney pie**

350 g raw flaky pastry
400 g raw stewing steak
200 g raw kidney

100 ml water
2 level teaspoons salt
15 g flour

Make the pastry. Prepare steak and kidney, cut into pieces and roll in seasoned flour. Place in a pie dish with water. Cover with pastry. Bake pie for 20 minutes at Mark 6, 200° C, then lower the heat to Mark 2, 150° C and cover with greaseproof paper. Cook for 2–2$\frac{1}{2}$ hours more.

### 426 Beef steak pudding

*Suet crust*
200 g flour
100 g suet
1½ level teaspoon baking powder
½ level teaspoon salt
130 ml water

500 g raw stewing steak
130 g onion (peeled and chopped)
50 g flour
25 ml water or stock
1 level teaspoon salt; pepper

Make the suet crust pastry, and line a pudding basin, leaving sufficient for a lid. Cut the meat into slices and roll in the seasoned flour. Put into the basin with the onion. Add a little water and cover with the remaining pastry. Steam for about 3 hours.

### 427 Beef stew

250 g raw stewing steak
75 g onion
75 g carrot
15 g dripping

300 ml water or stock
15 g flour
1 level teaspoon salt; pepper

Melt the dripping in a casserole and brown the pieces of meat. Remove the meat and brown the onion. Add the flour and cook the roux. Gradually blend in the water, add the meat, carrots and seasoning, bring to the boil and finish cooking at Mark 4, 180° C, for about 2 hours.

### 428 Bolognese sauce

25 g oil
75 g onion
75 g carrot
50 g celery
200 g minced beef

10 g tomato paste
200 g canned tomatoes
250 ml water or stock
1 level teaspoon salt; pepper, herbs

Brown the onion, carrot and celery in oil. Add the minced beef stirring thoroughly to brown. Add the tomatoes, stock and seasoning and simmer for 45 minutes with the lid on.

### 429 Curried meat

250 g cooked meat
200 g onion, peeled and chopped
50 g oil
75 g apple, peeled and chopped
50 g sultanas

15 g desiccated coconut
20 g flour
20 g curry powder
400 ml water
2 level teaspoons salt

Fry the onions in the oil. Add the apple, sultanas and coconut, then the flour and curry powder and fry for a minute or two. Add the water and bring to the boil. Simmer for 5 minutes. Add the cooked meat, cut into pieces and heat thoroughly.

### 430 Hot pot

250 g raw stewing steak
250 g potatoes
150 g onions

100 g carrots
125 ml stock
2 level teaspoons salt; pepper

Cut the steak into small pieces and arrange in layers with slices of carrot and onion. Add water and seasoning. Cover with a layer of sliced potatoes. Cover and bake at Mark 4, 180° C, for 2½ hours, removing the lid for the last 30 minutes to brown the potatoes.

### 431 Irish stew

250 g neck of mutton (weighed with bone)
250 g potato
125 g onion

350 ml water
1 level teaspoon salt; pepper

**Meat dishes**
*continued*

Cut up the meat, potato and onion and put into a saucepan. Add water and bring to the boil. Skim well and allow to simmer slowly for 1½ hours.

### 433 Moussaka

250 g minced beef
250 g aubergines or potatoes
150 g onions
30 g oil
100 ml water or stock
20 g tomato paste
1 level teaspoon salt

*Sauce*
150 ml milk
15 g flour
15 g oil
50 g cheese, grated
½ egg

Fry the sliced onions in the oil until soft and remove from pan. Fry the aubergines until transparent then brown the meat. Arrange layers of aubergines, meat and onions in a casserole. Add the tomato paste and the seasoned stock. Pour the cheese sauce over the top, and cooked for 1 hour at Mark 5, 190° C.

### 434 Shepherd's pie

350 g cooked minced beef
100 g onion boiled and chopped
150 ml water
500 g boiled potato
50 ml milk
20 g margarine
2 level teaspoons salt; pepper

Mix the beef and onion, moisten with water and add seasoning. Place in a pie dish. Mash the potato with the milk and margarine. Pile on top of the meat and bake in the oven for 25 minutes to brown. Mark 5, 190° C.

**Fish dishes**

### 548 Fish pie

200 g cooked white fish
400 g mashed potato

*Sauce*
150 ml milk
15 g margarine
15 g flour
½ level teaspoon salt

Flake the fish and mix with the white sauce. Pipe a potato border round a dish, pour in the fish mixture. Brown in the oven, Mark 6, 200° C, for 30 minutes.

### 549 Kedgeree

200 g smoked fillet, steamed
50 g rice
25 g margarine
2 eggs
½ level teaspoon salt; pepper

Boil the rice. Hard boil one egg. Melt the margarine and stir in the flaked fish, rice, seasoning and one beaten egg. Stir in chopped hard boiled egg and heat thoroughly.

**Vegetable dishes**

### 571 Beans, mung cooked, dahl

120 g dry beans
30 g butter
35 g onion
1 level teaspoon ginger
1 level teaspoon turmeric
½ level teaspoon garlic
2 level teaspoon salt
spices
chilli powder
840 ml water for cooking

Soak the beans in water for a few minutes; strain. Add the 840 ml water, salt and turmeric, bring to the boil and simmer for 40 minutes. Cook the chopped onions in the butter, with the garlic, ginger, spices and chilli powder. Add to the cooked dahl and simmer for 5 minutes.

Vegetable dishes *continued*

### 605 **Lentils** masur dahl, cooked

110 g dry lentils
20 g butter
30 g onion
1 level teaspoon ginger
½ level teaspoon garlic
1 level teaspoon salt
1 level teaspoon spices and seasonings
turmeric
680 ml water for cooking

Soak the lentils for 10–15 minutes; strain. Add the 680 ml water, bring to the boil, add salt and turmeric and simmer for 40 minutes. Cook the chopped onions in the butter, with the garlic, ginger, spices and seasonings. Add to the cooked dahl and simmer for 5 minutes.

### 631 **Peas, chick** cooked, dahl

110 g dry peas, whole
20 g butter
60 g onion
50 g tomatoes
2 level teaspoons ginger
½ level teaspoon garlic
1 level teaspoon salt
1 level teaspoon spices and seasonings
turmeric
500 ml water for cooking

Soak the peas overnight in cold water; strain. Cook the chopped onion in the butter, with the ginger, garlic and seasonings. Add the tomatoes. Mix, add the spices and finally the strained peas. Add the water and simmer for 1½ hours.

Preserves, sauces and soups

### 852 **Lemon curd**

300 g sugar (including some sugar lumps)
100 g butter
4 lemons (juice = 150 ml)
4 eggs

Wash lemons and rub a few sugar lumps over the rind to extract the flavour. Squeeze lemons. Melt butter, lemon juice and all the sugar in a double pan. Add the eggs one by one and cook slowly, stirring all the time, until the mixture coats the back of a spoon. Pour into jars and cover.

### 854 **Marzipan**

300 g ground almonds
150 g caster sugar
150 g icing sugar
1 egg
20 ml lemon juice

Mix almonds and sugar, add beaten egg and knead all ingredients until smooth.

### 920 **Bread sauce**

250 ml milk
50 g fresh breadcrumbs
5 g margarine
1 small onion
2 cloves
mace
½ level teaspoon salt

Put the milk and the onion, stuck with cloves, in a saucepan and bring to the boil. Add the breadcrumbs, and simmer for about 20 minutes over gentle heat. Remove the onion, stir in the margarine and season.

### 922 **Cheese sauce**

350 ml milk
25 g flour
25 g margarine
75 g cheese
½ level teaspoon salt
pepper, cayenne

Melt the fat in a pan. Add the flour and cook gently for a few minutes stirring all the time. Add the milk and cook until the mixture thickens, stirring continually. Add the grated cheese and seasoning. Reheat to soften the cheese and serve immediately.

### 923 Chutney, apple

500 g cooking apples
400 g onions
100 g raisins
400 ml vinegar
450 g sugar
1 level teaspoon salt
2 level teaspoons curry powder
½ level teaspoon mustard
½ level teaspoon pepper
½ level teaspoon ground ginger

Peel and core the apples and peel the onions and chop into small pieces. Mix all the ingredients except the sugar and boil gently till soft. Add the sugar and boil for a further 30 minutes. Pour into jars and tie down.

### 924 Chutney, tomato

1 kg tomatoes
125 g cooking apples
500 g onions
100 g sultanas
450 ml vinegar
500 g sugar
1 level teaspoon salt
½ level teaspoon mustard
¼ level teaspoon pepper
2 level teaspoons curry powder

Peel the tomatoes, chop the apples and onions into small pieces. Mix all the ingredients except the sugar and boil gently until soft. Add the sugar and boil for a further 30 minutes. Pour into jars and tie down.

### 925 French dressing

25 ml vinegar
75 g olive oil
½ level teaspoon salt
½ level teaspoon pepper

Shake the ingredients together in a screw-topped jar or bottle.

### 926 Mayonnaise

1 egg yolk
125 g oil
¼ level teaspoon salt
¼ level teaspoon made mustard
20 ml vinegar
pepper

Beat yolk and seasoning in a bowl. Whisk oil in very gradually to form a thick emulsion, adding the vinegar.

### 927 Onion sauce

*White sauce*
350 ml milk
25 g flour
25 g margarine
200 g cooked onion
1 level teaspoon salt
pepper

Make the white sauce and add the chopped onion and seasoning.

### 933 Tomato sauce

400 g tomatoes
25 g carrot
50 g onion
25 g bacon, streaky
15 g margarine
250 ml stock
25 g flour
½ level teaspoon salt
herbs (bouquet garni)

Fry the chopped vegetables gently with the margarine and bacon. Stir in the flour, blended with some of the stock, then the rest of the stock and the herbs. Simmer for 40 minutes, then sieve or liquidise if desired. Reheat, adjust seasoning and serve.

### 934 and 935 White sauce sweet or savoury

350 ml milk
25 g flour
25 g margarine
30 g sugar
*or*
½ level teaspoon salt

Melt the fat in a pan. Add the flour and cook for a few minutes, stirring constantly. Add the milk and salt or sugar and cook gently until the mixture thickens.

## 943 Lentil soup

| | |
|---|---|
| 100g lentils | 25g margarine |
| 25g carrot | 25g flour |
| 50g turnip | 1 litre stock |
| 50g onion | 125ml milk |
| 1 ham bone | herbs (bouquet garni) |
| | salt and pepper to taste |

Melt the dripping and toss the lentils and sliced vegetables in it over a gentle heat. Add the stock, seasoning, herbs and ham bone and bring to the boil. Simmer for 2–2½ hours stirring at intervals. Remove the bone. Sieve or liquidise and return to the pan with the flour blended to a smooth cream with the milk. Simmer for 5 minutes, and adjust seasoning.

# Appendix 5: Key to the use of amino acid and fatty acid numbers

This key shows the relationship between the numbers in section 1 and the numbers in sections 2 and 3. Primarily it is intended for use in the calculation of amino acid and fatty acid composition per 100g of food.

**Description of the key**

The number in the first column is the code number assigned in section 1; this is followed by the name of the item. A name given in bold italics *does not* appear in section 1 of the tables and is usually a grouped item appearing in one of the other sections.

The following columns give the appropriate code numbers in the amino acid section and fatty acid sections respectively.

In many cases amino acids or fatty acids have not been measured in a particular foodstuff; where it is reasonable to assume that little error would result from the use of values for a related food the code number of this food is given in parentheses.

The value zero indicates that no protein or fat is present in the food.

A dash means that it is not possible to give any guidance about which is the most appropriate value to use. Where fruits and vegetables are concerned a dash in the fatty acid column for all practical purposes can be regarded as zero. This generalisation applies for many foods and the symbol ∅ is used where little or no error would result from ignoring this food in amino acid or fatty acid calculations.

The symbol 'a' indicates that the value for fatty acids will depend on the fat used in cooking and that no general guidance can be given.

The symbol 'R' indicates that the values have been derived from calculations from a recipe. The appropriate items to use in calculating amino acids and fatty acids are given in part 2 of this key.

**Calculation of amino acids and fatty acids per 100 g food**

Amino acids per 100 g are obtained by multiplying the total nitrogen (g/100 g, given in section 1) by the amino acids composition (mg amino acid per g N) of the appropriate item in section 2 as indicated in the key.

For example:

Item 252 **Beef rump steak** grilled, lean and fat
Total N = 4.36 g/100 g
Corresponding item in amino acid section, 2237

| | Amino acids | | | |
|---|---|---|---|---|
| | Ile | Leu | Lys | etc |
| Amino acids in 2237 (mg/gN) | 320 | 500 | 570 | |
| Amino acids in 252 (mg/100 g) = (4.36 × values in 2237) | 1395 | 2180 | 2485 | etc |

The values for cooked dishes are based on the information given in part 2 of the key. The amino acids in the ingredients are multiplied by the amount of total nitrogen contributed by the ingredients to 100 g of the dish.

For example:

Item 116 **Pancakes**

| Ingredients | Item in section 2 | Total N contributed by ingredients |
|---|---|---|
| Flour | 2011 | 0.43 |
| Milk | 2123 | 0.32 |
| Egg | 2165 | 0.25 |

The amino acids in the cooked dish are derived as follows:

| | Amino acids | | | |
|---|---|---|---|---|
| | Ile | Leu | Lys | etc |
| From flour (0.43 × values in 2011) | 103 | 189 | 52 | |
| milk (0.32 × values in 2123) | 112 | 205 | 163 | |
| egg (0.25 × values in 2165) | 88 | 130 | 98 | |
| Amino acids in item 116 (mg/100 g) = | 303 | 524 | 313 | etc |

Fatty acids per 100 g are calculated in a similar way using the compositions given in section 3, ***except*** that the factor giving the proportion of fatty acids in the total fat must also be used in the calculation (see p 17).

For example:

Item 252 **Beef rump steak** grilled, lean and fat
Fat 12.1 g/100 g; factor 0.953
Corresponding item in fatty acid section 3240

| | Fatty acids | | | |
|---|---|---|---|---|
| | 14:0 | 15:0 | 16:0 | etc |
| Fatty acids in item 3240 (g/100 g total fatty acids) | 3.2 | 0.6 | 26.9 | |
| Fatty acids in item 252 (g/100 g) = (12.1 × 0.953 × values in 3240/100) | 0.37 | 0.07 | 3.10 | |

For cooked dishes the values in the fatty acid section are multiplied by values for the fatty acids contributed by the ingredients of the dish.

For example:

Item 116 **Pancakes**

| Ingredient | Item in section 3 | Fat contributed | Factor |
|---|---|---|---|
| Flour | 3008 | 0.29 | 0.67 |
| Milk | 3123 | 2.20 | 0.945 |
| Eggs | 3165 | 1.39 | 0.830 |
| Lard | 3185 | 12.42 | 0.956 |

The fatty acids in the cooked dish are derived as follows:

| | Fatty acids | | |
|---|---|---|---|
| | 14:0 | 16:0 | 18:0 |
| From flour (0.29 × 0.67 × values in 3008/100) | Tr | 0.03 | Tr |
| milk (2.20 × 0.945 × values in 3123/100) | 0.23 | 0.54 | 0.23 |
| eggs (1.39 × 0.830 × values in 3165/100) | Tr | 0.33 | 0.11 |
| lard (12.42 × 0.956 × values in 3185/100) | 0.19 | 3.18 | 1.85 |
| Fatty acids in 116 (g/100g) | 0.42 | 4.08 | 2.19 |

# Appendix 5 (part 1): Key to the use of amino acid and fatty acid numbers

| | | Food names | Amino acids: tables section 2 | Fatty acids: tables section 3 |
|---|---|---|---|---|
| **Cereals** | 1 | **Arrowroot** | — | — |
| | 2 | **Barley** pearl, raw | 2002 | 3002 |
| | 3 | boiled | 2002 | 3002 |
| | 4 | **Bemax** | 2009 | 3207 |
| | 5 | **Bran** wheat | 2005 | 3005 |
| | 6 | **Cornflour** | 2006 | 3198 |
| | 7 | **Custard powder** | 2006 | 3198 |
| | 8 | ***Flour general*** | — | 3008 |
| | 9 | wholemeal (100%) | 2009 | 3008 |
| | 10 | brown (85%) | 2010 | 3008 |
| | 11 | white (72%) breadmaking | 2011 | 3008 |
| | 12 | household plain | 2011 | 3008 |
| | 13 | self raising | 2011 | 3008 |
| | 14 | patent (40%) | 2011 | 3008 |
| | 15 | **Macaroni** raw | 2011 | 3008 |
| | 16 | boiled | 2011 | 3008 |
| | 17 | **Oatmeal** raw | 2017 | 3017 |
| | 18 | **Porridge** | 2017 | 3017 |
| | 19 | **Rice** polished, raw | 2019 | 3019 |
| | 20 | boiled | 2019 | 3019 |
| | 21 | **Rye** flour (100%) | 2021 | 3021 |
| | 22 | **Sago** raw | — | — |
| | 23 | **Semolina** raw | 2011 | 3008 |
| | 24 | **Soya** flour, full fat | 2024 | 3205 |
| | 25 | low fat | 2024 | 3205 |
| | 26 | **Spaghetti** raw | 2011 | 3008 |
| | 27 | boiled | 2011 | 3008 |
| | 28 | canned in tomato sauce | 2011 | — |
| | 29 | **Tapioca** | — | — |
| | 30 | **Bread** wholemeal | 2009 | 3030 |
| | 31 | brown | 2010 | 3030 |
| | 32 | Hovis | 2010 | (3030) |
| | 33 | white | 2011 | 3033 |
| | 34 | white, fried | 2011 | a |
| | 35 | toasted | 2011 | 3033 |
| | 36 | dried crumbs | 2011 | 3033 |
| | 37 | currant | 2011 | 3033 |
| | 38 | malt | 2009 | — |
| | 39 | soda | R | R |
| | 40 | **Rolls** brown, crusty | 2010 | 3030 |
| | 41 | soft | 2010 | (3030) |
| | 42 | white crusty | 2011 | (3033) |
| | 43 | soft | 2011 | (3033) |
| | 44 | starch reduced | 2011 | (3008) |
| | 45 | **Chapatis** with fat | 2010 | a |
| | 46 | without fat | 2010 | 3008 |
| | 47 | **All-bran** | 2005 | 3005 |
| | 48 | **Cornflakes** | 2006 | 3198 |
| | 49 | **Grapenuts** | 2002 | — |

| | | Food names | Amino acids: tables section 2 | Fatty acids: tables section 3 |
|---|---|---|---|---|
| **Cereals** *continued* | 50 | **Muesli** | (2017) | (3017) |
| | 51 | **Puffed wheat** | 2009 | 3008 |
| | 52 | **Ready Brek** | 2017 | 3017 |
| | 53 | **Rice Krispies** | 2019 | 3019 |
| | 54 | **Shredded Wheat** | 2009 | 3008 |
| | 55 | **Special K** | — | — |
| | 56 | **Sugar Puffs** | 2009 | 3008 |
| | 57 | **Weetabix** | 2009 | 3008 |
| | | **Biscuits** | | |
| | 58 | **Chocolate** full coated | 2011 | 3058 |
| | 59 | **Cream crackers** | 2011 | — |
| | 60 | **Crispbread** rye | 2021 | 3060 |
| | 61 | wheat, starch reduced | 2011 | 3061 |
| | 62 | **Digestive** plain | 2010 | — |
| | 63 | chocolate | — | 3063 |
| | 64 | **Ginger nuts** | (2011) | 3064 |
| | 65 | **Home made** | R | R |
| | 66 | **Matzo** | (2011) | 3066 |
| | 67 | **Oatcakes** | (2017) | 3067 |
| | 68 | **Sandwich** | (2011) | 3068 |
| | 69 | **Semi-sweet** | (2011) | 3069 |
| | 70 | **Short-sweet** | (2011) | 3070 |
| | 71 | **Shortbread** | R | R |
| | 72 | **Wafers** filled | (2011) | 3072 |
| | 73 | **Water biscuits** | (2011) | — |
| | 74 | **Fancy iced cakes** | (2011) | 3074 |
| | 75 | **Fruit cake** rich | R | R |
| | 76 | rich, iced | R | R |
| | 77 | plain | — | 3077 |
| | 78 | **Gingerbread** | R | R |
| | 79 | **Madeira cake** | (2011) | 3079 |
| | 80 | **Rock cakes** | R | R |
| | 81 | **Sponge cake** with fat | R | R |
| | 82 | **Sponge cake** without fat | R | R |
| | 83 | jam filled | | 3083 |
| | 84 | **Currant buns** | 2011) | — |
| | 85 | **Doughnuts** | (2011) | — |
| | 86 | **Eclairs** | R | R |
| | 87 | **Jam tarts** | R | R |
| | 88 | **Mince pies** | R | R |
| | 89 | **Pastry, choux** raw | R | R |
| | 90 | cooked | R | R |
| | 91 | **flaky** raw | 2011 | R |
| | 92 | cooked | 2011 | R |
| | 93 | **shortcrust** raw | 2011 | R |
| | 94 | cooked | 2011 | R |
| | 95 | **Scones** | R | R |
| | 96 | **Scotch pancakes** | R | R |
| | 97 | **Apple crumble** | R | R |
| | 98 | **Bread and butter pudding** | R | R |
| | 99 | **Cheesecake** | R | R |
| | 100 | **Christmas pudding** | R | R |
| | 101 | **Custard** egg | R | R |
| | 102 | made with powder | 2123 | 3123 |
| | 103 | **Custard tart** | R | R |
| | 104 | **Dumpling** | R | R |

| | | Food names | Amino acids: tables section 2 | Fatty acids: tables section 3 |
|---|---|---|---|---|
| **Cereals** *continued* | 105 | **Fruit pie** individual | — | — |
| | 106 | pastry top | R | R |
| | 107 | **Ice cream** dairy | 2123 | 3107 |
| | 108 | non-dairy | 2123 | 3108 |
| | 109 | **Jelly** packet, cubes | 2959 | 0 |
| | 110 | made with water | 2959 | 0 |
| | 111 | made with milk | R | 3123 |
| | 112 | **Lemon meringue pie** | R | R |
| | 113 | **Meringues** | 2166 | 0 |
| | 114 | **Milk pudding** | R | R |
| | 115 | canned, rice | (R) | (R) |
| | 117 | **Queen of puddings** | R | R |
| | 116 | **Pancakes** | R | R |
| | 118 | **Sponge pudding** steamed | R | R |
| | 119 | **Suet pudding** steamed | R | R |
| | 120 | **Treacle tart** | R | R |
| | 121 | **Trifle** | R | R |
| | 122 | **Yorkshire pudding** | R | R |
| **Milk** | 123 | ***Milk, cows'*** | 2123 | 3123 |
| | 124 | fresh, whole, summer | 2123 | 3123 |
| | 125 | fresh, whole, winter | 2123 | 3123 |
| | 126 | ***Milk, fresh, whole, Channel Islands*** | 2123 | 3123 |
| | 127 | Channel Islands, summer | 2123 | 3123 |
| | 128 | Channel Islands, winter | 2123 | 3123 |
| | 129 | sterilised | 2123 | 3123 |
| | 130 | longlife (UHT treated) | 2123 | 3123 |
| | 131 | fresh, skimmed | 2123 | 3123 |
| | 132 | condensed, whole, sweetened | 2123 | 3123 |
| | 133 | condensed, skimmed, sweetened | 2123 | 3123 |
| | 134 | evaporated, whole, unsweetened | 2123 | 3123 |
| | 135 | dried, whole | 2123 | 3123 |
| | 136 | dried, skimmed | 2123 | 3123 |
| | 137 | **Milk, goats'** | — | 3137 |
| | 138 | **human** mature | 2138 | 3138 |
| | 139 | transitional | (2138) | (3138) |
| | 140 | **Butter** salted | 2123 | 3123 |
| | 141 | ***Cream, single*** | 2123 | 3123 |
| | 142 | single, summer | 2123 | 3123 |
| | 143 | winter | 2123 | 3123 |
| | 144 | ***Cream, double*** | 2123 | 3123 |
| | 145 | double, summer | 2123 | 3123 |
| | 146 | winter | 2123 | 3123 |
| | 147 | ***Cream, whipping*** | 2123 | 3123 |
| | 148 | whipping, summer | 2123 | 3123 |
| | 149 | winter | 2123 | 3123 |
| | 150 | sterilised, canned | 2123 | 3123 |
| | 151 | **Cheese** Camembert type | 2123 | 3123 |
| | 152 | Cheddar type | 2123 | 3123 |
| | 153 | Danish Blue type | 2123 | 3123 |
| | 154 | Edam type | 2123 | 3123 |
| | 155 | Parmesan type | 2123 | 3123 |
| | 156 | Stilton type | 2123 | 3123 |
| | 157 | cottage | 2123 | 3123 |
| | 158 | cream | 2123 | 3123 |
| | 159 | processed | 2123 | 3123 |
| | 160 | cheese spread | 2123 | 3123 |

| | | Food names | Amino acids: tables section 2 | Fatty acids: tables section 3 |
|---|---|---|---|---|
| **Milk** *continued* | 161 | **Yogurt** low fat, natural | 2161 | 3123 |
| | 162 | flavoured | 2161 | 3123 |
| | 163 | fruit | 2161 | 3123 |
| | 164 | hazelnut | 2161 | 3123 |
| | 165 | **Eggs** whole, raw | 2165 | 3165 |
| | 166 | white, raw | 2166 | 0 |
| | 167 | yolk, raw | 2167 | 3165 |
| | 168 | dried | 2165 | 3165 |
| | 169 | boiled | 2165 | 3165 |
| | 170 | fried | 2165 | a |
| | 171 | poached | 2165 | 3165 |
| | 172 | omelette | 2165 | 3165 |
| | 173 | scrambled | 2165 | 3165 |
| | 174 | **Cauliflower cheese** | R | R |
| | 175 | **Cheese pudding** | R | R |
| | 176 | **Cheese soufflé** | R | R |
| | 177 | **Macaroni cheese** | R | R |
| | 178 | **Pizza** cheese and tomato | R | R |
| | 179 | **Quiche Lorraine** | R | R |
| | 180 | **Scotch egg** | R | R |
| | 181 | **Welsh rarebit** | R | R |
| **Fats and Oils** | 182 | **Cod liver oil** | 0 | |
| | 183 | **Compound cooking fat** | 0 | 3183 |
| | 184 | **Dripping, beef** | 0 | 3184 |
| | 185 | **Lard** | 0 | 3185 |
| | 186 | **Low fat spread** | 0 | 3186 |
| | 187 | **Margarine** | 2123 | a |
| | | **hard** animal and vegetable oils | 2123 | 3188 |
| | | vegetable oils only | 2123 | 3189 |
| | | **soft** animal and vegetable oils | 2123 | 3190 |
| | | vegetable oils only | 2123 | 3191 |
| | | **polyunsaturated** vegetable oils only | 2123 | 3192 |
| | 193 | **Suet** block | — | 3194 |
| | 194 | shredded | — | 3194 |
| | 195 | **Vegetable oils** | 0 | a |
| | 196 | coconut | 0 | 3196 |
| | 197 | cottonseed | 0 | 3197 |
| | 198 | maize, corn | 0 | 3198 |
| | 199 | olive | 0 | 3199 |
| | 200 | palm | 0 | 3200 |
| | 201 | peanut, groundnut | 0 | 3201 |
| | 202 | rapeseed (high erucic acid) | 0 | 3202 |
| | 203 | rapeseed (low erucic acid) | 0 | 3203 |
| | 204 | safflowerseed | 0 | 3204 |
| | 205 | soyabean | 0 | 3205 |
| | 206 | sunflowerseed | 0 | 3206 |
| | 207 | wheatgerm | 0 | 3008 |
| **Meat** | 208 | **Bacon, dressed carcase** raw | 2210 | 3209 |
| | 210 | **lean** average raw | 2210 | 3209 |
| | 211 | **fat** average raw | 2210 | 3209 |
| | 212 | **fat** average cooked | 2210 | 3209 |
| | 213 | **collar joint** raw | 2210 | 3209 |
| | 214 | boiled lean and fat | 2210 | 3209 |
| | 215 | boiled lean only | 2210 | 3209 |

| | | Food names | Amino acids: tables section 2 | Fatty acids: tables section 3 |
|---|---|---|---|---|
| **Meat** *continued* | 216 | **Gammon joint** raw | 2210 | 3209 |
| | 217 | boiled, lean and fat | 2210 | 3209 |
| | 218 | boiled, lean only | 2210 | 3209 |
| | 219 | **Gammon rashers** grilled, lean and fat | 2210 | 3209 |
| | 220 | lean only | 2210 | 3209 |
| | 221 | **Bacon rashers raw**, back | 2210 | 3209 |
| | 222 | middle | 2210 | 3209 |
| | 223 | streaky | 2210 | 3209 |
| | 225 | **fried,** average lean | 2210 | 3209 |
| | 226 | back, lean and fat | 2210 | 3209 |
| | 227 | middle, lean and fat | 2210 | 3209 |
| | 228 | streaky, lean and fat | 2210 | 3209 |
| | 230 | **grilled,** average lean | 2210 | 3209 |
| | 231 | back, lean and fat | 2210 | 3209 |
| | 232 | middle, lean and fat | 2210 | 3209 |
| | 233 | streaky, lean and fat | 2210 | 3209 |
| | 235 | **Beef, dressed carcase** raw | 2237 | 3240 |
| | 237 | **lean** average, raw | 2237 | 3240 |
| | 240 | **fat** average, raw | (2237) | 3240 |
| | 241 | **fat** average, cooked | 2237 | 3240 |
| | 242 | **brisket** raw, lean and fat | 2237 | 3240 |
| | 243 | boiled, lean and fat | 2237 | 3240 |
| | 244 | **forerib** raw, lean and fat | 2237 | 3240 |
| | 245 | roast, lean and fat | 2237 | 3240 |
| | 246 | lean only | 2237 | 3240 |
| | 247 | **mince** raw | 2237 | 3240 |
| | 248 | stewed | 2237 | 3240 |
| | 249 | **rump steak** raw, lean and fat | 2237 | 3240 |
| | 250 | fried, lean and fat | 2237 | 3240 |
| | 251 | lean only | 2237 | 3240 |
| | 252 | grilled, lean and fat | 2237 | 3240 |
| | 253 | lean only | 2237 | 3240 |
| | 254 | **silverside** salted, boiled, lean and fat | 2237 | 3240 |
| | 255 | lean only | 2237 | 3240 |
| | 256 | **sirloin** raw, lean and fat | 2237 | 3240 |
| | 257 | roast, lean and fat | 2237 | 3240 |
| | 258 | lean only | 2237 | 3240 |
| | 259 | **stewing steak** raw, lean and fat | 2237 | 3240 |
| | 260 | stewed, lean and fat | 2237 | 3240 |
| | 261 | **topside** raw, lean and fat | 2237 | 3240 |
| | 262 | roast, lean and fat | 2237 | 3240 |
| | 263 | lean only | 2237 | 3240 |
| | 264 | **Lamb, dressed carcase** raw | 2266 | 3269 |
| | 266 | **lean** average, raw | 2266 | 3269 |
| | 269 | **fat** average, raw | 2266 | 3269 |
| | 270 | cooked | 2266 | 3269 |
| | 271 | **breast** raw, lean and fat | 2266 | 3269 |
| | 272 | roast, lean and fat | 2266 | 3269 |
| | 273 | lean only | 2266 | 3269 |
| | 274 | **chops, loin** raw, lean and fat | 2266 | 3269 |
| | 275 | grilled, lean and fat | 2266 | 3269 |
| | 276 | lean and fat (with bone) | 2266 | 3269 |
| | 277 | lean only | 2266 | 3269 |
| | 278 | lean only (with fat and bone) | 2266 | 3269 |

**Meat**
*continued*

| | Food names | Amino acids: tables section 2 | Fatty acids: tables section 3 |
|---|---|---|---|
| 279 | **Lamb cutlets** raw, lean and fat | 2266 | 3269 |
| 280 | grilled, lean and fat | 2266 | 3269 |
| 281 | lean and fat (with bone) | 2266 | 3269 |
| 282 | lean only | 2266 | 3269 |
| 283 | lean only (with fat and bone) | 2266 | 3269 |
| 284 | **leg** raw, lean and fat | 2266 | 3269 |
| 285 | roast, lean and fat | 2266 | 3269 |
| 286 | lean only | 2266 | 3269 |
| 287 | **scrag and neck** raw, lean and fat | 2266 | 3269 |
| 288 | stewed, lean and fat | 2266 | 3269 |
| 289 | lean only | 2266 | 3269 |
| 290 | lean only (with fat) | 2266 | 3269 |
| 291 | **shoulder** raw, lean and fat | 2266 | 3269 |
| 292 | roast, lean and fat | 2266 | 3269 |
| 293 | lean only | 2266 | 3269 |
| 294 | **Pork, dressed carcase** raw | 2296 | 3299 |
| 296 | **lean** average, raw | 2296 | 3299 |
| 299 | **fat** average, raw | (2296) | 3299 |
| 300 | cooked | (2296) | 3299 |
| 301 | **belly** rashers, raw | 2296 | 3299 |
| 302 | grilled, lean and fat | 2296 | 3299 |
| 303 | **chops, loin** raw | 2296 | 3299 |
| 304 | grilled, lean and fat | 2296 | 3299 |
| 305 | lean and fat (with bone) | 2296 | 3299 |
| 306 | lean only | 2296 | 3299 |
| 307 | lean only (with bone) | 2296 | 3299 |
| 308 | **leg** raw, lean and fat | 2296 | 3299 |
| 309 | roast, lean and fat | 2296 | 3299 |
| 310 | lean only | 2296 | 3299 |
| 311 | **Veal, cutlet** fried | 2237 | 3240 |
| 312 | **fillet** raw | 2237 | 3240 |
| 313 | roast | 2237 | 3240 |
| 314 | **Chicken** raw, meat only | 2314 | 3314 |
| 315 | meat and skin | (2314) | 3314 |
| 316 | light meat | 2314 | 3314 |
| 317 | dark meat | 2314 | 3314 |
| 318 | boiled, meat only | 2314 | 3314 |
| 319 | light meat | 2313 | 3314 |
| 320 | dark meat | 2314 | 3314 |
| 321 | roast, meat only | 2314 | 3314 |
| 322 | meat and skin | 2314 | 3314 |
| 323 | light meat | 2314 | 3314 |
| 324 | dark meat | 2314 | 3314 |
| 325 | wing quarter (with bone) | 2314 | 3314 |
| 326 | leg quarter (with bone) | 2314 | 3314 |
| 327 | **Duck** raw, meat only | 2327 | 3328 |
| 328 | meat with fat and skin | (2327) | 3328 |
| 329 | roast, meat only | 2327 | 3328 |
| 330 | meat with fat and skin | (2327) | 3328 |
| 331 | **Goose** roast | (2327) | — |
| 332 | **Grouse** roast | (2327) | 3332 |
| 333 | roast (with bone) | (2327) | 3332 |
| 334 | **Partridge** roast | (2327) | 3334 |
| 335 | roast (with bone) | (2327) | 3334 |
| 336 | **Pheasant** roast | (2327) | 3336 |
| 337 | roast (with bone) | (2327) | 3336 |

| | | Food names | Amino acids tables section 2 | Fatty acids tables section 3 |
|---|---|---|---|---|
| **Meat** *continued* | 338 | **Pigeon** roast | (2327) | — |
| | 339 | roast (with bone) | (2327) | — |
| | 340 | **Turkey** raw, meat only | 2340 | 3340 |
| | 341 | meat and skin | 2340 | 3340 |
| | 342 | light meat | 2340 | 3340 |
| | 343 | dark meat | 2340 | 3340 |
| | 344 | roast, meat only | 2340 | 3340 |
| | 345 | meat and skin | 2340 | 3340 |
| | 346 | light mat | 2340 | 3340 |
| | 347 | dark meat | 2340 | 3340 |
| | 348 | **Hare** stewed | 2350 | 3350 |
| | 349 | stewed (with bone) | 2350 | 3350 |
| | 350 | **Rabbit** raw | 2350 | 3350 |
| | 351 | stewed | 2350 | 3350 |
| | 352 | stewed (with bone) | 2350 | 3350 |
| | 353 | **Venison** roast | (2237) | — |
| | 354 | **Brain, calf** and **lamb** raw | 2354 | — |
| | 355 | **calf** boiled | 2354 | — |
| | 356 | **lamb** boiled | 2354 | 3356 |
| | 357 | ***Heart, lamb and ox*** | 2357 | — |
| | 358 | **Heart, lamb** raw | 2357 | 3358 |
| | 359 | **sheep** roast | 2357 | 3358 |
| | 360 | **ox** raw | 2357 | 3360 |
| | 361 | stewed | 2357 | 3360 |
| | 362 | **pig** raw | 2357 | — |
| | 361 | ***Kidney, lamb, ox and pig*** | 2363 | — |
| | 364 | **Kidney, lamb** raw | 2363 | 3364 |
| | 365 | fried | 2363 | a |
| | 366 | **ox** raw | 2363 | 3366 |
| | 367 | stewed | 2363 | 3366 |
| | 368 | **pig** raw | 2363 | 3368 |
| | 369 | stewed | 2363 | 3368 |
| | 370 | ***Liver, all species*** | 2370 | — |
| | 371 | **Liver, calf** raw | 2370 | 3371 |
| | 372 | fried | 2370 | a |
| | 373 | **chicken** raw | 2370 | 3373 |
| | 374 | fried | 2370 | a |
| | 375 | **lamb** raw | 2370 | 3375 |
| | 376 | fried | 2370 | a |
| | 377 | **ox** raw | 2370 | 3377 |
| | 378 | stewed | 2370 | 3377 |
| | 379 | **pig** raw | 2370 | 3379 |
| | 380 | stewed | 2370 | 3379 |
| | 381 | **Oxtail** raw | 2381 | 3240 |
| | 382 | stewed | 2381 | 3240 |
| | 383 | stewed (with bone) | 2381 | 3240 |
| | 384 | **Sweetbread, lamb** raw | 2384 | 3384 |
| | 385 | fried | 2384 | a |
| | 386 | ***Tongue, lamb and ox*** | 2386 | — |
| | 387 | **Tongue, lamb** raw | 2386 | 3399 |
| | 388 | **sheep** stewed | 2386 | 3399 |
| | 389 | **ox** pickled, raw | 2386 | — |
| | 390 | boiled | 2386 | — |
| | 391 | **Tripe** dressed | 2391 | 3391 |
| | 392 | stewed | 2391 | 3391 |
| | 393 | **Beef, corned** | 2393 | 3240 |

| | | Food names | Amino acids: tables section 2 | Fatty acids : tables section 3 |
|---|---|---|---|---|
| **Meat** *continued* | 394 | **Ham** | 2394 | 3394 |
| | 395 | **Ham and pork** chopped | 2395 | 3395 |
| | 396 | **Luncheon meat** | 2396 | 3396 |
| | 397 | **Stewed steak with gravy** | 2397 | 3240 |
| | 398 | **Tongue, lamb and ox,** canned | 2398 | — |
| | 399 | ***Tongue, lamb*** | — | 3399 |
| | 400 | **Veal, jellied** | 2400 | — |
| | 401 | **Black pudding** fried | 2401 | — |
| | 402 | **Faggots** | 2402 | — |
| | 403 | **Haggis** boiled | 2403 | — |
| | 404 | **Liver sausage** | 2404 | 3404 |
| | 405 | **Frankfurters** | 2405 | (3299) |
| | 406 | **Polony** | 2406 | — |
| | 407 | **Salami** | 2407 | (3299) |
| | 408 | **Sausages, beef** raw | 2408 | 3408 |
| | 409 | fried | 2408 | a |
| | 410 | grilled | 2408 | 3408 |
| | 411 | **Sausages, pork** raw | 2411 | 3411 |
| | 412 | fried | 2411 | a |
| | 413 | grilled | 2411 | 3411 |
| | 414 | **Saveloy** | 2414 | — |
| | 415 | **Beefburgers** raw | 2415 | (3240) |
| | 416 | fried | 2415 | (3240) |
| | 417 | **Brawn** | 2417 | — |
| | 418 | **Meat paste** | 2418 | (3299) |
| | 419 | **White pudding** | 2419 | — |
| | 420 | **Cornish pastie** | 2420 | — |
| | 421 | **Pork pie** individual | 2421 | — |
| | 422 | **Sausage roll** flaky pastry | R | R |
| | 423 | short pastry | R | R |
| | 424 | **Steak and kidney pie** with pastry top only | R | R |
| | 425 | individual | 2425 | 3425 |
| | 426 | **Beefsteak pudding** | R | R |
| | 427 | **Beef stew** | R | R |
| | 428 | **Bolognese sauce** | R | R |
| | 429 | **Curried meat** | R | R |
| | 430 | **Hot pot** | R | R |
| | 431 | **Irish stew** | R | R |
| | 432 | **Irish stew** (with bone) | R | R |
| | 433 | **Moussaka** | R | R |
| | 434 | **Shepherds' pie** | R | R |
| **Fish** | 435 | ***White and fatty fish all species*** | 2435 | — |
| | 438 | **Cod** raw, fresh fillets | 2435 | 3438 |
| | 439 | frozen steaks | 2435 | 3438 |
| | 440 | baked | 2435 | 3438 |
| | 441 | baked (with bones and skin) | 2435 | 3438 |
| | 442 | fried in batter | 2435 | a |
| | 443 | grilled | 2435 | 3438 |
| | 444 | poached | 2435 | 3438 |
| | 445 | poached (with bones and skin | 2435 | 3438 |
| | 446 | steamed | 2435 | 3438 |
| | 447 | steamed (with bones and skin) | 2435 | 3438 |
| | 448 | **Cod smoked** raw | 2435 | 3438 |
| | 449 | poached | 2435 | 3438 |
| | 450 | **dried** salt, boiled | 2435 | 3438 |

**Fish**
*continued*

| | Food names | Amino acids: tables section 2 | Fatty acids: tables section 3 |
|---|---|---|---|
| 451 | **Haddock, fresh** raw | 2435 | 3451 |
| 452 | fried | 2435 | a |
| 453 | fried (with bone) | 2435 | a |
| 454 | steamed | 2435 | 3451 |
| 455 | steamed (with bones) | 2435 | 3451 |
| 456 | **smoked** steamed | 2435 | 3451 |
| 457 | steamed (with bones and skin) | 2435 | 3451 |
| 458 | **Halibut** raw | 2435 | 3458 |
| 459 | steamed | 2435 | 3458 |
| 460 | steamed (with bones and skin) | 2435 | 3458 |
| 461 | **Lemon sole** raw | 2435 | 3461 |
| 462 | fried | 2435 | a |
| 463 | fried (with bone) | 2435 | a |
| 464 | steamed | 2435 | 3461 |
| 465 | steamed (with bones and skin) | 2435 | 3461 |
| 466 | **Plaice** raw | 2435 | 3466 |
| 467 | fried in batter | 2435 | a |
| 468 | fried in crumbs | 2435 | a |
| 469 | steamed | 2435 | 3466 |
| 470 | steamed (with bones and skin) | 2435 | 3466 |
| 471 | **Saithe** raw | 2435 | 3471 |
| 472 | steamed | 2435 | 3471 |
| 473 | steamed (with bones and skin) | 2435 | 3471 |
| 474 | **Whiting** raw | 2435 | 3474 |
| 475 | fried | 2435 | a |
| 476 | fried (with bones) | 2435 | a |
| 477 | steamed | 2435 | 3474 |
| 478 | steamed (with bones and skin) | 2435 | 3474 |
| 480 | **Eel** raw | 2435 | — |
| 481 | stewed | 2435 | — |
| 482 | **Herring** raw | 2435 | 3482 |
| 483 | fried | 2435 | a |
| 484 | **Herring** fried (with bones) | 2435 | a |
| 485 | grilled | 2435 | 3482 |
| 486 | grilled (with bones) | 2435 | 3482 |
| 487 | **Bloater** grilled | 2435 | 3482 |
| 488 | grilled (with bones) | 2435 | 3482 |
| 489 | **Kipper** baked | 2435 | 3482 |
| 490 | baked (with bones) | 2435 | 3482 |
| 491 | **Mackerel** raw | 2435 | 3491 |
| 492 | fried | 2435 | a |
| 493 | fried (with bones) | 2435 | a |
| 494 | **Pilchards** canned in tomato sauce | 2435 | 3494 |
| 495 | **Salmon** raw | 2435 | (3498) |
| 496 | steamed | 2435 | (3498) |
| 497 | steamed (with bones and skin) | 2435 | (3498) |
| 498 | canned | 2435 | 3498 |
| 499 | smoked | 2435 | (3498) |
| 500 | **Sardines** canned in oil, fish only | 2435 | (3501) |
| 501 | fish plus oil | 2435 | 3501 |
| 502 | canned in tomato sauce | 2435 | 3502 |
| 503 | ***Sprats, raw*** | — | 3503 |
| 504 | **Sprats** fried | 2435 | a |
| 505 | fried (with bones) | 2435 | a |
| 506 | **Trout, brown** steamed | 2435 | — |
| 507 | steamed (with bones) | 2435 | — |

| | | Food names | Amino acids tables section 2 | Fatty acids tables section 3 |
|---|---|---|---|---|
| **Fish** *continued* | 508 | **Tuna** canned in oil | 2435 | 3508 |
| | 509 | **Whitebait** fried | 2435 | a |
| | 510 | ***Dogfish, raw*** | 2435 | 3510 |
| | 511 | **Dogfish** fried in batter | 2435 | — |
| | 512 | fried (with waste) | 2435 | a |
| | 513 | ***Skate, raw*** | 2435 | 3513 |
| | 514 | **Skate** fried in batter | 2435 | a |
| | 515 | fried (with waste) | 2435 | a |
| | 516 | ***Crustacea, all kinds*** | 2516 | — |
| | 517 | ***Crab, raw*** | — | 3517 |
| | 518 | **Crab** boiled | 2516 | 3517 |
| | 519 | boiled (with shell) | 2516 | 3517 |
| | 520 | canned | 2516 | 3517 |
| | 521 | **Lobster** boiled | 2516 | 3517 |
| | 522 | boiled (with shell) | 2516 | 3517 |
| | 523 | **Prawns** boiled | 2516 | 3517 |
| | 524 | boiled (with shell) | 2516 | 3517 |
| | 525 | **Scampi** fried | 2516 | a |
| | 526 | ***Shrimps, raw*** | — | 3526 |
| | 527 | **Shrimps** boiled | 2516 | 3526 |
| | 528 | boiled (with shell) | 2516 | 3526 |
| | 529 | canned | 2516 | 3526 |
| | 530 | ***Molluscs all kinds*** | 2530 | — |
| | 531 | **Cockles** boiled | 2530 | — |
| | 532 | **Mussels** raw | 2530 | 3532 |
| | 533 | boiled | 2530 | 3532 |
| | 534 | boiled (with shell) | 2530 | 3532 |
| | 535 | **Oysters** raw | 2530 | 3535 |
| | 536 | raw (with shell) | 2530 | 3535 |
| | 537 | ***Scallops raw*** | | 3537 |
| | 538 | **Scallops** steamed | 2530 | 3537 |
| | 539 | **Whelks** boiled | 2530 | — |
| | 540 | boiled (with shell) | 2530 | — |
| | 541 | **Winkles** boiled | 2530 | — |
| | 542 | boiled (with shell) | 2530 | — |
| | 543 | **Fish cakes** frozen | — | — |
| | 544 | fried | — | — |
| | 545 | **Fish fingers** frozen | R | a |
| | 546 | fried | R | a |
| | 547 | **Fish paste** | — | — |
| | 548 | **Fish pie** | R | R |
| | 549 | **Kedgeree** | R | R |
| | 550 | **Roe, cod** hard, raw | — | 3550 |
| | 551 | fried | — | a |
| | 552 | **herring** soft, raw | — | — |
| | 553 | fried | — | a |
| **Vegetables** | 554 | **Ackee** canned | — | — |
| | 555 | **Artichokes, globe** boiled | — | ø |
| | 556 | boiled (as served) | — | ø |
| | 557 | **Jerusalem** boiled | — | ø |
| | 558 | **Asparagus** boiled | 2558 | ø |
| | 559 | boiled (as served) | 2558 | ø |
| | 560 | **Aubergine** raw | — | ø |
| | 561 | **Beans, French** boiled | 2561 | ø |
| | 562 | **runner** raw | 2561 | 3562 |

| | Food names | Amino acids: tables section 2 | Fatty acids: tables section 3 |
|---|---|---|---|
| **Vegetables** *continued* | | | |
| 563 | boiled | 2561 | 3562 |
| 564 | **broad** boiled | 2564 | — |
| 565 | **butter** raw | 2565 | — |
| 566 | boiled | 2565 | — |
| 567 | **haricot** raw | 2567 | — |
| 568 | boiled | 2567 | — |
| 569 | **baked** canned in tomato sauce | 2567 | 3569 |
| 570 | **mung** green gram, raw | — | — |
| 571 | cooked, dahl | — | — |
| 572 | **red kidney** raw | 2572 | — |
| 573 | **Beansprouts** canned | — | Ø |
| 574 | **Beetroot** raw | 2574 | Ø |
| 575 | boiled | 2574 | Ø |
| 576 | **Broccoli tops** raw | 2576 | Ø |
| 577 | boiled | 2576 | Ø |
| 578 | **Brussels sprouts** raw | 2578 | Ø |
| 579 | boiled | 2578 | Ø |
| 580 | **Cabbage, red** raw | 2585 | Ø |
| 581 | **Savoy** raw | 2585 | Ø |
| 582 | boiled | 2585 | Ø |
| 583 | **spring** boiled | 2585 | Ø |
| 584 | **white** raw | 2585 | Ø |
| 585 | **winter** raw | 2585 | Ø |
| 586 | boiled | 2585 | Ø |
| 587 | **Carrots, old** raw | 2587 | Ø |
| 588 | boiled | 2587 | Ø |
| 589 | **young** boiled | 2587 | Ø |
| 590 | canned | 2587 | Ø |
| 591 | **Cauliflower** raw | 2591 | Ø |
| 592 | boiled | 2591 | Ø |
| 593 | **Celeriac** boiled | — | Ø |
| 594 | **Celery** raw | 2594 | Ø |
| 595 | boiled | 2594 | Ø |
| 596 | **Chicory** raw | — | Ø |
| 597 | **Cucumber** raw | 2597 | 3597 |
| 598 | **Endive** raw | — | Ø |
| 599 | **Horseradish** raw | — | Ø |
| 600 | **Laverbread** | — | Ø |
| 601 | **Leeks** raw | — | Ø |
| 602 | boiled | — | Ø |
| 603 | **Lentils** raw | 2603 | — |
| 604 | split, boiled | 2603 | — |
| 605 | masur dahl, cooked | 2603 | — |
| 606 | **Lettuce** | 2606 | |
| 607 | **Marrow** raw | — | Ø |
| 608 | boiled | — | Ø |
| 609 | **Mushrooms** raw | 2609 | 3609 |
| 610 | fried | 2609 | a |
| 611 | **Mustard and cress** raw | — | Ø |
| 612 | **Okra** raw | — | Ø |
| 613 | **Onions** raw | 2613 | Ø |
| 614 | boiled | 2613 | Ø |
| 615 | fried | 2613 | Ø |
| 616 | **spring** raw | 2613 | Ø |
| 617 | **Parsley** raw | — | Ø |

**Vegetables**
*continued*

| | Food names | Amino acids: tables section 2 | Fatty acids: tables section 3 |
|---|---|---|---|
| 618 | **Parsnips** raw | — | ∅ |
| 619 | boiled | — | ∅ |
| 620 | **Peas** fresh, raw | 2620 | 3621 |
| 621 | boiled | 2620 | 3621 |
| 622 | frozen, raw | 2620 | 3621 |
| 623 | boiled | 2620 | 3621 |
| 624 | canned, garden | 2620 | 3621 |
| 625 | processed | 2620 | 3621 |
| 626 | dried, raw | 2620 | 3621 |
| 627 | boiled | 2620 | 3621 |
| 628 | split, dried raw | 2620 | 3621 |
| 629 | boiled | 2620 | 3621 |
| 630 | **chick** Bengal gram raw | 2630 | — |
| 631 | cooked dahl | 2630 | — |
| 632 | channa dahl | 2630 | — |
| 633 | **red** pigeon, raw | 2633 | — |
| 634 | **Peppers, green,** raw | — | 3634 |
| 635 | boiled | — | 3634 |
| 636 | **Plantain** green, raw | — | ∅ |
| 637 | boiled | — | ∅ |
| 638 | ripe, fried | — | a |
| 639 | **Potatoes, old** raw | 2639 | 3639 |
| 640 | boiled | 2639 | 3639 |
| 641 | mashed | 2639 | a |
| 642 | baked | 2639 | 3639 |
| 643 | baked (with skin) | 2639 | 3639 |
| 644 | roast | 2639 | a |
| 645 | chips | 2639 | a |
| 646 | frozen | 2639 | a |
| 647 | frozen, fried | 2639 | a |
| 648 | **new** boiled | 2639 | 3639 |
| 649 | canned | 2639 | 3639 |
| 650 | **instant** powder | 2639 | 3639 |
| 651 | made up | 2639 | 3639 |
| 652 | **Potato crisps** | 2639 | a |
| 653 | **Pumpkin** raw | — | ∅ |
| 654 | **Radishes** raw | — | ∅ |
| 655 | **Salsify** boiled | — | ∅ |
| 656 | **Seakale** boiled | — | ∅ |
| 657 | **Spinach** boiled | 2657 | 3657 |
| 658 | **Spring greens** boiled | 2669 | ∅ |
| 659 | **Swedes** raw | — | ∅ |
| 660 | boiled | — | ∅ |
| 661 | **Sweetcorn, on-the-cob** raw | 2006 | 3198 |
| 662 | boiled | 2006 | 3198 |
| 663 | canned, kernels | 2006 | 3198 |
| 664 | **Sweet potatoes** raw | 2664 | 3664 |
| 665 | boiled | 2664 | 3664 |
| 666 | **Tomatoes** raw | 2666 | ∅ |
| 667 | fried | 2666 | a |
| 668 | canned | 2666 | ∅ |
| 669 | **Turnips** raw | 2669 | 3669 |
| 670 | boiled | 2669 | 3669 |
| 671 | **Turnip tops** boiled | 2671 | ∅ |
| 672 | **Watercress** raw | — | ∅ |

| | | Food names | Amino acids: tables section 2 | Fatty acids: tables section 3 |
|---|---|---|---|---|
| **Vegetables** *continued* | 673 | **Yam** raw | 2673 | ∅ |
| | 674 | boiled | 2673 | ∅ |
| **Fruit** | 675 | **Apples, eating** | 2675 | 3675 |
| | 676 | (with skin and core) | 2675 | 3675 |
| | 677 | **cooking** raw | 2675 | 3675 |
| | 678 | baked without sugar | 2675 | 3675 |
| | 679 | baked (with skin) | 2675 | 3675 |
| | 680 | stewed, without sugar | 2675 | 3675 |
| | 681 | with sugar | 2675 | 3675 |
| | 682 | **Apricots** fresh, raw | 2682 | ∅ |
| | 683 | raw (with stones) | 2682 | ∅ |
| | 684 | stewed without sugar | 2682 | ∅ |
| | 685 | stewed without sugar (with stones) | 2682 | ∅ |
| | 686 | with sugar | 2682 | ∅ |
| | 687 | with sugar (with stones) | 2682 | ∅ |
| | 688 | dried, raw | 2682 | ∅ |
| | 689 | stewed, without sugar | 2682 | ∅ |
| | 690 | with sugar | 2682 | ∅ |
| | 691 | canned | 2682 | ∅ |
| | 692 | **Avocado pears** | 2692 | 3692 |
| | 693 | **Bananas** raw | 2693 | 3693 |
| | 694 | raw (with skin) | 2693 | 3693 |
| | 695 | **Bilberries** raw | — | ∅ |
| | 696 | **Blackberries** raw | — | ∅ |
| | 697 | stewed, without sugar | — | ∅ |
| | 698 | with sugar | — | ∅ |
| | 699 | **Cherries, eating** raw | — | ∅ |
| | 700 | raw (with stones) | — | ∅ |
| | 701 | **cooking** raw | — | ∅ |
| | 702 | raw (with stones) | — | ∅ |
| | 703 | stewed without sugar | — | ∅ |
| | 704 | without sugar (with stones) | — | ∅ |
| | 705 | with sugar | — | ∅ |
| | 706 | with sugar (with stones) | — | ∅ |
| | 707 | **Cranberries** raw | — | ∅ |
| | 708 | **Currants, black** raw | — | ∅ |
| | 709 | stewed without sugar | — | ∅ |
| | 710 | with sugar | — | ∅ |
| | 711 | **red** raw | — | ∅ |
| | 712 | stewed without sugar | — | ∅ |
| | 713 | with sugar | — | ∅ |
| | 714 | **white** raw | — | ∅ |
| | 715 | stewed without sugar | — | ∅ |
| | 716 | with sugar | — | ∅ |
| | 717 | **dried** | 2736 | ∅ |
| | 718 | **Damsons** raw | — | ∅ |
| | 719 | raw (with stones) | — | ∅ |
| | 720 | stewed without sugar | — | ∅ |
| | 721 | without sugar (with stones) | — | ∅ |
| | 722 | with sugar | — | ∅ |
| | 723 | with sugar (with stones) | — | ∅ |
| | 724 | **Dates** dried | 2724 | ∅ |
| | 725 | dried (with stones) | 2724 | ∅ |
| | 726 | **Figs, green** raw | 2726 | ∅ |

**Fruit**
*continued*

| | Food names | Amino acids: tables section 2 | Fatty acids: tables section 3 |
|---|---|---|---|
| 727 | **dried** raw | 2726 | ∅ |
| 728 | stewed without sugar | 2726 | ∅ |
| 729 | with sugar | 2726 | ∅ |
| 730 | **Fruit pie filling** canned | — | ∅ |
| 731 | **Fruit salad** canned | — | ∅ |
| 732 | **Gooseberries, green** raw | — | ∅ |
| 733 | stewed without sugar | — | ∅ |
| 734 | with sugar | — | ∅ |
| 735 | **ripe** raw | — | ∅ |
| 736 | **Grapes, black** raw | 2736 | ∅ |
| 737 | raw (whole grapes) | 2736 | ∅ |
| 738 | **white** raw | 2736 | ∅ |
| 739 | raw (whole grapes) | 2736 | ∅ |
| 740 | **Grapefruit** raw | (2773) | ∅ |
| 741 | raw (whole fruit) | (2773) | ∅ |
| 742 | canned | (2773) | ∅ |
| 743 | **Greengages** raw | — | ∅ |
| 744 | raw (with stones) | — | ∅ |
| 745 | stewed without sugar | — | ∅ |
| 746 | without sugar (with stones) | — | ∅ |
| 747 | with sugar | — | ∅ |
| 748 | with sugar (with stones) | — | ∅ |
| 749 | **Guavas** canned | (2773) | ∅ |
| 750 | **Lemons** whole | (2773) | ∅ |
| 751 | juice, fresh | — | ∅ |
| 752 | **Loganberries** raw | — | ∅ |
| 753 | stewed without sugar | — | ∅ |
| 754 | with sugar | — | ∅ |
| 755 | canned | — | ∅ |
| 756 | **Lychees** raw | — | ∅ |
| 757 | canned | — | ∅ |
| 758 | **Mandarin oranges** canned | (2773) | ∅ |
| 759 | **Mangoes** raw | — | ∅ |
| 760 | canned | — | ∅ |
| 761 | **Medlars** raw | — | ∅ |
| 762 | **Melons, Canteloupe** raw | 2762 | ∅ |
| 763 | raw (with skin) | 2762 | ∅ |
| 764 | **yellow, Honeydew** raw | (2762) | ∅ |
| 765 | raw (with skin) | (2762) | ∅ |
| 766 | **watermelon** raw | 2766 | ∅ |
| 767 | raw (with skin) | 2766 | ∅ |
| 768 | **Mulberries** raw | — | ∅ |
| 769 | **Nectarines** raw | (2779) | ∅ |
| 770 | raw (with stones) | (2779) | ∅ |
| 771 | **Olives** in brine | — | 3199 |
| 772 | in brine (with stones) | — | 3199 |
| 773 | **Oranges** raw | 2773 | ∅ |
| 774 | raw (with peel and pith) | 2773 | ∅ |
| 775 | **Orange juice** fresh | 2773 | ∅ |
| 776 | **Passion fruit** raw | — | ∅ |
| 777 | raw (with skin) | — | ∅ |
| 778 | **Paw-paw** canned | — | ∅ |
| 779 | **Peaches** fresh, raw | 2779 | ∅ |
| 780 | raw (with stones) | 2779 | ∅ |
| 781 | dried, raw | 2779 | ∅ |

| | | Food names | Amino acids tables section 2 | Fatty acids tables section 3 |
|---|---|---|---|---|
| **Fruit** *continued* | 782 | stewed without sugar | 2779 | ∅ |
| | 783 | with sugar | 2779 | ∅ |
| | 784 | canned | 2779 | ∅ |
| | 785 | **Pears, eating** | 2785 | ∅ |
| | 786 | (with skin and core) | 2785 | ∅ |
| | 787 | **cooking** raw | 2785 | ∅ |
| | 788 | stewed without sugar | 2785 | ∅ |
| | 789 | with sugar | 2785 | ∅ |
| | 790 | canned | 2785 | ∅ |
| | 791 | **Pineapple** fresh | 2791 | ∅ |
| | 792 | canned | 2791 | ∅ |
| | 793 | **Plums, Victoria, dessert** raw | — | ∅ |
| | 794 | raw (with stones) | — | ∅ |
| | 795 | **cooking** raw | — | ∅ |
| | 796 | raw (with stones) | — | ∅ |
| | 797 | stewed without sugar | — | ∅ |
| | 798 | without sugar (with stones) | — | ∅ |
| | 799 | with sugar | — | ∅ |
| | 800 | with sugar (with stones) | — | ∅ |
| | 801 | **Pomegranate juice** | — | ∅ |
| | 802 | **Prunes** dried, raw | — | ∅ |
| | 803 | raw (with stones) | — | ∅ |
| | 804 | stewed without sugar | — | ∅ |
| | 805 | without sugar (with stones) | — | ∅ |
| | 806 | stewed with sugar | — | ∅ |
| | 807 | (with stones) | — | ∅ |
| | 808 | **Quinces** raw | — | ∅ |
| | 809 | **Raisins** dried | 2736 | ∅ |
| | 810 | **Raspberries** raw | — | ∅ |
| | 811 | stewed without sugar | — | ∅ |
| | 812 | with sugar | — | ∅ |
| | 813 | canned | — | ∅ |
| | 814 | **Rhubarb** raw | — | ∅ |
| | 815 | stewed without sugar | — | ∅ |
| | 816 | with sugar | — | ∅ |
| | 817 | **Strawberries** raw | 2817 | ∅ |
| | 818 | canned | 2817 | ∅ |
| | 819 | **Sultanas** dried | 2736 | ∅ |
| | 820 | **Tangerines** raw | (2773) | ∅ |
| | 821 | raw (with peel and pips) | (2773) | ∅ |
| **Nuts** | 822 | **Almonds** | 2822 | 3822 |
| | 823 | (nuts with shells) | 2822 | 3822 |
| | 824 | **Barcelona nuts** | (2830) | (3830) |
| | 825 | (nuts with shells) | (2830) | (3830) |
| | 826 | **Brazil nuts** | 2826 | 3826 |
| | 827 | (nuts with shells) | 2826 | 3826 |
| | 828 | **Chestnuts** | — | 3828 |
| | 829 | (nuts with shells) | — | 3828 |
| | 830 | **Cob or hazel nuts** | 2830 | 3830 |
| | 831 | (nuts with shells) | 2830 | 3830 |
| | 832 | **Coconut** fresh | 2832 | 3832 |
| | 833 | milk | — | ∅ |
| | 834 | desiccated | 2832 | 3832 |

| | | Food names | Amino acids tables section 2 | Fatty acids tables section 3 |
|---|---|---|---|---|
| **Nuts** *continued* | 835 | **Peanuts** fresh | 2835 | 3835 |
| | 836 | (nuts with shells) | 2835 | 3835 |
| | 837 | roasted and salted | 2835 | 3835 |
| | 838 | **Peanut butter** smooth | 2838 | 3838 |
| | 839 | **Walnuts** | 2839 | 3839 |
| | 840 | (nuts with shells) | 2839 | 3839 |
| **Sugars** | 841 | **Glucose** liquid | 0 | 0 |
| | 842 | **Sugar,** Demerara | 0 | 0 |
| | 843 | white | 0 | 0 |
| | 844 | **Syrup,** golden | 0 | 0 |
| | 845 | **Treacle,** black | 0 | 0 |
| | 846 | **Cherries,** glacé | 0 | 0 |
| | 847 | **Honey** comb | — | — |
| | 848 | in jar | — | — |
| | 849 | **Jam** fruit with edible seeds | — | — |
| | 850 | stone fruit | — | — |
| | 851 | **Lemon curd** starch based | — | — |
| | 852 | home made | 2165 | R |
| | 853 | **Marmalade** | 2773 | 0 |
| | 854 | **Marzipan** | 2822 | 2822 |
| | 855 | **Mincemeat** | — | — |
| | 856 | **Boiled sweets** | 0 | 0 |
| | 857 | **Chocolate** milk | 2857 | 3857 |
| | 858 | plain | 2858 | 3858 |
| | 859 | fancy and filled | — | — |
| | 860 | Bounty Bar | — | — |
| | 861 | Mars Bar | — | — |
| | 862 | **Fruit gums** | — | ∅ |
| | 863 | **Liquorice allsorts** | — | — |
| | 864 | **Pastilles** | — | ∅ |
| | 865 | **Peppermints** | ∅ | ∅ |
| | 866 | **Toffees, mixed** | — | — |
| **Beverages** | 867 | **Bournvita** | — | — |
| | 868 | **Cocoa powder** | 2868 | 3868 |
| | 869 | **Coffee and chicory essence** | (2872) | ∅ |
| | 870 | **Coffee** ground, roasted | — | — |
| | 871 | infusion 5 min | (2872) | ∅ |
| | 872 | instant | 2872 | ∅ |
| | 873 | **Drinking chocolate** | 2868 | 3873 |
| | 874 | **Horlicks malted milk** | — | — |
| | 875 | **Ovaltine** | — | — |
| | 876 | **Tea, Indian** | — | ∅ |
| | 877 | infusion | ∅ | ∅ |
| | 878 | **Coca-cola** | ∅ | ∅ |
| | 879 | **Grapefruit juice** canned, unsweetened | (2773) | ∅ |
| | 880 | sweetened | (2773) | ∅ |
| | 881 | **Lemonade** | 0 | 0 |
| | 882 | **Lime juice cordial** | ∅ | 0 |
| | 883 | **Lucozade** | ∅ | 0 |
| | 884 | **Orange drink** | ∅ | 0 |
| | 885 | **Orange juice** canned, unsweetened | 2773 | ∅ |
| | 886 | sweetened | 2773 | ∅ |
| | 887 | **Pineapple juice** canned | 2791 | ∅ |

| | | Food names | Amino acids tables section 2 | Fatty acids tables section 3 |
|---|---|---|---|---|
| **Beverages** *continued* | 888 | **Ribena** undiluted | — | ∅ |
| | 889 | **Rosehip syrup** undiluted | — | ∅ |
| | 890 | **Tomato juice** canned | 2666 | ∅ |
| | 891 | **Brown ale** bottled | (2895) | ∅ |
| | 892 | **Canned** bitter | (2895) | ∅ |
| | 893 | **Draught** bitter | (2895) | ∅ |
| | 894 | mild | (2895) | ∅ |
| | 895 | **Keg** | 2895 | ∅ |
| | 896 | **Lager** bottled | 2896 | ∅ |
| | 897 | **Pale ale** bottled | (2895) | ∅ |
| | 898 | **Stout** bottled | (2895) | ∅ |
| | 899 | **Stout** extra | (2895) | ∅ |
| | 900 | **Strong ale** | (2895) | ∅ |
| | 901 | **Cider** dry | ∅ | 0 |
| | 902 | sweet | ∅ | 0 |
| | 903 | vintage | ∅ | 0 |
| | 904 | **Wine, red** | ∅ | 0 |
| | 905 | **rosé** | ∅ | 0 |
| | 906 | **white** dry | ∅ | 0 |
| | 907 | medium | ∅ | 0 |
| | 908 | sweet | ∅ | 0 |
| | 909 | sparkling | ∅ | 0 |
| | 910 | **Port** | ∅ | 0 |
| | 911 | **Sherry** dry | ∅ | 0 |
| | 912 | medium | ∅ | 0 |
| | 913 | sweet | ∅ | 0 |
| | 914 | **Vermouth** dry | ∅ | 0 |
| | 915 | sweet | ∅ | 0 |
| | 916 | **Advocaat** | 2165 | 3165 |
| | 917 | **Cherry brandy** | ∅ | 0 |
| | 918 | **Curaçao** | ∅ | 0 |
| | 919 | **Spirits 70% proof** | 0 | 0 |
| **Sauces** | 920 | **Bread sauce** | R | R |
| | 921 | **Brown sauce** bottled | — | — |
| | 922 | **Cheese sauce** | R | R |
| | 923 | **Chutney,** apple | 2675 | ∅ |
| | 924 | tomato | 2666 | ∅ |
| | 925 | **French dressing** | — | 3199 |
| | 926 | **Mayonnaise** | 2165 | a |
| | 927 | **Onion sauce** | R | R |
| | 928 | **Piccalli** | — | — |
| | 929 | **Pickle** sweet | — | — |
| | 930 | **Salad cream** | — | — |
| | 931 | **Tomato ketchup** | 2666 | ∅ |
| | 932 | **Tomato pureé** | 2666 | ∅ |
| | 933 | **Tomato sauce** | R | R |
| | 934 | **White sauce** savoury | R | R |
| | 935 | sweet | R | R |
| **Soups** | 937 | **Bone and vegetable broth** | — | — |
| | 938 | **Soup chicken, cream of** canned | — | — |
| | 939 | condensed | — | — |
| | 940 | condensed, as served | — | — |

| | | Food names | Amino acids tables section 2 | Fatty acids tables section 3 |
|---|---|---|---|---|
| **Soups** *continued* | 941 | **chicken noodle** dried | — | — |
| | 942 | dried, as served | — | — |
| | 943 | **lentil** | R | R |
| | 944 | **minestrone** dried | — | — |
| | 945 | dried, as served | — | — |
| | 946 | **mushroom, cream of** canned | — | — |
| | 947 | **oxtail** canned, ready to serve | — | — |
| | 948 | dried | — | — |
| | 949 | dried, as served | — | — |
| | 950 | **tomato, cream of** canned | — | — |
| | 951 | condensed | — | — |
| | 952 | condensed, as served | — | — |
| | 953 | dried | — | — |
| | 954 | dried, as served | — | — |
| | 955 | **vegetable** canned | | — |
| **Miscellaneous** | 956 | **Baking powder** | 2011 | ∅ |
| | 957 | **Bovril** | 2957 | ∅ |
| | 958 | **Curry powder** | — | — |
| | 959 | **Gelatin** | 2959 | ∅ |
| | 960 | **Ginger, ground** | — | — |
| | 961 | **Marmite** | 2961 | ∅ |
| | 962 | **Oxo cubes** | — | — |
| | 963 | **Mustard powder** | — | — |
| | 964 | **Pepper** | — | — |
| | 965 | **Salt, block** | 0 | 0 |
| | 966 | **table** | 0 | 0 |
| | 967 | **Vinegar** | 0 | ∅ |
| | 968 | **Yeast** bakers, compressed | 2968 | — |
| | 969 | dried | 2968 | — |

# Appendix 5 (part 2): Key extension to calculation of amino acid and fatty acid composition of cooked dishes

| | Tables section 2 code | N contributed per 100 g | Tables section 3 code | Fat contributed per 100 g |
|---|---|---|---|---|
| 39 **Soda bread** | 2011 | 1.17 | 3008 | 0.81 |
| | 2123 | 0.20 | 2123 | 1.49 |
| 65 **Biscuits** home made | 2011 | 0.85 | 3008 | 0.6 |
| | 2165 | 0.24 | 3165 | 1.4 |
| | 2123 | 0.01 | 3187 | 20.0 |
| 71 **Shortbread** | 2011 | 1.06 | 3008 | 0.7 |
| | 2123 | 0.02 | 3123 | 25.3 |
| 75 **Fruit cake, rich** | 2011 | 0.26 | 3008 | 0.2 |
| | 2165 | 0.23 | 3165 | 1.3 |
| | | | 3187 | 9.5 |
| | 2736 | 0.13 | | |
| 76 **Fruit cake, rich, iced** | 2011 | 0.17 | 3008 | 0.1 |
| | 2165 | 0.21 | 3165 | 1.0 |
| | | | 3187 | 6.4 |
| | 2736 | 0.09 | | |
| | 2822 | 0.24 | 3822 | 4.0 |
| 78 **Gingerbread** | 2011 | 0.66 | 3008 | 0.4 |
| | 2165 | 0.25 | 3165 | 1.4 |
| | 2123 | 0.06 | 3123 | 0.4 |
| | | | 3187 | 10.4 |
| 80 **Rock cakes** | 2011 | 0.64 | 3008 | 0.4 |
| | 2123 | 0.05 | 3123 | 0.3 |
| | 2165 | 0.18 | 3165 | 1.0 |
| | | | 3187 | 14.6 |
| | 2736 | 0.05 | | |
| 81 **Sponge cake, with fat** | 2011 | 0.49 | 3058 | 0.4 |
| | 2165 | 0.56 | 3165 | 3.1 |
| | 2123 | 0.01 | 3187 | 23.0 |
| 82 **Sponge cake, without fat** | 2011 | 0.50 | 3008 | 0.3 |
| | 2165 | 1.14 | 3165 | 6.4 |
| 86 **Eclairs** | 2011 | 0.25 | 3008 | 0.2 |
| | 2123 | 0.07 | 3123 | 13.6 |
| | 2165 | 0.28 | 3165 | 1.6 |
| | | | 3187 | 5.8 |
| | 2858 | 0.13 | 3858 | 2.8 |
| 87 **Jam tarts** | 2011 | 0.56 | 3008 | 0.4 |
| | | | 3187 | 6.5 |
| | | | 3185 | 8.0 |
| | 2682 | 0.05 | | |
| 88 **Mince pies** | 2011 | 0.70 | 3008 | 0.5 |
| | | | 3187 | 8.2 |
| | | | 3185 | 10.0 |
| | 2736 | 0.04 | 3675 | 2.0 |

| | Tables section 2 code | N contributed per 100 g | Tables section 3 code | Fat contributed per 100 g |
|---|---|---|---|---|
| 89 **Pastry, choux** raw | 2011 | 0.43 | 3008 | 0.3 |
| | 2165 | 0.49 | 3165 | 2.7 |
| | | | 3187 | 10.0 |
| 90 **Pastry, choux** cooked | 2011 | 0.66 | 3008 | 0.5 |
| | 2165 | 0.76 | 3165 | 4.2 |
| | | | 3187 | 5.4 |
| 91 **Pastry, flaky** raw | 2011 | 0.77 | 3008 | 0.5 |
| | | | 3187 | 13.6 |
| | | | 3185 | 16.5 |
| 92 **Pastry, flaky** cooked | 2011 | 1.02 | 3008 | 0.7 |
| | | | 3187 | 17.9 |
| | | | 3185 | 21.4 |
| 93 **Pastry, shortcrust** raw | 2011 | 1.03 | 3008 | 0.7 |
| | | | 3187 | 12.2 |
| | | | 3185 | 14.9 |
| 94 **Pastry, shortcrust** cooked | 2011 | 1.20 | 3008 | 0.8 |
| | | | 3187 | 14.1 |
| | | | 3185 | 17.3 |
| 95 **Scones** | 2011 | 1.10 | 3008 | 0.7 |
| | 2123 | 0.20 | 3123 | 1.5 |
| | | | 3187 | 12.4 |
| 96 **Scotch pancakes** | 2011 | 0.71 | 3008 | 0.5 |
| | 2123 | 0.22 | 3123 | 1.6 |
| | 2165 | 0.20 | 3165 | 1.1 |
| | | | 3187 | 8.4 |
| 97 **Apple crumble** | 2011 | 0.29 | 3008 | 0.2 |
| | | | 3187 | 6.7 |
| | 2675 | 0.03 | | |
| 98 **Bread and butter pudding** | 2011 | 0.15 | 3033 | 0.2 |
| | 2123 | 0.47 | 3123 | 5.7 |
| | 2165 | 0.36 | 3165 | 1.9 |
| | 2736 | 0.01 | | |
| 99 **Cheesecake** | 2011 | 0.26 | (3069) | 3.2 |
| | 2123 | 0.21 | 3123 | 24.2 |
| | 2165 | 0.22 | 3165 | 1.2 |
| | | | 3187 | 6.3 |
| 100 **Christmas pudding** | 2011 | 0.46 | 3008 | 0.1 |
| | | | 3033 | 0.4 |
| | 2165 | 0.23 | 3165 | 1.3 |
| | | | 3194 | 8.5 |
| | 2736 | 0.11 | | |
| | 2822 | 0.08 | 3822 | 1.3 |
| 101 **Custard, egg** | 2123 | 0.52 | 3123 | 3.8 |
| | 2165 | 0.39 | 3165 | 2.2 |
| 102 **Custard powder** | 2123 | 0.60 | 3123 | 4.4 |
| 103 **Custard tart** | 2011 | 0.51 | 3008 | 0.4 |
| | 2123 | 0.26 | 3123 | 1.9 |
| | 2165 | 0.20 | 3165 | 1.1 |
| | | | 3187 | 6.1 |
| | | | 3185 | 7.4 |

| | Tables section 2 code | N contributed per 100 g | Tables section 3 code | Fat contributed per 100 g |
|---|---|---|---|---|
| 104 **Dumpling** | 2011 | 0.51 | 3008 | 0.4 |
| | | | 3194 | 11.3 |
| 106 **Fruit pie, pastry top** | 2011 | 0.28 | 3008 | 0.2 |
| | | | 3187 | 3.3 |
| | 2675 | 0.06 | 3185 | 4.1 |
| 111 **Jelly, made with milk** | 2959 | 0.25 | | |
| | 2123 | 0.22 | 3123 | 1.6 |
| 112 **Lemon meringue pie** | 2011 | 0.38 | 3008 | 0.3 |
| | 2165 | 0.37 | 3165 | 2.0 |
| | | | 3187 | 6.8 |
| | | | 3185 | 5.5 |
| 114 **Milk pudding** | see type | 0.09 | | |
| | 2123 | 0.57 | 3123 | 4.2 |
| 116 **Pancakes** | 2011 | 0.43 | 3008 | 0.3 |
| | 2123 | 0.32 | 3123 | 2.2 |
| | 2165 | 0.25 | 3165 | 1.4 |
| | | | 3185 | 12.4 |
| 117 **Queen of puddings** | 2011 | 0.14 | 3033 | 0.2 |
| | 2123 | 0.25 | 3123 | 5.7 |
| | 2165 | 0.38 | 3165 | 2.0 |
| 118 **Sponge pudding** steamed | 2011 | 0.60 | 3008 | 0.4 |
| | 2123 | 0.05 | 3123 | 0.3 |
| | 2165 | 0.34 | 3165 | 1.9 |
| | | | 3187 | 13.8 |
| 119 **Suet pudding** steamed | 2011 | 0.61 | 3008 | 0.2 |
| | | | 3033 | 0.4 |
| | 2123 | 0.16 | 3123 | 1.1 |
| | | | 3194 | 16.4 |
| 120 **Treacle tart** | 2011 | 0.65 | 3008 | 0.4 |
| | | | 3033 | 0.1 |
| | | | 3187 | 6.1 |
| | | | 3185 | 7.4 |
| 121 **Trifle** | 2011 | 0.07 | | |
| | 2123 | 0.29 | 3123 | 4.2 |
| | 2165 | 0.16 | 3165 | 0.9 |
| | 2682 | 0.01 | | |
| | 2822 | 0.04 | 3822 | 1.0 |
| 122 **Yorkshire pudding** | 2011 | 0.48 | 3008 | 0.3 |
| | 2123 | 0.36 | 3123 | 2.7 |
| | 2165 | 0.28 | 3165 | 1.6 |
| | | | 3184 | 5.5 |
| 172 **Omelette** | 2165 | 1.64 | 3165 | 9.7 |
| | 2123 | 0.01 | 3123 | 3.5 |
| 173 **Scrambled eggs** | 2165 | 1.59 | 3165 | 8.9 |
| | 2123 | 0.08 | 3123 | 13.8 |
| 174 **Cauliflower cheese** | 2011 | 0.05 | | |
| | 2123 | 0.69 | 3123 | 5.4 |
| | | | 3187 | 2.6 |
| | 2591 | 0.16 | | |

| | | Tables section 2 code | N contributed per 100 g | Tables section 3 code | Fat contributed per 100 g |
|---|---|---|---|---|---|
| 175 | **Cheese pudding** | 2011 | 0.16 | 3008 | 0.2 |
| | | 2123 | 1.01 | 3123 | 8.1 |
| | | 2165 | 0.46 | 3165 | 2.5 |
| 176 | **Cheese soufflé** | 2011 | 0.15 | 3008 | 0.2 |
| | | 2123 | 0.94 | 2123 | 7.7 |
| | | 2165 | 0.69 | 3165 | 3.9 |
| | | | | 3187 | 7.20 |
| 177 | **Macaroni cheese** | 2011 | 0.36 | 3008 | 0.3 |
| | | 2123 | 0.83 | 3123 | 6.6 |
| | | | | 3187 | 2.8 |
| 178 | **Pizza, cheese and tomato** | 2011 | 0.50 | 3008 | 0.3 |
| | | 2123 | 0.94 | 3123 | 7.6 |
| | | | | 3199 | 3.5 |
| | | 2968 | 0.05 | | |
| | | 2666 | 0.04 | | |
| 179 | **Quiche Lorraine** | 2011 | 0.41 | 3008 | 0.3 |
| | | 2123 | 1.02 | 3123 | 8.1 |
| | | 2165 | 0.39 | 3165 | 2.2 |
| | | 2210 | 0.55 | 3209 | 6.7 |
| | | | | 3187 | 4.8 |
| | | | | 3185 | 5.9 |
| 180 | **Scotch eggs** | 2011 | 0.17 | 3008 | 0.1 |
| | | 2165 | 0.85 | 3165 | 4.7 |
| | | 2411 | 0.84 | 3411 | 16.1 |
| 181 | **Welsh rarebit** | 2011 | 0.6 | 3033 | 0.9 |
| | | 2123 | 1.9 | 3123 | 22.7 |
| 422 | **Sausage roll, flaky pastry** | 2011 | 0.64 | 3008 | 0.4 |
| | | | | 3187 | 11.3 |
| | | | | 3185 | 13.8 |
| | | 2411 | 0.57 | 3411 | 10.7 |
| 423 | **Sausage roll, short pastry** | 2011 | 0.74 | 3008 | 0.5 |
| | | | | 3187 | 8.8 |
| | | | | 3185 | 10.8 |
| | | 2411 | 0.62 | 3411 | 11.7 |
| 424 | **Steak and kidney pie, pastry top** | 2011 | 0.35 | 3008 | 0.2 |
| | | | | 3187 | 5.6 |
| | | | | 3185 | 6.8 |
| | | 2237 | 1.53 | 3240 | 5.0 |
| | | 2363 | 0.59 | 3366 | 0.6 |
| 426 | **Beef steak pudding** | 2011 | 0.37 | 3008 | 0.2 |
| | | 2237 | 1.38 | 3240 | 4.5 |
| | | | | 3194 | 7.4 |
| | | 2613 | 0.02 | | |
| 427 | **Beef stew** | 2011 | 0.05 | | |
| | | | | 3184 | 2.7 |
| | | 2237 | 1.47 | 3240 | 4.8 |
| | | 2613 | 0.03 | | |

| | | Tables section 2 code | N contributed per 100g | Tables section 3 code | Fat contributed per 100g |
|---|---|---|---|---|---|
| 428 | **Bolognese sauce** | | | 3198 | 4.7 |
| | | 2237 | 1.14 | 3240 | 6.2 |
| | | 2587 | 0.02 | | |
| | | 2595 | 0.01 | | |
| | | 2666 | 0.08 | | |
| 429 | **Curried meat** | 2011 | 0.30 | 3008 | 0.3 |
| | | | | 3198 | 5.6 |
| | | 2237 | 1.40 | 3240 | 3.1 |
| | | 2613 | 0.03 | | |
| | | 2736 | 0.02 | | |
| | | 2832 | 0.02 | 2832 | 1.1 |
| 430 | **Hot pot** | 2237 | 1.29 | 3240 | 4.2 |
| | | 2587 | 0.02 | | |
| | | 2639 | 0.14 | | |
| | | 2613 | 0.04 | | |
| 431 | **Irish stew** | 2266 | 0.65 | 3269 | 7.3 |
| | | 2639 | 0.15 | | |
| | | 2613 | 0.03 | | |
| 432 | **Irish stew** (with bone) | 2266 | 0.59 | 3269 | 6.7 |
| | | 2639 | 0.14 | | |
| | | 2613 | 0.04 | | |
| 433 | **Moussaka** | 2011 | 0.03 | | |
| | | 2123 | 0.34 | 3123 | 2.72 |
| | | 2237 | 0.91 | 3240 | 4.9 |
| | | 2613 | 0.03 | | |
| | | 2639 | 0.10 | | |
| | | 2666 | 0.02 | | |
| | | 2165 | 0.06 | 3165 | 0.3 |
| | | | | 3198 | 5.5 |
| 434 | **Shepherd's pie** | 2123 | 0.02 | 3123 | 0.2 |
| | | | | 3187 | 1.4 |
| | | 2237 | 1.11 | 3240 | 4.5 |
| | | 2613 | 0.01 | | |
| | | 2639 | 0.10 | | |
| 545 | **Fish fingers** frozen | 2435 | 1.24 | a | a |
| | | 2011 | 0.78 | | |
| 546 | fried | 2435 | 1.66 | a | a |
| | | 2011 | 0.50 | | |
| 548 | **Fish pie** | 2011 | 0.03 | | |
| | | 2123 | 0.11 | 3123 | 1.5 |
| | | | | 3187 | 3.9 |
| | | 2435 | 0.85 | 3438 | 0.2 |
| | | 2638 | 0.14 | | |
| 549 | **Kedgeree** | 2019 | 0.04 | 3019 | 0.1 |
| | | 2165 | 0.42 | 3165 | 2.3 |
| | | | | 3187 | 4.3 |
| | | 2435 | 1.57 | 3451 | 0.4 |
| 852 | **Lemon curd** | | | 3123 | 10.7 |
| | homemade | 2165 | 0.53 | 3165 | 2.8 |

| | Tables section 2 code | N contributed per 100 g | Tables section 3 code | Fat contributed per 100 g |
|---|---|---|---|---|
| 920 **Bread sauce** | 2011 | 0.25 | 3033 | 0.3 |
| | 2123 | 0.45 | 3123 | 3.3 |
| | | | 3187 | 1.4 |
| 922 **Cheese sauce** | 2011 | 0.10 | 3008 | 0.1 |
| | 2123 | 1.21 | 3123 | 9.5 |
| | | | 3187 | 5.0 |
| 927 **Onion sauce** | 2011 | 0.08 | 3008 | 0.1 |
| | 2123 | 0.35 | 3123 | 2.5 |
| | | | 3187 | 3.8 |
| | 2613 | 0.03 | | |
| 933 **Tomato sauce** | 2011 | 0.10 | | |
| | | | 3187 | 1.3 |
| | 2210 | 0.14 | 3209 | 1.1 |
| 934 **White sauce, savoury** | 2011 | 0.11 | | |
| | 2123 | 1.21 | 3123 | 9.5 |
| | | | 3187 | 5.0 |
| 935 **White sauce, sweet** | 2011 | 0.68 | | |
| | 2123 | 0.55 | 3123 | 4.1 |
| | | | 3187 | 6.2 |
| 943 **Lentil soup** | 2011 | 0.06 | | |
| | 2123 | 0.09 | 3123 | 0.7 |
| | | | 3187 | 2.8 |
| | 2587 | 0.03 | | |
| | 2603 | 0.53 | | |

# Appendix 6: Key to references and sources of data

The following key shows the sources of the data for virtually all the new entries in the tables. It identifies all the new analyses carried out at the Laboratory of the Government Chemist and the Dunn Nutritional Laboratory, and gives references to values derived from the literature. Where a food or nutrient does not appear in this key it means either that the values are used unchanged from the third edition or that no information is available.

The following symbols are used in the key.

Bold type : new analytical data

* from the Laboratory of the Government Chemist

+ from the Dunn Nutritional Laboratory

| | | | |
|---|---|---|---|
| Prox | Proximate constituents | Cl | Chloride |
| DF | Dietary fibre | Vit A | Retinol and carotene |
| N | Total nitrogen | Vit D | Vitamin D |
| CHO | Carbohydrate | Thi | Thiamin |
| Na | Sodium | Rib | Riboflavin |
| K | Potassium | Nic | Nicotinic acid |
| Ca | Calcium | Vit C | Vitamin C |
| Mg | Magnesium | Vit E | Vitamin E |
| P | Phosphorus | Vit $B_6$ | Vitamin $B_6$ |
| Fe | Iron | Vit $B_{12}$ | Vitamin $B_{12}$ |
| Cu | Copper | Folic | Folic acid |
| Zn | Zinc | Pant | Pantothenic acid |
| S | Sulphur | | |

The numbers given after the nutrient refer to the number of the reference. The literature in mainly confined to the period 1960–1976, though a few earlier publications are included where relevant. Emphasis has been given to papers reporting original work, although comprehensive review papers and food tables of other countries are included where appropriate. The coverage is of necessity selective, and while a much larger number of references were consulted during the course of the revision, only those that proved to be of direct use are included in this key.

# Section 1: Proximate and inorganic constituents and vitamins

*Food no*

**Cereals and cereal products**

2 **DF⁺** Rib 307 Vit E 279 Vit $B_6$ 229 Folic 131 Pant 229
3 Vitamins *calculated from raw*
4 Vitamins *manufacturer's data on carton*
5 **Prox⁺ DF⁺** Inorganics 29 Thi, Rib, Nic, Vit $B_6$, Pant, Biotin 97 Vit E 279 Folic 49
6 Zn 216 Folic 126
7 **Na⁺** Cl *Na × 1.5*
9 **Prox* DF⁺ K* Ca* Mg* P* Fe* Cu* Zn* Thi* Rib* Nic*** Vit E 279 Vit $B_6$ 155 **Folic*** Pant and Biotin 155
10 **Prox* DF⁺ K* Ca* Mg* P* Fe* Zn* Thi* Rib* Nic*** Vit $B_6$ 155 **Folic*** Pant 155
11 **Prox* DF⁺ K* Ca* Mg* P* Fe* Zn* Thi* Rib* Nic*** Vit E 279 Vit $B_6$ 155 **Folic*** Pant and Biotin 155
12 **Prox* DF⁺ K* Ca* Mg* P* Fe* Zn* Thi* Rib* Nic*** Vit E 279 Vit $B_6$ 155 **Folic*** Pant and Biotin 155
13 **Prox* DF⁺ Na* K* Ca* Mg* P* Fe* Cu* Zn* Thi* Rib* Nic* Folic***
15 **Water⁺ N⁺** Rib 307 Vit $B_6$ 229 Folic 131
16 Water, N *calculated from raw* Thi, Rib, Nic 307
17 **DF⁺** Vit E 128, 278, 279 Folic 137
18 DF *calculated* Folic 137
19 **DF⁺** Zn 216 Vit E 128, 278 Folic 131
20 DF *calculated* Zn 216 Folic 137
21 Na 307 Cu 238 Vit E 279 Folic 131
24 **Sugars⁺ Starch⁺ DF⁺** Na 307 Rib 307 Vit $B_6$ 229 Pant 229
25 Sugars, starch, DF *calculated from raw* Na 307 Rib 307 Vit $B_6$ 229 Pant 229
26 **Water⁺ N⁺** Rib 307 Vit $B_6$ 229 Folic 131
27 *Calculated from raw*
30 **Water* DF⁺ Na* K* Fe* Thi* Rib* Nic* Vit $B_6$*** The remaining nutrients *calculated* (*except* sugars and S *from 3rd edition*)
31 **DF⁺** The remaining nutrients *calculated* (*except* sugars and S *from 3rd edition*)
32 **DF⁺** Remaining nutrients *manufacturer's and British Baking Industries Research Association analytical data*
33 Water 163 **DF⁺** Fat 163 Na 163 K 163 Ca 163 Fe 163 Thi 163 Rib 163 Nic 163 Vit $B_6$ 163 Folic (free) 163 Remaining nutrients *calculated* (*except* sugars, N and S *from 3rd edition*)
34 Fat 145
40–43 Prox 172 Ca, Fe, S 172 Rest of inorganics *calculated* Thi, Rib, Nic, Vit $B_6$ 172
44 Na *manufacturer's data*
45 **Prox* DF⁺ Inorganics* Thi* Rib* Nic* Folic***
46 **Water⁺ Fat⁺** remainder *calculated*
47 **All nutrients*** *except* **DF⁺**
48 **All nutrients*** *except* **DF⁺**
49 **Prox* DF⁺ Inorganics* Thi* Rib* Nic* Folic* Vit E*** Vits A, D and $B_{12}$ *manufacturers' data*

| | | |
|---|---|---|
| Cereals and cereal products *continued* | *Food no* | |
| | 50 | **All nutrients*** *except* **DF**+ |
| | 51 | **All nutrients*** *except* **DF**+ |
| | 52 | **All nutrients*** *except* **DF**+ |
| | 53 | **All nutrients*** *except* **DF**+ |
| | 54 | **All nutrients*** *except* **DF**+, protein *manufacturers' data*, starch *calculated* |
| | 55 | **All nutrients*** *except* **DF**+ |
| | 56 | **All nutrients*** *except* **DF**+ |
| | 57 | **All nutrients*** *except* **DF**+ sugars *manufacturers' data* |
| | 58 | **All nutrients*** *except* **DF**+ |
| | 60 | **All nutrients*** *except* **DF**+ Folic, Pant and Biotin *calculated* |
| | 63 | **All nutrients*** *except* **DF**+ |
| | 64 | **All nutrients*** *except* **DF**+ |
| | 66 | **All nutrients*** *except* **DF**+ |
| | 67 | **All nutrients*** *except* **DF**+ Folic 137 Pant and Biotin *calculated* |
| | 68 | **All nutrients*** *except* **DF**+ |
| | 69 | **All nutrients*** *except* **DF**+ Folic 137 |
| | 70 | **All nutrients*** *except* **DF**+ Folic 137 |
| | 72 | **All nutrients*** *except* **DF**+ |
| | 74 | **All nutrients*** *except* **DF**+ |
| | 77 | **All nutrients*** *except* **DF**+ |
| | 79 | **All nutrients*** *except* **DF**+ |
| | 83 | **All nutrients*** *except* **DF**+ |
| | 105 | **All nutrients*** *except* **DF**+ |
| | 107 | **All nutrients*** |
| | 108 | **All nutrients*** |
| | 115 | **All nutrients*** |
| Milk and milk products | 124–125 | Water 164 Lactose 164 Protein 164 Fat 164, 207 **Na*** and 73 **K*** and 73, 87 **Ca*** and 164, 196, 249 **Mg*** and 196 **P*** and 249 **Fe*** and 196 **Cu*** and 218, 238, 269 **Zn*** and 18, 216, 269 Cl 249 Vit A 291 Vit D 291 **Rib*** and 52, 249 **Vit C** (boiled Milk)* and 258 Vit E 208, 291 Vit $B_6$ (boiled milk) 152 Vit $B_{12}$ (boiled milk) 152, 223 Folic 47, 94, 152, 199, 219, 223 |
| | 127–128 | Water 248 Lactose 248 Protein 248 Fat 207 Vit A 291 Vit D 291 Rib 249, 292 |
| | 129 | Thi 266 Rib 164 Nic 164 Vit C 266 Vit $B_6$ 266 Vit $B_{12}$ 266 Folic 266 |
| | 130 | Vit A 48, 93 Thi 48, 93, 111, 266 Rib 93 Nic 93 Vit C 48, 93, 266, 294 Vit E 93 Vit $B_6$ 48, 93, 111, 266 Vit $B_{12}$ 48, 93, 111, 266 Folic 48, 93, 266 Pant 93 Biotin 93 |
| | 132 | **Prox* Na* K* Ca* Mg* P* Fe* Cu* Zn* Vit A* Thi* Rib* Nic* Vit C* Vit E* Vit $B_6$* Folic*** |
| | 134 | **Prox* Na* K* Ca* Mg* P* Fe* Cu* Zn* Vit A* Thi* Rib* Nic* Vit C* Vit E* Vit $B_6$* Folic*** |
| | 135 | **Prox* Na* K* Ca* Mg* P* Cu* Zn* Cl* Vit A* Thi* Rib* Nic* Vit E* Vit $B_6$*** Folic 92, 94 |
| | 136 | **Prox* Na* K* Ca* Mg* P* Fe* Cu* Zn* Thi* Rib* Nic* Vit C* Vit E* Vit $B_6$* Vit $B_{12}$* Folic*** |
| | 137 | Prox 164, 233 Na, K, Ca, Mg, P 233 Fe 18 Cu 18, 238 Zn 18 Vit A 164 Vit D 164 Thi 121, 164 Rib 121, 164 Nic 121, 164 Vit C 121, 164, 223 Vit $B_6$ 229 Vit $B_{12}$ 223 Folic 94, 223 Pant 121, 164 Biotin 164 |
| | 138 | **All*** (*except* S and Vit D) |
| | 140 | **Water**+ **Fat**+ **Na**+ Zn 269 Vit A 291 Vit D 125, 291 Vit E 291 |

| | Food no | |
|---|---|---|
| **Milk and milk products** *continued* | 150 | **Prox* Na* Cl*** |
| | 151 | Ca 164 Zn 281 Rib 121 Nic 121, 272 Vit $B_6$ 151, 272 Vit $B_{12}$ 7, 50, 186 Folic 272 Pant 272 Biotin 272 |
| | 152 | Mg 87 P 87 Zn 108 Thi 121, 164 Rib 121, 164 Nic 121, 164, 272 Vit $B_6$ 272 Vit $B_{12}$ 7, 50, 186, 187 Folic 131, 272 Pant 272 Biotin 272 |
| | 153 | Thi 121 Rib 121 Nic 121, 272 Vit $B_6$ 121, 151, 272 Vit $B_{12}$ 7, 50, 121, 186, 187 Folic 272 Pant 272 Biotin 272 |
| | 154 | Nic 272 Vit $B_6$ 272 Vit $B_{12}$ 121 Folic 272 Pant 272 Biotin 272 |
| | 155 | Thi 121 Rib 121 Nic 272 Vit $B_6$ 272 |
| | 157 | **Prox* Inorganics* Thi* Rib* Nic* Vit $B_6$* Folic*** |
| | 158 | **Prox* Inorganics*** |
| | 159 | **Prox* Inorganics* Vit A* Thi* Rib* Nic* Folic*** |
| | 161–164 | **Prox* Inorganics* Thi* Rib* Nic* Vit C* Vit E* Vit $B_6$*** Vit $B_{12}$ 7, 186, 187 **Folic*** |
| **Eggs** | 165 | Prox 293 Na 293 K 293 Ca 293 Fe 293 Cu 161, 238 Zn 161 Vit A 293 Thi 293 Rib 293 Nic 293 Vit E 293 Vit $B_6$ 246 Vit $B_{12}$ 293 Folic 53, 293 Pant 293 |
| | 166 | Cu 269 Zn 270 Rib *calculated from whole egg* Vit $B_6$ 246 Vit $B_{12}$ 186 Folic 53, 131 |
| | 167 | Cu 238 Zn 270 Vit A, Rib, Vit $B_{12}$ Pant *calculated from whole egg* Vit $B_6$ 246 Folic 53, 131 |
| | 168 | Zn 281 Vit A, Vit $B_{12}$ *calculated from whole* Vit $B_6$ 246 Pant 229 |
| | 169 | Folic 53 |
| **Fats and oils** | 182 | Vit A *B.P. specification* Vit D *B.P. specification* Vit E 42, 179, 215 |
| | 186–187 | Water 301 Fat 301 Na 301 Vit A 301 Vit D 301 Vit E 301 |
| | 194 | **Water* Fat* Carbohydrate* Retinol* Carotene* Vit E*** |
| | 196 | Vit E 127, 278, 279 |
| | 197 | Vit E 127, 278, 279 |
| | 198 | Vit E 57, 75, 127, 278, 279 |
| | 199 | Vit E 57, 127, 278, 279 |
| | 200 | Vit E 278 |
| | 201 | Vit E 127, 179, 278 |
| | 202 | Vit E 127, 278 |
| | 204 | Vit E 25, 127, 278, 279 |
| | 205 | Vit E 25, 127, 278, 279 |
| | 206 | Vit E 278 |
| | 207 | Vit E 127, 278, 279 |

**Meat and meat products**

For all items marked *, analyses were made for water, total N, fat, Na, K, Ca, Mg, P, Fe, Cu, Zn, S, Cl, thiamin, riboflavin, nicotinic acid, vitamin E, vitamin $B_6$, vitamin $B_{12}$, folic acid, pantothenic acid and biotin. Where no analyses were made of a particular cut of meat, the values were calculated from a related cut or raw analyses, and they are given in parenthesis. Retinol, carotene and vitamin C were analysed in liver. The composition of carcase meat was obtained by applying the equations of Callow, 1948 (51) to recent dissection data on tissue proportions—Cuthbertson 1974a and b, 1975 (69, 70, 71). Where no information is given for poultry and offal items, they are the values retained from the 3rd edition.

| | |
|---|---|
| 213–223 | * |
| 226–228 | * |

**Meat and meat products**
*continued*

| *Food no* | |
|---|---|
| 231–233 | * |
| 242–263 | * |
| 271–275 | * |
| 277 | * |
| 279–280 | * |
| 282 | * |
| 284–289 | * |
| 291–293 | * |
| 301–304 | * |
| 306 | * |
| 308–310 | * |
| 312 | **Fe*** |
| 313 | Fe *calculated from raw* |
| 314 | * |
| 315 | **Prox*** in skin **Inorganics*** in skin Thi, Rib and Nic in skin 260 Other B vitamins in skin *not accounted for.* |
| 316–321 | * |
| 322 | **Prox*** in skin Inorganics in skin *calculated* |
| 323–324 | * |
| 325–326 | Plate waste determined on 10 samples. |
| 327 | * |
| 328 | **Prox*** in skin Inorganics in skin *calculated* |
| 329 | * |
| 330 | **Prox*** in skin Inorganics in skin *calculated* |
| 331 | Cu 238 Vit $B_6$ 188 |
| 332 | Thi, Rib and Nic 255 |
| 336 | Thi, Rib and Nic 255 |
| 338 | Nic 154 Vit E 44 |
| 340 | * |
| 341 | **Prox*** in skin Inorganics in skin *calculated* |
| 342–344 | * |
| 345 | **Prox*** in skin Inorganics in skin *calculated* |
| 346–347 | * |
| 350 | * |
| 351 | Vitamins *calculated from raw* |
| 353 | Thi 114 |
| 354 | * Vit A 162 Vit C 162 |
| 355 | * Vit C *calculated from raw* |
| 356 | * Vit C *calculated from raw* |
| 358 | * Vit A 162 Vit C 162 |
| 359 | Vitamins *calculated from raw* |
| 360 | * Vit A 162 Vit C 162 |
| 361 | * Vit C *calculated from raw* |
| 362 | Vit A 162 Vit C 162 |
| 364 | * Vit A 162, 193 Vit C 162 |
| 365 | * Vitamins A and C *calculated from raw* |
| 366 | * Vit A 162, 193 Vit C 162 |
| 367 | * Vitamins A and C *calculated from raw* |
| 368 | * Vit A 162, 193 Vit C 162 |
| 369 | * Vitamins A and C *calculated from raw* |
| 371 | * **CHO*** **Vit A*** **Vit C*** |
| 372 | * **CHO*** **Vit A*** **Vit C*** |
| 373 | * **CHO*** **Vit A*** Vit D 96 **Vit C*** |

**Meat and meat products** *continued*

*Food no*

374 * CHO* Vit A *calculated from raw* Vit C*
375 * CHO* Vit A* Vit C*
376 * CHO* Vit A *calculated from raw* Vit C*
377 * CHO* Vit A* Vit C*
378 * CHO* Vit A *calculated from raw* Vit C*
379 * CHO* Vit A* Vit C*
380 * CHO* Vit A *calculated from raw* Vit C*
381 *
382 *
384 * Vit A 162 Vit C 162
385 * CHO* Vit C *calculated from raw*
387 * Vit C 162
388 Vitamins *calculated from raw*
389 * Vit C 162
390 Vitamins *calculated from raw*
391 * Vit C 162
392 * Vit C *calculated from raw*
393–421 *
425 *

**Fish and fish products**

438 Prox* Inorganics* Thi* Rib* Nic* Vit E* Vit $B_6$* Vit $B_{12}$* Folic* Biotin 217
439 Prox* Inorganics* (*except* S) S *calculated* Thi* Rib* Nic* Vit $B_6$ Vit $B_{12}$* Folic*
440 Prox* Inorganics* (*except* S) S *calculated* Thi* Rib* Nic* Vit E* Vit $B_6$* Vit $B_{12}$* Folic*
443 Prox* Inorganics* (*except* S) S *calculated* Thi* Rib* Nic* Vit $B_6$* Vit $B_{12}$* Folic*
444 Prox* Inorganics* (*except* S) S *calculated* Thi* Rib* Nic* Vit E* Vit $B_6$* Vit $B_{12}$* Folic*
448 Prox* Inorganics* (*except* S) S *calculated* Thi* Rib* Nic* Vit $B_6$* Vit $B_{12}$* Folic*
449 Prox* Inorganics* (*except* S) S *calculated* Thi* Rib* Nic* Vit $B_6$* Vit $B_{12}$* Folic*
451 Ca, P, Fe 276 Cu 238 Zn 108 Thi, Rib, Nic 217 Folic 131 Biotin 217
458 Prox 273 Inorganics *calculated* Vit E 38 Folic 131 Pant 190 Biotin 217
461 Prox 273 Inorganics *calculated* Thi, Rib, Nic, Vit $B_{12}$ 217 Folic 131
466 Prox* Inorganics* (*except* S) S *calculated* Thi* and 217 Rib* and 217 Nic* Vit $B_6$* Vit $B_{12}$* Folic* Pant 217
467 Prox* Inorganics* (*except* S) S *calculated* Thi* Rib* Nic*
468 Prox* Inorganics* (*except* S) S *calculated* Thi* Rib* Nic* Vit $B_6$* Vit $B_{12}$* Folic*
471 Water* 217 Remainder of Prox and Inorganics *calculated* Thi, Rib 217 Nic 34 Vit E 38 Vit $B_6$ 217 Vit $B_{12}$ 217 Pant 34 Biotin 217
480 Zn 281 Vit D 68 Nic, Vit $B_6$, Vit $B_{12}$, Pant 217
482 Prox* Inorganics* (*except* S) S *calculated* Thi* and 217 Rib* and 217 Nic* and 217 Vit E* Vit $B_6$* Vit $B_{12}$* Folic* Biotin 217
485 Prox* Inorganics* (*except* S) S *calculated* Thi* Rib* Nic* Vit E* Vit $B_6$* Vit $B_{12}$* Folic*
491 Prox 273 Inorganics (*except* Cu and Zn) *calculated* Cu 238 Zn 210 Rib, Vit $B_{12}$, Pant, Biotin 217
494 Prox* Inorganics* Retinol* Vit D* Thi* Rib* Nic* Vit E* Vit $B_{12}$ 7
495 Water 66 Remainder of Prox and Inorganics (*except* Cu and Zn) *calculated* Cu and Zn 276 Thi, Vit $B_6$, Vit $B_{12}$ 217 Folic 131 Pant and Biotin 217

**Fish and fish products** *continued*

*Food no*

498 **Prox* Inorganics*** (*except* S) S *calculated* **Thi* Rib* Nic* Vit E* Vit $B_6$* Vit $B_{12}$* Folic***

499 **Prox* Inorganics* Thi* Rib* Nic***

500 **Prox* Inorganics*** (*except* S) S *calculated* **Retinol* Thi* Rib* Nic* Vit E* Vit $B_6$* Vit $B_{12}$* Folic***

501 *Calculated on the proportions 0.83 fish; 0.17 olive oil*

502 **Prox* Inorganics*** (*except* S) S *calculated* **Retinol* Thi* Rib* Nic* Vit E* Vit $B_6$* Vit $B_{12}$* Folic***

508 **Prox* Inorganics*** (*except* S) Vit D 220 **Thi* Rib* Nic* Vit E*** Vit $B_6$ 220 Vit $B_{12}$ 7 Folic 131 Pant and Biotin 220

511 **Prox* Inorganics*** (*except* S) S *calculated* **Thi* Rib* Nic* Vit E***

514 **Prox* Inorganics*** (*except* S) S *calculated* **Thi* Rib* Nic* Vit E***

518 Cu and Zn 210 Folic 131 Biotin 217

520 **Prox* Inorganics*** (*except* Zn and S) Zn 210 **Thi* Rib* Nic***

521 Cu 238 Zn 216 Thi 217 Vit E 3 Vit $B_{12}$ 217 Folic 131 Pant and Biotin 190

523 Cu and Zn 210

525 **Prox* Inorganics*** (*except* S) **Thi* Rib* Nic***

527 Zn 210 Vit $B_{12}$ 217 Biotin 190

529 **Prox* Inorganics*** (*except* S) **Thi* Rib* Nic* Vit $B_6$* Vit $B_{12}$* Folic*** Pant 289

531 Cu and Zn 210

532 Cu and Zn 210 Vit E 3, 38

533 Fe and Cu *calculated*

535 Cu and Zn 210 Vit E 3 Folic 126

538 Folic 131 Pant and Biotin 190

539 Zn 210 Vit E 38

541 Cu and Zn 210

543 **Prox* Inorganics*** (*except* S) **Thi* Rib* Nic***

544 **Prox* Inorganics*** (*except* S) **Thi* Rib* Nic***

545 **Prox* Inorganics*** (*except* S) **Thi* Rib* Nic* Vit $B_6$* Vit $B_{12}$* Folic***

546 **Prox* Inorganics*** (*except* S) **Thi* Rib* Nic* Vit $B_6$* Vit $B_{12}$* Folic***

547 **Prox* Inorganics*** (*except* S) **Thi* Rib* Nic* Vit E***

550 Prox 217 Retinol 242 Vit E 166 Vit $B_6$ 36 Vit $B_{12}$ 217 Pant and Biotin 35

552 Prox 217 Vit C 192 Vit $B_{12}$ and Pant *as cod milt* 34

**Vegetables**

The ranges which are given for carotene and vitamin C were derived in the main from data collected for the 3rd edition and no further information is given here.

554 **Prox* Inorganics*** (*except* S) **Thi* Rib* Nic* Vit C* Vit $B_6$* Folic***

555 Thi, Rib, Nic, Vit C, Vit $B_6$, Folic, Pant, Biotin 64

557 Zn 270 Vit E 31

558 Zn 254 Vit E 31 Folic 131

560 Carotene, Vit C, Thi, Rib, Nic 243 Vit $B_6$ 229 Folic 131, 176

562 **Prox* DF$^+$ Inorganics* Vit E* Folic***

563 **Prox* DF$^+$ Inorganics* Vit E* Folic***

564 Fat 134 Carotene 78, 134 Vit E 31

565 Fat 55 Zn 216 Vit $B_6$ 229 Folic 131 Pant 229

567 Fat 307 Zn 216 Vit $B_6$ and Pant 229

569 **Prox* DF$^+$ Inorganics* Thi* Rib* Nic* Vit C$^+$ Vit E* Vit $B_6$* Folic***

570 Water, Protein, Fat 55 CHO 306 Na and K 107 Ca 243 Mg and P 107 Fe 243 Cu, S, Cl 107 Carotene, Thi, Rib, Nic, Vit C 243 Folic 107

**Vegetables** *continued*

*Food no*

572 Water, Protein, Fat 55 CHO *as haricot beans* Ca 55 P 107 Fe 55 Carotene 243 Thi, Rib, Nic 55 Vit C 243 Vit $B_6$ and Pant 229

573 **Prox* DF⁺ Inorganics*** Carotene 243 **Thi* Rib* Nic* Vit C*** and 243 **Vit $B_6$* Folic***

574 Zn 108, 305 Vit E 31 Folic 131

575 Folic 137

576 **Prox* DF⁺ Inorganics* Vit C* Vit E*** Vit $B_6$ 244 **Folic***

577 **Prox* DF⁺ Inorganics* Vit C* Vit E*** Vit $B_6$ 244 **Folic***

578 **Prox* DF⁺ Inorganics* Vit C* Vit E* Folic***

579 **Prox* DF⁺ Inorganics*** (*except* S) **Vit C* Vit E* Folic***

580 Carotene 307 Other vitamins *as winter cabbage ex* Vit $B_6$ 244

581 Vit C 227

583 Carotene 253 Vit C 227 Folic 53

584 **Prox* DF⁺ Inorganics* Vit C* Vit E* Folic***

585–586 **Prox* DF⁺ Inorganics* Vit C* Vit E*** Vit $B_6$ 244 **Folic*** Pant 229

587–588 Zn 216 Vit E 31 Vit $B_6$ 229 Folic 53, 131

590 Zn 216 Folic 53

591–592 **Prox* DF⁺ Inorganics* Vit C* Vit E* Folic***

593 Thi, Rib, Nic, Vit C 134 Vit $B_6$ 229

594–595 Zn 108 Vit E 31 Folic 131

596 Zn 254 Carotene, Thi, Rib, Nic, Vit C 134 Vit $B_6$ 229 Folic 131

597 Zn 108, 270 Vit E 31 Folic 131, 137

598 Nic 134 Folic 53

599 Carotene, Thi, Rib, Nic 134 Vit $B_6$ 229

600 **Prox* DF⁺ Inorganics* Thi* Rib* Nic* Vit C* Vit E* Folic***

601 Vit E 31

602 Vit E 31, 32 Folic 137

603 Fat 243 Zn 216 Carotene, Rib, Nic, Vit C 243 Vit $B_6$ 229 Folic 176

604 **Water⁺ Fat⁺**

605 **Water⁺**

606 **Prox* DF⁺ Inorganics*** Vit E 31, 57 **Folic*** Pant 229

607 **Prox* Inorganics*** Carotene 224 **Folic***

609 Zn 270 Vit E 31 Folic 131

610 Folic 137

611 Vit C 119

612 Water, Protein, Fat 243 CHO 306 Na 107 K 107, 134 Ca 243 Mg and P 107, 134 Fe 243 Cu, S, Cl 107 Carotene, Thi, Rib, Nic, Vit C 243 Vit $B_6$ 229 Folic 107 Pant 229

613 Zn 108, 270 Vit E 31 Folic 131 Pant 229

614 Folic 53 Pant 229

616 Folic 131

617 Zn 270 Vit E 31

618 Zn 254 Rib 134 Vit E 31 Folic 131

620 Zn 231 Vit E 31 Pant 229

621 Dried peas Vit C 264

622–625 **Prox* DF* Inorganics* Thi* Rib* Nic* Vit C* Vit E* Vit $B_6$* Folic***

626 Fat 307 Zn 216 Vit $B_6$ 229 Folic 131 Pant 229

627 Fat 307

628–629 Fat 307

630 Water, Protein, Fat *Data from* 243 CHO *calculated* Na, K 107 Ca *data from* 243 P 107, 177, 178 Fe *Data from* 243 Cu, S, Cl, 107 Carotene 107 Thi, Rib, Nic 243 Vit C 107 Folic 107

631 **Water⁺ Fat⁺**

**Vegetables**
*continued*

*Food no*

632 **Prox* DF+ Inorganics* Thi* Rib* Nic* Folic***

633 Water, Protein, Fat 243 CHO *calculated* Na and K 107 Ca 243 Mg and P 107 Fe 243 Cu, S, Cl 107 Carotene, Thi, Rib, Nic, Vit C 243 Folic 107

634–635 **Prox* DF+ Inorganics*** Carotene 243 **Thi* Rib* Nic* Vit C* Vit E* Vit $B_6$* Folic*** Pant 229

636 Water, Protein, Fat 243 CHO 157, 306 Ca 243 Mg and P 107 Fe 243 Cu and S 107 Carotene, Thi, Rib, Nic, Vit C 243 Vit $B_6$ 229 Folic 107 Pant 229

637–638 **Prox* DF+ Inorganics* Thi* Rib* Nic* Vit C* Folic***

639 **Fe*** and 144 Zn 216, 231, 305 Vit E 31 Vit $B_6$ 229 Folic 53, 131

640–642 Fe and Zn *calculated from raw* Vit $B_6$ 229 Folic 53, 131

644–645 **Fat+** Fe and Zn *calculated from raw*

646–647 **Prox* DF+ Inorganics* Thi* Rib* Nic* Vit C* Vit $B_6$* Folic***

648 Fe and Zn *calculated from raw*

649 **Prox* DF+ Inorganics* Thi* Rib* Nic* Vit C* Vit E* Vit $B_6$* Folic***

650 **Prox* DF+ Inorganics* Thi* Rib* Nic* Vit C* Folic***

652 **Prox* DF+ Inorganics* Thi* Rib* Nic* Vit C* Vit E* Vit $B_6$* Folic***

653 Vit $B_6$ and Pant 229

654 Zn 254, 270 Vit E 31 Folic 131

657 Zn 108, 216, 270 Vit E 31 Vit $B_6$ 229 Folic 131, 137

658 Vitamins *calculated*

659–660 Vit E 31 Folic 53

661–662 **Prox* DF+ Inorganics*** Carotene 307 **Thi* Rib* Nic*** Vit C 307 **Vit E* Vit $B_6$* Folic*** Pant 229

663 **Prox* DF+ Inorganics*** Carotene 307 **Thi* Rib* Nic*** Vit C 307 **Folic***

664 Water 243 Remainder of prox and inorganics *calculated from boiled* Vit $B_6$ 229 Folic 131

665 Vitamins *calculated from raw*

666 Zn 216, 231 **Vit C*** and 45, 298, 299 **Vit E* Folic*** Pant 229

668 **Prox* DF+ Inorganics* Thi* Rib* Nic* Vit C* Vit E* Vit $B_6$* Folic***

669 Vit E 31 Folic 131 Pant 229

671 Vit $B_6$ and Pant 229

672 Zn 254 Rib 134 Vit E 31 Vit $B_6$ 229 Folic 137

673 Water, protein, fat 243 CHO 134, 306 Ca 134 Fe, Cu, Zn *calculated from boiled* Carotene, Thi, Rib, Nic, Vit C 243 Pant 229

674 **Prox* DF+ Inorganics* Thi* Rib* Nic* Vit C* Folic***

**Fruit**

The ranges which are given for carotene and vitamin C were derived in the main from data collected for the 3rd edition, and no further information is given here.

675 Cu Zn 240 Vit C 17, 20, 54, 84, 156, 159, 224, 247 Vit E 31

677 Vit C 54, 159, 247, 310

682 Zn 231 Nic 307 Vit $B_6$ 229

688 Zn 254 Vit $B_6$ 229 Folic 131

691 Zn 108 **Vit C+** Folic 137

692 **Prox*** Na 237 Fe 277 Vit C 243 **Vit E*** Vit $B_6$ 229 **Folic*** Pant 229 Biotin 277

693 Zn 108, 216 Vit E 43 Vit $B_6$ 229 Folic 53, 131 Pant 229

695 Prox 281 Inorganics 281 *except* Zn 108 Vitamins 281 *except* Folic 131

696 Vit E 31

699 Zn 108, 254, 281 Rib 247 Vit E 31 Folic 131 Pant 229

707 Thi, Rib 107 Vit $B_6$ 229 Folic 131 Pant 229

708 Vit E 31

**Fruit**
*continued*

*Food no*

| | |
|---|---|
| 711 | Carotene 107 Vit E 31 |
| 717 | Folic 131 |
| 718 | Vit E 31 |
| 724 | Zn 254 Vit $B_6$ 229 Folic 131, 137 |
| 726 | Zn 254 Vit $B_6$ 229 Pant 229 |
| 727 | Zn 254 Vit $B_6$ 229 Folic 131 Pant 229 |
| 730 | **Prox* Inorganics* Thi* Rib* Nic*** |
| 731 | **Fe**$^+$ |
| 732 | Zn 254 Vit E 31 |
| 734 | **Vit C**$^+$ in canned |
| 735 | Zn 254 Vit E 31 |
| 736–738 | Zn 281 Folic 31 Biotin 241 |
| 740 | Zn 231 Vit $B_6$ 229 Folic 53, 131, 284 Pant 229 |
| 742 | **Prox* DF**$^+$ **Inorganics* Folic*** |
| 749 | **Prox* DF**$^+$ **Inorganics*** Carotene, Thi, Rib, Nic *estimated from raw* 243 **Vit C*** Vit C in raw 243 Vit $B_6$ 229 |
| 750 | Vitamins 26 |
| 751 | Vitamins 26 Folic 131 |
| 756 | Prox 243 Na, K, Ca 307 Mg and P 107 Fe 243 S and Cl 107 Thi, Rib, Nic 243, Vit C 107, 243, 307 |
| 757 | **Prox* DF**$^+$ **Inorganics* Vit C*** |
| 758 | **Prox* DF**$^+$ **Inorganics* Vit C*** Vit $B_6$ 26 **Folic*** |
| 759 | Water and Protein 243 CHO 72 Na and K 307 Ca 243 Mg and P 307 Cu 315 Carotene, Thi, Rib, Nic, Vit C 243 Pant 229 |
| 760 | **Prox* DF**$^+$ **Inorganics* Vit C*** |
| 761 | Vit C 24 |
| 762–764 | Zn 108 Carotene, Rib 307 Vit E 31, 43 Vit $B_6$ 229 Folic 131 |
| 766 | Prox 243 Na and K 134, 315 Ca 134, 243, 315 Mg and P 134, 315 Fe 134, 243, 315 Cu 315 Carotene and Thi 243 Rib and Nic 134, 243 Vit C 243 Folic 131 Pant 229 |
| 768 | Thi 224 Vit C 24, 243 |
| 769 | Folic 131 |
| 771 | Carotene 307 |
| 773 | Zn 108, 216 Vit $B_6$ 229 Folic 49, 53, 131, 284 |
| 775 | Zn 108, 216, 231 Vit $B_6$ 229 Folic 49, 284 |
| 776 | Carotene, Thi, Rib, Nic 243 |
| 778 | **Prox* DF**$^+$ **Inorganics*** Thi, Rib, Nic *based on* 243 **Vit C*** |
| 779 | Zn 216, 231 Folic 131 |
| 781 | Rib and Nic 307 Vit $B_6$ 229 |
| 784 | **Fe**$^+$ |
| 785–787 | Zn 86 Vit E 31 Folic 131 Pant 229 |
| 790 | **Fe**$^+$ |
| 791 | Zn 254, 281 Vit $B_6$ 229 Folic 131 Pant 229 |
| 792 | **K**$^+$ **Fe**$^+$ **Vit C**$^+$ Vit $B_6$ 229 Folic 131 Pant 229 |
| 793 | Zn 254, 281 Folic 131 |
| 801 | Thi, Rib, Nic, Vit C 243 |
| 802 | Vit $B_6$ 229 Folic 131 Pant 229 |
| 808 | Thi, Rib, Nic, Vit C 243 |
| 809 | Zn 254 Rib 307 Vit $B_6$ 229 Folic 131 Pant 229 |
| 810 | Vit E 31 Vit $B_6$ and Pant 229 |
| 813 | Prox and inorganics 78 Thi, Nic, Vit $B_6$, Pant 78 |
| 814 | Rib, Nic 134 Vit E 31 Vit $B_6$ 229 Folic 131 |
| 816 | **Vit C**$^+$ in canned |

**Fruit** *continued*

*Food no*

817 Zn 254 Vit E 31 Vit $B_6$ 229 Folic 131 Pant 229

818 **Prox**$^*$ **DF**$^+$ **Inorganics**$^*$ **Vit C**$^*$ Vit $B_6$ 229 **Folic**$^*$ Pant 229

819 Vit E 30

820 Zn 270 Vit $B_6$ 229 Folic 131, 284 Pant 229

**Nuts**

822 Zn 269 Thi and Rib 307 Vit E 181, 279 Vit $B_6$ 229 Folic 131 Pant 229

826 Zn 269 Rib, Nic 307 Vit E 181 Vit $B_6$ and Pant 229

828 Rib 307 Vit E 181 Vit $B_6$ 229, 245 Pant 229

830 Zn 270 Rib 307 Vit E 181 Vit $B_6$ 229 Folic 131 Pant 229

832 Zn 270 Vit E 181 Vit $B_6$ 229 Folic 131 Pant 229

833 Thi, Rib, Nic, Vit C 307 Vit $B_6$ 229, 245 Pant 229

834 Thi, Rib, Nic 307

835 Zn 216, 270 Vit E 181, 279 Folic 131, 137

837 **Na**$^+$ Cl *calculated* Vit $B_6$ 229

838 **Prox**$^*$ **DF**$^+$ **Inorganics**$^*$ **Thi**$^*$ **Rib**$^*$ **Nic**$^*$ **Vit E**$^*$ **Vit** $\mathbf{B_6}^*$ **Folic**$^*$

839 Zn 108, 270 Vit E 181, 279 Vit $B_6$ 229 Folic 131 Pant 229

**Sugars, preserves and confectionery**

849 **Vit C**$^*$ in blackcurrant jam

851 **Prox**$^*$ **DF**$^+$ **Inorganics**$^*$

853 **DF**$^+$ Folic 137

855 **Prox**$^*$ **DF**$^+$ **Inorganics**$^*$

857 **Prox**$^*$ **Inorganics**$^*$ **Thi**$^*$ **Rib**$^*$ **Nic**$^*$ **Vit E**$^*$

858 **Prox**$^*$ **Inorganics**$^*$ **Thi**$^*$ **Rib**$^*$ **Nic**$^*$ **Vit E**$^*$

**Beverages**

867 Water, Protein, Fat *manufacturers' data* **CHO**$^+$ Inorganics *manufacturers' data*

868 **Prox**$^*$ **Inorganics**$^*$ **Thi**$^*$ **Rib**$^*$ **Nic**$^*$ **Vit E**$^*$ **Vit** $\mathbf{B_6}^*$ **Folic**$^*$

869 **Prox**$^*$ **Thi**$^*$ **Rib**$^*$ **Nic**$^*$

872 **Water**$^*$ **Nitrogen**$^*$ **Inorganics**$^*$ **Thi**$^*$ **Rib**$^*$ **Nic**$^*$ and 225, 287 Pant and Biotin 287

873 **Prox**$^*$ **Inorganics**$^*$ **Thi**$^*$ **Rib**$^*$ **Nic**$^*$ **Vit E**$^*$ **Vit** $\mathbf{B_6}^*$ **Folic**$^*$

874 Prox, Inorganics, Retinol, Vit D, Thi, Rib, Nic *manufacturers' data*

875 Prox *manufacturers' data* **Na**$^+$ **K**$^+$ **Fe**$^+$ Vit D, Thi *manufacturers' data on label*

876 Purine N 12 CHO 209, 282 Fat 209, 282 Zn 282 Carotene, Thi, Rib, Nic, Vit C, Pant 282

**Soft drinks, fruit and vegetable juices**

878 **Water**$^*$ **CHO**$^+$ *and manufacturers' data* **Inorganics**$^*$ *except* Fe *manufacturers' data*

879 **Prox**$^*$ **Inorganics**$^*$ **Vit C**$^*$ **Folic**$^*$

880 **Prox**$^*$ **Inorganics**$^*$ **Vit C**$^*$

883 Prox, Inorganics and Vit C *manufacturers' data*

884 Prox and Inorganics *manufacturers' data* **Vit C**$^+$

885 **Prox**$^*$ **Inorganics**$^*$ **Vit C**$^*$ **Folic**$^*$

886 **Prox**$^*$ **Inorganics**$^*$ **Vit C**$^*$

888 Prox and inorganics *manufacturers' data* **Vit C**$^+$

889 **Water**$^*$ **CHO**$^*$ **Na**$^*$ **K**$^*$ **Vit C**$^*$ **Folic**$^*$

890 **Water**$^*$ **Protein**$^*$ **CHO**$^+$ **Inorganics**$^*$ **Vit C**$^*$ **Folic**$^*$

**Alcholic beverages**

891 **Thi**$^*$ **Rib**$^*$ **Nic**$^*$ **Vit** $\mathbf{B_6}^*$ **Vit** $\mathbf{B_{12}}^*$ **Folic**$^*$

892 **Inorganics**$^*$

893 **Thi**$^*$ **Rib**$^*$ **Nic**$^*$ **Vit** $\mathbf{B_6}^*$ **Vit** $\mathbf{B_{12}}^*$ **Folic**$^*$

895 **Alcohol**$^*$ **Solids**$^*$ **Nitrogen**$^*$ **Inorganics**$^*$ **Thi**$^*$ **Rib**$^*$ **Nic**$^*$ **Vit** $\mathbf{B_6}^*$ **Vit** $\mathbf{B_{12}}^*$ **Folic**$^*$

| | Food no | |
|---|---|---|
| Alcoholic beverages *continued* | 896 | **Alcohol* Solids* Nitrogen* CHO + Inorganics* Thi* Rib* Nic* Vit $B_6$* Vit $B_{12}$* Folic*** |
| | 897–900 | **Thi* Rib* Nic* Vit $B_6$* Vit $B_{12}$* Folic*** |
| | 901–902 | Thi, Rib, Nic, Pant 109 |
| | 904 | **Thi* Rib* Nic* Vit $B_6$* Vit $B_{12}$* Folic*** |
| | 905–906 | **Prox* Inorganics* Thi* Rib* Nic* Vit $B_6$* Vit $B_{12}$* Folic*** |
| | 907–910 | **Thi* Rib* Nic* Vit $B_6$* Vit $B_{12}$* Folic*** |
| | 911 | **K + Thi* Rib* Nic* Vit $B_6$* Vit $B_{12}$* Folic*** |
| | 912 | **Prox* Inorganics* Thi* Rib* Nic* Vit $B_6$* Vit $B_{12}$* Folic*** |
| | 913 | **K + Thi* Rib* Nic* Vit $B_6$* Vit $B_{12}$* Folic*** |
| | 914–915 | **Prox* Inorganics* Thi* Rib* Nic* Vit $B_6$* Vit $B_{12}$* Folic*** |
| | 916–918 | **Prox*** |
| Sauces and pickles | 928 | **Prox* Inorganics* Thi* Rib* Nic*** |
| | 929 | **Prox* Inorganics* Thi* Rib* Nic*** |
| | 930 | Prox *manufacturers' data* |
| | 932 | **Water + Na +** |
| Soups | 938 | **Prox* Inorganics* Thi* Rib* Nic* Vit $B_6$*** |
| | 939 | **Prox* Cl* Rib* Nic*** |
| | 940 | *Calculated from soup as purchased* |
| | 941 | **Prox* Inorganics* Thi* Rib* Nic*** |
| | 944 | **Prox* DF + Inorganics* Thi* Rib* Nic*** |
| | 946 | **Prox* Inorganics* Thi* Rib* Nic* Vit $B_6$*** |
| | 947 | **Prox* Inorganics* Thi* Rib* Nic* Vit $B_6$*** |
| | 948 | **Prox* DF + Inorganics* Thi* Rib* Nic* Vit $B_6$*** |
| | 950 | **Prox* Inorganics* Carotene* Thi* Rib* Nic* Vit $B_6$* Folic*** |
| | 951 | **Prox* Cl* Rib* Nic*** |
| | 952 | *Calculated from soup as purchased* |
| | 953 | **Prox* DF + Inorganics* Thi* Rib* Nic* Folic*** |
| | 955 | **Prox* Inorganics* Carotene* Thi* Rib* Nic* Vit $B_6$* Folic*** |
| Miscellaneous | 957 | **Prox* Inorganics* Thi* Rib* Nic* Vit $B_6$* Vit $B_{12}$* Folic*** |
| | 959 | Water 307 **Nitrogen +** |
| | 961 | **Prox* Inorganics* Thi* Rib* Nic* Vit $B_6$* Vit $B_{12}$* Folic*** |
| | 968 | Water, Fat 243 **CHO + DF +** Na, K 307 Ca 243 Mg, P 307 Fe 243 Thi, Rib, Nic 307 Vit $B_6$ and Pant 229 |
| | 969 | Water, Fat 243 **Nitrogen +** and 295 Na, K 307 Ca 243 Mg and P 307 Fe 243 Cu 184, 238 Zn 76 184, 270 Thi 307 Rib and Nic 243 Vit E 77 Vit $B_6$ 229 Folic 49, 267, 286 Pant 229 Biotin 116 |

# Section 2: Amino acids

As the new analytical values are marked with an asterisk in section 2, this key refers only to the literature sources.

| | | Food no | |
|---|---|---|---|
| **Cereals** | 2002 | 91 | |
| | 2005 | 91 | |
| | 2006 | 91, 257 | |
| | 2009 | 91, 173 | |
| | 2010 | 91 | |
| | 2011 | 91, 163 | |
| | 2017 | 91, 262 | |
| | 2019 | 91 | |
| | 2021 | 91, 230 | |
| | 2024 | 91 | |
| **Milk** | 2123 | 91, 174, 311 | |
| | 2166–2167 | *Calculated from whole egg, using data of Lunven* 195 | |
| **Meat** | | All values new analytical data | |
| **Fish** | 2435 | 16, 19, 37, 63, 83, 91 | |
| | 2516 | 91 | |
| | 2530 | 91 | |
| **Vegetables** | 2558 | 78 | |
| | 2561 | 91 | |
| | 2564 | 91 | |
| | 2565 | 91 | |
| | 2567 | 91 | |
| | 2572 | 91 | |
| | 2574 | 91 | |
| | 2576 | 91 | |
| | 2578 | 91 | |
| | 2585 | 91 | |
| | 2587 | 91 | |
| | 2591 | 91 | |
| | 2594 | 91 | |
| | 2597 | 91 | |
| | 2603 | 91 | |
| | 2606 | 91 | |
| | 2609 | 78, 91, 205 | |
| | 2613 | 91 | |
| | 2620 | 91 | |
| | 2630 | 91 | |
| | 2633 | 91 | |
| | 2639 | 91, 149 | |
| | 2657 | 91 | |
| | 2664 | 91 | |
| | 2666 | 78, 91 | |
| | 2669 | 91 | |
| | 2671 | 91 | |
| | 2673 | 91, 95 | |

| | Food no | |
|---|---|---|
| **Fruit** | 2675 | 91 |
| | 2682 | 91, 124 |
| | 2692 | 91 |
| | 2693 | 91 |
| | 2724 | 10, 11, 91 |
| | 2726 | 91 |
| | 2736 | 91 |
| | 2762 | 230 |
| | 2766 | 204 |
| | 2773 | 91 |
| | 2779 | 91 |
| | 2785 | 204 |
| | 2791 | 204, 230 |
| | 2817 | 91 |
| **Nuts** | 2822 | 91 |
| | 2826 | 91 |
| | 2830 | 91 |
| | 2832 | 91 |
| | 2835 | 91 |
| | 2839 | 91, 230 |
| **Miscellaneous** | 2959 | 82 |

# Section 3: Fatty acids

As the new analytical values are marked with an asterisk in section 3, this key refers only to the literature sources.

| | *Food no* | |
|---|---|---|
| **Cereals** | 3002 | 21, 189, 252 |
| | 3005 | *as whole wheat* |
| | 3008 | 46, 89, 128, 141, 221, 275 |
| | 3017 | 21, 128, 189 |
| | 3019 | 128 |
| | 3021 | 21, 189, 275 |
| **Milk and eggs** | 3123 | 104, 110, 115, 138, 139, 213, 235, 236, 258, 261, 285 |
| | 3137 | 104, 129, 233 |
| | 3138 | *For range* 142, 165, 256, 283, 312 |
| | 3165 | 234, 250, 293 |
| **Fats and oils** | 3183 | *Data from manufacturer* 301 |
| | 3184 | *Taken as beef fat* |
| | 3185 | *Taken as pork fat* |
| | 3186 | *Data from manufacturer* 301 |
| | 3188–3192 | *Data from manufacturer* 301 |
| | 3196–3198 | 39, 62, 211 |
| | 3199 | 39, 130 |
| | 3200 | 39, 61, 62, 211 |
| | 3201 | 41, 62, 98, 313 |
| | 3202–3203 | 39, 62, 211, 212 |
| | 3204–3206 | 39, 62 |
| **Meat** | 3240 | 14, 15, 60, 103, 123, 132, 133, 135, 232, 251, 288 |
| | 3269 | 67, 102, 103, 135, 232 |
| | 3299 | 13, 59, 60, 103, 132, 194, 232 |
| | 3332 | 135 |
| | 3334 | 135 |
| | 3336 | 135 |
| | 3340 | 58, 90, 135, 222 |
| **Fish** | 3438 | 1, 8, 146 |
| | 3451 | 23, 28 |
| | 3458 | 28, 226 |
| | 3461 | 171 |
| | 3466 | 171 |
| | 3471 | 171 |
| | 3474 | 171 |
| | 3482 | 4, 6, 80, 112, 180 |
| | 3491 | 5, 117 |
| | 3503 | 118 |
| | 3510 | 171 |
| | 3513 | 171 |
| | 3517 | 170 |
| | 3526 | 169 |

| | Food no | |
|---|---|---|
| **Fish** | 3532 | 101 |
| ***continued*** | 3535 | 22, 28, 113 |
| | 3537 | 101 |
| | 3550 | 2, 146 |
| **Vegetables** | 3562 | 275 |
| | 3569 | 275 |
| | 3597 | 160 |
| | 3609 | 275 |
| | 3620 | 275 |
| | 3634 | 160, 296 |
| | 3639 | 100 |
| | 3657 | 275 |
| | 3664 | 27, 303 |
| | 3669 | 185 |
| **Fruit** | 2675 | 99 |
| | 3692 | 277 |
| | 3693 | 105 |
| **Nuts** | 3822 | 98 |
| | 3826 | 98 |
| | 3828 | 98 |
| | 3830 | 98, 130, 147, 200 |
| | 3832 | 39, 62, 211 |
| | 3835 | 41, 62, 98, 313 |
| | 3839 | 98, 130, 200 |

# Section 4: Cholesterol

As the new analytical values are marked in table 4.1, this key refers only to the literature sources and values calculated from recipes.

| | *Food no* | |
|---|---|---|
| **Cereal products** | | All the items given (except for ice cream which was analysed) show the contributions from eggs and milk products which were calculated from the recipes. |
| **Milk and milk products** | 4123 | 74, 88, 175 |
| | 4126 | *Calculated from fat content* |
| | 4129 | *As fresh whole milk* |
| | 4130 | *As fresh whole milk* |
| | 4131 | 175 |
| | 4132 | *Calculated from fat content* |
| | 4133 | *Calculated from fat content* |
| | 4134 | *Calculated from fat content* |
| | 4135 | 175 |
| | 4140 | 74, 175 |
| | 4141 | *Calculated from fat content* |
| | 4144 | *Calculated from fat content* |
| | 4147 | *Calculated from fat content* |
| | 4150–4151 | *Calculated from fat content* |
| | 4153–4156 | *Calculated from fat content* |
| | 4159–4160 | *Calculated from fat content* |
| **Eggs** | 4165 | The value given is that of Tolan et al 1974 (293). This is a little lower than some other quoted values e.g., 81, 88, 153, 297, 309 |
| | 4167 | *Calculated from whole egg* |
| | 4168 | *Calculated from whole egg* |
| | 4169 | *As raw egg* |
| | 4171 | *As raw egg* |
| **Egg and cheese dishes** | 4172–4181 | *Calculated from recipes* |
| **Meat and meat products** | | Virtually all the values are new analytical data and the cooked dishes are calculated from the recipes. |
| **Fish and fish products** | 4438 | 88, 153 |
| | 4440 | *Calculated from raw cod* |
| | 4443 | *Calculated from raw cod* |
| | 4444 | *Calculated from raw cod* |
| | 4446 | *Calculated from raw cod* |
| | 4451 | 88, 153 |
| | 4454 | *Calculated from raw haddock* |
| | 4458 | 88, 274 |
| | 4459 | *Calculated from raw halibut* |
| | 4461 | *As other white fish* |
| | 4464 | *Calculated from raw lemon sole* |

| | Food no | |
|---|---|---|
| **Fish and fish products** ***continued*** | 4466 | 153 |
| | 4469 | *Calculated from raw plaice* |
| | 4471 | *As other white fish* |
| | 4472 | *Calculated from raw saithe* |
| | 4477 | *Calculated from raw whiting* 274 |
| | 4482 | 88, 153 |
| | 4485 | *Calculated from raw herring* |
| | 4487 | *As herring* |
| | 4489 | *As herring* |
| | 4491 | 88, 274 |
| | 4498 | 153 |
| | 4500 | 88, 274 |
| | 4501 | *Calculated from fish only* |
| | 4517 | 88, 168, 271, 274, 290 |
| | 4520 | *As fresh crab* |
| | 4521 | 88, 168, 271, 274 |
| | 4523 | 271 |
| | 4525 | 271 |
| | 4526 | 88, 153, 168, 271, 274, 290 |
| | 4531 | 271 |
| | 4532 | 153 |
| | 4535 | 88, 271, 290 |
| | 4537 | 88, 271, 290 |
| | 4539 | 140, 271 |
| | 4541 | 140, 271 |
| | 4552 | 153 |
| **Products containing eggs** | | *Calculated from the recipes* |

## References to Sections 1–4


1 Ackman, R. G., and Burgher, R. D. (1964) Cod flesh: component fatty acids as determined by gas–liquid chromatography. *J. Fish. Res. Bd Can.* **21**, 367–371

2 Ackman, R. G., and Burgher, R. D. (1964) Cod roe: component fatty acids as determined by gas–liquid chromatography. *J. Fish. Res. Bd Can.* **21**, 469–476

3 Ackman, R. G., and Cormier, M. G. (1967) α-tocopherol in some Atlantic fish and shellfish with particular reference to live-holding without food. *J. Fish. Res. Bd Can.* **24**, 357–373

4 Ackman, R. G., and Eaton, C. A. (1966) Some commercial Atlantic herring oils; fatty acid composition. *J. Fish. Res. Bd Can.* **23**, 991–1006

5 Ackman, R. G., and Eaton, C. A. (1971) Mackerel lipids and fatty acids. *Can. Inst. Food Technol. J.* **4**, 169–174

6 Ackman, R. G., Eaton, C. A., and Hingley, J. (1975) Fillet fat and fatty acid details for Newfoundland winter herring. *Can. Inst. Food Sci. Technol. J.* **8**, 155–159

7 Adams, J. F., McEwan, F., and Wilson, A. (1973) The vitamin $B_{12}$ content of meals and items of diet. *Brit. J. Nutr.* **29**, 65–72

8 Addison, R. F., Ackman, R. G., and Hingley, J. (1968) Distribution of fatty acids in cod flesh lipids. *J. Fish. Res. Bd Can.* **25**, 2083–2090

9 Alderman, G., and Stranks, M. H. (1967) The iodine content of bulk herd milk in summer in relation to estimated dietary iodine intake of cows. *J. Sci. Food Agric.* **18**, 151–153

10 Al-Aswad, M. B. (1971) The amino acids content of some Iraqi dates. *J. Food Sci.*, **36**, 1019–1020

11 Al-Rawi, N., Markakis, P., and Bauer, D. H. (1967) Amino acid composition of Iraqi dates. *J. Sci. Food Agric.* **18**, 1–2

12 Al-Samarrae, W., Ma, M. C. F., and Truswell, A. S. (1975) Mexthylxanthine consumption from coffee and tea. *Proc. Nutr. Soc.* **34**, 18A–19A

13 Anderson, B. A. (1976) Comprehensive evaluation of fatty acids in foods. VII. Pork products. *J. Amer. diet. Ass.* **69**, 44–49

14 Anderson, B. A., Kinsella, J. A., and Watt, B. K. (1975) Comprehensive evaluation of fatty acids in foods. II. Beef products. *J. Amer. diet. Ass.* **67**, 35–41

15 Anderson, D. B., Breidenstein, B. B., Kauffman, R. G., Cassens, R. G., and Bray, R. W. (1971) Effect of cooking on fatty acid composition of beef lipids. *J. Food Technol.* **6**, 141–152

16 Anon. (1958–1959) Amino acids in the edible parts of food fishes. *Ann. Rep. Fish. Res. Bd Can.* 132

17 Anon. (1968) Vitamin C in Tasmanian apples. *Food Technol. Aust.* **20**, 73

18 Archibald, J. G. (1958) Trace elements in milk: a review. Parts I and II. *Dairy Sci. Abstr.* **20**, 711–725 and 799–807

19 Arnesen, G. (1969) Total and free amino acids in fishmeals and vacuum-dried codfish organs, flesh, bones, skin and stomach contents. *J. Sci. Food Agric.* **20**, 218–220

20 Askew, H. O., and Kidson, E. B. (1947) Changes in vitamin C content and acidity of apples during cool storage. *N. Z. J. Sci. Technol.* [A] **28**, 344–351

21 Aylward, F., and Showler, A. J. (1962) Plant lipids. IV The glycerides and phosphatides in cereal grains. *J. Sci. Food Agric.* **13**, 492–499

22 Bannatyne, W. R., and Thomas, J. (1969) Fatty acid composition of New Zealand shellfish lipids. *N. Z. J. Sci.* **12**, 207–212

23 Beare, J. L. (1962) Fatty acid composition of food fats. *J. agric. Food Chem.* **10**, 120–123

24 Bicknell, F., and Prescott, F. (1942) *The vitamins in medicine*. Heinemann, London

25 Bieri, J. G., and Evarts, R. P. (1975) Vitamin E adequacy of vegetable oils. *J. Amer. diet. Ass.* **66**, 134–139

26 Birdsall, J. J., Derse, P. H., and Teply, L. J. (1961) Nutrients in California lemons and oranges. II Vitamin, mineral, and proximate composition. *J. Amer. diet. Ass.* **38**, 555–559

27 Boggess, T. S., Marion, J. E., Woodroof, J. G., and Dempsey, A. H. (1967) Changes in lipid composition of sweet potatoes as affected by controlled storage. *J. Food Sci.* **32**, 554–558

28 Bonnet, J. C., Sidwell, V. D., and Zook, E. G. (1974) Chemical and nutritive values of several fresh and canned finfish, crustaceans and mollusks. 2. Fatty acid composition. *Marine Fish Rev.* **36**, (2), 8–14

29 Booth, R. G., Carter, R. H., Jones, C. R., and Moran, T. (1946) The chemical composition of wheat and wheat products. In *The nation's food*, edited by A. L. Bacharach and T. Rendle. Society of Chemical Industry, London, pp. 162–182

30 Booth, V. H. (1963) Determination of tocopherols in plant tissues. *Analyst* **88**, 627–632

31 Booth, V. H., and Bradford, M. P. (1963a) Tocopherol contents of vegetables and fruits. *Brit. J. Nutr.* **17**, 575–581

32 Booth, V. H., and Bradford, M. P. (1963) The effect of cooking on $\alpha$-tocopherol in vegetables. *Int. Z. Vitaminforsch.* **33**, 276–278

33 Bowen, H. J. M. (1959) The determination of chlorine, bromine and iodine in biological material by activation analysis. *Biochem. J.* **73**, 381–384

34 Braekkan, O. R. (1958) Vitaminer i norsk fisk. 3. Vitaminer i forskjellige organer fra de viktigste torskefisker (Gadidae) fanget langs Norsketysten. *Fiskdir. Skr. Ser. Teknol. Undersøkelser* **3** (6), 32 pp

35 Braekkan, O. R. (1958) Vitamins and the reproductive cycle of ovaries in cod (*Gadus morrhua*). *Fiskdir. Skr. Teknol. Undersøkelser* **3** (7), 19 pp

36 Braekkan, O. R., and Boge, G. (1962) Vitamin $B_6$ and the reproductive cycle of ovaries in cod (*Gadus morrhua*). *Nature, Lond.* **193**, 394–395

37 Braekkan, O. R., and Boge, G. (1962) A comparative study of amino acids in the muscle of different species of fish. *Fiskdir. Skr. Ser. Teknol. Undersøkelser* **4** (3), 19 pp

38 Braekkan, O. R., Lambertsen, G., and Myklestad, H. (1963) Alpha-tocopherol in some marine organisms and fish oils. *Fiskdir. Skr. Ser. Teknol. Undersøkelser* **4** (8), 11 pp

39 Brignoli, C. A., Kinsella, J. E., and Weihrauch, J. L. (1976) Comprehensive evaluation of fatty acids in foods. V. Unhydrogenated fats and oils. *J. Amer. diet. Ass.* **68**, 224–229

40 Broadhead, G. D., Pearson, I. B., and Wilson, G. M. (1965) Seasonal changes in iodine metabolism. 1. Iodine content of cows' milk. 2. Fluctuation in urinary iodine excretion. *Brit. med. J.* **i**, 343–348

41 Brown, D. F., Cater, C. M., Mattil, K. F., and Darroch, J. G. (1975) Effect of variety, growing location and their interaction on the fatty acid composition of peanuts. *J. Food Sci.* **40**, 1055–1060

42 Brown, F. (1953) Occurrence of vitamin E in cod and other fish-liver oils. *Nature, Lond.* **171**, 790–791

43 Bunnell, R. H., Keating, J. Quaresimo, A., and Parman, G. K. (1965) Alpha-tocopherol content of foods. *Amer. J. clin. Nutr.* **17**, 1–10

44 Bunyan, J., Edwin, E. E., Diplock, A. T., and Green, J. (1961) Ubiquinone and tocopherol in birds. *Nature, Lond.* **190**, 637

45 Burge, J., Mickelsen, O., Nicklow, C., and Marsh, G. L. (1975) Vitamin C in tomatoes: comparison of tomatoes developed for mechanical or hand harvesting. *Ecol. Food Nutr.* **4**, 27–31

46 Burkwall, M. P., and Glass, R. L. (1965) The fatty acids of wheat and its milled products. *Cereal Chem.* **42**, 236–246

47 Burton, H., Ford, J. E., Franklin, J. G., and Porter, J. W. G. (1967) Effects of repeated heat treatments on the levels of some vitamins of the B-complex in milk. *J. Dairy Res.* **34**, 193–197

48 Burton, H., Ford, J. E., Perkin, A. G., Porter, J. W. G., Scott, K. J., Thompson, S. Y., Toothill, J., and Edwards-Webb, J. D. (1970) Comparison of milks processed by the direct and indirect methods of ultra-high temperature sterilization. IV. The vitamin content of milks sterilized by different processes. *J. Dairy Res.* **37**, 529–533

49 Butterfield, S., and Calloway, D. H. (1972) Folacin in wheat and selected foods. *J. Amer. diet. Ass.* **60**, 310–314

50 Callieri, D. A. (1959) Studies on the vitamin $B_{12}$, cyanocobalamin-binding capacity, desoxyribosides, and methionine in some commercial milk products and cheese. *Acta chem. scand.* **13**, 737–749

51 Callow, E. H. (1948) Comparative studies of meat. 2. The changes in the carcass during growth and fattening, and their relation to the chemical composition of the fatty and muscular tissues. *J. agric. Sci., Camb.* **38**, 174–199

52 Causeret, J. (1959) Ebullition domestique et teneur en riboflavine du lait de vache. *Lait* **39**, 159–165

53 Chanarin, I. (1975) The folate content of foodstuffs and the availability of different folate analogues for absorption. *Getting the most out of food* No. 10. Van den Berghs and Jurgens Ltd, London, pp. 41–64

54 Chappell, G. (1940) The distribution of vitamin C in foods sold on the open market. *J. Hyg., Camb.* **40**, 699–732

55 Chatfield, C. (1949) *Food composition tables for international use.* FAO Nutrition Studies No 3. Food and Agriculture Organization, Rome

56 Chilean Iodine Educational Bureau. (1952) *Iodine content of foods:* annotated bibliography 1825–1951. Chilean Iodine Educational Bureau, London

57 Christie, A. A., Dean, A. C., and Millburn, B. A. (1973) The determination of vitamin E in food by colorimetry and gas–liquid chromatography. *Analyst* **98**, 161–167

58 Chung, R. A., Lien, Y. C., and Munday, R. A. (1967) Fatty acid composition of turkey meat as affected by dietary fat, cholesterol and diethylstilbestrol. *J. Food Sci.* **32**, 169–172

59 Chung, R. A., and Lin, C. C. (1965) The fatty acid content of pork cuts and variety meats as affected by different dietary lipids. *J. Food Sci.* **30**, 860–864

60 Chung, R. A., McKay, J. A., and Ramey, C. L. (1966) Fatty acid changes in beef, pork, and fish after deep-fat frying in different oils. *Food Technol.* **20**, 691–693

61 Clegg, A. J. (1973) Composition and related nutritional and organoleptic aspects of palm oil. *J. Amer. Oil Chem. Soc.* **50**, 321–323

62 Codex Alimentarius Commission (1976) *Report of the eighth session of the Codex Committee on Fats and Oils.* London, 24–28 November 1975. Alinorm 76/19. Food and Agriculture Organization and World Health Organization

63 Connell, J. J., and Howgate, P. F. (1959) The amino acid composition of some British food fishes. *J. Sci. Food Agric.* **10**, 241–244

64 Cook, B. B., and Sundaram, S. (1963) Nutrients in raw vs cooked globe artichokes. *J. Amer. diet. Ass.* **42**, 231–233

65 Coombs, T. L. (1972) The distribution of zinc in the oyster *Ostrea edulis* and its relation to enzymic activity and to other metals. *Marine Biol.* **12**, 170–178

66 Cowey, C. B., Daisley, K. W., and, Parry, G. (1962) Study of amino acids, free or as components of protein, and of some B-vitamins in the tissues of the Atlantic Salmon, *Salmo salar,* during spawning migration. *Comp. Biochem. Physiol.* **7**, 29–38

67 Cramer, D. A., Barton, R. A., Shorland, F. B., and Czochanska, Z. (1967) A comparison of the effects of white clover (*Trifolium repens*) and of perennial ryegrass (*Lolium perenne*) on fat composition and flavour of lamb. *J. agric. Sci., Camb.* **69**, 367–373

68 Cunningham, M. M. (1935) The vitamin D content of some New Zealand fish oils. With a note on the prophylactic method of biological assay. *N. Z. J. Sci. Technol.* **17**, 563–567

69 Cuthbertson, A. (1974a) Personal communication

70 Cuthbertson, A. (1974b) Personal communication

71 Cuthbertson, A. (1975) Personal communication

72 Dako, D. Y., Watson, J. D., and Amoakwa-Adu, M. (1974) Available carbohydrates in Ghanaian foodstuffs. 1. Distribution of sugars in fruits. *Plant Foods for Man* **1**, 121–125

73 Dawes, S. N. (1970) Sodium and potassium in cow's milk. II. Bulk milk, *N. Z. J. Sci.* **13**, 69–77

74 de Man, J. M. (1964) The free and ester cholesterol content of milk and dairy products. *Z. Ernährwiss.* **5**, 1–4

75 Dean, A. C. (1971) Separation of dimeric tocopherol products from vitamin E in food by dry-column chromatography. *Chemy Ind.* (24), 677–678

76 Dewar, W. A. (1967) The zinc and manganese contents of some British poultry foods. *J. Sci. Food Agric.* **18**, 68–71

77 Diplock, A. T., Green, J., Edwin, E. E., and Bunyan, J. (1961) Tocopherol, ubiquinones and ubichromenols in yeasts and mushrooms. *Nature, Lond.* **189**, 749–750

78 Doesburg, J. J., and Meijer, A. (1964) Analyse van Nederlandse Blikconserven. II. Groete- en vruchtenprodukten. *Voeding* **25**, 258–301

79 Dong, F. M., and Oace, S. M. (1975) Folate concentration and pattern in bovine milk. *J. agric. Food Chem.* **23**, 534–538

80 Drozdowski, B., and Ackman, R. G. (1969) Isopropyl alcohol extraction of oil and lipids in the production of fish protein concentrate from herring. *J. Amer. Oil Chem. Soc.* **46**, 371–376

81 Dua, P. N., Dilworth, B. C., Day, E. J., and Hill, J. E. (1967) Effect of dietary vitamin A and cholesterol on cholesterol and carotenoid content of plasma and egg yolk. *Poult. Sci.* **46** 530–531

82 Eastoe, J. E. (1955) The amino acid composition of mammalian collagen and gelatin. *Biochem. J.* **61**, 589–600

83 Ellinger, G. M., and Boyne, E. (1965) Amino acid composition of some fish products and casein. *Brit. J. Nutr.* **19**, 587–592

84 Eric, B., le Compte, J., and Reeve, R. F. (1970) Organoleptic assessment of irradiated Granny Smith apples from Western Australia. *Food Technol. Aust.* **22**, 298–300

85 Exler, J., Kinsella, J. E., and Watt, B. K. (1975) Lipids and fatty acids of important finfish: new data for nutrient tables. *J. Amer. Oil Chem. Soc.* **52**, 154–159

86 Faust, M., Shear, C. B., and Brooks, H. J. (1969) Mineral element gradients in pears. *J. Sci. Food Agric.* **20**, 257–258

87 Feeley, R. M., Criner, P. E., Murphy, E. W., and Toepfer, E. W. (1972) Major mineral elements in dairy products. *J. Amer. diet. Ass.* **61**, 505–510

88 Feeley, R. M., Criner, P. E., and Watt, B. K. (1972) Cholesterol content of foods. *J. Amer. diet. Ass.* **61**, 134–149

89 Fisher, N., Broughton, M. E., Peel, D. J., and Bennett, R. (1964) The lipids of wheat. II. Lipids of flours from single varieties of widely varying baking quality. *J. Sci. Food Agric.* **15**, 325–341

90 Fishwick, M. J. (1968) Changes in the lipids of turkey muscle during storage at chilling and freezing temperatures. *J. Sci. Food Agric.* **19**, 440–445

91 Food and Agriculture Organization (1970) *Amino-acid content of foods and biological data on proteins*. FAO Nutrition Studies No 24, Food and Agriculture Organization, Rome

92 Ford, J. E., Porter, J. W. G., Scott, K. J., Thompson, S. Y., le Marquand, J., and Truswell, A. S. (1974) Comparison of dried milk preparations for babies on sale in 7 European countries. II. Folic acid, vitamin $B_6$, thiamin, riboflavin and vitamin E. *Archs Dis. Childh.* **49**, 874–877

93 Ford, J. E., Porter, J. W. G., Thompson, S. Y., Toothill, J., and Edwards-Webb, J. (1969) Effects of ultra-high-temperature (UHT) processing and of subsequent storage on the vitamin content of milk. *J. Dairy Res.* **36**, 447–454

94 Ford, J. E., and Scott, K. J. (1968) The folic acid activity of some milk foods for babies. *J. Dairy Res.* **35**, 85–90

95 Francis, B. J., Halliday, D., and Robinson, J. M. (1975) Yams as a source of edible protein. *Trop. Sci.* **17**, 103–110

96 Fraser, D. R. (1976) Personal communication

97 Fraser, J. R. (1958) Flour survey 1950–1956. *J. Sci. Food Agric.* **9**, 125–136

98 Fristrom, G. A., Stewart, B. C., Weihrauch, J. L., and Posati, L. (1975) Comprehensive evaluation of fatty acids in foods. IV. Nuts, peanuts and soups. *J. Amer. diet. Ass.* **67**, 351–355

99 Galliard, T. (1968) Aspects of the lipid metabolism in higher plants. II. The identification and quantitative analysis of lipids from the pulp of pre- and post-climacteric apples. *Phytochemistry* **7**, 1915–1922

100 Galliard, T. (1973) Lipids of potato tubers. I. Lipid and fatty acid composition of tubers from different varieties of potato. *J. Sci. Food Agric.* **24**, 617–622

101 Gardner, D., and Riley, J. P. (1972) The component fatty acids of the lipids of some species of marine and freshwater molluscs. *J. mar. biol. Ass., UK* **52**, 827–838

102 Garton, G. A., and Duncan, W. R. H. (1969) Composition of adipose tissue triglycerides of neonatal and year-old lambs. *J. Sci. Food Agric.* **20**, 39–42

103 Giam, I., and Dugan, L. R. (1965) The fatty acid composition in free and bound lipids in freeze-dried meats. *J. Food Sci.* **30**, 262–265

104 Glass, R. L., Troolin, H. A., and Jenness, R. (1967) Comparative biochemical studies of milks. 4. Constituent fatty acids of milk fats. *Comp. Biochem. Biophys.* **22**, 415–425

105 Goldstein, J. L., and Wick, E. L. (1969) Lipids in ripening banana fruit. *J. Food Sci.* **34**, 482–484

106 Gontzea, I., and Sutzescu, P. (1968) *Natural antinutritive substances in foodstuffs and forages*. S. Karger, Basel.

107 Gopalan, C., Ramastri, B. V., and Balasubramanian, S. C. (1971) *Nutritive value of Indian foods*. Nat. Inst. Nutr., Indian Counc. Med. Res., Hyderabad

108 Gormican, A. (1970) Inorganic elements in foods used in hospital menus. *J. Amer. diet. Ass.* **56**, 397–403

109 Goverd, K. A., and Carr, J. G. (1974) The content of some B-group vitamins in single-variety apple juices and commercial ciders. *J. Sci. Food Agric.* **25**, 1185–1190

110 Gray, I. K. (1973) Seasonal variations in the composition and thermal properties of New Zealand milk fat. I. Fatty-acid composition. *J. Dairy Res.* **40**, 207–214

111 Gregory, M. E., and Burton, H. (1965) The effect of ultra-high temperature heat treatment on the content of thiamine, vitamin $B_6$ and vitamin $B_{12}$ of milk. *J. Dairy Res.* **32**, 13–17

112 Gruger, E. H. (1967) Fatty acid composition. In *Fish oils: their chemistry, technology, stability, nutritional properties and uses*, edited by M. E. Stansby. Avi Publications, Westport, pp 3–30.

113 Gruger, E. H., Nelson, R. W., and Stansby, M. E. (1964) Fatty acid composition of oils from 21 species of marine fish, freshwater fish and shellfish. *J. Amer. Oil Chem. Soc.* **41**, 662–667

114 Guild, L., and Raines, R. (1972) Thiamin content and retention in venison. *J. Amer. diet. Ass.* **60**, 42–44

115 Hall, A. J. (1970) Seasonal and regional variations in the fatty acid composition of milk. *Diary Inds.* **35**, 20–24

116 Hardinge, M. G., and Crooks, H. (1961) Lesser known vitamins in foods. *J. Amer. diet. Ass.* **38**, 240–245

117 Hardy, R., and Keay, J. N. (1972) Seasonal variations in the chemical composition of Cornish mackerel *Scomber scombrus* L with detailed reference to the lipids. *J. Food Technol.* **7**, 125–137

118 Hardy, R., and Mackie, P. (1969) Seasonal variation in some of the lipid components of sprats (*Sprattus sprattus*). *J. Sci. Food Agric.* **20**, 193–198

119 Harkett, P. J. (1973) Personal communication

120 Harrison, M. T., McFarlane, S., Harden, R. McG., and Wayne, E. (1965) Nature and availability of iodine in fish. *Amer. J. clin. Nutr.* **17**, 73–77

121 Hartman, A. M., and Dryden, L. P. (1965) *Vitamins in milk and milk products.* American Dairy Science Association, Champaign, Illinois

122 Hartmann, B. G., and Hillig, F. (1934) Acid constituents of food products, with special reference to citric, malic and tartaric acids. *J. Ass. off. agric. Chem.* **27**, 522–531

123 Hecker, A. L., Cramer, D. A., and Hougham, D. F. (1975) Compositional and metabolic growth effects in the bovine. Muscle, subcutaneous and serum total fatty acids. *J. Food Sci.*, **40**, 144–149

124 Hegazi, S. M., and Salem, S. A. (1972) Amino acid pattern of the Egyptian apricot fruits (Hamawy). *J. Sci. Food Agric.* **23**, 497–499

125 Henry, K. M., Hosking, Z. D., Thompson, S. Y., Toothill, J., Edwards-Webb, J., and Smith, L. P. (1971) Factors affecting the concentration of vitamins in milk. III. Effect of season and solar radiation on the vitamin D potency of butter. *J. Dairy Res.* **38**, 209–216

126 Herbert, V. (1963) A palatable diet for producing experimental folate deficiency in man. *Amer. J. clin. Nutr.* **12**, 17–20

127 Herting, D. C., and Drury, E-J. E. (1963) Vitamin E content of vegetable oils and fats. *J. Nutr.* **81**, 335–342

128 Herting, D. C., and Drury, E-J. E. (1969) Alpha-tocopherol content of cereal grains and processed cereals. *J. agric. Food Chem.* **17**, 785–790

129 Hilditch, T. P., and Jasperson, H. (1944) The component acids of milk fats of the goat, ewe and mare. *Biochem. J.* **38**, 443–447

130 Hilditch, T. P., and Williams, P. N. (1964) *The chemical constitution of natural fats.* 4th edition. Chapman and Hall, London

131 Hoppner, K., Lampi, B., and Perrin, D. E. (1972) The free and total folate activity in foods available on the Canadian market. *Can. Inst. Food Sci. Technol. J.* **5**, 60–66

132 Hornstein, I., Crowe, P. F., and Heimberg, M. J. (1961). Fatty acid composition of meat tissue lipids. *J. Food Sci.* **26**, 581–586

133 Hornstein, I., Crowe, P. F., and Hiner, R. (1967) Composition of lipids in some beef muscles. *J. Food Sci.* **32**, 650–655

134 Howard, F. D., MacGillivray, J. H., and Yamaguchi, M. (1962) Nutrient composition of fresh California-grown vegetables. *Calif. agric. exp. Sta. Bull.* No. 788

135 Hubbard, A. W., and Pocklington, W. D. (1968) Distribution of fatty acids in lipids as an aid to the identification of animal tissues. 1. Bovine, porcine, ovine, and some avian species. *J. Sci. Food Agric.* **19**, 571–577

136 Hulme, A. C. (editor) (1971) *The biochemistry of fruits and their products*, vol. 2. Academic press, London and New York

137 Hurdle, A. D. F., Barton, D., and Searles, I. H. (1968) A method for measuring folate in food and its application to a hospital diet. *Amer. J. clin. Nutr.* **21**, 1202–1207

138 Hutton, K., Seeley, R. C., and Armstrong, D. G. (1969) The variation throughout a year in the fatty acid composition of milk fat from two dairy herds. *J. Dairy Res.* **36**, 103–113

139 Huyghebaert, A., and Hendrickx, H. (1970) The relation between the fatty acid composition and iodine value and refractive index of butterfat. *Milchwissenschaft* **25**, 506–510

140 Idler, D. R., and Wiseman, P. (1971) Sterols of molluscs. *Int. J. Biochem.* **2**, 516–528

141 Inkpen, J. A., and Quackenbush, F. W. (1969) Extractable and 'bound' fatty acids in wheat and wheat products. *Cereal Chem.* **46**, 580–587

142 Insull, W., and Ahrens, E. H. (1959) The fatty acids of human milk from mothers on diets taken *ad libitum*. *Biochem. J.* **72**, 27–33

143 Iverson, J. L., Firestone, D., and Horwitz, W. (1963) Fatty acid composition of oil from roasted and unroasted peanuts by gas–liquid chromatography. *J. Ass. off. agric. Chem.* **46**, 718–725

144 Jacobs, A., and Greenman, D. A. (1969) Availability of food iron. *Brit. med. J.* **i**, 673–676

145 Jamieson, M. M., Oxenham, J., and Robertson, J. (1961) Fat absorption by white bread during frying. *Proc. Nutr. Soc.* **20**, xxii–xxiii

146 Jangaard, P. M., Ackman, R. G., and Sipos, J. C. (1967) Seasonal changes in fatty acid composition of cod liver, flesh, roe and milt lipids. *J. Fish. Res. Bd Can.* **24**, 613–627

147 Jart, A. (1963) The fatty acid composition of filbert oil. *Acta chem. scand.* **11**, 1186–1187

148 Johansen, O., and Steinnes, E. (1976) Determination of iodine in plant material by a neutron activation method. *Analyst* **101**, 455–457

149 Kaldy, M. S., and Markakis, P. (1972) Amino acid composition in selected potato varieties. *J. Food Sci.* **37**, 375–377

150 Kaplan, E., Holmes, J. H., and Sapeika, N. (1974) Caffeine content of tea and coffee. *S. Afr. med. J.* **48**, 510–511

151 Karlin, R. (1961) Sur le taux de vitamine $B_6$ dans les fromages: variations au cours de la maturation. *Int. Z. Vitaminforsch.* **31**, 176–184

152 Karlin, R. (1969) Sur la teneur en folates des laits de grand mélange. Effets de divers traitements thermiques sur les taux de folates, $B_{12}$ et $B_6$ de ces laits. *Int. Z. Vitaminforsch.* **39**, 359–371

153 Keller, G. H. M., and van de Bovenkamp, P. (1974) Cholesterolgehalte van voedingsmiddelen. *Voeding* **35**, 409–411

154 Kellog, W. L., Denton, C. A., and Bird, H. R. (1947) Nicotinic acid content of squab and pigeon tissues. *Poult. Sci.* **26**, 435–436

155 Kent-Jones, D. W. (1958) The case for fortified flour. *Proc. Nutr. Soc.* **17**, 38–43

156 Kenworthy, A. L., and Harris, N. (1963) Composition of McIntosh, Red Delicious and Golden Delicious apples as related to environment and season. *Quart. Bull. Mich. agric. exp. Sta.* **46**, 293–334

157 Ketiku, A. O. (1973) Chemical composition of unripe (green) and ripe plantain (*Musa paradisiaca*). *J. Sci. Food Agric.* **24**, 703–707

158 Keys, O. H. (1943) Vitamin C in applies and other materials. *N. Z. J. Sci. Technol.* [B] **24**, 146–148

159 Kieser, M. E., and Pollard, A. (1947) Vitamin C in English apples. *Nature, Lond.* **159**, 65

160 Kinsella, J. E. (1971) Composition of the lipids of cucumber and peppers. *J. Food Sci.* **36**, 865–866

161 Kirkpatrick, D. C., and Coffin, D. E. (1975) Trace metal content of chicken eggs. *J. Sci. Food Agric.* **26**, 99–103

162 Kizlaitis, L., Steinfeld, M. I., and Siedler, A. J. (1962) Nutrient content of variety meats. 1. Vitamin A, vitamin C, iron and proximate composition. *J. Food Sci.* **27**, 459–462

163 Knight, R. A., Christie, A. A., Orton, C. R., and Robertson, J. (1973) Studies on the composition of food. 4. Comparison of nutrient content of retail white bread made conventionally and by the Chorleywood Bread Process. *Brit. J. Nutr.* **30**, 181–188

164 Kon, S. K. (1972) *Milk and milk products in human nutrition.* FAO Nutrition Studies, No 27, 2nd edition. Food and Agriculture Organization, Rome

165 Krámer, M., Szöke, K., Lindner, K., and Tarján, R. (1965) The effect of different factors on the composition of human milk. 3. Effect of dietary fats on lipid composition of human milk. *Nutritio Dieta* **7**, 71–79

166 Kringstad, H., and Folkvord, S. (1949) The nutritive value of cod roe and cod liver. *J. Nutr.* **38**, 489–502

167 Kritchevsky, D. (1963) Sterols. In *Comprehensive biochemistry*, edited by M. Florkin and E. H. Stotz, vol. 10. Elsevier, Amsterdam, London and New York. pp 1–22

168 Kritchevsky, D., Tepper, S. A., Ditullo, N. W., and Holmes, W. L. (1967) The sterols of seafood. *J. Food Sci.* **32**, 64–66

169 Krzeczkowski, R. A. (1970) Fatty acids in raw and processed Alaska pink shrimp. *J. Amer. Oil Chem. Soc.* **47**, 451–452

170 Krzeczkowski, R. A., Tenney, R. D., and Kelley, C. (1971) Alaska king crab: fatty acid composition, carotenoid index and proximate analysis. *J. Food Sci.* **36**, 604–606

171 Laboratory of the Government Chemist (1964) Unpublished data

172 Laboratory of the Government Chemist (1967) Composition of bread rolls. In *Report of the Government Chemist 1966*. Ministry of Technology, HMSO, London. pp 43–44

173 Laboratory of the Government Chemist (1969) Unpublished data

174 Laboratory of the Government Chemist (1975) Unpublished data

175 Lacroix, D. E., Mattingly, W. A., Wong, N. P., and Alford, J. A. (1973) Cholesterol, fat and protein in dairy products. *J. Amer. diet. Ass.* **62**, 275–279

176 Lakshmiah, N., and Ramasastri, B. V. (1969) Folic acid content of some Indian foods of plant origin. *J. Nutr. Diet., India* **6**, 200–203

177 Lal, B. M., Prakash, V., and Verma, S. C. (1963) The distribution of nutrients in the seed parts of Bengal gram. *Experienta* **19**, 154–155

178 Lal, B. M., Rohewal, S. S., Verma, S. C., and Prakash, V. (1963) Chemical composition of some pure strains of Bengal gram (*Cicer arietinum* L.). *Ann. Biochem. exp. Med.* **23**, 543–548

179 Lambertsen, G., and Braekkan, O. R. (1959) The spectrophotometric determination of α-tocopherol. *Analyst* **84**, 706–711

180 Lambertsen, G., and Braekkan, O. R. (1965) The fatty acid composition of herring oils. *Fiskdir. Skr. Ser. Teknol. Undersøkelser* **4** (13), 14 pp

181 Lambertsen, G., Myklestad, H., and Braekkan, O. R. (1962) Tocopherols in nuts. *J. Sci. Food Agric.* **13**, 617–620

182 Lambertsen, G., Myklestad, H., and Braekkan, O. R. (1964) The determination of α- and γ-tocopherols in margarine. *J. Food Sci.* **29**, 164–167

183 Lange, W. (1950) Cholesterol, phytosterol and tocopherol content of food products and animal tissues. *J. Amer. Oil Chem. Soc.* **27**, 414–422

184 Larkin, D., Page, M., Bartlet, J. C., and Chapman, R. A. (1954) The lead, zinc and copper content of foods. *Foods Res.* **19**, 211–218

185 Lepage, M. (1967) Identification and composition of turnip root lipids. *Lipids* **2**, 244–250

186 Lichtenstein, H., Beloian, A., and Murphy, E. W. (1961) Vitamin $B_{12}$-microbiological assay methods and distribution in selected foods. *U.S. Dept. Agric. Home Econ. Res. Rep.* No 13. Washington DC

187 Lichtenstein, H., Beloian, A., and Reynolds, H. (1959) Comparative vitamin $B_{12}$ assay of foods of animal origin by *Lactobacillus leichmanii* and *Ochromonas malhamensis*. *J. agric. Food Chem.* **7**, 771–774

188 Lieck, H., and Søndergaard, H. (1958) The content of vitamin $B_6$ in Danish foods. *Int. Z. Vitaminforsch.* **29**, 68–77

189 Lindberg, P., Bingefors, S., Lannek, N., and Tanhuanpää, E. (1964) The fatty acid composition of Swedish varieties of wheat, barley, oats and rye. *Acta agric. scand.* **14**, 3–11

190 Loughlin, M. E., and Teeri, A. E. (1960) Nutritive value of fish. II. Biotin, folic acid, pantothenic acid and free amino acids of various salt-water species. *Food Res.* **25**, 479–483

191 Love, R. M. (1970) *The chemical biology of fishes.* Academic Press, London and New York

192 Love, R. M., Lovern, J. A., and Jones, N. R. (1959) *The chemical composition of fish tissues.* DSIR Food Investigation Special Report No 69. HMSO, London

193 Lowe, J. S., Morton, R. A., and Vernon, J. (1957) Unsaponifiable constituents of kidney in various species. *Biochem. J.* **67**, 228–234

194 Luddy, F. E., Herb, S. F., Magidman, P., Spinelli, A. M., and Wasserman, A. E. (1970) Color and the lipid composition of pork muscles. *J. Amer. Oil Chem. Soc.* **47**, 65–68

195 Lunven, P., Le Clement de St Marcq, C., Carnovale, E., and Fratoni, A. (1973) Amino acid composition of hen's egg. *Brit. J. Nutr.* **30**, 189–194

196 Macy, I. G., Kelly, H. J., and Sloan, R. E. (1953) *The composition of milks.* National Academy of Science and National Research Council Publication No 254. Washington DC

197 Marion, W. W., Maxon, S. T., and Wangen, R. M. (1970) Lipid and fatty acid composition of turkey liver, skin and depot tissue. *J. Amer. Oil Chem. Soc.* **47**, 391–392

198 Mason, E. M., O'Donovan, E. M., and Kilbride, D. (1945) *An enquiry into the cause of goitre in County Tipperary.* An investigation of iodine content of foodstuff, soil and drinking water of that county compared with others of less goitrous counties in Ireland. Unpublished report to the Medical Research Council of Ireland, quoted by Chilean Iodine Educational Bureau 1952

199 Matoth, Y., Pinkas, A., and Sroka, Ch. (1965) Studies on folic acid in infancy. III. Folates in breast fed infants and their mothers. *Amer. J. clin. Nutr.* **16**, 356–359

200 Mattson, F. H., and Volpenhein, R. A. (1963) The specific distribution of unsaturated fatty acids in the triglycerides of plants. *J. Lipid Res.* **4**, 392–396

201 McCance, R. A., Sheldon, W., and Widdowson, E. M. (1934) Bone and vegetable broth. *Archs Dis. Childh.* **9**, 251–258

202 McCance, R. A., and Widdowson, E. M. (1935) Phytin in human nutrition. *Biochim. J.* **29**, 2694–2699

203 McCance, R. A., and Widdowson, E. M. (1942) Mineral metabolism of healthy adults on white and brown bread dietaries. *J. Physiol.* **101**, 44–85

204 McCarthy, M. A., Orr, M. L., and Watt, B. K. (1968) Phenylalanine and tyrosine in vegetables and fruits. *J. Amer. diet. Ass.* **52**, 130–134

205 McKellar, R. L., and Kohrman, R. E. (1975) Amino acid composition of the Morel mushroom. *J. agric. Food Chem.* **23**, 464–467

206 Merrill, A. L., and Watt, B. K. (1955) *Energy value of foods—basis and derivation. US* Department of Agriculture. Agriculture Handbook No 74, Washington DC

207 Milk Marketing Board Joint Milk Quality Committee (1973) *Milk compositional and hygienic quality control.* England and Wales. A progress report. Milk Marketing Board, Thames Ditton

208 Millar, K. R., and Sheppard, A. D. (1972) $\alpha$-tocopherol and selenium levels in human and cows' milk. *N. Z. J. Sci.* **15**, 3–15

209 Millin, D. J., and Rustidge, D. W. (1967) Tea manufacture. *Process Biochem.* **2**, 9–13

210 Ministry of Agriculture, Fisheries and Food, Working Party on the Monitoring of Foodstuffs for Heavy Metals. Unpublished papers

211 Ministry of Agriculture, Fisheries and Food (1974) Personal communication

212 Ministry of Agriculture, Fisheries and Food (1975) Personal communication

213 Moore, J. H., and Williams, D. L. (1965) A note on the effect of a commercial drying process on the long chain fatty acids of milk. *J. Dairy Res.* **32**, 19–20

214 Moore, T. (1957) *Vitamin A.* Elsevier, London

215 Moore, T., Sharman, I. M., and Ward, R. J. (1959) Cod-liver oil as both source and antagonist of vitamin E. *Brit. J. Nutr.* **13**, 100–110

216 Murphy, E. W., Willis, B. W., and Watt, B. K. (1975) Provisional tables on the zinc content of foods. *J. Amer. diet. Ass.* **66**, 345–355

217 Murray, J., and Burt, J. R. (1969) The composition of fish. *Torry Advisory Note* No 38. Torry Research Station, Aberdeen

218 Murthy, G. K., Rhea, U. S., and Peeler, J. T. (1972) Copper, iron, manganese, strontium and zinc content of market milk. *J. Dairy Sci.* **55**, 1666–1674

219 Naiman, J. L., and Oski, F. A. (1964) The folic acid content of milk. Revised figures based on an improved assay method. *Pediatrics* **34**, 274–276

220 Neilands, J. B., Strong, F. M., and Elvehjem, C. A. (1947) The nutritive value of canned foods 25. Vitamin content of canned fish products. *J. Nutr.* **34**, 633–643

221 Nelson, J. H., Glass, R. L., and Geddes, W. F. (1963) The triglycerides and fatty acids of wheat. *Cereal Chem.* **40**, 343–351

222 Neudoerffer, T. S., and Lea, C. H. (1967) Effects of dietary polyunsaturated fatty acids on the composition of the individual lipids of turkey breast and leg muscle. *Brit. J. Nutr.* **21**, 691–714

223 Nicol, D. J., and Davis, R. E. (1967) The folate and vitamin $B_{12}$ content of infant milk foods with particular reference to goats' milk. *Med. J. Aust.* **ii**, 212–214

224 Nobile, S., and Woodhill, J. M. (1973) A survey of the vitamin content of some 2,000 foods as they are consumed by selected groups of the Australian population. *Food Technol. Aust.* **25**, 80–100

225 Okungbowa, P., Ma, M. C. F., and Truswell, A. S. (1977) Niacin in instant coffee. *Proc. Nutr. Soc.* **36**, 26A

226 Olley, J., and Duncan, W. R. H. (1965) Lipids and protein denaturation in fish muscle. *J. Sci. Food Agric.* **16**, 99–104

227 Olliver, M. (1947) The cabbage as a source of ascorbic acid in the human diet. *Chemy Ind.* No 18, 235–240

228 Orr, J. B. (1931) *Report to the Nutrition Committee of the Medical Research Council on the correlation between iodine supply and the incidence of endemic goitre.* Medical Research Council Special Report Series No 154. HMSO, London

229 Orr, M. L. (1969) Pantothenic acid, vitamin $B_6$ and vitamin $B_{12}$ in foods. US Department of Agriculture Home Economics Research Report No 36. Washington DC

230 Orr, M. L., and Watt, B. K. (1957) *Amino acid content of foods.* US Department of Agriculture Home Economics Research Report No 4. Washington DC

231 Osis, D., Kramer, L., Waitrowski, E., and Spencer, H. (1972) Dietary zinc intake in man. *Amer. J. clin. Nutr.* **25**, 582–588

232 Ostrander, J., and Dugan, L. R. (1962) Some differences in composition of covering fat, intermuscular fat, and intramuscular fat of meat animals. *J. Amer. Oil Chem. Soc.* **39**, 178–181

233 Parkash, S., and Jenness, R. (1968) The composition and characteristics of goats' milk: a review. *Dairy Sci. Abstr.* **30**, 67–87

234 Parkinson, T. L. (1966) The chemical composition of eggs. *J. Sci. Food Agric.* **17**, 101–111

235 Parodi, P. W. (1970) Fatty acid composition of Australian butter and milk fat. *Aust. J. Dairy Technol.* **25**, 200–205

236 Parodi, P. W. (1972) Observations on the variation in fatty acid composition of milkfat. *Aust. J. Dairy Technol.* **27**, 90–94

237 Pearson, D. (1975) Seasonal English market variations in the composition of South African and Israeli avocados. *J. Sci. Food Agric.* **26**, 207–213

238 Pennington, J. T., and Calloway, D. H. (1973) Copper content of foods. *J. Amer. diet. Ass.* **63**, 143–153

239 Pennock, J. F., Neiss, G., and Mahler, H. R. (1962) Biochemical studies on the developing avian embryo. 5. Ubiquinone and some other unsaponifiable lipids. *Biochem. J.* **85**, 530–537

240 Perring, M. A. (1968) Recent work at the Ditton Laboratory on the chemical composition and storage characteristics of apples in relation to orchard factors. *Rep. E. Malling Res. Sta. for 1967*, 191–198

241 Peynaud, E., and Lafourcade, S. (1958) Evolution des vitamines B dans le raisin. *Qualitas Pl. Mater. Veg.* **3**, 404–414

242 Plack, P. A., Kon, S. K., and Thompson, S. Y. (1959) Vitamin $A_1$ aldehyde in the eggs of the herring (*Clupae harengus* L.) and other marine teleosts. *Biochem. J.* **71**, 467–476

243 Platt, B. S. (1962) *Tables of representative values of foods commonly used in tropical countries.* Medical Research Council Special Report Series No 302. HMSO, London

244 Polansky, M. M. (1969) Vitamin $B_6$ components in fresh and dried vegetables. *J. Amer. diet. Ass.* **54**, 118–121

245 Polansky, M. M., and Murphy, E. W. (1966) Vitamin $B_6$ components in fruit and nuts. *J. Amer. diet. Ass.* **48**, 109–111

246 Polansky, M. M., and Toepfer, E. W. (1969) Vitamin $B_6$ components in some meats, fish, dairy products and commercial infant formulas. *J. agric. Food Chem.* **17**, 1394–1397

247 Pollard, A. (1950) Vitamins in fruit juices and related products. In *Recent advances in fruit juice production* edited by V. L. S. Charley. Commonwealth Bureau of Horticulture and Plant Crops Technical Communication No 21. pp 125–144

248 Porter, J. W. G. (1975) *Milk and dairy foods.* The value of foods series, general editors P. Fisher and A. E. Bender. Oxford University Press

249 Porter, J. W. G. (1976) Personal communication

250 Posati, L. P., Kinsella, J. E., and Watt, B. K. (1975) Comprehensive evaluation of fatty acids in foods. III. Eggs and egg products. *J. Amer. diet. Ass.* **67**, 111–115

251 Pothoven, M. A., Beitz, D. C., and Zimmerli, A. (1974) Fatty acid compositions of bovine adipose tissue and of *in vitro* lipogenesis. *J. Nutr.* **104**, 430–433

252 Price, P. B., and Parsons, J. G. (1974) Lipids of six cultivated barley (*Hordeum vulgare* L) varieties. *Lipids* **9**, 560–566

253 Pyke, M. (1942) The vitamin content of vegetables. *J. Soc. chem. Ind., Lond.* **61**, 149–151

254 Randoin, L., Le Gallic, P., Dupuis, Y., and Bernardin, A. (1961) *Tables de composition des aliments.* Institut Scientifique d'Hygiène Alimentaire. J. Lanore, Paris

255 Räsänen, L., Ahlstrom, A., and Kytovuori, P. (1972) Nutritional value of game birds. *Soumen Kemistilehti B.* **45**, 314–316

256 Read, W. W. C., and Sarrif, A. (1965) Human milk lipids, 1. changes in fatty acid composition of early colostrum. *Amer. J. clin. Nutr.* **17**, 177–179

257 Reiners, R. A., Morgan, R. E., and Shroder, J. D. (1970) Note on the amino acid composition of the protein in commercial corn starch. *Cereal Chem.* **47**, 205–206

258 Renner, E., and Baier, D. (1971) Einfluss von Temperatur und Sauerstoff auf den Gehalt an Ascorbinsäure und ungesättigten Fettsäuren in Milch. *Dt. Molk.-Ztg* **92**, 75–78

259 Renner, E., and Baier, D. (1971) Einfluss des Lichtes auf den Gehalt der Milch an Ascorbinsäure und ungesättigten Fettsäuren. *Dt. Molk-Ztg* **92**, 541–543

260 Rice, E. E., Strandine, E. J., Squires, E. M., and Lyddon, B. (1946) The distribution and comparative content of certain B-complex vitamins in chicken muscles. *Arch. Biochem.* **10**, 251–260

261 Richardson, T., and McGann, T. C. A. (1964) Fatty acids in Irish butterfat. *Irish J. agric. Res.* **3**, 151–157

262 Robbins, G. S., Pomeranz, Y., and Briggle, L. W. (1971) Amino acid composition of oat groats. *J. agric. Food Chem.* **19**, 536–539

263 Roberson, S., Marion, J. E., and Woodroof, J. G. (1966) Composition of commercial peanut butters. *J. Amer. diet. Ass.* **49**, 208–210

264 Robertson, J., and Sissons, D. J. (1966) The effects of maturity, processing, storage in the pod and cooking on the vitamin C content of fresh peas. *Nutrition, Lond.* **20**, 21–27

265 Rodgers, K., and Poole, D. B. (1958) The estimation of iodine in biological materials: a modification of the method of Ellis and Duncan. *Biochem. J.* **70**, 463–471

266 Rolls, B. A., and Porter, J. W. G. (1973) Some effects of processing and storage on the nutritive value of milk and milk products. *Proc. Nutr. Soc.* **32**, 9–15

267 Schertel, M. E., Boehne, J. W., and Libby, D. A. (1965) Folic acid derivatives in yeast. *J. biol. Chem.* **240**, 3154–3158

268 Schlettwein-Gsell, D., and Mommsen-Straub, S. (1972) Ubersicht Spurenelemente in Lebensmitteln. VII. Magnesium. *Int. Z. Vitaminforsch.* **42**, 324–352

269 Schroeder, H. A. (1971) Losses of vitamins and trace minerals resulting from processing and preservation of foods. *Amer. J. clin. Nutr.* **24**, 562–573

270 Schroeder, H. A., Nason, A. P., Tipton, I. H., and Balassa, J. J. (1967) Essential trace elements in man: zinc. Relation to environmental cadmium. *J. chron. Dis.* **20**, 179–210

271 Schulze, A., and Truswell, A. S. (1977) Sterols in British shellfish. *Proc. Nutr. Soc.* **36**, 25A

272 Shahani, K. M., Hathaway, I. L., and Kelly, P. L. (1962) B-complex vitamin content of cheese. II. Niacin, pantothenic acid, pyridoxine, biotin and folic acid. *J. Dairy Sci.* **45**, 833–841

273 Sidwell, V. D., Bonnet, J. C., and Zook, E. G. (1973) Chemical and nutritive values of several fresh and canned finfish, crustaceans and mollusks. 1. Proximate composition, calcium and phosphorus. *Marine Fish. Rev.* **35** (12), 16–19

274 Sidwell, V. D., Foncannon, P. R., Moore, N. S., and Bonnet, J. C. (1974) Composition of the edible portion of raw (fresh or frozen) crustaceans, finfish and mollusks. 1. Protein, fat, moisture, ash, carbohydrate, energy value, and cholesterol. *Marine Fish. Rev.* **36** (3), 21–35

275 Sinclair, A. J. (1974) Personal communication

276 Skramstad, K. H. (1969) Mineralstoffer i fisk. *Tidsskr. Hermetikkind* **55**, 14–20

277 Slater, G. G., Shankman, S., Shepherd, J. S., and Alfin-Slater, R. B. (1975) Seasonal variation in the composition of California Avocados. *J. agric. Food. Chem.* **23**, 468–474

278 Slover, H. T. (1971) Tocopherols in foods and fats. *Lipids* **6**, 291–296

279 Slover, H. T., Lehmann, J., and Valis, R. J. (1969) Vitamin E in foods: determination of tocols and tocotrienols. *J. Amer. Oil Chem. Soc.* **46**, 417–420

280 Smith, C. L., Kelleher, J., Losowsky, M. S., and Morrish, N. (1971) The content of vitamin E in British diets. *Brit. J. Nutr.* **26**, 89–96

281 Souci, S. W., Fauchman, W., and Kraut, H. (1962, 1964) *Die Zusammensetzung der Lebensmittel, Nährwert-Tabellen.* Wissenschaftliche Verlagsgesellschaft mbH., Stuttgart

282 Stagg, G. V., and Millin, D. J. (1975) The nutritional and therapeutic value of tea—a review. *J. Sci. Food Agric.* **26**, 1439–1459

283 Stevens, J. F. (1970) Faecal fatty acid patterns in the neonate. *J. med. Lab. Technol.* **27**, 327–331

284 Streiff, R. R. (1971) Folate levels in citrus and other juices. *Amer. J. clin. Nutr.* **24**, 1390–1392

285 Stull, J. W., and Brown, W. H. (1964) Fatty acid composition of milk. II. Some differences in common dairy breeds. *J. Dairy Sci.* **47**, 1412

286 Tamura, T., and Stokstad, E. L. R. (1973) The availability of food folate in man. *Brit. J. Haematol.* **25**, 513–532

287 Teply, L. J. (1958) Nutritional study of instant coffee powder. *Food Technol.* **12**, 485–486

288 Terrell, R. N., Lewis, R. W., Cassens, R. G., and Bray, R. W. (1967) Fatty acid compositions of bovine subcutaneous fat depots determined by gas–liquid chromatography. *J. Food Sci.* **32**, 516–520

289 Thomas, M. H., and Colloway, D. H. (1961) Nutritional value of dehydrated foods. *J. Amer. diet. Ass.* **39**, 105–116

290 Thompson, M. H. (1964) Cholesterol content of various species of shellfish. 1. Method of analysis and preliminary survey of variables. *US Fish. Wildlife Serv. Fish. Ind. Res.* **2**, 11–15

291 Thompson, S. Y., Henry, K. M., and Kon, S. K. (1964) Factors affecting the concentration of vitamins in milk. 1. Effect of breed, season and geographical location on fat-soluble vitamins. *J. Dairy Res.* **31**, 1–25

292 Thompson, S. Y., and Kon, S. K. (1964) Factors affecting the concentration of vitamins in milk. 2. Effect of breed, season and geographical location on riboflavin. *J. Dairy Res* **31**, 27–30

293 Tolan, A., Robertson, J., Orton, C. R., Head, M. J., Christie, A. A., and Millburn, B. A. (1974) Studies on the composition of food. 5. The chemical composition of eggs produced under battery, deep litter and free range conditions. *Brit. J. Nutr.* **31**, 185–200

294 Toothill, J., Thompson, S. Y., and Edwards-Webb, J. (1970) Observations on the use of 2,4-dinitrophenylhydrazine and 2,6-dichlorophenolindophenol for determination of vitamin C in raw and in heat-treated milk. *J. Dairy Res.* **37**, 29–45

295 Trevelyan, W. E. (1975) Determination of uric acid precursors in dried yeast and other forms of single cell protein. *J. Sci. Food Agric.* **26**, 1673–1680

296 Tsatsaronis, G. C., and Kehayoglou, A. H. (1971) Fatty acid composition of Capsicum oils by gas–liquid chromatography. *J. Amer. Oil Chem. Soc.* **48**, 365–367

297 Turk, D. E., and Barnett, B. D. (1971) Cholesterol content of market eggs. *Poult. Sci.* **50**, 1303–1306

298 Twomey, D. G., and Goodchild, J. (1970) Variations in the vitamin C content of imported tomatoes. *J. Sci. Food Agric.* **21**, 313

299 Twomey, D. G., and Ridge, B. D. (1970) Note on L-ascorbic acid content of English early tomatoes. *J. Sci. Food Agric.* **21**, 314

300 Underwood, E. J. (1971) *Trace elements in human and animal nutrition*, 3rd edition. Academic Press, London and New York

301 Van den Berghs and Jurgens Ltd (1976) Personal communication

302 Vought, R. L., and London, W. T. (1964) Dietary sources of iodine. *Amer. J. clin. Nutr.* **14**, 186–192

303 Walter, W. M., Hansen, A. P., and Purcell, A. E. (1971) Lipids of cured Centennial sweet potatoes. *J. Food Sci.* **36**, 795–797

304 Wangen, R. M., Marion, W. W., and Hotchkiss, D. K. (1972) Influence of age on the fatty acid composition of breast and thigh muscles of male turkeys. *Agric. Biol. Chem.* **36**, 2081–2086

305 Warren, H. V. (1972) Variations in the trace element contents of some vegetables. *J. Roy. Coll. gen. Practnrs* **22**, 56–60

306 Watson, J. D., Dako, D. Y., and Amoakwa-Adu, M. (1975) Available carbohydrates in Ghanaian foodstuffs. 2. Sugars and starch in staples and other foodstuffs. *Plant Foods for Man*, **1**, 169–176

307 Watt, B. K., and Merrill, A. L. (1963) *Composition of foods—raw, processed, prepared.* US Department of Agriculture, Agriculture Handbook No 8. Washington DC

308 Wayne, E. J., Koutras, D. A., and Alexander, W. D. (1964) *Clinical aspects of iodine metabolism.* Blackwells, Oxford

309 Weiss, J. F., Naber, E. C., and Johnson, R. M. (1964) Effect of dietary fat and other factors on egg yolk cholesterol. 1. The 'cholesterol' content of egg yolk as influenced by dietary unsaturated fat and the method of determination. *Arch. Biochem. Biophys.* **105**, 521–526

310 West, C., and Zilva, S. S. (1944) Synthesis of vitamin C in stored apples. *Biochem. J.* **38**, 105–108

311 Williams, A. P., Bishop, D. R., Cockburn, J. E., and Scott, K. J. (1976) Composition of ewe's milk. *J. Dairy Res.* **43**, 325–329

312 Woodruff, C. W., Bailey, M. C., Davis, J. T., Rogers, N., and Coniglio, J. G. (1964) Serum lipids in breast-fed infants and in infants fed evaporated milk. *Amer. J. clin. Nutr.* **14**, 83–90

313 Worthington, R. E., Hammons, R. O., and Allison, J. R. (1972) Varietal differences and seasonal effects on fatty acid composition and stability of oil from 82 peanut genotypes. *J. agric. Food Chem.* **20**, 727–730

314 Zanobini, A., Firenzouli, A. M., and Bianchi, A. (1974) Isolamento e dosaggio della vitamina D in avocado (*Persea gratissima*). *Boll. Soc. Ital. Biol. sper.* **50**, 887–891

315 Zook, E. G., and Lehmann, J. (1968) Mineral composition of fruits. II. Nitrogen, calcium, magnesium, phosphorus, potassium, aluminum, boron, copper, iron, manganese and sodium. *J. Amer. diet. Ass.* **52**, 225–231

# Index of foods

*** Foods are indexed by food number *not* page number**

* **Foods are indexed by food number *not* page number**

*** Foods are indexed by food number *not* page number**

*** Foods are indexed by food number *not* page number**

* **Foods are indexed by food number *not* page number**

*** Foods are indexed by food number *not* page number**

*** Foods are indexed by food number *not* page number**





Printed in England for Her Majesty's Stationery Office by McCorquodale Printers Ltd. London
HM 7816 Dd 587267 K60 1/78 McC3339/3